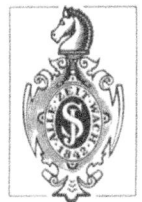

Basil S. Lewis Asher Kimchi (Eds.)

Heart Failure Mechanisms and Management

With 136 Figures

Springer-Verlag Berlin Heidelberg GmbH

BASIL S. LEWIS, MD
Director
Department of Cardiology
Lady Davis Carmel Hospital
34362 Haifa, Israel

ASHER KIMCHI, MD
Assistant Clinical Professor of Medicine
University of California, Los Angeles
Attending Physician
Division of Cardiology
Cedars-Sinai Medical Center
Los Angeles, CA 90048, USA

ISBN 978-3-540-53145-6

Library of Congress Cataloging-in-Publication Data. Heart failure mechanisms and management/B.S. Lewis, A. Kimchi (eds.). p. cm. Includes bibliographical references. ISBN 978-3-540-53145-6   ISBN 978-3-642-58231-8 (eBook)
DOI 10.1007/978-3-642-58231-8
1. Congestive heart failure. 2. Heart failure. I. Lewis, B.S. (Basil S.) II. Kimchi. A (Asher) [DNLM: 1. Heart Failure, Congestive-physiopathology. 2. Heart Failure, Congestive-therapy.   WG 370 H43653]   RC685.C53H44 1991   616. 1′2-dc20   DNLM/DLC
for Library of Congress   90–10423   CIP

© Springer-Verlag Berlin Heidelberg 1991
Originally published by Springer-Verlag Berlin Heidelberg New York in 1991

The use of registered names, trademarks, etc. in this publication does not imply, even in the absence of a specific statement, that such names are exempt from the relevant protective laws and regulations and therefore free for general use.

Product Liability: The Publisher can give no guarantee for information about drug dosage and application thereof contained in this book. In every individual case the respective user must check its accuracy by consulting other pharmaceutical literature.

Typesetting: International Typesetters Inc., Makati, Philippines
27/3130-543210 — Printed on acid-free paper

To the memory of our parents,
Bluma and Philip Lewis
and Rivka and Yaacov Kimchi.

To our wives and children
Noga, Yair, Noam, and Eran Lewis
and Becky, Eyal, and Eitan Kimchi.

Preface

Following remarkable advances in medical care, the past decade has witnessed a significant improvement in the survival of patients with many different forms of heart disease. In the majority of cases, however, the advances have been palliative and not curative. The result has been the production of an ever-increasing population of patients with heart disease, many of whom suffer from myocardial dysfunction and latent or overt heart failure. Heart failure is now a major cause of morbidity and mortality in cardiac patients.

This book aims to combine in a single volume data relating to both pathophysiological mechanisms and the clinical management of the patient with heart failure. It includes chapters dealing with molecular, biochemical, and pathophysiological aspects of heart failure, ventricular function and its assessment, and the clinical aspects of heart failure in different cardiac disorders, including ischemic heart disease, valvular heart disease, and the cardiomyopathies. There are sections on pharmacotherapy, the role of arrhythmias, exercise physiology, and neurohumoral mechanisms. The book also deals with newer interventional techniques, newer surgical procedures and some current problems relating to cardiac assist devices and heart and heart-lungs transplantation.

The publication of this volume was initiated at the 1st International Symposium on Heart Failure — Mechanisms and Management, organized by the International Society of Heart Failure, and held in Jerusalem, Israel. We are grateful to the large number of contributing authors for their ideas and the discussion presented in the book. We are deeply indebted to Schwarz Pharma AG and Bayer AG for their educational grant which enabled publication of this volume and to Chava Scharf, Isis Rivlin, and Kelly Morse for their outstanding secretarial assistance in its preparation. We also thank our families and friends, who provided endless help and encouragement in the planning of this book.

BASIL S. LEWIS
ASHER KIMCHI

Contents

Molecular and Biochemical Aspects

Pathophysiological Aspects of Heart Failure

Ventricular Function in Heart Failure

Cardiomyopathies

Pharmacotherapy of Heart Failure

Inotropic Drugs in the Management of Heart Failure

Angiotensin Converting Enzyme Inhibitors

Nitrate Therapy

Calcium Antagonists

Cardiac Arrhythmias in Heart Failure

Exercise Physiology and Exercise Therapy in Heart Failure

Neurohumoral Mechanisms

Newer Interventional Techniques

Newer Surgical Techniques in the Patient with Heart Failure

Cardiac Assist Devices, Heart Transplantation

List of Contributors

ABRAMS, J.
Division of Cardiology, University of New Mexico, School of Medicine
Albuquerque, NM 87131, USA

ALPERT, J.S.
Division of Cardiovascular Medicine, University of Massachusetts
Medical Center, 55 Lake Avenue North, Worcester, MA 01655, USA

ANDERSON, S.D.
Hallstrom Institute of Cardiology, Royal Prince Albert Hospital
University of Sydney, 2050 Camperdown, N.S.W., Australia

ANGOLI, L.
Divisione di Cardiologia, Policlinico S. Matteo, 27100 Pavia, Italy

ANTIMISIARIS, M.
Section of Cardiology 691/111E, Veterans Administration Medical Center
of West Los Angeles, Wilshire and Sawtelle Boulevards, Los Angeles, CA 90073, USA

ANVERSA, P.
Department of Pathology, New York Medical College
Valhalla, NY 10595, USA

ARBEL, Y.
Cardiac Unit, Meir General Hospital, 44281 Kfar Saba, Israel

AUPETIT, B.
Department of Cardiothoracic Surgery, Groupe Hospitalier
Pitie-Salpetriere, 47 et 83, Boulevard de l'Hôpital
75634 Paris Cedex, France

BAKST, A.
Cardiac Unit, Meir General Hospital, 44281 Kfar Saba, Israel

BARLOW, C.W.
Department of Cardiology, University of the Witwatersrand
York Road, Parktown, Johannesburg 2193, South Africa

BARLOW, J.B.
Department of Cardiology, University of the Witwatersrand
York Road, Parktown, Johannesburg 2193, South Africa

BEKER, B.
Cardiac Unit, Meir General Hospital, 44281 Kfar Saba, Israel

BENOTTI, J.R.
Cardiac Catheterization Laboratories, Division of Cardiovascular Medicine
University of Massachusetts Medical School, Worcester, MA 01655, USA

BERNOTAT-DANIELOWSKI, S.
Max-Planck-Institut, Abteilung für experimentelle Kardiologie
Benekestr. 2, W-6350 Bad Nauheim, FRG

BERTRAND, M.E.
Service de Cardiologie B et Hémodynamique, Hôpital Cardiologique
Université de Lille, Boulevard du Professeur Leclerc, 59037 Lille, France

BESA, G.
Division of Thoracic and Cardiovascular Surgery, ULSS 25, 37100 Verona, Italy

BLEESE, N.
Kerckhoff-Klinik, Abteilung für Thorax- und Cardiovascular-Chirurgie
Benekestr. 2-6, W-6350 Bad Nauheim, FRG

BLEIFELD, W.
II. Medizinische Klinik, Abteilung Kardiologie, Universitätskrankenhaus Eppendorf
Martinistr. 52, W-2000 Hamburg 20, FRG

BOEWER, V.
Zentralinstitut für Herz-Kreislauf-Forschung,
Wiltbergstr. 50, O-1115 Berlin-Buch, FRG

BORS, V.
Department of Cardiothoracic Surgery, Groupe Hospitalier
Pitie-Salpetriere, 47 et 83, Boulevard de l'Hôpital
75634 Paris Cedex, France

BRAMUCCI, E.
Divisione di Cardiologia, Policlinico S. Matteo, 27100 Pavia, Italy

BUB, A.
Institut für Anatomie und Zellbiologie III, Universität Heidelberg
Im Neuenheimer Feld 307, W-6900 Heidelberg, FRG

BURNS, D.
Cardiovascular Division, University of Minnesota, Box 488-UMHC
420 Delaware Street SE, Minneapolis, MN 55455, USA

BURNS, D.E.
Minneapolis Heart Institute, 920 East 28th Street, Suite 40
Minneapolis, MN 55407, USA

CABROL, A.
Department of Cardiothoracic Surgery, Groupe Hospitalier
Pitie-Salpetriere, 47 et 83, Boulevard de l'Hôpital
75634 Paris Cedex, France

CABROL, C.
Department of Cardiothoracic Surgery, Groupe Hospitalier
Pitie-Salpetriere, 47 et 83, Boulevard de l'Hôpital
75634 Paris Cedex, France

CARLSON, T.A.
Minneapolis Heart Institute, 920 East 28th Street, Suite 40
Minneapolis, MN 55407, USA

CARLYLE, P.
Cardiovascular Division, University of Minnesota, Box 488-UMHC
420 Delaware Street SE, Minneapolis, MN 55455, USA

CECONI, C.
Cattedra di Cardiologia, c/o Spedali Civili, 25100 Brescia, Italy

CHAPPUIS, F.P.
Clinique Scientifique, Centre de Cardiologie HCUG
Hôpital Cantonal Universitaire de Genève, 24 Rue Micheli-du-Crest
1211 Geneva 4, Switzerland

CHATTERJEE, K.
Cardiology Division, Moffitt Hospital, Room 1186 University of California,
San Francisco, CA 94143-0124, USA

CHEKANOV, V.S.
Bakulev Institute of Cardiovascular Surgery, AMS USSR, Leninsky Pr. 8
Moscow 117931, USSR

CHOMETTE, G.
Department of Cardiothoracic Surgery, Groupe Hospitalier
Pitie-Salpetriere, 47 et 83, Boulevard de l'Hôpital
75634 Paris Cedex, France

CHOONG, C.Y.P.
Hallstrom Institute of Cardiology, Royal Prince Albert Hospital
University of Sydney, 2050 Camperdown, N.S.W., Australia

CIOFFI, P.
Divisione di Cardiologia, Policlinico S. Matteo, 27100 Pavia, Italy

CLEMSON, B.
Division of Cardiology, The Milton S. Hershey Medical Center
The Pennsylvania State University, P.O. Box 850, Hershey, PA 17033, USA

COHN, J.N.
Cardiovascular Division, University of Minnesota, Box 488-UMHC
420 Delaware Street SE, Minneapolis, MN 55455, USA

DANESI, R.
Cattedra di Cardiologia, c/o Spedali Civili, 25100 Brescia, Italy

DAVIS, D.
Division of Cardiology, The Milton S. Hershey Medical Center
The Pennsylvania State University, P.O. Box 850, Hershey, PA 17033, USA

DE SERVI, S.
Divisione di Cardiologia, Policlinico S. Matteo, 27100 Pavia, Italy

DEAN, H.
Cardiac Unit, Meir General Hospital, 44281 Kfar Saba, Israel

DEI CAS, L.
Cattedra di Cardiologia, c/o Spedali Civili, 25100 Brescia, Italy

DI SEGNI E.
The Heart Institute, Chaim Sheba Medical Center
52621 Tel Hashomer, Israel

DESRUENNES, M.
Department of Cardiothoracic Surgery, Groupe Hospitalier
Pitie-Salpetriere, 47 et 83, Boulevard de l'Hôpital
75634 Paris Cedex, France

DORSAZ, P.A.
Cardiology Center, University Hospital, 1211 Geneva 4, Switzerland

ELBORN, J.S.
Royal Victoria Hospital, Belfast BT112 6BA, Northern Ireland

ELKAYAM, U.
Department of Medicine, Section of Cardiology, LAC-USC Medical Center
University of Southern California School of Medicine, Los Angeles, CA 90033, USA

ERLEMEIER, H.-H.
II. Medizinische Klinik, Abteilung Kardiologie, Universitätskrankenhaus Eppendorf
Martinistr. 52, W-2000 Hamburg 20, FRG

ESSOP, R.
Department of Cardiology, Baragwanath Hospital
P.O. Bertsham 2013, South Africa

FEELISCH, M.
Abteilung Pharmakologie, Schwarz Pharma AG
Mittelstr. 11-13, W-4019 Monheim, FRG

FELLER, S.M.
Rockefeller University, Box 41, 1230 York Avenue, New York, NY 10021, USA

FERRARI, R.
Cattedra di Cardiologia, c/o Spedali Civili, 25100 Brescia, Italy

FINKELSTEIN, S.
Cardiovascular Division, University of Minnesota, Box 488-UMHC
420 Delaware Street SE, Minneapolis, MN 55455, USA

FORSSMANN, W.-G.
Niedersächsisches Institut für Peptid-Forschung GmbH (IPF)
Feodor-Lynen-Str. 5, W-3000 Hannover 61, FRG

FÖRSTER, A.
Universitätsklinik für Innere Medizin, Bereich Medizin (Charité)
der Humboldt-Universität zu Berlin, O-1040 Berlin, FRG

FOURRIER, J.L.
Service de Cardiologie B et Hémodynamique, Hôpital Cardiologique
Université de Lille, Boulevard du Professeur Leclerc, 59037 Lille, France

FROEDE, R.
Max-Planck-Institut, Abteilung für experimentelle Kardiologie
Benekestr. 2, W-6350 Bad Nauheim, FRG

GAGELMANN, M.
Institut für Anatomie und Zellbiologie III, Universität Heidelberg
Im Neuenheimer Feld 307, W-6900 Heidelberg, FRG

GANDJBAKHCH, I.
Department of Cardiothoracic Surgery, Groupe Hospitalier
Pitie-Salpetriere, 47 et 83, Boulevard de l'Hôpital
75634 Paris Cedex, France

GHIO, S.
Divisione di Cardiologia, Policlinico S. Matteo, 27100 Pavia, Italy

GOBEL, F.L.
Minneapolis Heart Institute, 920 East 28th Street, Suite 40
Minneapolis, MN 55407, USA

GOLDENBERG, I.F.
Minneapolis Heart Institute, 920 East 28th Street, Suite 40
Minneapolis, MN 55407, USA

GOMMEAUX, A.
Service de Cardiologie B et Hèmodynamique, Hôpital Cardiologique
Université de Lille, Boulevard du Professeur Leclerc, 59037 Lille, France

GOODWIN, J.F.
2 Pine Grove, Lake Road, Wimbledon, London SW19 7HE, UK

GORDON, M.
Minneapolis Heart Institute, 920 East 28th Street, Suite 40
Minneapolis, MN 55407, USA

GUAINI, T.
Cattedra di Cardiologia, c/o Spedali Civili, 25100 Brescia, Italy

GULBA, D.
Abteilung für Kardiologie, Medizinische Hochschule Hannover
Konstanty-Gutschow-Str. 8, W-3000 Hannover 61, FRG

HARDING, S.E.
National Heart and Lung Institute, Dovehouse Street
London SW3 6LY, UK

HARIGAYA, S.
Biological Research Laboratory, Tanabe Seiyaku Co. Ltd.
Kawagishi 2-2-50, Toda, Saitama 335, Japan

HECKER, H.
Abteilung für Kardiologie, Medizinische Hochschule Hannover
Konstanty-Gutschow-Str. 8, W-3000 Hannover 61, FRG

HEIN, S.
Max-Planck-Institut, Abteilung für experimentelle Kardiologie
Benekestr. 2, W-6350 Bad Nauheim, FRG

HESS, O.M.
Division of Cardiology, Medical Policlinic, University Hospital
Rämistr. 100, 8091 Zürich, Switzerland

HOSHIYAMA, M.
Biological Research Laboratory, Tanabe Seiyaku Co. Ltd.
Kawagishi 2-2-50, Toda, Saitama 335, Japan

HUGENHOLTZ, P.G.
SocAR S.A., 22, rue Juste-Olivier, 1260 Nyon, Switzerland

HUNN, D.
Minneapolis Heart Institute, 920 East 28th Street, Suite 40
Minneapolis, MN 55407, USA

JOHNSON, K.
Minneapolis Heart Institute, 920 East 28th Street, Suite 40
Minneapolis, MN 55407, USA

JORGENSEN, C.R.
Minneapolis Heart Institute, 920 East 28th Street, Suite 40
Minneapolis, MN 55407, USA

JOST, P.
Abteilung für Kardiologie, Medizinische Hochschule Hannover
Konstanty-Gutschow-Str. 8, W-3000 Hannover 61, FRG

JOST, S.
Abteilung für Kardiologie, Medizinische Hochschule Hannover
Konstanty-Gutschow-Str. 8, W-3000 Hannover 61, FRG

JOYCE, L.D.
Minneapolis Heart Institute, 920 East 28th Street, Suite 40
Minneapolis, MN 55407, USA

JUGDUTT, B.I.
Division of Cardiology, 2C2.43 Walter Mackenzie Health Sciences Centre
University of Alberta, Edmonton, Alberta, Canada, T6G 2R7

KASS, D.A.
Division of Cardiology, Johns Hopkins Medical Institutions
Baltimore, MD 21205, USA

KAYANAKIS, J.-G.
Cardiologic Center Paulmy, 64100 Bayonne, France

KELLY, D.T.
Hallstrom Institute of Cardiology, Royal Prince Albert Hospital
University of Sydney, 2050 Camperdown, N.S.W., Australia

KIMCHI, A.
Cedars-Sinai Medical Towers, 8635 W. Third Street, Suite 1080W
Los Angeles, CA 90048, USA

KLEIN, H.O.
Cardiac Unit, Meir General Hospital, 44281 Kfar Saba, Israel

KRAKOVSKY, A.A.
Bakulev Institute of Cardiovascular Surgery, AMS USSR, Leninsky Pr. 8
Moscow 117931, USSR

KRAYENBÜHL, H.P.
Division of Cardiology, Medical Policlinic, University Hospital
Rämistr. 100, 8091 Zürich, Switzerland

KUBO, S.
Cardiovascular Division, University of Minnesota, Box 488-UMHC
420 Delaware Street SE, Minneapolis, MN 55455, USA

KULICK, D.L.
Department of Medicine, Section of Cardiology, LAC-USC Medical Center
University of Southern California School of Medicine, Los Angeles, CA, USA

LABLANCHE, J.M.
Service de Cardiologie B et Hémodynamique, Hôpital Cardiologique
Université de Lille, Boulevard du Professeur Leclerc, 59037 Lille, France

LEE, G.
Western Heart Institute, Department of Cardiovascular Medicine
St. Mary's Hospital and Medical Center, 450 Stanyan Street,
San Francisco, CA 94117, USA

LEE, M.H.
Xintec Corporation, 900 Alice Street, Oakland, CA 94607, USA

LEGER, P.
Department of Cardiothoracic Surgery, Groupe Hospitalier
Pitie-Salpetriere, 47 et 83, Boulevard de l'Hôpital
75634 Paris Cedex, France

LEJEMTEL, T.H.
Division of Cardiology, Department of Medicine, Albert Einstein College
of Medicine, Bronx, NY 10461, USA

LEUENBERGER, U.
Division of Cardiology, The Milton S. Hershey Medical Center
The Pennsylvania State University, P.O. Box 850, Hershey, PA 17033, USA

LEVASSEUR, J.P.
Department of Cardiothoracic Surgery, Groupe Hospitalier
Pitie-Salpetriere, 47 et 83, Boulevard de l'Hôpital
75634 Paris Cedex, France

LEVI, A.
Cardiac Unit, Meir General Hospital, 44281 Kfar Saba, Israel

LEWIS, B.S.
Department of Cardiology, Lady Davis Carmel Hospital
7 Michal Street, 34362 Haifa, Israel

LICHTLEN, P.R.
Abteilung für Kardiologie, Medizinische Hochschule Hannover
Konstanty-Gutschow-Str. 8, W-3000 Hannover 61, FRG

MADISON, C.
Minneapolis Heart Institute, 920 East 28th Street, Suite 40
Minneapolis MN 55407, USA

MADISON, J.D.
Minneapolis Heart Institute, 920 East 28th Street, Suite 40
Minneapolis, MN 55407, USA

MALL, G.
Institut für Pathologie, Universität Heidelberg, Im Neuenheimer Feld 220
W-6900 Heidelberg, FRG

MARCUS, R.H.
University of Chicago, Department of Medicine, 5841 South Maryland Avenue
Box 410, Room W-607, Chicago, IL 60637, USA

MARMOR, A.
Cardiac Unit, Rebecca Sieff Hospital, P.O. Box 1429, 13113 Zefat, Israel

MASON, D.T.
Western Heart Institute, St. Mary's Hospital and Medical Center
450 Stanyan Street, San Francisco, CA 94117, USA

MAUGHAN, W.L.
Division of Cardiology, Johns Hopkins Medical Institutions
Baltimore, MD 21205, USA

McDONALD, K.
Cardiovascular Division, University of Minnesota, Box 488-UMHC
420 Delaware Street SE, Minneapolis, MN 55455, USA

McLAY, J.
Department of Clinical Pharmacology, Ninewells Hospital
and Medical School, Dundee, Scotland

McMURRAY, J.
Department of Cardiology, Western Infirmary, Glasgow, Scotland

McVEIGH, G.
Cardiovascular Division, University of Minnesota, Box 488-UMHC
420 Delaware Street SE, Minneapolis, MN 55455, USA

MENEGATTI, G.
Institute of Cardiology, P.A. Stefani, 37126 Verona, Italy

METRA, M.
Cattedra di Cardiologia, c/o Spedali Civili, 25100 Brescia, Italy

MICHOROWSKI, B.L.
Division of Cardiology, 2C2.43 Walter Mackenzie Health Sciences Centre
University of Alberta, Edmonton, Alberta, Canada, T6G 2R7

MIRSKY, I.
Department of Medicine, Brigham and Women's Hospital
75 Francis Street, Boston, MA 02115, USA

MONRAD, E.S.
Division of Cardiology, Medical Policlinic, University Hospital
Rämistr. 100, 8091 Zürich, Switzerland

MOONEY, M.R.
Minneapolis Heart Institute, 920 East 28th Street, Suite 40
Minneapolis, MN 55407, USA

MORANDO, G.
Institute of Cardiology, P.A. Stefani, 37126 Verona, Italy

MUSCH, T.
Division of Cardiology, The Milton S. Hershey Medical Center
The Pennsylvania State University, P.O. Box 850, Hershey, PA 17033, USA

NAGAO, T.
Department of Toxicology and Pharmacology, Faculty of Pharmaceutical Sciences
University of Tokyo, Bunkyo-ku, Tokyo 113, Japan

NAYLER, W.G.
Department of Medicine, University of Melbourne, Austin Hospital
Heidelberg, Victoria, 3084, Australia

NICHOLLS, D.P.
Royal Victoria Hospital, Belfast BT112 6BA, Northern Ireland

NOACK, E.
Institut für Pharmakologie, Heinrich-Heine-Universität
W-4000 Düsseldorf, FRG

NODARI, S.
Cattedra di Cardiologia, c/o Spedali Civili, 25100 Brescia, Italy

NÖTGES, A.
Abteilung Kardiologie I, Herz-Kreislauf-Klinik Bevensen
Rönstedter Str. 25, W-3118 Bad Bevensen, FRG

OCKENE, I.S.
Division of Cardiovascular Medicine, University of Massachusetts
Medical School, Worcester, MA 01655, USA

OLSEN, E.G.J.
Department of Histopathology, Cardiovascular Division
Royal Brompton & National Heart Hospital, Sydney Street, London SW3 6NP, UK

OPIE, L.H.
Heart Research Unit, University of Cape Town, Medical School
Observatory, 7925, South Africa

PAVIE, A.
Department of Cardiothoracic Surgery, Groupe Hospitalier
Pitie-Salpetriere, 47 et 83, Boulevard de l'Hôpital
75634 Paris Cedex, France

PEDERSEN, W.
Minneapolis Heart Institute, 920 East 28th Street, Suite 40
Minneapolis, MN 55407, USA

PIATTI, L.
Divisione di Cardiologia, Policlinico S, Matteo, 27100 Pavia, Italy

POCOCK, W.A.
Department of Cardiology, University of the Witwatersrand
York Road, Parktown, Johannesburg 2193, South Africa

POOLE-WILSON, P.A.
National Heart and Lung Institute, Dovehouse Street
London SW3 6LY, UK

PRITZKER, MR.
Minneapolis Heart Institute, 920 East 28th Street, Suite 40
Minneapolis, MN 55407, USA

RAFFLENBEUL, W.
Abteilung für Kardiologie, Medizinische Hochschule Hannover
Konstanty-Gutschow-Str. 8, W-3000 Hannover 61, FRG

REISIN, L.
Heart Institute, Barzilai Hospital, Ahskelon, Israel

RILEY, M.
Royal Victoria Hospital, Belfast BT112 6BA, Northern Ireland

RINK, D.L.
Xintec Corporation, 900 Alice Street, Oakland, CA 94607, USA

RINK, J.L.
Xintec Corporation, 900 Alice Street, Oakland, CA 94607, USA

ROSENDORFF, C.
University of the Witwatersrand Medical School, 7 York Road
Johannesburg 2193, South Africa

ROUBIN, G.S.
Hallstrom Institute of Cardiology, Royal Prince Albert Hospital
University of Sydney, 2050 Camperdown, N.S.W., Australia

RUTISHAUSER, W.
Cardiology Center, University Hospital, 1211 Geneva 4, Switzerland

SARELI, P.
Department of Cardiology, Baragwanath Hospital
P.O. Bertsham 2013, South Africa

SASAKI, Y.
Biological Research Laboratory, Tanabe Seiyaku Co. Ltd.
Kawagishi 2-2-50, Toda, Saitama 335, Japan

SASAYAMA, S.
Toyama Medical and Pharmaceutical University
2630 Sugitani, Toyama 930-01, Japan

SCHAPER, JUTTA
Max-Planck-Institut, Abteilung für experimentelle Kardiologie
Benekestr. 2, W-6350 Bad Nauheim, FRG

SCHNEEWEISS, A.
Sauerberg 12, W-6208 Bad Schwalbach 7, FRG

SCHNEIDER, J.
Division of Cardiology, Medical Policlinic, University Hospital
Schmelzbergstr. 12, 8091 Zürich, Switzerland

SCHOENBAUM, M.L.
Section of Cardiology 691/111E, Veterans Administration Medical Center
of West Lost Angeles, Wilshire and Sawtelle Boulevards, Los Angeles, CA 90073, USA

SCHROEDER, J.S.
Stanford University School of Medicine, Division of Cardiology
300 Pasteur Drive, Stanford, CA 94305-5246, USA

SHABETAI, R.
Cardiology Section, San Diego Veterans Administration Medical Center
La Jolla, CA 92161, USA

SHEN, W.F.
Hallstrom Institute of Cardiology, Royal Prince Albert Hospital
University of Sydney, 2050 Camperdown, N.S.W., Australia

SINGH, B.N.
Section of Cardiology 691/111E, Veterans Administration Medical Center
of West Los Angeles, Wilshire and Sawtelle Boulevards,
Los Angeles, CA 90073, USA

SINN, R.
Abteilung Kardiologie I, Herz-Kreislauf-Klinik Bevensen
Rönstedter Str. 25, W-3118 Bad Bevensen, FRG

SINOWAY, L.
Division of Cardiology, The Milton S. Hershey Medical Center
The Pennsylvania State University, P.O. Box 850, Hershey, PA 17033, USA

SONNENBLICK, E.H.
Division of Cardiology, Department of Medicine
Albert Einstein College of Medicine, Bronx, NY 10461, USA

SOUFER, R.
Department of Diagnostic Radiology, Yale University, School of Medicine
333 Cedar Street, New Haven, CT 06510, USA

SPECCHIA, G.
Divisione di Cardiologia, Policlinico S. Matteo, 27100 Pavia, Italy

STANFORD, C.F.
Royal Victoria Hospital, Belfast BT112 6BA, Northern Ireland

STEVENSON, L.W.
UCLA Cardiomyopathy and Transplant Center, UCLA Medical Center
Los Angeles, CA 90024, USA

STRUTHERS, A.D.
Department of Clinical Pharmacology, Ninewells Hospital and Medical School
Dundee, Scotland

SZEFNER, J.
Department of Cardiothoracic Surgery, Groupe Hospitalier
Pitie-Salpetriere, 47 et 83, Boulevard de l'Hôpital
75634 Paris Cedex, France

TAKANAKA, C.
Fujihigashi 4057-5, Shimouchi, Seki-Shi, Gifu-ken, 501-32, Japan

TRABER, U.
Abteilung Kardiologie I, Herz-Kreislauf-Klinik Bevensen
Rönstedter Str. 25, W-3118 Bad Bevensen, FRG

TURINA, M.
Clinic of Cardiovascular Surgery, University Hospital
Rämistr. 100, 8091 Zürich, Switzerland

TURRI, M.
Institute of Cardiology, P.A. Stefani, 37126 Verona, Italy

TYMCHAK, W.J.
Division of Cardiology, 2C2.43 Walter Mackenzie Health Sciences Centre
University of Alberta, Edmonton, Alberta, Canada, T6G 2R7

VAISSIER, E.
Department of Cardiothoracic Surgery, Groupe Hospitalier
Pitie-Salpetriere, 47 et 83, Boulevard de l'Hôpital
75634 Paris Cedex, France

VALANTINE, H.A.
Stanford University School of Medicine, Division of Cardiology
300 Pasteur Drive, Stanford, CA 94305-5246, USA

VASSANELLI, C.
Institute of Cardiology, P.A. Stefani, 37126 Verona, Italy

WALKER, M.
Minneapolis Heart Institute, 920 East 28th Street, Suite 40
Minneapolis, MN 55407, USA

WALLUKAT, G.
Zentralinstitut für Herz-Kreislauf-Forschung, Wiltbergstr. 50
O-1115 Berlin-Buch, FRG

WENGER, N.K.
Emory University School of Medicine, 69 Butler Street, S.E.
Atlanta, GA 30303, USA

WOLF, R.
Abteilung Kardiologie I, Herz-Kreislauf-Klinik Bevensen
Rönstedter Str. 25, W-3118 Bad Bevensen, FRG

WOLLENBERGER, A.
Zentralinstitut für Herz-Kreislauf-Forschung, Wiltbergstr. 50
O-1115 Berlin-Buch, FRG

WORTHINGTON, M.G.
Heart Research Unit, University of Cape Town, Medical School
Observatoŕy, 7925, South Africa

YABANA, H.
Biological Research Laboratory, Tanabe Seiyaku Co. Ltd.
Kawagishi 2-2-50, Toda, Saitama 335, Japan

ZANOLLA, L.
Institute of Cardiology, P.A. Stefani, 37126 Verona, Italy

ZARDINI, P.
Institute of Cardiology, P.A. Stefani, 37126 Verona, Italy

ZARET, B.L.
Section of Cardiovascular Medicine, Yale University, School of Medicine
333 Cedar Street, New Haven, CT 06510, USA

ZELIS, R.
Division of Cardiology, The Milton S. Hershey Medical Center
The Pennsylvania State University, P.O. Box 850, Hershey, PA 17033, USA

ZUCKER, I.H.
Department of Physiology and Biophysics, University of Nebraska
College of Medicine, 42nd and Dewey Avenue, Omaha, NB 68105, USA

Molecular and Biochemical Aspects

Autonomic Receptor Function in Congestive Heart Failure

C. ROSENDORFF

The major determinants of cardiac output (preload, myocardial contractility, afterload and heart rate) may all be modulated by the sympathetic nervous system. This has led to the notion, supported by much good data, that abnormalities in sympathetic neural and receptor function might contribute to the development or maintenance of cardiac dysfunction in patients with congestive heart failure. Most of the studies have been based on measurements of plasma or tissue catecholamine concentrations, or on observations of the effects of altering the sympathetic status in humans or other animals by neurophysiological or pharmacological means.

The pharmacological approach has depended heavily on the concept of receptors as the initial recognition sites for neurotransmitters, hormones and drugs (collectively known as ligands). Recently, it has become possible to identify some of the central and peripheral nervous system pathways involved in the control of normal cardiac output, including descending central autonomic fibres from the hypothalamus to the medulla and the reflex baroreceptor pathway, both of which probably share a common efferent component terminating in heart, vascular smooth muscle and adrenal medulla. Our knowledge of the central neurohumoral transmitters involved in these pathways is still sketchy; it is likely that there is a larger variety of transmitters involved than we had previously thought. Both at synapses and at the peripheral neuroeffector junction, it has become possible to identify and measure the biochemical effects [such as transmembrane ion fluxes and cyclic adenosine monophosphate (cAMP) generation] of receptor activation. Recently, we have been able to characterize the receptors themselves, to measure their concentrations, binding affinities, distribution, coupling to biochemical responses, regulation and changes in disease. This has led naturally to studies on the receptor-controlled membrane and intracellular events which used to be called "excitation-contraction coupling".

Adrenergic Receptors

The effects of sympathetic nerve stimulation or of circulating catecholamines are mediated by membrane-bound protein adrenoceptors (Fig. 1). These receptors bind reversibly with epinephrine and/or norepinephrine, as well as with other exogenous catecholamines and catecholamine analogues. They are specific and

B.S. Lewis, A. Kimchi (Eds.)
Heart Failure Mechanisms and Management
© Springer-Verlag Berlin Heidelberg 1991

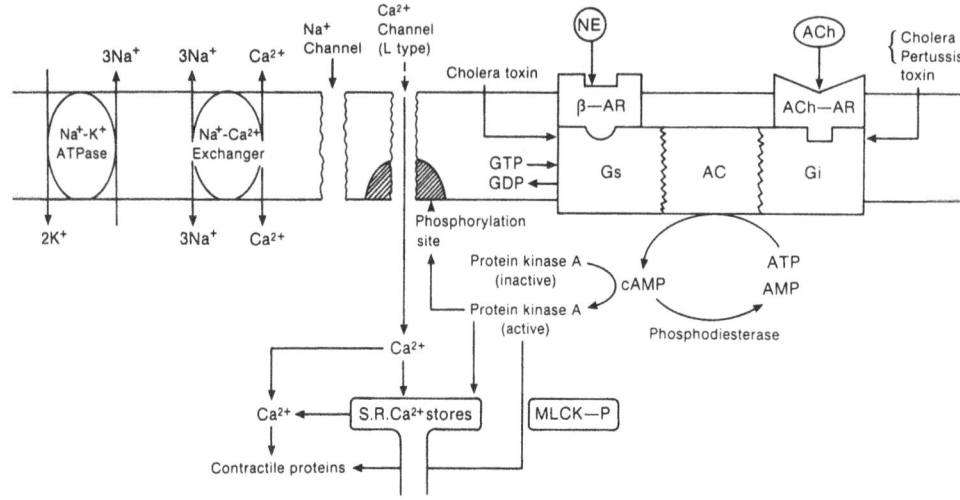

Fig. 1. Main receptor and ion channel mechanisms in the cardiac myocyte. Norepinephrine (*NE*) released from sympathetic nerve terminals or in the circulation binds to and activates beta-adreno-ceptors (*β-AR*). Beta-adrenoceptors and acetylcholine (muscarinic) receptors (*ACh-AR*) activate the alpha subunit of the GNP-binding regulatory membrane proteins G_s and G_i, respectively, which in turn stimulate (G_s) or inhibit (G_i) adenylate cyclase (*AC*). AC catalyses the production of cAMP, which in turn activates protein kinase A. cAMP is broken down by cAMP phosphodiesterase III. Active protein kinase A phosphorylates sites on the Ca^{2+} channel, the sarcoplasmic reticulum (*S.R.*), specifically phospholamban, and the contractile proteins (especially myosin light chain, *MLCK-P*) (phosporylated form of Myosin light chain kinase) and their regulatory elements (especially troponin I). Ca^{2+} released from the sarcoplasmic reticulum, mainly by the transsarcolemmal influx of Ca^{2+}, activates contractile proteins. The sites of action of some important inotropic agents are shown. Alpha$_2$-receptor activity (not shown) is probably also via G_i proteins. Pathways mediating alpha$_1$-receptor activity are shown in Fig. 2

saturable, and relay signals so that a characteristic intracellular response follows. There are two main types of adrenoceptors, alpha and beta based on the relative potency series of agonists [1-4].

Beta-receptors may be divided into beta$_1$ and beta$_2$ subtypes. Cardiac receptors are chiefly the beta$_1$ subtype [5]. Receptor density varies through the heart, with the highest concentration of beta$_1$-receptors in the sinus node, followed closely by the ventricles, and the least in the atria. Beta$_2$-receptors seem to be mainly in the sinus node and, to a lesser extent, in the atria [5,6]. Hence, selective beta$_2$-agonists, such as salbutamol, cause tachycardia, whereas selective beta$_1$-agonists such as dobutamine have a dominant inotropic activity.

Alpha-receptor subtypes have been defined [2,7,8] based on the development of selective agonists and antagonists. In the heart the myocytic alpha receptors are almost exclusively the alpha$_1$ subtype [9]. Stimulation of the alpha$_1$-receptors results in a positive inotropic effect [10]. However, it is likely that there are also prejunctional alpha$_2$-receptors on sympathetic nerve terminals, mediating feedback inhibition of norepinephrine release. Clonidine might therefore be expected to inhibit the effects of sympathetic stimulation on the heart; however, this effect is difficult to isolate from the central sympathetic inhibitory effect of clonidine and the consequent reduction in ventricular afterload.

In contrast to the alpha$_2$-receptor negative feedback system, presynaptic beta-receptors increase norepinephrine release from sympathetic nerve terminals [11,12]. It has been suggested that norepinephrine is released under beta-receptor control initially and, when the concentration of the transmitter reaches a threshold, it triggers the negative feedback mechanism on the presynaptic alpha$_2$-receptors resulting in an inhibition of release [11]. In support of this idea, it has been found that beta-receptors have a much lower threshold to norepinephrine than alpha-receptors in a variety of vascular beds [13–15].

Other presynaptic modulators are dopamine receptors (DA$_2$) and serotonin (5-HT$_1$) receptors which inhibit and stimulate norepinephrine release, respectively.

Muscarinic Receptors

Although both preganglionic and postganglionic parasympathetic nerve terminals release acetylcholine, the preganglionic receptors are nicotinic receptors, while postganglionic receptors within heart muscle are muscarinic receptors. Therefore, drugs such as nicotine and dimethylphenylpiperazinium, which are nicotinic agonists, suppress sinoatrial pacemaker activity [16]. However, these effects are inhibited by both atropine, a muscarinic receptor antagonist, and hexamethionium, a nicotinic receptor antagonist. Thus, stimulation of the vagal response by nicotine can be inhibited either directly at the preganglionic nicotinic receptor site by hexamethionium or at the postganglionic muscarinic receptor site by atropine.

The effects of muscarinic receptor activation include the following:

1. Activation of the guanosine triphosphate (GTP)-inhibitory protein (Gi) which couples the muscarinic receptor to adenylate cyclase [17].
2. Efflux of K^+ from cells, resulting in hyperpolarization of the cell membrane, reflecting changes in transmembrane K^+ permeability.
3. Decrease of Ca^{2+} movement into cells. The acetylcholine-mediated increase in the outward K^+ current tends to shorten the action potential duration, including the plateau phase, during which the Ca^{2+} current flows into the cell. Since the contractile force is related to the level of free ionized Ca^{2+} in the cell, the negative inotropic effect of vagal stimulation may be caused by either a direct inhibitory effect of acetylcholine on Ca^{2+} entry, or an indirect effect on Ca^{2+} entry due to a decrease in action potential duration. There may also be an acetylcholine-stimulated atropine-inhibitable efflux of Ca^{2+} from atrial cells [18]. Recently, the genes and/or the cDNA for both subtypes of the beta-adrenegic receptor [19], both subtypes of the alpha adrenergic receptor [20–22] and the muscarinic receptor [23] have been cloned and sequenced. The receptors all have a remarkable similar topology of seven transmem-

brane spanning hydrophobic segments with, in addition, fairly high sequence homology. The extracellular domain is the site of high-affinity ligand binding, while the intracellular domain mediates signal transduction, particularly receptor/G-protein interactions (see below).

Membrane Related Modulation of Receptor Activity

Much of the excitement in this field in recent years has been due to the development of techniques for the quantitation of adrenergic receptors, both concentration and affinity, for agonists and antagonists. The most commonly used technique is radioligand binding.

Changes in adrenergic responsiveness may be due to changes in adrenoreceptor number or affinity, or in the coupling or transduction of receptor activation to intracellular events. A number of studies have described changes in adrenoceptor number and affinity in cardiovascular disease, particularly congestive heart failure and hypertension [24].

Several reports have demonstrated that the density of ventricular myocardial beta-adrenoceptors is reduced in both animal models and in patients with congestive heart failure, regardless of aetiology [25,26], and that this decrease in beta-adrenoceptor number is associated with a reduced sensitivity of myocardial contractile responses to beta-adrenergic stimulation [25]. This decrease in beta-receptor-mediated response is not related to a deficit in the adenylase cyclase-cAMP system because cAMP formation and contractile responses to histamine, forskolin and sodium fluoride are not decreased in congestive heart failure when compared with normal myocardial tissue [25,27].

What is the mechanism of the down-regulation of myocardial $beta_1$ adrenoceptors? The most widely accepted explanation relates to excessive sympathetic tone. Patients with congestive heart failure are known to have high levels of circulating norepinephrine, as well as increased plasma renin activity and arginine vasopressin. The elevated levels of plasma norepinephrine are probably a marker for the increased release of norepinephrine into synaptic clefts. When the heart is normal, vasoconstriction induced by the sympathetic nervous system, the renin-angiotensin system and by vasopressin might be an appropriate mechanism to support the blood pressure. However, in congestive heart failure these effects may be counterproductive, leading both to a further decrement in pump performance [owing to an increase in afterload and left ventricular (LV) wall stress] and to a down-regulation of cardiac myocytic beta-receptors.

Both chronotropic and inotropic responses are mediated by both $beta_1$- and $beta_2$-adrenoreceptors in the myocardium, although $beta_1$-adrenoceptors are present in greater concentrations [5,29]. The $beta_1$-receptor population is more sensitive to down-regulation [30]. This down-regulatory process can be a rapid, dynamic one. In rats, almost half the myocardial beta-adrenoceptors are "lost" within 10 min of incubation with isoproternol [31], and 85% of these "lost" receptors return to the cell surface when the beta-agonist is removed. The recycling of the beta-adrenoceptor to the cell surface is inhibited by monesin and colchicine, implying that the Golgi apparatus and the microtubules are somehow involved in this process [27].

Recently, Limas et al. [32] found that sera from patients with idiopathic dilated cardiomyopathy reduced the number of beta-receptors on rat cardiac membranes, and this decrease can be prevented by preincubating the sera with anti-human Ig-G, indicating the presence of autoantibodies. We do not know whether this finding will be extended to sera from patients with congestive cardiac failure of other causes, and, if so, whether this is an alternative or an additional explanation of the beta-adrenoceptor down-regulation.

In a study on hearts from normal subjects and patients with idiopathic dilated cardiomyopathy [33], it was found that sarcolemmal $alpha_1$-adrenoreceptor-binding sites were almost double in number in the diseased hearts than in the normal ones. In the failing hearts the $alpha_1$-receptors were shown to be coupled to a GTP-binding protein.

There are probably changes in muscarinic receptor function too. In dogs with experimental heart failure, ligand-binding studies using ^{3}H-quinuclidinyl benzilate and LV sarcolemma showed that muscarinic receptor density in heart failure declined 36% from control, with a loss of high-affinity agonist-binding sites. The functional efficacy of the muscarinic receptor was consequently impaired, as assessed by significantly smaller inhibition of adenylate cyclase by the muscarinic agonist methacholine [17].

Receptor-Contraction Coupling Mechanisms

When suitable agonists, such as norepinephrine released from a sympathetic nerve terminal, bind with the beta-adrenoceptor on the cardiac myocyte membrane, there is activation of a guanosine nucleotide regulatory protein, or G-protein (sometimes referred to as the N-protein), by the opening up of a nucleotide-binding site of the G-protein to allow occupancy by GTP, which, in turn, causes the G-protein to stimulate adenylate cyclase (Fig. 1) [34-37]. A switching-off mechanism for the process is provided by the intrinsic GTP-ase activity of the G-protein which hydrolyses the attached GTP to GDP. It is now recognized that there are stimulatory and inhibitory forms of the G-protein (designated G_s and G_i, respectively).

Activation of the catalytic moiety of adenylate cyclase stimulates cAMP formation. cAMP activates protein kinase A, which, in turn, may catalyse the phosphorylation of a site in the Ca^{2+} channel to increase transmembrane Ca^{2+} influx. Other reactions affected by protein kinases may include the phosphorylation of myosin light chain kinase and myosin itself.

When a suitable agonist, such as circulating norepinephrine or norepinephrine released from a sympathetic nerve terminal, binds to the $alpha_1$-adrenoreceptor in the myocardiac cell membrane, there is binding with another G-protein which, in turn, activates the catalytic moiety of phospholipase C, situated on the inside of the cell membrane phospholipid bilayer (Fig. 2). The activated enzyme breaks down inositol lipids in the plasma membrane, particularly phosphatidylinositol-4,5-bisphosphate (PIP_2), with the production of two second messengers, inositol-1,4,5-trisphosphate (IP_3) and diacylglycerol, which, in turn, activates a phospholipid-dependent protein kinase C (PKC). IP_3 stimulates the release of Ca^{2+} from stores in the sarcoplasmic reticulum to activate the cellular contractile proteins, but, also, may affect the kinetics of transmembrane Ca^{2+} influx.

PKC has a whole lot of interesting actions, one of which is the phosphorylation activation of a 50 kDa protein which results ultimately in the mobilization of arachidonate and the formation of prostaglandins, guanylate cyclase and cytoplasmic cGMP. Another action is on Na^+-proton exchange, with implications for cell growth, development and cell division.

There is a paucity of data on the way, qualitatively or quantitatively, the schema is altered in congestive heart failure. The subsensitivity of beta-adrenergic responses in failing human hearts may be explained by down-regulation of $beta_1$-receptors. Recently, it has been shown that the activity of a 40 000 molecular weight pertussis toxin substrate, probably the alpha subunit of the inhibitory G-protein (alpha-G_1), is increased by 36% in failing human hearts when compared with nonfailing controls, associated with a 30% decrease in basal as well as 5'-guanylylimidodiphosphate-stimulated adenylate cyclase activity [38]. Further studies, in which antibodies were used to examine failing hearts,

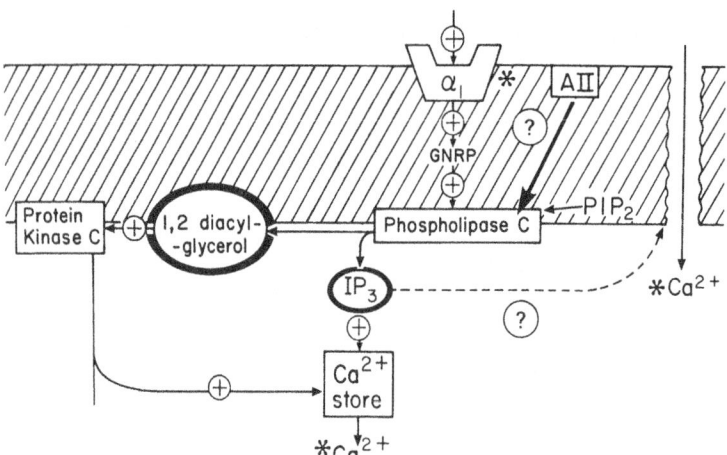

Fig. 2. Pathways mediating alpha$_1$-adrenoceptor activity. Norepinephrine released from sympathetic nerve terminals or in the circulation binds to and activates alpha$_1$-adrenoceptors (α_1) which, via a guanine nucleotide regulatory protein, activates phospholipase C. This enzyme catalyses the conversion of phosphatidylinositol biophosphate (*PIP$_2$*) to 1,2-diacylglycerol and inositol trisphosphate (*IP$_3$*). 1,2-Diacylglycerol activates protein kinase C, which, in turn, has a number of important actions, including Na^+-H^+ exchange, phosphorylation of antiphospholipase-A$_2$, and phosphorylation of the myosin light chain. IP$_3$ stimulates Ca^{2+} release from the sarcoplasmic reticulum and may open transsarcolemmal Ca^{2+} channels

have indicated that minor decreases in the amount of the active (alpha) moiety of G_s may be associated with prominent changes in functional activity of this protein in terms of its ability to be activated by GTP [39].

These studies have given rise to an attempt by Horn et al. [40] to use peripheral blood mononuclear leucocytes (MNL) as a "tissue" to examine changes in the concentration of G_s in patients with congestive heart failure. Patients with congestive heart failure (New York Heart Association class III) had 80% less $alpha_s$ than controls, and these levels increased 2.5 fold after treatment with angiotensin-converting enzyme inhibitors. Although these are potentially very important observations, a number of questions regarding these data have been raised [41]. These include the possibility that these effects may be the result of raised plasma catecholamine levels, and that the method used (cholera toxin labelling) is not an adequate means to quantitate amounts of G-proteins. There are also some conceptual questions, such as: is congestive heart failure a symptom complex that involves cells throughout the body, as would be implied by a decrease in G_s in MNL; how could treatment with ACE inhibitors increase levels of G_s?

The consequence of an enhanced G_i activity, with or without some defect of G_s, is a deficient production of cAMP. In a study on myocardium in vitro from patients with end-stage cardiac failure [42], peak isometric force generated in response to increased extracellular Ca^{2+} reached control levels, but the time course of contraction and rate of relaxation were greatly prolonged. The inotropic effectiveness of the beta-adrenergic agonist isoproterenol and the phosphodiesterase inhibitors milrinone, caffeine and isobutylmethylxanthine was markedly reduced. In contrast, the effectiveness of inotropic stimulation with acetylstrophanthidin and the adenylate cyclase activator forskolin was preserved. After a minimally effective dose of forskolin was given to elevate intracellular cAMP levels, the inotropic responses of muscles from the failing hearts to phosphodiesterase inhibitors were markedly potentiated. These data suggest that an abnormality in cAMP production may be a fundamental defect present in patients with end-stage heart failure, and that this can greatly diminish the effectiveness of agents that depend on cAMP for production of a positive inotropic effect.

A predicted consequence of decreased cAMP concentration is abnormal intracellular Ca^{2+} handling in these heart cells. The same authors [43] have provided evidence that this is so; in heart muscle from patients with end-stage cardiac failure, contractions and Ca^{2+} transients of muscles from failing hearts were markedly prolonged, and there was a diminished capacity to restore low resting Ca^{2+} levels during diastole. On a more pragmatic level, the elucidation of these membrane-linked and intracellular receptor-contraction coupling events has clarified the mechanisms of action of more traditional drugs for heart failure and has made possible the development of new forms of therapy.

Cellular/Molecular Basis of Action of Inotropic Drugs

There is considerable interest in the development of new orally active positive inotropic agents, and a number of different drug candidates have been identified to act through different cellular and biochemical mechanisms [44], by inhibiting Na^+-K^+-ATPase (cardiac glycosides), stimulating beta-adrenoceptors (beta-agonists, e.g. dopamine), stimulating adenylate cyclase (forskolin), inhibiting phosphodiesterase (e.g. amrinone, milinone), activating Ca^{2+} ion channels (e.g. Bay K-8644) or by enhancing the Ca^{2+} sensitivity of the myocardial contractile proteins (e.g. sulmazole). Table 1 lists a selection of compounds that affect Ca^{2+} availability to initiate and maintain contractility.

The mechanisms of action of some of these agents is still uncertain. For example, amrinone, milronone (listed as phosphodiesterase inhibitors) and pimobendan (a "calcium sensitizer") are also A_1 adenosine receptor antagonists [65,66]. Sulmazole (calcium sensitizer) seems to stimulate the myocyte by three

Table 1. Inotropic agents

Mode of action	Compound	Reference
Inhibition of Na^+-K^+-ATPase	Cardiac glycosides	
Stimulation of beta-adrenoceptors	Dopamine	[45]
	Ibopamine	[46]
	Dobutamine	[47]
	Butopamine	[48]
	Denopamine	[49]
	Prenalterol	[50]
	Xamoterol	[51]
Stimulation of adenylate cyclase	Forskolin	[52]
cAMP phosphodiesterase III inhibitors	Amrinone	[53]
	Milrinone	[53]
	Enoximone	[54]
	Piroximone	[54]
	OPC-8212	[55]
	Imazodan	[56]
Activators of Ca^{2+} ion channels	Bay K-8644	[57]
	CGP 28 392	[58]
Agents that enhance the Ca^{2+} sensitivity of myocardial contractile proteins ("calcium sensitizers")	Sulmazole	[59]
	Isomazole	
	UN-LZ97,98	
	BM 14,478	[60]
	MCI-154	[61]
	DPI 201–106	[62]
	Pimobendan	[63,64]
	UD-CG 212	

additional mechanisms: (a) inhibition of cAMP phosphodiesterase; (b) antagonism of endogenous adenosine at A_1 receptors; and (c) blockade of the inhibitory guanine nucleotide regulatory protein G_i [66]. DPI 201–106 appears also to open Na^+ channels, and pimobendan and UD-DG 212 both also have a selective cAMP phosphodiesterase III inhibitor activity.

Dopamine and dopamine analogues are useful in the therapy of congestive heart failure by virtue of their ability to behave as agonists at beta-adrenoreceptors in the heart, as well as by reducing ventricular afterload by DA_1-receptor mediated vasodilatation. However, relatively specific DA_2-receptor agonists such as lergotrile, pergolide, bromocriptine and DPDA (*N,N*-di-n-propyldopamine) are negatively chronotropic but have no effect on myocardial contractility [67].

Conclusion

The cardiovascular adaptations to volume or pressure overload are short, intermediate and longer term. Short-term responses are beat-to-beat and depend on relationships between the loading characteristics of the heart and muscle shortening such as those described in the Frank-Starling ventricular function curve. Intermediate-term effects are usually reflex or endocrine mediated, while longer-term adaptations refer to changes in the rates of gene expression. It is in this last area that research advances have been so spectacular in the past few years.

Autonomic receptors, particularly alpha- and beta-adrenergic receptors have been recognized and characterized at many levels of the sympathetic nervous system, not only by the methods of classical pharmacology, but also by radioligand-binding methods. The genes encoding adrenergic receptors have been cloned and sequenced, and we now know much more of the complex transduction mechanisms which link membrane receptors with the contractile proteins of the heart cells.

In congestive heart failure there is down-regulation of beta-receptors in cardiac myocytes. There is also an increase of the G_i inhibitory protein and, possibly a decrease of the G_s stimulatory protein, both resulting in a defect of cAMP formation. This, in turn, will adversely affect intracellular Ca^{2+} handling by the cell. Also, in heart failure, there is an increase in $alpha_1$-receptors, of unknown significance, and a decline in muscarinic receptor density with impaired muscarinic functional efficiency.

It is likely that, as the cascade of receptor-contractile coupling is clarified, more cellular abnormalities related to receptors and their activity will come to light in heart failure. There are profound implications of these developments for understanding the mechanism of action of inotropic drugs and for the development of new forms of therapy for heart failure.

References

1. Ahlquist RP (1948) A study of adrenotropic receptors. Am J Physiol 153:586-600
2. Berthelson S, Pettinger WA (1977) A functional basis for classification of alpha-adrenergic receptors. Life Sci 21:596-606
3. Hoffman BB, Lefkowitz RJ (1980) Radioligand binding studies of adrenergic receptors: new insights into molecular and physiological regulation. Ann Rev Pharmacol Toxicol 20:581-608
4. Motulsky HJ, Insel PA (1982) Adrenergic receptors in man. N Engl J Med 307:18-29
5. Stiles GL, Taylor S, Lefkowitz RJ (1983) Human cardiac beta-adrenergic receptors: subtype heterogenicity delineated by direct ligand binding. Life Sci 33:467-473
6. Hedberg A, Minnerman KP, Molinoff PB (1980) Differential distribution of beta-1 and beta-2 adrenergic receptors in cat and guinea-pig heart. J Pharmacol Exp Ther 212:503-508
7. Hoffman BB, Lefkowitz RJ (1980) Alpha-adrenergic receptor subtypes. N Engl J Med 302:1390-1395
8. Bylund DB, U'Pritchard DC (1983) Characterisation of alpha$_1$ and alpha$_2$-adrenergic receptors. Int Rev Neurobiol 24:343-431
9. U'Prichard DC, Snyder SH (1979) Distinct alpha-noradrenergic receptors differentiated by binding and physiological relationships. Life Sci 24:79-88
10. Scholz H, Bruckner R (1982) Effects of beta- and alpha-adrenoceptor stimulating agents on mechanical activity, electrophysiological parameters and cyclic nucleotide levels in the heart. In: Caldarera CR, Harris P (eds) Advances in studies on heart metabolism. CLUEB, Bologna
11. Adler-Graschinsky E, Langer SZ (1975) Possible role of a beta-adrenoreceptor in the regulation of noradrenaline release by nerve stimulation through a positive feed-back mechanism. Br J Pharmacol 53:43-40
12. Kawasaki H, Clive WH, Su C (1982) Enhanced presynaptic beta-adrenoreceptor-mediated modulation of vascular adrenergic neurotransmission in spontaneously hypertensive rats. J Pharmacol Exp Ther 223:721-728
13. Rosendorff C, Cranston WI (1971) Effects of intrahypothalamic and intraventricular noradrenaline and 5-hydroxytryptamine on hypothalamic blood flow in the conscious rabbit. Circ Res 28:492-502
14. Bomzon L, Rosendorff C, Scriven DRL, Farr J (1975) The effect of noradrenaline, adrenergic blocking agents and tyramine on the intrarenal distribution of blood flow in the baboon. Cardiovasc Res 9:314-322
15. Rosendorff C, Hoffman JIE, Verrier E, Rouleau JR, Boerboom LE (1981) Cholesterol sensitizes coronary vessels to norepinephrine. Circ Res 48:320-329
16. Pappano AJ (1976) Onset of chronotropic effects of nicotinic drugs and tyramine on the sino-atrial pacemaker in chick embryo heart; relationship to the development of autonomic neuroeffector transmission. J Pharmacol Exp Ther 196:676-684
17. Vatner DE, Lee DL, Schwarz KR, Longabaugh JP, Fujii AM, Vatner SF, Homcy CJ (1988) Impaired cardiac muscarinic receptor function in dogs with heart failure. J Clin Invest 81:1836-1842
18. Prokopczuk A, Pytkowski B, Lawartowski B (1981) Effect of acetylcholine on calcium efflux from atrial myocardium. Eur J Pharmacol 70:1-6
19. Frielle T, Collins S, Daniel KW, Caron MG, Lefkowitz RJ, Kobilka BK (1987) Cloning of the cDNA for the human beta-adrenergic receptor. Proc Natl Acad Sci USA 84:7920-7924
20. Kobilka BK, Matsui HG, Kobilka TA, Yang-Feng TL, Francke U, Caron MG, Lefkowitz RJ, Regan JW (1987) Cloning, sequencing, and expression of the gene coding for the human platelet alpha$_2$-adrenergic receptor. Science 238:650-656
21. Regan JW, Kobilka TS, Yang-Feng TL, Caron MG, Lefkowitz RJ, Kobilka BK (1988) Cloning and expression of a human kidney cDNA for an alpha$_2$-adrenergic receptor subtype. Proc Natl Acad Sci USA 85:6301-6305
22. Cotecchia S, Schwinn DA, Randall RR, Lefkowtiz RJ, Caron MG, Kobilka BK (1988) Molecular cloning and expression of the cDNA for the hamster alpha$_1$-adrenergic receptor. Proc Natl Acad Sci USA 85:7159-7163

23. Peralta EG, Winslow JW, Peterson GL, Smith DH, Ramachandran J, Schimerlik MI, Capon DJ, Ashkenazi A (1987) Primary structure and biochemical properties of an M2 muscarinic receptor: Muscarinic subtypes are distinct gene products. Science 236:600–605

24. Rosendorff C, Susanni E, Hurwitz ML, Ross FP (1985) Adrenergic receptors in hypertension: radioligand binding studies. J Hypertension 3:571–581

25. Bristow MR, Ginsburg R, Minobe W et al. (1982) Decreased catecholamine sensitivity and beta-adrenergic-receptor density in failing human hearts. N Engl J Med 307:205–211

26. Ruffolo RR, Kopia GA (1986) Importance of receptor regulation in the pathophysiology and therapy of congestive heart failure. Am J Med [Suppl 2B] 80:67–72

27. Baumann G, Mercader D, Busch U et al. (1983) Effects of the H_2-receptor agonist impromidine in human myocardium from patients with heart failure due to mitral an aortic valve disease. J Cardiovasc Pharmacol 5:618–625

28. Francis GS, Cohn JN (1986) The autonomic nervous system in congestive heart failure. Ann Rev Med 37:235–247

29. Williams RS (1983) Selectivity of prenalterol for adrenergic receptor subtypes: a potential mechanism of inotropic selectivity. J Cardiovasc Pharmacol 5:266–271

30. Bristow MR, Ginsburg R, Umans V, Fowler M, Minobe W, Rasmussen R, Zera P, Menlove R, Shah P, Jamieson S, Stinson EB (1986) $Beta_1$- and $beta_2$-adrenergic receptor subpopulations in nonfailing and failing human ventricular myocardium: compiling of both receptor subtypes to muscle contraction and selective $beta_1$-receptor down regulation in heart failure. Circ Res 59:297–309

31. Limas CJ, Limas C (1984) Rapid recovery of cardiac beta-adrenergic receptors after isoproterenol-induced "down"-regulation. Circ Res 55:524–531

32. Limas CJ, Goldenberg IF, Limas C (1989) Autoantibodies against beta-adrenoceptors in human idiopathic dilated cardiomyopathy. Circ Res 64:97–103

33. Vago T, Bevilaqua M, Norbiato G, Baldi G, Chebat E, Bertora P, Baroldi G, Accinni R (1989) Identification of $alpha_1$-adrenergic receptors on sarcolemma from nomal subjects and patients with idiopathic dilated cardiomyopathy: characteristics and linkage to GTP-binding protein. Circ Res 64:474–481

34. Harris P, Harding SE (1986) The molecular actions of beta-agonists in the cardiac sarcolemma. J Cardiovasc Pharmacol [Suppl 3] 8:S10–S11

35. Weiss ER, Kelleher DJ, Woon CW, Soparkar S, Osawa S, Heasley LE, Johnson GL (1988) Receptor activation of G-proteins. FASEB J 2:2841–2848

36. Shenolikar S (1988) Protein phosphorylation: hormones, drugs, and bioregulation. FASEB J 2:2753–2764

37. Rosenthal W, Herscheller J, Trautwein W, Schultz G (1988) Control of voltage dependent Ca^{2+} channels by G protein-coupled receptors. FASEB J 2:2784–2790

38. Feldman AM, Cates AE, Veazey WB, Herschberger RE, Bristow MR, Baughman KL, Baumgartner WA, Van Dop C (1988) Increase of the 40 000-mol wt pertussis toxin substrate (G-protein) in the failing human heart. J Clin Invest 82:189–197

39. Ransnas LA, Hjalmarson A, Insel PA (1988) Dilated cardiomyopathy is associated with an impaired activation of the stimulatory G-protein, G_s, by GTP in heart membranes (abstract). Circulation 78(Suppl II):11–178

40. Horn EM, Corwin SJ, Steinberg SF, Chow YK, Neuberg GW, Cannon PJ, Powers ER, Bilezikian JP (1988) Reduced lymphocyte stimulatory guanine nucleotide regulatory protein and beta-adrenergic receptors in congestive heart failure and reversal with angiotensin converting enzyme inhibitor therapy. Circulation 78:1373–1379

41. Insel PA, Ransnas LA (1988) G-proteins and cardiovascular disease. Circulation 78:1511–1513

42. Feldman MD, Copelas L, Gwathmey JK, Phillips P, Warren SE, Schoen FJ, Grossman W, Morgan JP (1987) Deficient production of cyclic AMP: pharmacologic evidence of an important cause of contractile dysfunction in patients with end-stage heart failure. Circulation 75:331–339

43. Gwathmey JK, Copelas L, MacKinnon R, Schoen FJ, Feldman MD, Grossman W, Morgan JP (1987) Abnormal intracellular calcium handling in myocardium from patients with end-stage heart failure. Circ Res 61:70–76

44. Wetzel B, Hauel N (1988) New cardiotonic agents — a promising approach for the treatment of heart failure. Trends Pharmacol Sci 9:116–170

45. Maskin CS, Kugler J, Sonnenblick EH, Le Jemtel TH (1983) Acute inotropic stimulation with dopamine in severe congestive heart failure: beneficial hemodynamic effect at rest but not during maximal exercise. Am J Cardiol 52:1028-1032
46. Cantelli J, Lolli C, Bomba E, Brunelli D, Bracchetti D (1986) Ibopamine. Curr Ther Res Clin Exp 39:900-911
47. Chatterjee K, Bendersky R, Parmley WW (1982) Dobutamine in heart failure. Eur Heart J [Suppl D] 3:107-114
48. Thompson MJ, Juss P, Unverferth DV, Fasola A, Leier CV (1980) Hemodynamic effects of intravenous butopamine in congestive heart failure. Clin Pharmacol Ther 28:324-334
49. Ikeo T, Nagao T, Murata S, Yabana H, Sato M, Nakajima H (1986) Cardiovascular effects of the new positive inotropic agent denopamine with special reference to species difference and the effect on the failing heart. Arzneimittelforsch 36:1063-1068
50. Lambertz H, Meyer J, Erbel R (1984) Long-term hemodynamic effects of prenalterol in patients with severe congestive heart failure. Circulation 69:298-305
51. Molajo AO, Bennett DH (1985) Effect of xamoterol (ICI 118587), a new beta adrenoceptor partial agonist, on resting haemodynamic variables and exercise tolerance in patients with left ventricular dysfunction. Br Heart J 54:17-21
52. Bristow MR, Ginsburg R, Strosberg A, Montgomery W, Minobe W (1984) Pharmacology and inotropic potential of forskolin in the human heart. J Clin Invest 74:212-223
53. Alousi AA, Johnson DC (1986) Pharmacology of the bipyridines: amrinone and milrinone. Circulation 73 III:10-24
54. Maskin CS, Weber KT, Janicki JS (1987) Long-term oral enoximone therapy in chronic cardiac failure. Am J Cardiol 60:63C-67C
55. Iijima T, Taira N (1987) Membrane current changes responsible for the positive inotropic effect of OPC-8212, a new positive inotropic agent, in single ventricular cells of the guinea pig heart. J Pharmacol Exp Ther 240:657-662
56. Bristol JA, Sircar J, Moos WH, Evans DB, Weishaar RE (1984) Cardiotonic agents 1. 4,5-dihydro-6-[4-(1H-imidazol-1-yl) phenyl]-3 (2H)-pyridazinones: novel positive inotropic agents for the treatment of congestive heart failure. J Med Chem 27:1099-1101
57. Schramm M, Bechem M, Franchowiak G, Gro R, Thomas G (1985) One enantiomer of the positive inotropic dihydropyridine Bay K 8644 is a calcium-antagonist. J Mol Cell Cardiol 17[Suppl 3]:201
58. Laurent S, Kim D, Smith TW, Marsh JD (1985) Inotropic effect, binding properties, and calcium flux effects of the calcium channel agonist CGP 28392 in intact cultured embryonic chick ventricular cells. Circ Res 56:676-682
59. Hagemeijer F, Segers A, Schelling A (1984) Cardiovascular effects of sulmazol administered intravenously to patients with severe heart failure. Eur Heart J 5:158-167
60. Freund P, Muller-Bechmann B, Strein K, Kling L, Ruegg JC (1987) Ca^{2+}-sensitizing effects of BM 14,478 on skinned cardiac muscle fibres of guinea pig papillary muscle. Eur J Pharmacol 136:243-246
61. Kitada Y, Narimatsu A, Matsumura N, Endo M (1987) Contractile proteins: possible targets for the cardiotonic action of MCI-154, a novel cardiotonic agent? Eur J Pharmacol 134:229-231
62. Scholtysik G, Salzmann R, Berthold R, Herzig JW, Quast U, Markstein R (1985) DPI 201-106, a novel cardioactive agent. Combination of cAMP-independent positive inotropic, negative chronotropic, action potential prolonging and coronary dilatory properties. Naunyn Schmiedebergs Arch Pharmacol 329:316-325
63. Anon (1986) Pimobendan. Drugs Future 11:625-626
64. Fritsche R, Scheld HH, Van Meel JCA, Hehrlein W (1986) Effect of pimobendan on calcium sensitivity of skinned fibres isolated from human papillary muscles. Br J Pharmacol 89:751P
65. Paton DM, Manuel JM (1988) Mechanisms of action of the new cardiotonic drugs. Trends Pharmacol Sci 9:431-432
66. Parsons WJ, Rankumar V, Stiles GL (1988) The new cardiotonic agent sulmazole is an A_1 adenosine receptor antagonist and functionally blocks the inhibitory regulator, Gi. Mol Pharmacol 33:441-448
67. Cavero I, Massingham R, Lefevre-Borg F (1982) Peripheral dopamine receptors, potential targets for a new class of antihypertensive agents. Life Sci 31:1059-1069

Beta-Adrenoceptors in Heart Failure: A Mechanism or a cAMP Follower?

S.E. Harding and P.A. Poole-Wilson

Introduction

In the myocardium of many patients with symptoms of heart failure there is a decrease in beta-adrenoceptor number, accompanied by a reduction in responsiveness to beta-agonists [3,5,8,10,16]. The hypothesis that this results simply from exposure to high circulating catecholamines is in dispute. The role of beta-adrenoceptor desensitisation in the progression of heart failure and the therapeutic implications are the subject of considerable debate.

Plasma Catecholamines in Heart Failure

Plasma noradrenaline is elevated in heart failure [17], and the concentration in patients at rest is related to the severity of heart failure and to mortality [12]. In mild untreated heart failure plasma noradrenaline is increased, but decreases with treatment as the expanded body fluid compartments are normalised [2]. By contrast, plasma renin is not raised but increases after treatment with a diuretic [2]. In severe heart failure, plasma noradrenaline is increased in both treated and untreated patients [1]. Plasma adrenaline is unchanged in both mild and severe untreated heart failure. Thus in man stimulation of the sympathetic nervous system is an early response to heart failure.

Elevation of plasma noradrenaline is widely regarded as an indicator of sympathetic activity. However, the plasma concentration depends not only on the overspill of noradrenaline from synapses, but also on the metabolism of noradrenaline in the liver and elsewhere. Liver function and blood flow are reduced in heart failure and may contribute in a minor way to the observed increase of plasma concentrations.

Plasma noradrenaline increases on exercise in both normal persons and in patients with heart failure [17]. For intermediate levels of exercise, the increase in patients with heart failure is greater. However, at peak exercise normal persons have higher plasma noradrenaline concentrations. The sympathetic system is stimulated earlier during exercise in heart failure, but the maximum stimulation possible is less.

B.S. Lewis, A. Kimchi (Eds.)
Heart Failure Mechanisms and Management
© Springer-Verlag Berlin Heidelberg 1991

Myocardial Catecholamines in Heart Failure

Noradrenaline is reduced in the myocardium of humans with heart failure, but the clinical features of heart failure precede the reduction [11,24]. The reduction is attributed either to defective synthesis linked to reduced activity of tyrosine hydroxylase [21] or to an abnormality of transport of dopamine across the membrane of the noradrenergic granule [28]. However, although most patients do have low noradrenaline and high dopamine, many do not. There is no simple relation between plasma noradrenaline concentrations and myocardial concentrations [24].

Desensitisation of Beta-Receptors in Heart Failure

Desensitisation is a general term and may be due either to uncoupling of the receptor from the effector or to a decrease in the receptor density at the sarcolemma (down-regulation). Down-regulated receptors can be either reversibly sequestered away from the cell membrane (internalisation) or irreversibly degraded. Beta-adrenoceptor desensitisation in the myocardium of patients with symptoms of heart failure has been confirmed by a number of independent methods. These methods include in vivo assessment of cardiac function after treatment with beta-agonists, isometric force measurements in atrial or ventricular muscle strips, and adenylate cyclase or radioligand binding assays of sarcolemmal membrane fractions [3,5,8,13]. Although the general finding of beta-adrenoceptor desensitisation is consistent, there are problems in quantitation of the effect with each of these methods. The measurement of in vivo myocardial response in the presence of altered loading conditions and heart size is notoriously difficult. The sensitivity of intact muscle strips in vitro can be modified by release of tissue noradrenaline or adenosine [19]. Assays which use sarcolemmal preparations can be affected by the presence of non-myocyte membranes [29] or by a decrease in surface membrane protein/intracellular protein ratio during hypertrophy.

Homologous or Heterologous Desensitisation?

The simple hypothesis put forward is that beta-adrenoceptor desensitisation may result from prolonged exposure to the raised plasma noradrenaline that is found in these patients. This hypothesis is as yet unproven because the nature of the changes in the adenylate cyclase cascade (Fig. 1) that occur in heart failure are not agreed upon. It is known that infusion of a beta-agonist will result in beta-adrenoceptor desensitisation, and that this desensitisation is initially homologous. In homologous desensitisation, only responses to agonists acting through the beta-adrenoceptor are reduced; this is due to the action of the

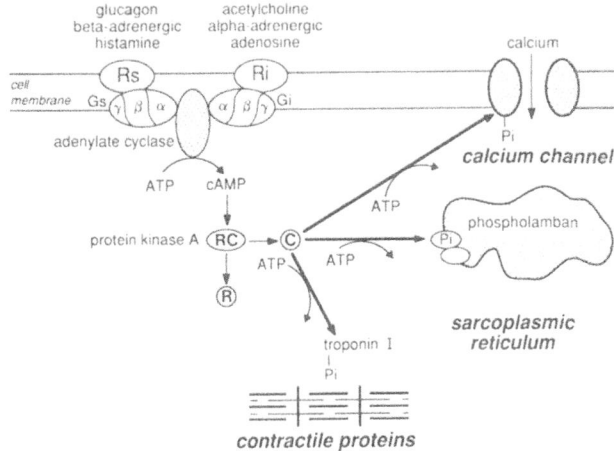

Fig. 1. The beta-receptor pathway. *Rs*, stimulatory receptor; *Ri*, inhibitory receptor; *Gs*, stimulatory guanine-nucleotide binding protein; *Gi*, inhibitory guanine-nucleotide binding protein; *R*, regulatory subunit of protein kinase A; *C*, catalytic subunit of protein kinase A

beta-adrenoceptor kinase (BARK), which phosphorylates only the agonist-oc-cupied form of the receptor. With heterologous desensitisation there are alte-rations in distal parts of the adenylate cyclase pathway. A pattern of change consistent with homologous desensitisation has been found in failing heart by Bristow et al. [4–6] who report that responses to the positive inotropic agents calcium, forskolin, histamine and vasoactive intestinal peptide (VIP) are pre-served at the time as those to beta-adrenoceptor agonists are lost. Other evidence that points to circulating noradrenaline as a desensitising agent is the preferential down-regulation of beta$_1$- rather than beta$_2$-receptors in heart failure [8] (noradrenaline is primarily a beta$_1$-agonist), and the fact that heart failure of varying aetiologies produces the same effect [5,16]. The finding that beta-adrenoceptor desensitisation is observed in all chambers of the heart studied [7] would also support this conclusion, but evidence is conflicting on this point [5].

Evidence against a homologous desensitisation has been found in several studies. Bohm et al. [3] have shown that the effects of histamine and a phos-phodiesterase inhibitor were attenuated in heart failure. Another study [10], on papillary muscles obtained during mitral valve replacement, found reduced responsiveness of a wide variety of inotropic agents relative to calcium. It has been suggested that there is a reduction in basal cAMP in the failing heart, and that this is due to deficiencies in production separate from the beta-adrenoceptor [15]. There have also been several reports that the inhibitory guanine-nucleotide binding protein (G$_i$) is raised in heart failure [14,23]. Animal models of heart failure have given conflicting results, some failing to show any beta-adrenoceptor desensitisation [20,31].

The reasons for the variability in the pattern of desensitisation in the adenylate cyclase cascade is not known. It may be that the extent of exposure to raised catecholamines is an important determinant of the effect. In cultured rat heart cells an apparent homologous desensitisation will turn to a heterologous form with increased concentration of noradrenaline [25]. The underlying cause, a reduction in basal cAMP levels leading to a decreased maximal cAMP production by both isoprenaline and forskolin, is the same at both stages. In the early phase, however, forskolin still generates enough cAMP to produce a maximal response, while isoprenaline does not. This produces an apparent difference in the degree of subsensitivity to the two agents. After more severe exposure to noradrenaline, the depression in cAMP generation is sufficient to affect responses to both isoprenaline and forskolin.

We also suggest the possibility that the alpha-adrenergic effects of noradrenaline may alter parts of the beta-adrenoceptor/adenylate cyclase cascade. Alpha-adrenergic stimulation results in breakdown of phosphatidylinositol bisphosphate (PIP_2) to inositol trisphosphate (IP_3) and diacylglycerol (DAG) [26]. DAG will then activate protein kinase C (PKC) [9]. It has been shown that PKC directly phosphorylates sites on receptors that stimulate adenylate cyclase [27], and that the subsensitivity produced is in addition to any homologous desensitisation caused by the receptor's own agonist [30]. VIP (vasoactive intestinal peptide), HI (histamine) and ANP (atrial natriuretic peptide) receptors have all been shown to down-regulate in response to raised PKC [18,22,30]. There exist, therefore, possibilities for crosstalk between the alpha- and beta-adrenoceptor pathways. Desensitisation to a dual agonist may well be more complex than that to a pure beta-adrenoceptor effector.

Beta-Blockade in Heart Failure

Several groups have reported benefit of beta-blockade in patients with heart failure. At first sight this is a paradoxical result because the negative inotropic effect of beta-blockade might be expected to make the heart failure worse. Possible mechanisms include a reduction of heart rate resulting in better myocardial perfusion and possibly a reduced oxygen consumption. Diastolic relaxation may be improved or be more complete because of the longer diastolic time. Myocardial ischaemia may be relieved as in angina pectoris, and any effect of "stunned" or "hibernating" heart be overcome. Oxygen consumption may be lessened and a direct toxic effect of catecholamines on the heart muscle prevented. Beta-adrenoceptor desensitisation may be prevented so that during exercise, when the increase in plasma catecholamines is sufficient to partially overcome the blockade, the heart is able to respond to the beta-stimulation. Partial agonists, such as xamoteral (Corwin), may have the benefits of beta-blockers without completely depriving resting muscle of inotropic support. Further trials are necessary to determine whether the benefit of beta-blockade is a real phenomenon and in which group of patients the benefit is greatest. It might be expected that beta-blockade would be of value in patients with small hearts, myocardial hypertrophy, a degree of diastolic dysfunction and coronary artery disease as the cause of heart failure.

Conclusion

The sympathetic system is stimulated in heart failure and is an early and important compensatory response. During the development of symptoms, the receptors in the heart are diminished in number, the myocardial noradrenaline content reduced and the response of the myocardium to sympathetic stimulation limited. To what extent this is merely a manifestation of myocardial disease or an important mechanism detemining cardiac function is less certain. The matter needs to be resolved because the role of many therapeutic strategies and new pharmaceutical agents in heart failure rests on an understanding of the importance of the sympathetic system in heart failure.

References

1. Anand IS, Ferrari R, Kalra GS, Wahi PL, Poole-Wilson PA, Harris P (1989) Edema of cardiac origin: studies of body water and sodium, renal function, hemodynamics and plasma hormones in untreated congestive heart failure. Circulation 80:299–305
2. Bayliss J, Norell M, Capena-Anson R, Sutton G, Poole-Wilson PA (1987) Untreated heart failure: clinical and neuroendocrine effects of introducing diuretics. Br Heart J 57:17–22
3. Bohm M, Beuckelmann D, Brown L, Feiler G, Lorenz B, Nabauer M, Kemkes B, Erdmann E (1988) Reduction of beta-adrenoceptor density and evaluation of positive inotropic responses in isolated, diseased human myocardium. Eur Heart J 9:844–852
4. Bristow MR, Ginsburg R, Gilbert EM, Hershberger RE (1987) Heterogeneous regulatory changes in cell surface membrane receptors coupled to a positive inotropic response in the failing human heart. Basic Res Cardiol 82 (Suppl 2):369–377
5. Bristow MR, Ginsburg R, Minobe W, Cubicciotti RS, Sageman WS, Lurie K, Billingham ME, Harrison DC, Stinson EB (1982) Decreased catecholamine sensitivity and beta-adrenergic receptor density in failing human hearts. N Engl J Med 307:205–211
6. Bristow MR, Ginsburg R, Strosberg A, Montgomery W, Minobe W (1984) Pharmacology and inotropic potential of forskolin in the human heart. J Clin Invest 74:212–223
7. Brodde OE (1988) The functional importance of beta 1 and beta 2 adrenoceptor in the human heart. A symposium: Focus on heart failure – current experiences in basic research and clinical studies on dopexamine hydrochloride (Dopacard). September 12–13, 1987, Paris, France. Proceedings. Am J Cardiol 62:1C–88C
8. Brodde OE, Schuler S, Kretsch R, Brinkmann M, Borst HG, Hetzer R, Reidmeister JC, Warnecke H, Zerkowski HR (1986) Regional distribution of beta-adrenoceptors in the human heart: coexistence of functional beta$_1$- and beta$_2$-adrenoceptors in both atria and ventricles in severe congestive cardiomyopathy. J Cardiovasc Pharmacol 8:1235–1242
9. Bronfman M, Morales MN, Orellana A (1988) Diacylglycerol activation of protein kinase C is modulated by long-chain ACYL-CoA. Biochem Biophys Res Commun 152:987–992
10. Brown L, Lorenz B, Erdmann E (1986) Reduced positive inotropic effects in diseased human ventricular myocardium. Cardiovasc Res 20:516–520
11. Chidsey CA, Braunwald EB, Morrow AG, Mason DT (1963) Myocardial norepinephrine concentration in man; effects of reserpine and of congestive heart failure. N Engl J Med 269:653–658
12. Cohn JN, Levine TB, Olivari MT, Garberg V, Lura D, Francis GS, Simon AB, Rector T (1984) Plasma norepinephrine as a guide to prognosis in patients with chronic congestive heart failure. N Engl J Med 311:819–823
13. Erne P, Lipkin D, Maseri A (1988) Impaired beta-adrenergic receptor and normal postreceptor responsiveness in congestive heart failure. Am J Cardiol 61:1132–1134

14. Feldman AM, Cates AE, Veazey WB, Hershberger RE, Bristow MR, Baughman KL, Baumgartner WA, Van Dop C (1988) Increase of the 40,000-mol wt pertussis toxin substrate (G-protein) in the failing human heart. J Clin Invest 82:189–197
15. Feldman MD, Copelas BS, Gwathmey JK, Phillips P, Warren SE, Schoen FJ, Grossman W, Morgan JP (1987) Deficient production of cyclic AMP: pharmacologic evidence of an important cause of contractile dysfunction in patients with end-stage failure. Circulation 2:331–339
16. Fowler MB, Laser JA, Hopkins GL, Minobe W, Bristow MR (1986) Assessment of the B-adrenergic receptor pathway in the intact failing human heart: progressive receptor down-regulation and subsensitivity to agonist response. Circulation 74:1290–1302
17. Francis GS, Goldsmith SR, Ziesche SM, Cohn JN (1982) Response of norepinephrine and epinephrine to dynamic exercise in patients with congestive heart failure. Am J Cardiol 49:1152–1156
18. Hirata Y (1988) Heterologous down-regulation of vascular atrial natriuretic peptide receptors by phorbol esters. Biochem Biophys Res Commun 152:1097–1103
19. Hopwood AM, Harding SE, Harris P (1987) An antiadrenergic effect of adenosine on guinea-pig but not rabbit ventricles. Eur J Pharmacol 137:67–75
20. Karliner JS, Alabaster C, Stephens H, Barnes P, Dollery C (1981) Enhanced noradrenaline response in cardiomyopathic hamsters: possible relation to changes in adrenoceptors studied by radioligand binding. Cardiovasc Res 15:296–304
21. Levitt M, Spector S, Sjoerdsma A, Undenfriend S (1965) Elucidation of the rate limiting step in norepinephrine biosynthesis in the perfused guinea-pig heart. J Pharmacol Exp Ther 148:1–8
22. Mitsuhashi M, Payan DG (1988) Phorbol ester-mediated desensitization of histamine H1 receptors on a cultured smooth muscle cell line. Life Sci 43:1433–1440
23. Neumann J, Schmitz W, Scholz H, von Meyerinck L, Doring V, Kalmar P (1988) Increase in myocardial G_i-proteins in heart failure. Lancet 2:936–937
24. Pierpont GL, Francis GS, DeMaster EG, Olivari MT, Ring WT, Goldberg IF, Reynolds S, Cohn JN (1987) Heterologous myocardial catecholamine concentrations in patients with congestive heart failure. Am J Cardiol 60:316–321
25. Reithmann C, Werdan K (1988) Homologous vs. heterologous desensitization of the adenylate cyclase system in heart cells. Eur J Pharmacol 154:99–104
26. Scholz J, Schaefer B, Schmitz W, Scholz H, Steinfath M, Lohse M, Schwabe U, Puurunen J (1988) Alpha-1 adrenoceptor-mediated positive inotropic effect and inositol trisphosphate increase in mammalian heart. J Pharmacol Exp Ther 245:327–335
27. Sibley DR, Benovic JL, Caron MG, Lefkowitz RJ (1988) Phosphorylation of cell surface receptors: a mechanism for regulating signal transduction pathways. Endocr Rev 9:38–56
28. Sole MJ, Helke CJ, Jacobwitz DM (1982) Increased dopamine in the failing hamster heart: transvesicular transport of dopamine limits the rate of norepinephrine synthesis. Am J Cardiol 49:1682–1690
29. Tomlins B, Harding SE, Kirby MS, Poole-Wilson PA, Williams AJ (1986) Contamination of a cardiac sarcolemmal preparation with endothelial plasma membrane. Biochim Biophys Acta 856:137–143
30. Turner JT, Bollinger DW, Toews ML (1988) Vasoactive intestinal peptide receptor/adenylate cyclase system: differences between agonist- and protein kinase C-mediated desensitization and further evidence for receptor internalization. J Pharmacol Exp Ther 247:417–423
31. Vescovo G, Kirby MS, Harding SE, Wanless RB, Anand IS, Poole-Wilson PA (1987) Responses to isoprenaline and calcium in myocytes isolated from the hearts of adriamycin-treated rabbits. J Mol Cell Cardiol 19 (Suppl 3):312 (Abstract)

Anti-β-Adrenoceptor Autoantibodies with β-Adrenergic Agonistic Activity from Patients with Myocarditis and Dilated Cardiomyopathy

G. Wallukat, V. Boewer, A. Förster, and A. Wollenberger

There exists considerable evidence from both clinical and experimental studies for an involvement of the immune system in the pathogenesis of myocarditis and dilated cardiomyopathy (DCM), the latter being suspected to be in many cases a sequel of viral myocarditis [1]. This involvement of the immune system pertains to both humoral and cell-mediated immunity. The present communication will be confined to a consideration of certain aspects of the humoral side of immunity in myocarditis and DCM, specifically to effects of a group of heart-reactive immunoglobulins (autoantibodies) that circulate in the serum of patients with these diseases.

Immunoglobulins of these patients have been found by immunofluorescent staining to bind to a variety of structures of the myocardial cell [2,3], but only a few of the molecular constituents of these cellular structures have been identified as the respective autoantigens, such as the adenine nucleotide translocator [4] (a mitochondrial protein) and the cardiac myosin heavy chain [5] (likewise an intracellular protein). Recently Limas et al. [6] reported the results of a radioligand binding study showing the presence in the serum of patients with DCM of autoantibodies directed against the cardiac β_1-adrenergic receptor. The present work deals with the possible functional role of what presumably are the same anti-β-adrenoceptor autoantibodies, which we obtained not only from patients with DCM, but also from patients with myocarditis who were not in a state of heart failure. As a functional test system we used neonatal rat heart myocytes beating spontaneously in rocker culture (see below) and responsive to autonomous nerve transmitters and related hormones and drugs [7], as shown in the present experiments by their chronotropic response.

Methods

Based on previously detailed procedures [8,9], trypsin-dissociated cells from the heart ventricles of 1–2-day-old rats were cultured at 37°C in flasks attached to a rocking apparatus and containing Halle SM 20–1 culture medium equilibrated with air and supplemented with 10% decomplemented calf serum, 0.1 mU insulin, and 2 μM fluorodeoxyuridine. In a few experiments undecomplemented calf serum was used. The medium was replaced with fresh medium at the end of the 1st, 4th, 7th, and toward the end of the 8th day. After a lapse of 2 h, the vessels were

B.S. Lewis, A. Kimchi (Eds.)
Heart Failure Mechanisms and Management
© Springer-Verlag Berlin Heidelberg 1991

transferred to the heated stage of an inverted microscope, where ten small circular fields of the cell monolayer were observed through the holes of a metal template. The beats of a selected cell or synchronously contracting cell cluster in a given field were counted before and after addition of γ-globulin. Unless stated otherwise, the preincubation with the globulins lasted for about 60 min. The counting of beats in the presence of a given γ-globulin preparation or other substance tested was repeated twice in the course of the succeeding weeks, each time in a different culture, yielding counts of beats of up to 30 cells or cell clusters in a total of 30 fields per substance or substance mixture tested. The basal rate of beating on the 8th day of cultivation had previously been determined in our laboratory to average 136.4 ± 6.6 per minute (means ± SE, $n = 130$).

Specimens of the left ventricular musculature were obtained by endomyocardial biopsy. Cardiac contractile function was assessed by echocardiography and invasive techniques. The γ-globulin fraction was isolated by the ammonium sulfate precipitation method [10] from the serum of patients with biopsy-proven myocarditis and with idiopathic DCM as well as from the serum of healthy subjects and of patients with some other diseases (Table 1). The globulins were kept frozen at –20°C before being thawed and added to the culture vessels, at the bottom of which the heart myocytes were beating, to give final dilutions of 1:10–1:100, reckoned in terms of the serum volume from which they had been prepared. In a few experiments, aliquots of the dissolved immunoglobulins were mixed in a centrifuge tube with what was considered an excess of goat anti-human immunoglobin, IgM, or IgG antibody preparation, from which sodium azide had been removed by dialysis. The precipitated immune complex was centrifuged off, and the supernatant was used as in the case of the original γ-globulin fraction. Figures for the final dilution of the supernatant also refer to the original serum volume.

Table 1. Some characteristics of subjects at rest

Condition	n	Age (years)	Sex m	Sex f	LVEF (%)	LVEDP (Torr)	LVEDVI (ml/m²)
Dilated cardiomyopathy	18	43	17	1	36.8 ± 3.6	22.9 ± 2.0	127.9 ± 9.2
Myocarditis	14	32	4	10	59.3 ± 2.8	10.1 ± 0.9	71.4 ± 4.4
Chronic ischemic heart disease	6	52	3	3	–	–	–
Acute myocardial infarction	4	63	3	1	–	–	–
Allergic asthma	6				–	–	–
Hypertension[a]	6	42	5	1	–	–	–
Healthy persons	6	47	1	4	–	–	–

[a] No heart disease and chronically treated with a β-blocker.

LV, left ventricular; *EF*, ejection fraction; *EDP*, end diastolic pressure; *EDVI*, end diastolic volume index.

Anti-human γ-globulin was obtained from Staatliches Institut für Immun-präparate, anti-human IgM and anti-human IgG from Behringwerke AG, (−)- and (+)-propranolol from VEB Isis Chemie. The following drugs were kindly donated: bisoprolol by Merck AG, metoprolol by Ciba-Geigy AG, and ICI 118,551 by Imperial Chemical Industries PLC.

Results

Figure 1 indicates that the serum γ-globulin fraction of every one of the patients with myocarditis and DCM caused an increase in the frequency of beat of the cultured cardiomyocytes that was inhibitable by propranolol (see also Fig. 2), pointing to β-receptors as the target of the globulins. In contrast, the globulins from the patients with the other diseases listed and from the healthy persons lacked this stimulatory property. There was no overlap of the data of the myocarditis and DCM patients, on the one hand, with those of any member of the other groups on the other hand. Relative to the basal rate of beat, the acceleration by the myocarditic and cardiomyopathic γ-globulins was only moderate, but well

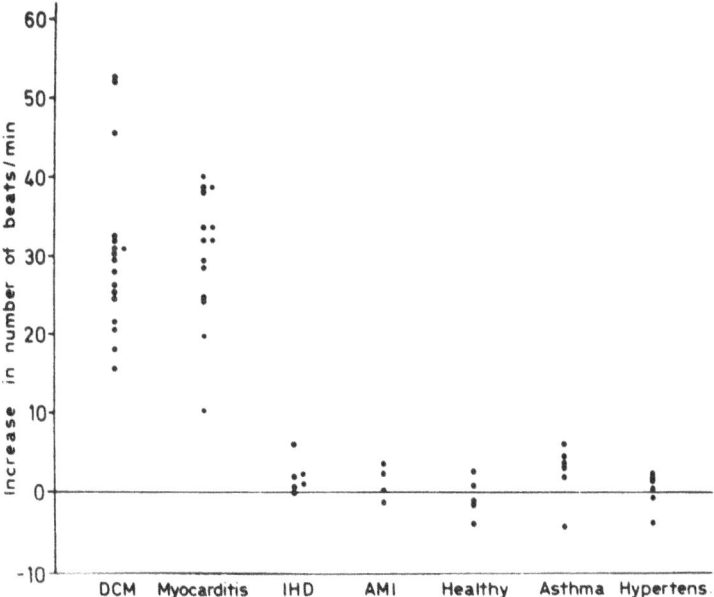

Fig. 1. Positive chronotropic response of rocker-cultured neonatal rat heart myocytes to the serum γ-globulin fraction of patients with myocarditis and DCM. This response was in every single case completely or nearly completely eliminated by 0.1 μM (−)-propranolol or 1 μM bisoprolol. No propranolol- or bisoprolol-sensitive chronotropic response to γ-globulins of patients with some other diseases and of healthy persons. Dilution of the globulins was 1:20. *IHD*, ischemic heart disease; *AMI*, acute myocardial infarction

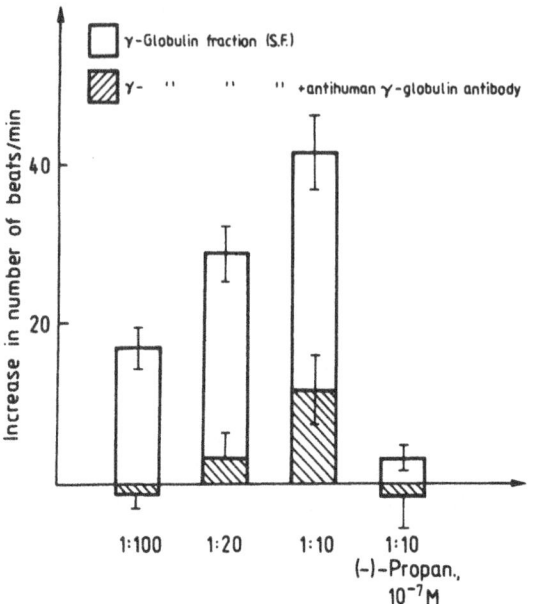

Fig. 2. Effect of goat anti-human γ-globulin antibodies on the beat-accelerating action of the serum γ-globulin fraction of a patient with acute myocarditis. *Open columns,* before immunoprecipitation; *hatched columns,* after immuno-precipitation

reproducible and approaching in magnitude, at a dilution of 1:20, that achieved by a maximally effective concentration of isoprenaline (Fig. 3).

The chronotropic responses of the myocarditic and cardiomyopathic γ-globulins were of identical magnitude (mean $\pm$ SD = 30.2 $\pm$ 8.3 and 30.0 $\pm$ 10.4, respectively). The corresponding values for the other groups were: ischemic heart disease: 2.5 $\pm$ 3.1; acute myocardial infarction: 1.2 $\pm$ 2.5; hypertension: 0.2 $\pm$ 2.5; asthma: 2.8 $\pm$ 1.7 healthy persons: -0.6 $\pm$ 2.5. One of the patients with ischemic heart disease had a myocardial infarction 2 years earlier. Hypertensive patients under chronic treatment with β-blockers were included in this study because of the possibility (see [11]) that anti-idiotypic antibodies to antibodies against serum albumin-linked β-blockers might be formed that would display β-adrenergic agonistic activity. This was obviously not the case. Patients with allergic asthma were also included because their serum may contain antibodies against the β_2-adrenoceptor [12] that inhibit the beat-accelerating action of the β_2-selective adrenergic agonist clenbuterol [13]. As shown in Fig. 1, however, the serum of such patients does not contain the stimulatory immunoglobulins possessed by the patients with myocarditis and DCM.

In the experiment shown in Fig. 2, removal of the chronotropic immuno-globulins with anti-human γ-globulin antibodies left the supernatant devoid of beat-accelerating activity at 100- and 20-fold dilutions, thereby providing evidence that antibodies were responsible for the chronotropic action. A residual stimulatory activity remained at a dilution of 1:10, probably because, as suggested by the effect of propranolol (Fig. 2), the amount of the anti-human γ-globulin added was insufficient for the complete removal of the agonistic immunoglo-bulins present at this low dilution. The concentration dependence of the action

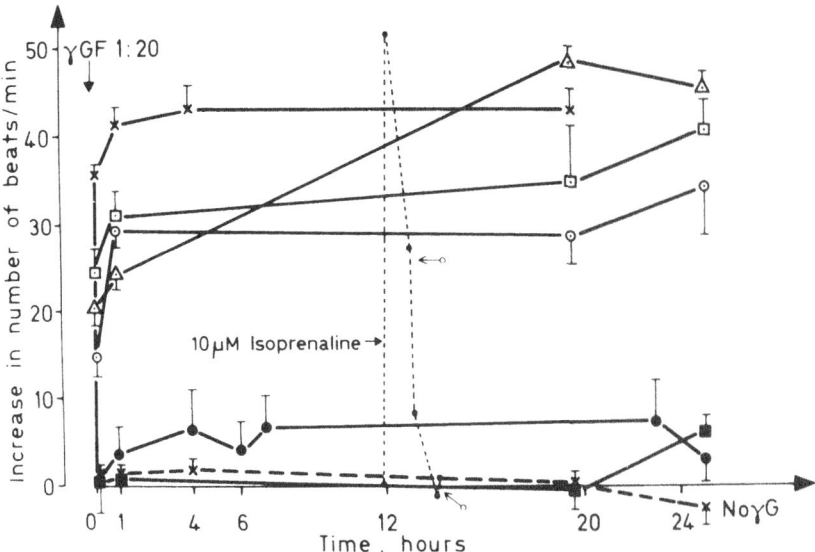

Fig. 3. Persistent chronotropic action of the serum γ-globulin fraction of patients with myocarditis and DCM on rocker-cultured neonatal rat heart myocytes. *Solid lines with triangles and open squares,* patients with DCM; *solid lines with crosses and open circles,* patients with myocarditis; *solid lines with solid squares,* patient with ischemic heart disease; *solid line with solid circles,* healthy control. *Arrows with small circle,* wash and addition of fresh medium containing 10 μM isoprenaline

of the stimulatory immunoglobulins, in this case from a patient with myocarditis, is clearly evident from Fig. 2.

From the data listed in Table 2, it may be gathered that the chronotropic action of the circulating immunoglobulins in DCM was due to autoantibodies of the IgG class since it was abolished by immunoprecipitation with anti-human IgG. Treatment with anti-human IgM, on the other hand, failed to alter the magnitude of the chronotropic response.

Table 3 indicates that the inhibition of the positive chronotropic response of the cultured heart myocytes to the myocarditis and DCM immunoglobulins by

Table 2. Effect of goat anti-human IgM and IgG antibodies on the beat-accelerating action of the serum γ-globulin fraction of patients with dilated cardiomyopathy (DCM)

Patient	Diagnosis	Dilution of supernatant	Increase in number of beats per minute following treatment of the γ-globulins with:	
			Anti-human IgM	Anti-human IgG
1	Severe DCM	1:20	39.8 ± 5.1	2.5 ± 2.2
2	Moderately severe DCM	1:20	34.2 ± 4.5	1.3 ± 1.3
3	Incipient postmyocarditic DCM	1:40	24.0 ± 4.4	4.0 ± 4.2

Table 3. Influence of adrenergic antagonists on the chronotropic response of neonatal rat heart myocytes to the γ-globulin fraction of patients with DCM and myocarditis

| | Phentol-amine 1 μM | ICI 118,551 0.1 μM | (+)-Prop-ranolol 0.1 μM | (−)-Prop-ranolol 0.1 μM | Bisoprolol | | Metoprolol | |
					0.1 μM	1 μM	0.65 μM	6.5 μM
Increase in frequency of beat (%)	106 ± 5	106 ± 16	93 ± 7	13 ± 6	43 ± 9	1 ± 5	70 ± 7	18 ± 6

One representative patient per antagonist; 30–60 min of exposure to the globulins at dilution 1:20. The results are expressed as a percentage of the responses in the absence of antagonist.

0.1 μM (−)-propranolol was stereoselective insofar as the same concentration of (+)-propranolol was ineffective. Since (−)-propranolol is well known to be two to three orders of magnitude more potent as a β-blocker than is the (+)-enantiomer, this finding provides additional support for the conclusion (see above) that the chronotropic autoantibodies in the serum of patients with myocarditis and DCM are directed against the β-adrenergic receptor. Phentolamine and ICI 118,551, at concentrations known to be fairly selective blockers of α_1- and β_2-adrenoceptors, respectively, did not antagonize the chronotropic action of the γ-globulin fraction from patients with myocarditis and DCM (Table 3), suggesting that the chronotropic autoantibodies were not directed against the chronotropic α_1- and β_2-receptors that are present on cultured neonatal rat ventricular myocytes [14,15]. One can presume from these preliminary findings, in confirmation and extension of the results of the radioligand binding experiments of Limas et al. [6] and in concordance with analogous data pertaining to Chagas' disease [16], that the β_1-adrenoceptors of rat heart myocytes are a target with which circulating autoantibodies found in human myocarditis and DCM can crossreact, thereby developing an agonistic β-adrenergic activity.

In sharp contrast to the chronotropic action of isoprenaline, which was subject to relatively rapid desensitization, the action of the immunoglobulins of the patients with myocarditis and DCM, which as a rule reached its peak after about 1 h, continued unabated at about peak levels for as long as 24 h (Fig. 3) and even for 2 or 3 days (not shown). Neither was this action reversed by washing and subsequent incubation for many hours in culture medium not containing the human immunoglobulins (not shown). At any time, however, it could rapidly be opposed by propranolol and β_1-blockers (Fig. 2 and legend of Fig. 1; Table 3).

Discussion

Patients with myocarditis and DCM can be differentiated from those with chronic ischemic heart disease and from other groups on the basis of the propranolol- and bisoprolol-sensitive positive chronotropic effect exerted by their serum γ-globulin fraction on spontaneously beating cultured neonatal rat heart myocytes – an effect mediated by β_1-adrenoceptors and not shared by the immunoglobulins from the subjects in the other investigated groups (Fig. 1). The discriminating power of this property appears to be high, as there was no overlap between the data for the patients with myocarditis and DCM on the one hand and those for the other subjects on the other hand. If these still preliminary findings can be confirmed in larger populations and if diluted serum can be used instead of the serum γ-globulin fraction, the present functional test could qualify as a diagnostic aid.

There was no difference between the myocarditic and cardiomyopathic patient groups with respect to the ability of their serum γ-globulin fraction to elicit an increase in the frequency of beat of cultured neonatal rat heart myocytes. In fact, the mean increases in the two groups were identical, which contrasts with the marked difference between them with respect to cardiac pump function. Neither was there, within the DCM group, a correlation between β-adrenergic activity of the anti-β-adrenoceptor antibodies and the hemodynamic data recognizable. In a cohort of DCM patients, a similar lack of correlation was seen between ejection fraction and ability of their sera to displace a labeled β-adrenoceptor ligand from its specific binding sites on cardiac membranes [6]. As regards the myocarditis group, it cannot be stated with any degree of assurance on the basis of the present data whether the present functional test is capable of distinguishing patients with healing or healed myocarditis from those in the acute stage of the disease, as well as from those having passed into postmyocarditic DCM. To answer this question data are required on a considerably greater number of patients. Should such differentiation prove to be possible, it might furnish a clue to whatever role such autoimmunity products as the agonistic anti-β-adrenoceptor autoantibodies might play in the transition from myocarditis to DCM.

Borda et al. [16] reported that only in the presence of complement did sera and IgG from patients with Chagas' disease exert chronotropic and inotropic effects on isolated rat atria. The small number of present experiments in which undecomplemented calf serum came to be used yielded results that did not differ from those obtained in medium containing decomplemented serum. It is conceivable that on incubation with complement toxic effects might have become manifest since complement-dependent cytolysis mediated by circulating antibodies from subsets of patients with myocarditis and DCM has been observed in isolated newborn or mature rat cardiomyocytes [2,3,17]. This point requires clarification in experiments to come.

The following features of the positive chronotropic response of our cultured cardiomyocytes to immunoglobulins of patients with myocarditis and DCM merit being recalled: (a) the response was selectively inhibited by (−)-propranolol and β_1-adrenergic antagonists, implicating β_1-adrenoceptors as a target of the immunoglobulins; (b) it approached in magnitude a maximally effective concentration of isoprenaline; and (c) it remained unweakened for 24 h or longer. Taken together, these features are of special interest in the context of the hypothesis [18] that an exaggerated chronic adrenergic may be of pathogenetic significance in DCM. Provided that the present findings can be extrapolated to the clinical setting, they could furnish at least a partial explanation for the beneficial effects that have been achieved in the treatment of DCM with β-blockers [19–21].

At first sight, it seems unreasonable to withhold from a failing heart, by administration of a β-blocker, the support that it can derive from the adrenergic nervous system. In the search for the rationale of this therapy it can be argued [22–24] that the sharply elevated plasma noradrenaline levels in DCM, together with an increased sympathetic nerve traffic, constitute a harmful adrenergic overloading of the heart that one should strive to overcome. This line of reasoning can now be strengthened by referring to present findings suggesting that in DCM the heart may steadily be exposed to immunoglobulins that are capable of stimulating its β-adrenoceptors without subsequent tachyphylaxis and whose action can effectively be opposed by β-blockers.

Summary

The serum γ-globulin fraction of patients with myocarditis and DCM increased the beating frequency of cultured neonatal rat heart myocytes in a concentration-dependent fashion and with an intrinsic activity approaching that of isoprenaline. This effect, exerted in DCM by IgG, was stereoselectively inhibited by $(-)$-propranolol and was also inhibited by the β_1-selective adrenergic antagonists bisoprolol and metoprolol, but not by the β_2-selective antagonist ICI 118,551 and the α-adrenergic blocker phentolamine, implicating β_1-adrenergic receptors as the target of the chronotropic immunoglobulins. No such immunoglobulins were present in the serum of healthy persons and of patients with chronic ischemic heart disease, acute myocardial infarction, allergic asthma, and hypertension treated with β-blockers. The positive chronotropic action of the myocarditis and DCM immunoglobulins, in sharp contrast to that of isoprenaline, was not reversed by washing and persisted for 24 h and longer without any weakening. Our findings are of interest in the context of the hypothesis that an excessive chronic adrenergic drive may be a pathogenetic factor in DCM. Provided that these findings can be extrapolated to the clinical setting, they could furnish at least a partial explanation for the beneficial effects that have been achieved in the treatment of this heart disease with β-blockers.

Acknowledgement. We are indebted to Prof. J. Witte and Drs. V. Homuth, P. Morgan, O. Titlbach, and J. Dehnert for providing sera of their patients.

References

1. Bolte H-D (ed) (1984) Viral heart disease. Springer, Berlin Heidelberg New York
2. Maisch B, Trostel-Soeder R, Stechemesser E, Berg PA, Kochsiek K (1982) Diagnostic relevance of humoral and cell-mediated immune reactions in patients with acute viral myocarditis. Clin Exp Immunol 48:533–545

3. Maisch B, Deeg P, Liebau G, Kochsiek K (1983) Diagnostic relevance of humoral and cytotoxic immune reactions in primary and secondary dilated cardiomyophathy. Am J Cardiol 52:1072–1078

4. Schultheiss H-P, Schulze K, Kühl U, Ulrich G, Klingenberg M (1986) The ADP/ATP carrier as a mitochondrial auto-antigen – facts and perspectives. Ann New York Acad Sci 488:44–64

5. Rose NR, Beisel KW, Herskowitz A, Neu N, Wolfgram LJ, Alvarez FL, Traystman MD, Craig SW (1987) Cardiac myosin and autoimmune myocarditis. Ciba Found Sympos 129:3–24

6. Limas CJ, Goldenberg IF, Limas C (1989) Autoantibodies against β-adrenoceptors in human idiopathic dilated cardiomyopathy. Circulation Res 64:97–103

7. Wollenberger A (1985) Seventy-five years of cardiac tissue and cell culture. Trends Pharmacol Sci 6:383–387

8. Halle W, Wollenberger A (1971) Myocardial and other muscle cell cultures. In: Schwartz A (ed) Methods in pharmacology, vol 1. Appleton-Century Crofts, New York, pp 191–246

9. Wallukat G, Wollenberger A (1980) Differential α- and β-adrenergic responsiveness of beating rat heart myocytes after stationary and non-stationary cultivation. Acta Biol Med Germ 39:K7-K13

10. Weir DM (1967) Handbook of experimental immunology. Davies, Philadelphia, pp 3–9

11. Guillet JG, Kaveri SV, Durieu O, Delavier C, Hoebeke J, Strosberg AD (1985) β-Adrenergic agonist activity of a monoclonal anti-idiotypic antibody. Proc Natl Acad Sci USA 82:1781–1784

12. Venter JC, Fraser CM, Harrison LC (1980) Autoantibodies to β_2-adrenergic receptors: a possible cause of adrenergic hyporesponsiveness in allergic rhinitis and asthma. Science 207:1361–1363

13. Wallukat G, Wollenberger A (1987) Effects of the serum gamma globulin fraction of patients with allergic asthma and dilated cardiomyopathy on chronotropic β adrenoceptor function in cultured neonatal rat heart myocytes. Biomed Biochim Acta 46:S634–S639

14. Kupfer LE, Robinson RB, Bilezikian JP (1982) Indentification of α_1-adrenergic receptors in cultured rat myocardial cells with a new iodinated α_1-adrenergic antagonist. [^{125}I] IBE 2254. Circulation Res 51:250–254

15. Wallukat G, Wollenberger A (1987) Involvement of β_2-adrenergic receptors in the potentiation of the chronotropic action of isoprenaline evoked in rocker-cultured neonatal rat heart cells by pyruvate and L(+)-lactate. In: Beamish RE, Panagia V, Dhalla NS (eds) Pharmacological aspects of heart disease. Nijhoff, Boston, pp 217–231

16. Borda E, Pascual J, Cossio P, Delavega M, Arana R, Sterin-Borda L (1984) A circulating IgG in Chagas' disease which binds to β-adrenoceptors of myocardium and modulates their activity. Clin Exp Immunol 57:679–686

17. Fukuta S, Yamakawa K, Hayashi Y, Iwamoto S, Umemoto S, Kusukawa R, Wada K (1984) Immunological study of heart diseases with special reference to the cytotoxicity of the heterophile antibody against cultured myocardial cells. Jpn Circ J 48:1354–1357

18. Fowles RE (1985) Progress of research in cardiomyopathy and myocarditis in the USA. In: Sekiguchi M, Olsen EGJ, Goodwin JF (eds) Myocarditis and related disorders. Springer, Berlin Heidelberg New York, pp 5–7

19. Waagstein F, Hjalmarson A, Varnauskas E, Wallentin I (1975) Effect of chronic beta-adrenergic receptor blockade in congestive cardiomyopathy. Br Heart J 37:1022–1036

20. Waagstein F, Hjalmarson A, Swedberg K, Wallentin I, Saunders R, Fletcher RD, Loeb HS, Hughes VC, Baker B (1983) Beta blockers in dilated cardiomyopathies: they work. Eur Heart J 4 (Suppl A): 173–178

21. Engelmeier RS, O'Connel JB, Walsh R, Rad N, Scanlon PJ, Gunnar RM (1985) Improvement in symptoms and exercise tolerance by metoprolol in patients with dilated cardiomyopathy: a double-blind, randomized placebo controlled trial. Circulation 72:536–546

22. Bristow MR, Kantrowitz NE, Ginsburg R, Fowler MB (1985) β-Adrenergic function in heart muscle disease and heart failure. J Mol Cell Cardiol 7 (Suppl 2): 41–52

23. Shanes JG (1987) β-Blockade – rational or irrational therapy for congestive heart failure? Circulation 76:971–973

24. Leimbach WN, Wallin BG, Victor RG, Aylward PE, Sundhoef G, Mark AL (1986) Direct evidence from intraneural recordings for increased central sympathetic outflow in patients with heart failure. Circulation 73:913–919

Pathophysiological Aspects of Heart Failure

Heart Failure:
Etiological Models and Therapeutic Challenges*

E.H. SONNENBLICK, T.H. LeJEMTEL, and P. ANVERSA

Despite therapeutic advances over the past 30 years, heart failure remains an increasing cause of morbidity and mortality. Approximately 1% of the American population suffers from congestive heart failure with an incidence of new cases of approximately 400 000 per year. New therapeutic approaches to control ventricular overloads, treat salt and water accumulation, and strengthen a weakened myocardium where possible have clearly reduced morbidity and improved quality of life. Nevertheless, with current therapy, only minor improvement in the high rate of mortality associated with heart failure has been observed (approximately 50% per year in patients with a primary hospital diagnosis of heart failure and as much as 50% in 5 years for patients in whom the diagnosis is made on an out-patient basis) [1]. These considerations argue for a careful reassessment of the therapeutic targets involved in the treatment of heart failure with reconsideration of the etiological models upon which such therapy is based [2,3].

In terms of initial definitions, *heart failure* can be reasonably considered in terms of two pathological problems: (a) *myocardial failure*; and (b) *congestive heart failure* (Fig. 1). Myocardial failure or dysfunction of the ventricle begins with various "work overloads" imposed on the heart. Pressure overloads such as hypertension and aortic stenosis are the most apparent and the extent of the overload is well expressed in terms of the LaPlace relation in which tension (T) in the wall is directly related to developed pressure (P) and ventricular radius (r), and inversely related to wall thickness (h), i.e., $T = Pr/2h$ [4]. In pressure overloads, hypertrophy generally occurs to an extent that will tend to normalize the tension in the wall of the ventricle. Less obvious, but as important as a pressure overload, is the work overload consequent to losing myocardium. This loss of myocardium may occur segmentally, as in the case of an acute myocardial infarction, or more diffusely, as occurs in dilated cardiomyopathies. In both of these latter circumstances, hypertrophy of the remaining nonischemic myocardial cells occurs in approximate proportion to the amount of myocardium that is lost [5]. However, since the developed pressure in the ventricle is not increased, one might term the hypertrophic growth in response to lost myocardium as "reactive hypertrophy." Although reactive hypertrophy and pressure overload hypertrophy may have a difference in initiating loads, the cellular alterations as well as their biochemical, mechanical, and electrophysiological consequences that ultimately alter ventricular performance are the same [6].

*Supported by Grants HL 18824 (EHS), HL 38132 (PA), HL 27219, HL 27219, and HL 37412.

B.S. Lewis, A. Kimchi (Eds.)
Heart Failure Mechanisms and Management
© Springer-Verlag Berlin Heidelberg 1991

1. CARDIAC FAILURE

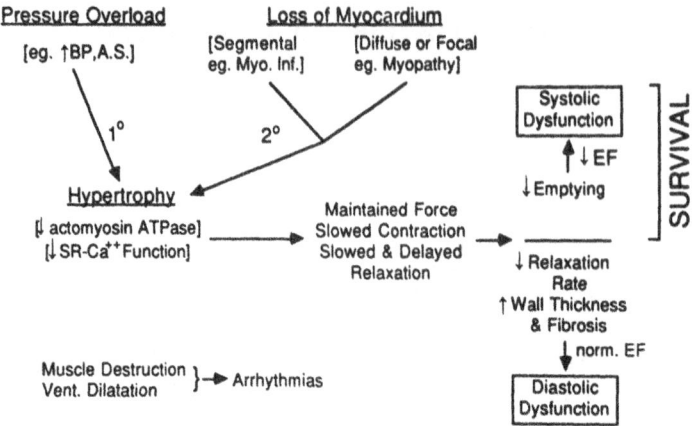

2. CONGESTIVE FAILURE

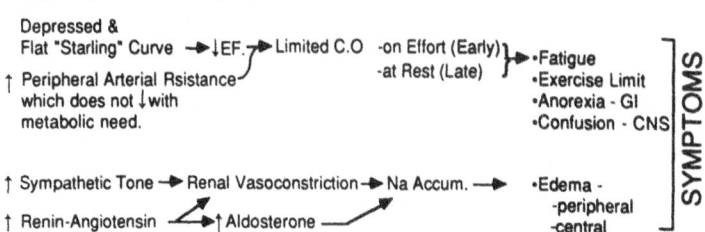

Fig. 1. The two components of heart failure; cardiac failure, and congestive failure

The LaPlace relation is important both in systole and diastole. With systolic overloads, myocellular enlargement occurs. In diastole, increased volume and filling pressure result in alterations in the structure of the ventricular wall over a period of time. These changes of cellular hypertrophy from systole and progressive alterations in the pressure-volume curve from diastole are the basis of *ventricular wall remodeling* [2,3] which is a fundamental process in the evolution of heart failure.

Myocellular hypertrophy initiates important adaptive alterations in the cardiac cell and ultimately ventricular performance. In response to the overload, synthesis of more fetal types of isoenzymes occurs, characterized by a shift from the VI to the V3 isoforms of myosin associated with a slowing of the Ca^{2+}-activated myosin ATPase [7]. At the same time, a slowing of the calcium pumps associated with the sarcoplasmic reticulum is observed. These chemical alterations, which appear to reflect a generalized adaptive process, are associated with alterations in the mechanics of myocardial contraction characterized by a slowing of the rate of contraction, a prolongation of the time to peak tension, and a delay in the rate of relaxation [5]. Peak developed tension may remain normal in that the prolongation of contraction compensates for the slowing of contraction. Prolongation of contraction and a delay in relaxation may then contribute to alterations in ventricular diastole as observed in the hypertrophied heart. Slowing of relaxation may reduce the normal elastic recoil of the ventricle in early diastolic filling and thus reduce the time of diastole so that diastolic filling time is constrained. This can contribute to the elevated filling pressures observed in the hypertrophied heart due to a thickened wall per se and any associated ventricular wall fibrosis. Constraints on the time for diastole may also serve to limit coronary blood flow and its reserve, an effect that will be magnified by any associated large vessel coronary obstructive disease. Since peak force production of the hypertrophied myocardium is normal, one would anticipate that ejection fraction for the overall ventricle would be reasonably well maintained, at least early in the process. With these considerations in mind, *diastolic dysfunction* of the hypertrophied left ventricle may be viewed as an early manifestation of the systolic dysfunction occurring as an adaptation to ventricular hypertrophy per se. Depending on many factors, including age and extent of the overload, stable hypertrophy may be maintained for very long periods of time. With ischemia and loss of cells, diastolic volume will tend to increase, and this leads to augmented wall tension. Further, as end-diastolic volume of the left ventricle increases, ejection fraction falls, resulting in ventricular failure. This evolution of ventricular failure will be discussed further (Fig. 2). The fall in ejection fraction is clearly correlated with mortality but is very poorly correlated, if at all, with symptoms [8]. This important dilemma will also be discussed subsequently.

In contrast to myocardial failure, congestive heart failure develops as a consequence of limited performance of the left ventricle and is characterized by limitations of cardiac output on demand which results ultimately in salt accumulation with congestion and edema, and in peripheral organ dysfunction with easy fatigue, anorexia, and even mental confusion. Associated with this limitation of the ventricular pumping capacity is the activation of neurohumoral systems

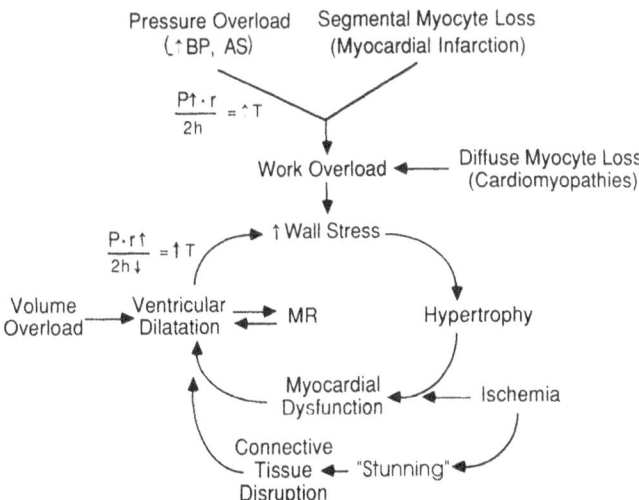

Fig. 2. Inter-relations of primary myocardial damage to the vicious cycle of myocardial dysfunction. Ventricular dilatation results in ventricular wall remodelling, characterized by myocellular elongation and hypertrophy, but also by relative myocyte slippage, the latter resulting in a decrease number of myocytes across the ventricular wall and a further increase in tension per cell [8a]

which contribute importantly to peripheral vascular alterations and the evolution of congestive heart failure (Fig. 1). Such alterations are correlated with limited exercise performance and morbidity but are very poorly correlated with mortality [8].

In the presence of sustained overloads, the evolution of myocardial hypertrophy to ventricular dysfunction with a progressively reduced ejection fraction involves alterations in the architecture of the ventricle, i.e., ventricular wall remodeling (Fig. 2). While a work overload may be associated with an adequate amount of ventricular hypertrophy that may serve to compensate totally for the added load, such compensation may be disrupted by further loss of cells or other concomitant disease processes. In this circumstance, the ventricle falls back on augmented diastolic volume to maintain cardiac output, and two consequences ensue owing to the LaPlace relation. In diastole, with increased diastolic filling pressure and volume, stretching of the ventricular wall occurs so that an augmented diastolic volume develops for any given filling pressure. In elastic structures, this would be characterized as "stress relaxation." As r and P are increased, diastolic wall tension rises. During systole, an augmented wall tension is also necessary for any given degree of pressure development so that additional left ventricular hypertrophy needs to occur to compensate for augmented tension. As diastolic volume enlarges, two processes occur. Myocytes elongate and increase their diameter. In addition, myocytes are displaced relative to one another (myocellular slippage), so that the number of cells across the wall becomes reduced [8a]. As the number of cells across the wall is reduced, the tension per cell is further increased. Since the process of hypertrophy is limited in the face of augmented diastolic volume, the basis for a vicious cycle is created. Another important consequence of augmented diastolic volume is the development of mitral insufficiency that is largely, if not totally, dependent on enlargement of the atroventricular mitral ring. This type of mitral insufficiency is highly dynamic and is readily altered by changes in diastolic ventricular volume.

Another important and largely unrecognized problem for compensation in the overloaded heart is the continued and unrecognized loss of myocardial cells that occurs with *aging* [9]. In rats, the loss of myocytes as a function of aging has been shown to be as great as 20%, and any such loss of cells would create an increasing load for the remaining myocardium. Moreover, aging also produces many of the same biochemical alterations that occur with pressure overloads per se [10], and the hypertrophy of pressure overload and aging are at least additive [11] in laying the basis for ventricular dysfunction.

Recurrent *ischemia* can alter ventricular function and structure to create further overloads for the myocardium by both overt and subtle mechanisms. With the loss of ischemic cells, reactive hypertrophy of the remaining myocardium occurs [5,6,12]. Following a large acute myocardial infarction, cardiac output is maintained by a compensatory increase in diastolic ventricular volume with increased fiber length in the remaining myocardium. The nonischemic myocytes hypertrophy in approximate proportion to the amount of myocardium that is lost [5]. The consequences of the increase in diastolic ventricular volume for the ultimate course of ventricular performance are immense [13,14]. Stretching of the wall in the nonischemic portion of the heart over a prolonged period of time mimics what is observed following sustained volume overloads [8a,13]. The diastolic pressure volume curve moves to the right with a greater diastolic volume being accommodated for any given filling pressure. With time, diastolic volume tends to increase progressively, and the ventricle becomes more spherical in shape. This process, which has the character of "stress relaxation" in the ventricular wall, is not only associated with increased fiber length but also with a *decrease* in the number of myocytes across the wall. Thus myocytes elongate, and hypertrophy slip relative to one another, resulting in ventricular wall remodeling. With the decrease in number of myocytes across the wall, an increased tension is created per cell, which in turn requires further myocellular hypertrophy. The augmented diastolic ventricular volume will also result in an increased systolic tension that will also increase the extent of myocellular hypertrophy. Thus, both diastole with ventricular wall remodeling and systole with increased systolic tension will combine to augment the amount of hypertrophy that is necessary to result in a balanced LaPlace relation. If the LaPlace relation is not balanced, continued diastolic ventricular enlargement occurs, and a progressive fall in ejection fraction is observed over a period of time [2,3].

Other consequences of ischemia may serve to amplify these events and could, under some circumstances, be a primary factor in the development of ventricular failure and dilatation. When coronary blood flow is restored, segmental dysfunction of temporarily ischemic myocardium persists for relatively long periods of time. This has been termed "stunning." We [16] have studied this phenomenon in a dog model in which the left anterior descending coronary artery was temporarily occluded for 5 min with a subsequent 10-min period of reperfusion, repeated 12 times. Mechanical contraction was largely lost in the area of ischemia, and, over the period of repeated ischemia, stretching of the ventricular wall was observed so that there was increased segment length for any given ventricular filling pressure. When the ultrastructure of the ventricular tissue in the stunned area was studied by electro microscopy, intracellular structure was totally normal. Nevertheless, and to our surprise, scanning electron microscopy revealed major damage and disruption of the intercellular connective tissue. The mechanisms involved in this pathological process are as yet unclear, but it is intriguing to note that oxygen-derived free radicals produced in "stunned" myocardium can activate collagenases that reside in the extracellular space [17]. This freeing of cells from one another would provide another basis for myocellular slippage and ventricular wall remodeling in recurrent ischemia, even without myocardial infarction. Whether this can account for ventricular dilatation in other pathological problems, such as cardiomyopathies where animal models demonstrate microvascular spasm and focal ischemia, is an intriguing possibility but unknown.

Alterations in the peripheral circulation and the associated adaptive mechanisms available to the failing ventricle may serve to amplify the central abnormalities of ventricular function (Fig. 3). Augmented diastolic ventricular volume, the Frank Starling mechanism, helps to maintain stroke volume within certain limits, but the augmented ventricular volume also increases ventricular

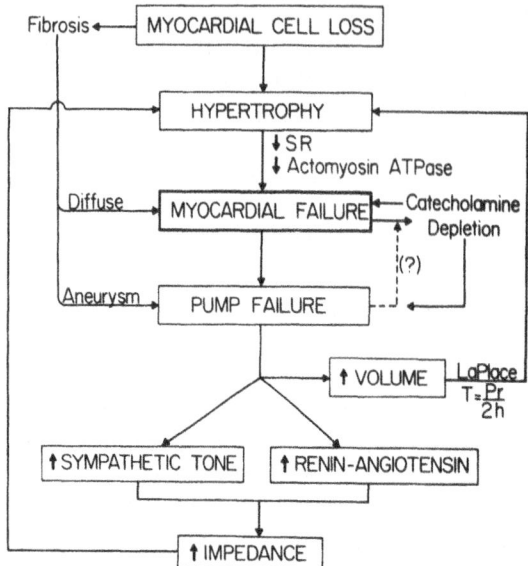

Fig. 3. Relations of central cardiac adaptations to peripheral adaptations and the negative feedbacks which ensue

wall tension that will reduce the extent of myocardial shortening for a given load and augment the amount of hypertrophy that is necessary to normalize the wall tension. Increased sympathetic tone and the activation of the renin-angiotensin system increase peripheral arterial impedence which, in turn, will also augment the ventricular wall tension necessary for the ventricle to function. This in turn will enhance the central cardiac hypertrophy.

The development of congestive heart failure commonly involves the important factor of time (Fig. 4). Following the acute damage sustained by the myocardium, as denoted in Fig. 4 by two acute myocardial infarctions, the ejection fraction is reduced very abruptly and maintained at the reduced level proportional to the size of the myocardial infarction. Nevertheless, with recovery from the acute events, resting cardiac output and the capacity to increase cardiac output on exercise may be quite well sustained with a reasonably normal maximal oxygen consumption during exercise (VO_2 max). Over a relatively long period of time, that may be measured in months or even years, during which the patient is generally asymptomatic, alterations in the left ventricular wall may be preceding, as outlined previously. Ventricular wall remodeling is occurring with a slowly increasing diastolic ventricular volume. Since the cardiac output and stroke volume are maintained relatively constant, the fall in ejection fraction that would occur would be relatively small and difficult, if not impossible, to measure. Cardiac output at rest may well remain normal with only a modest reduction in the cardiac output attained during exercise and a minor concomitant fall in the VO_2 max that is associated with little or no symptoms. At some point in time, increased salt accumulation may be triggered by mechanisms that are as yet undefined, leading to central and peripheral edema that is commonly treated with diuretics. Over a subsequent period of time, a modest fall in the resting cardiac

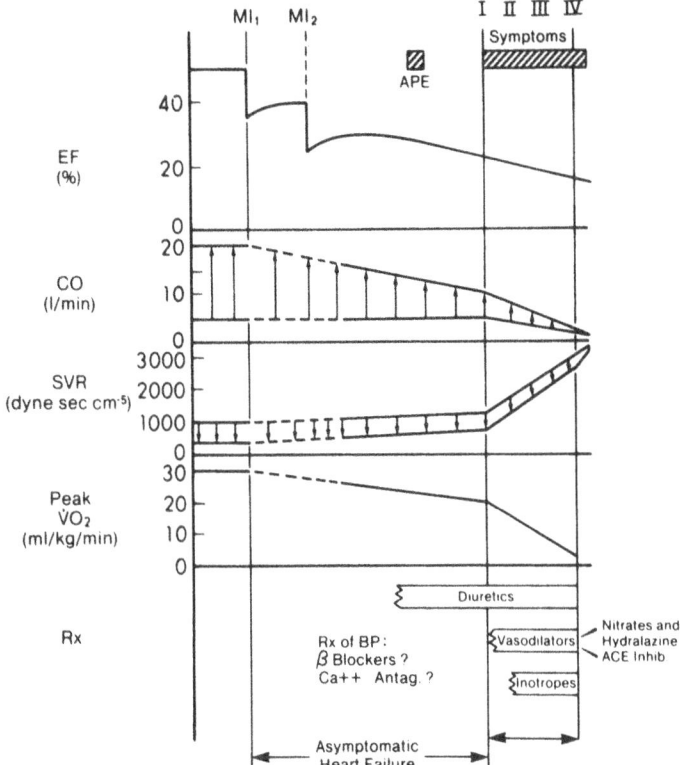

Fig. 4. The evolution of heart failure to congestive failure. Time is measured in months. MI_1 and MI_2 denote two acute myocardial infarctions. Cardiac output and peripheral vascular resistance are given at rest and with maximal exercise

output tends to occur, which may be accentuated by the use of diuretics. More importantly, the rise in cardiac output on exercise becomes increasingly limited with a failure of the peripheral resistance to fall normally in response to the metabolic stimulation of exercise [8]. At this point in time, the VO_2 max becomes increasingly limited and with associated central and peripheral congestion. Patient symptoms increase greatly with an associated worsening of clinical class. This occurs with little or no observable change in ejection fraction. Thus, symptoms are generated by alterations in the peripheral circulation without requiring a substantive further decline in ventricular function. The cause of the increase in peripheral impedence and the failure of this impedence to decline on metabolic demand have yet to be defined and may be multifactoral. One suggestion has been that augmented activity of the renin-angiotensin system with increased angiotensin II leads to smooth muscle hypertrophy in the peripheral arterioles, and this may limit the capacity for vascular dilatation. This may also help to explain why there is a substantial delay in clinical improvement on administration of angiotension-converting inhibitors to patients, since restoration of a capacity to dilate the periphery requires time. Whether there are other vascular endothelial factors involved remains to be determined. Nevertheless, a restoration of the capacity of the arterial vasculature to dilate in response to metabolic demand characterizes clinical improvement and enhanced exercise performance [8]. As noted previously, this need not involve a substantive alteration in the ejection fraction so that, while ejection fraction remains depressed, clinical class may be improved substantially.

Improvement in the mortality rate in heart failure requires preservation of myocardium and prevention of ventricular dilatation. This may reduce ventricular arrhythmias that increase the extent of risk. Preservation of myocardium may involve multiple considerations including inhibition of microvascular spasm, should it be shown to occur in humans as it does in some animal cardiomyopathies, and the use of beta-blockers in certain appropriate situations where cells may be further damaged by augmented levels of catecholamines. Catecholamines may also contribute to an increased heart rate which may not be sustainable by damaged myocytes. The control of ischemia will certainly be important in any of these settings.

The control of symptoms is more likely to be accomplished by limiting the accumulation of salt and restoring the capacity of the peripheral vasculature to respond to metabolic need. Inhibition of smooth muscle hypertrophy in the arterioles may be important in heart failure as it is in persistent hypertension. Nevertheless, such alterations in the peripheral circulation do not prevent the primary problems that occur in the myocardium, and these should not be mixed together relative to therapeutic ends. Morbidity and mortality differ in etiology, and therapy thus requires specific targeting to these problems.

References

1. McKee PA, Castelli WP, McNamara PM et al. (1971) The natural history of congestive heart failure: the Framingham study. N Engl J Med 285:1441–1446
2. Sonnenblick EH, Factor SM, Eng C, LeJemtel TH, Anversa P (1989) The primary etiology of heart failure: myocyte loss, reactive hypertrophy, dynamic ischemia, and ventricular wall remodelling. In: Dollery CT, Sherwood (eds) Cardiac and renal failure: an expanding role for the ACE inhibitors. Hanley and Belfers, Philadelphia
3. Sonnenblick EH, LeJemtel TH, Eng C, Factor SM, Anversa P (1989) The relationship of dynamic ischemia, ventricular wall remodelling and reactive hypertrophy to the development of cardiomyopathies: pathophysiological and therapeutic considerations. In: Sonnenblick EH, Lesch M, Laragh J (eds) New frontiers in cardiovascular therapy: focus on angiotensin converting enzyme inhibition. Excerpta Medica, New York, pp 167–175
4. Sonnenblick EH, Strobeck JE, Capasso JM, Factor SM (1983) Ventricular hypertrophy: models and methods. NIH workshop on hypertrophy, Sept 21–22, 1981, Bethesda, Maryland. In: Tarazi RC, Dunbar JB (eds) Perspectives in cardiovascular research, vol 8. Raven, New York, pp 13–20
5. Anversa P, Beghi C, Kikkawa Y, Olivetti G (1985) Myocardial response to infarction in the rat. Morphometric measurement of infarct size and myocyte cellular hypertrophy. Am J Pathol 118:484–492
6. Anversa P, Ricci R, Olivetti G (1986) Quantitative structural analysis of the myocardium during physiologic growth and induced cardiac hypertrophy: a review. J Am Coll Cardiol 7:1440–1449
7. Capasso JM, Strobeck ME, Sonnenblick EH (1981) Myocardial mechanical alterations during gradual onset, long-term hypertension in rats. Am J Physiol 241:435–441

8. Mancini DM, LeJemtel TH, Factor S, Sonnenblick EH (1980) Central and peripheral components of cardiac failure. Am J Med 80 [Suppl 2B]:2–13

8a. Olivetti G, Capasso JM, Sonnenblick EH, Anversa P (1990) Side to side slippage of myocytes participates in ventricular wall remodelling acutely after myocardial infarction in rats. Circ Res 67:23–84

9. Anversa P, Hiler B, Ricci R, Guideri G, Olivetti G (1986) Myocyte cell loss and myocyte hypertrophy in the aging rat heart: J Am Coll Cardiol 8:1441–1448

10. Capasso JM, Aronson RS, Sonnenblick EH (1982) Reversible alterations in excitation contraction coupling during myocardial hypertrophy in rat papillary muscle. Circ Res 51:189–195

11. Capasso JM, Malhotra A, Scheuer J, Sonnenblick EH (1986) Myocardial biochemical, contractile, and electrical performance after imposition of hypertension in young and old rats. Circ Res 58:445–460

12. Anversa P, Loud AV, Levicky V, Guideri G (1985) Left ventricular failure induced by myocardial infarction. I. Myocyte hypertrophy. Am J Physiol 248:H876–882

13. Fletcher PJ, Pfeffer MA, Braunwald E (1981) Left ventricular diastolic pressure – volume relations in rats with healed myocardial infarction. Circ Res 49:618–626

14. McKay RG, Pfeffer MA, Pasternak RC, Markis JE, Come PC, Nakao S, Alderman JD, Ferguson JJ, Safian RD, Grossman W (1986) Left ventricular remodelling after myocardial infarction: a corollary to infarct expansion. Circulation 74:693–702

15. Ross, J Jr, Sonnenblick EH, Taylor RR, Spotnitz HM, Covell JW (1971) Diastolic geometry and sarcomere lengths in the chronically dilated canine left ventricle. Circulation Res 28:49–61

16. Zhao M, Zang H, Robinson RF, Factor SM, Sonnenblick EH, Eng C (1987) Profound structural alterations of the estracellular collagen matrix in post-ischemic dysfunctional but viable myocardium. J Am Coll Cardiol 10:1322–1334

17. Bolli R (1988) Oxygen-derived free radicals and post ischemic myocardial dysfunction "stunned" myocardium. J Am Coll Cardiol 12:239–249

18. Factor SM, Minase T, Cho S, Fein F, Capasso JM, Sonnenblick EH (1984) Coronary microvascular abnormalities in the hypertensive-diabetic rat: a primary cause of cardiomyopathy? Am J Pathol 116:9–20

19. Factor SM, Sonnenblick EH (1985) The pathogenesis of clinical and experimental congestive cardiomyopathies: recent concepts. Prog Cardiovasc Dis 27:395–420

Vascular Compliance in Heart Failure: A Contributor to Impedance, and the Response to Vasodilator Drugs

J.N. Cohn, S. Finkelstein, S. Kubo, G. McVeigh, K. McDonald, D. Burns, and P. Carlyle

The load placed on the failing left ventricle is an important determinant of its performance and thus a critical factor in the symptoms and progression of left ventricular failure [1]. The load imposed by the vasculature has traditionally been characterized by the calculated systemic vascular resistance, which merely represents the ratio of mean arterial pressure to flow. In a pulsatile system, however, the mean pressure and flow provide little insight into the dynamic nature of the left ventricle and the response of the vasculature to pulsatile pressure. To understand the total impedance to flow imposed by the vasculature, therefore, knowledge of vascular resistance, which is confined largely to the arterioles, must be supplemented by knowledge of the arterial compliance, which exists at all levels of the arterial bed [2].

Attempts to assess vascular compliance in the intact circulation can take several forms. Direct measurement of the pressure: volume relationship of a specific artery is limited by the precision of noninvasive methodology for measuring artery volume and also by the concern that this artery may not be representative of the total vasculature. Fourier analysis of simultaneous high-fidelity pressure and flow signals has been utilized to describe impedance at various frequencies, and the arbitrary averaging of impedance moduli at lower frequencies has been taken as a measure of the characteristic impedance which should provide an assessment of vascular compliance [3]. This technique requires complex instrumentation and assumptions regarding the frequencies to be included in the characterisitc impedance calculation.

We have instead employed a time-domain analysis of compliance by analyzing the pressure decay during diastole from an intra-arterial recording, usually from the brachial artery. By independent measurement of stroke volume, calculation of vascular compliance can be made using a Windkessel model of the circulation. As previously described by Watt and Burrus [4], a modified Windkessel model including both a proximal and distal compliance in parallel with a resistance provides a satisfactory model of the circulation. Mathematical curve fitting with the aid of a computer-based Gauss-Newton curve-fitting technique allows solution of a third-order equation with minimal least squares error to describe the actual recorded diastolic wave form. The solution to the equation can then serve to solve the Windkessel model and provide values for both proximal (C_1) and distal (C_2) compliances [4–6].

The nature of the curve fitting that leads to this solution is of critical importance. The exponential decay of the arterial pressure after closure of the

B.S. Lewis, A. Kimchi (Eds.)
Heart Failure Mechanisms and Management
© Springer-Verlag Berlin Heidelberg 1991

aortic valve is a function of both the resistance to systolic run-off (the vascular resistance) and the mobilization of blood stored in the arterial capacitance vessels, particularly the large arteries consisting of the aorta and its primary branches. The rate of this exponential decay will therefore be increased by either a reduction in resistance or a decrease in proximal compliance. The distal compliance is a major site of sinusoidal waves that are superimposed on the exponential decay curve. These waves probably represent, at least in part, reflected waves that reverberate back from distal sites of resistance or compliance change. The frequency and amplitude of these sinusoidal waves are affected by changes in either resistance or distal compliance.

We have previously reported [7] that, in patients with heart failure, distal vascular compliance is strikingly reduced compared to that in normal control subjects. Proximal compliance was slightly lower than in normal subjects, but the difference did not reach statistical significance. The anatomic localization of this distal vascular compliance is not definable from the model system, but is likely to be in the smaller arteries that may also be involved in limiting maximal hyperemic blood flow in patients with heart failure [8].

Several mechanisms could account for this decrease in vascular compliance in heart failure. Neurohormonal stimulation, which is characteristic of heart failure [9], could play a role in contributing to constriction of the arteries. In studies in the awake dog, we have demonstrated [10] that, during infusion of both norepinephrine and angiotensin, distal vascular compliance is reduced. Therefore, the increased sympathetic nervous system activity and the increased plasma renin activity could be responsible for the decreased vascular distensibility. A possible role for increased sodium and water content of the arterial wall also must be considered. In addition, an abnormality in endothelial release of relaxing factor, a defect identified in some disease states, also could be present in patients with heart failure and might contribute to increased stiffness of the vessels.

In assessing the effect of disease states on vascular compliance, great attention must be paid to the influence of age. Both proximal and distal compliance are very age dependent [11], and thus changes in disease must carefully be dissociated from age-related effects. In the case of both heart failure and hypertension, our studies to date suggest that the reduction in distal vascular compliance is independent of the age-related reduction in compliance.

The response of the arterial bed to vasodilator drug therapy also can be assessed by monitoring vascular compliance. Sodium nitroprusside, which is known to dilate resistance vessels and lower systemic vascular resistance, also produces a striking increase in both proximal and distal vascular compliance. Indeed, this increase in compliance may be an important component of the impedance-reducing effect of nitroprusside in patients with heart failure. In preliminary studies we have noted a similar response of distal vascular compliance to the converting enzyme inhibitors.

Since vasodilator drugs may have dissimilar effects on resistance and compliance [5,6], and the dose response of these vascular effects may be different, it now becomes critical to assess each of these drugs for their relative resistance and compliance effects at the doses used clinically. Furthermore, monitoring of vascular compliance during drug titration might prove to be a valuable tool for selecting the optimal dose of vasodilator drugs for the treatment of left ventricular failure. Further studies are needed.

Conclusion

The development of a practical method for assessing vascular compliance has now made it possible to study the effect of disease and drugs on the stiffness of the arterial vasculature. The importance of this vascular parameter in a pulsatile system has too long been neglected in the evaluation of cardiovascular function. Additional studies should yield new insights into the systems that control arterial compliance and the role of arterial compliance in left ventricular dysfunction and hypertension.

References

1. Cohn JN (1973) Blood pressure and cardiac performance. Am J Med 55:351–361
2. Finkelstein SM, Collins VR (1982) Vascular hemodynamic impedance measurements. Prog Cardiovasc Dis 24:401–418
3. Milnor WR (1975) Arterial impedance as ventricular afterload. Circ Res 36:565
4. Watt TB, Burrus C (1976) Arterial pressure contour analysis for estimating human vascular properties. J Appl Physiol 40:171–176
5. Zobel LR, Finkelstein SM, Carlyle PF, Cohn JN (1980) Pressure pulse contour analysis in determining the effect of vasodilator drugs on vascular hemodynamic impedance characteristics in dogs. Am Heart J 100:81–88
6. Finkelstein SM, Collins VR, Cohn JN (1988) Arterial vascular compliance response to vasodilators by Fourier and pulse contour analysis. Hypertension 12:380–387
7. Finkelstein SM, Cohn JN, Collins RV, Carlyle PF, Shelley W (1985) Vascular hemodynamic impedance in congestive heart failure. Am J Cardiol 55:423–427
8. Zelis R, Flaim SF (1982) Alterations in vasomotor tone in congestive heart failure. Prog Cardiovasc Dis 24:437–459
9. Levine TB, Francis GS, Goldsmith SR, Simon A, Cohn JN (1982) Activity of the sympathetic nervous system and renin-angiotensin system assessed by plasma hormone levels and their relationship to hemodynamic abnormalities in congestive heart failure. Am J Cardiol 49:1659–1666
10. Mock JE, Finkelstein SM, Eaton J, Hatfield G, Cohn JN (1987) Vasoconstrictor drug effects on vascular compliance by pulse contour analysis. IEEE Eng Med Biol Soc Proc 9:878–880
11. Feske WI, Finkelstein SM, Mock JE, Francis GS, Cohn JN (1988) Reduced arterial compliance in hypertension. Hypertension 12:343

Cardiac and Baroreflex Control of the Circulation in Heart Failure*

I.H. ZUCKER

Neurohumoral abnormalities in heart failure include increased secretion of vasoactive hormones such as catecholamines [1], vasopressin [2,3], renin-angiotensin [4], and prostaglandins [5]. Alterations in autonomic function also occur in heart failure, especially as regards the arterial baroreflex control of heart rate [6–8]. It is generally assumed that the initial elevation in sympathetic tone that occurs in heart failure is mediated by unloading of the arterial baroreceptors due, in part, to a falling cardiac output. Although this idea fits with our current understanding of the reflex control of blood pressure, it is a simplification to think that the unloading of normally functioning reflexogenic areas of the circulation in a chronic disease state accounts for this observation. Heart failure results in an increase in catecholamine excretion and in plasma catechols [1,9], while at the same time specific organs such as the heart are depleted of catecholamines [10]. In addition, patients and experimental animals with heart failure are significantly hyporesponsive to administration of exogenous catecholamines [11–13]. This apparent paradox may have important implications in determining the mechanism(s) of the alterations in cardiovascular reflex function in heart failure.

The reflex control of cardiovascular function relies on the input from a variety of sensory endings which are distributed throughout the cardiovascular system. As with most sensory endings, discharge characteristics depend upon the environment that surrounds the receptor. It has long been appreciated that arterial baroreceptors reset as a function of the ambient arterial pressure. Arterial baroreflex control of heart rate is markedly attenuated in patients and experimental animals with heart failure [6,7]. Cardiac receptor control of the circulation is similarly altered in heart failure [2,14,15]. Undoubtedly much of the abnormal reflex control in heart failure is due to alterations in autonomic function in both the heart [6] and in the peripheral circulation [16]. However, abnormalities in the sensory endings themselves cannot be ruled out as a contributory factor in the abnormal cardiovascular reflexes observed in heart failure.

*Supported, in part, by NIH Grant Nos. HL 33359, HL 22594, and HL 38690.

B.S. Lewis, A. Kimchi (Eds.)
Heart Failure Mechanisms and Management
© Springer-Verlag Berlin Heidelberg 1991

Cardiac Receptors

The discharge characteristics and reflex effects of stimulation of atrial receptors with medullated fibers have been extensively studied since the early work of Bainbridge [17] and later of Henry et al. [18]. Although the influence of atrial receptors on mechanisms which control fluid balance in humans is currently under some doubt [19], these receptors exert a profound influence on urine flow, vasopressin secretion, heart rate, and peripheral sympathetic nerve activity in the dog and in other species. Since patients with heart failure generally have chronically distended atria as well as ventricles, it was of interest to determine if alterations in atrial receptor discharge could be observed after chronic elevations of left atrial pressure.

In a study by Greenberg et al. [14], it was shown that dogs with pulmonary artery stenosis and tricuspid avulsion had a reduced left atrial receptor discharge sensitivity compared to normal dogs. In a model of canine high-output heart failure, we subsequently showed similar results [15]. Dogs with aorta-vena caval fistulas (AVF) exhibited a lower atrial receptor discharge rate compared to sham dogs at most changes in left atrial pressure. The maximal slope in the dogs with chronic AVFs was lower than the sham-operated dogs. It is important to realize that the dogs with this model of congestive heart failure showed hemodynamic evidence of chronic congestive heart failure even though cardiac output was elevated. They had left ventricular end diastolic pressures in the range of 25-30 mmHg and heart rates in excess of 140 bpm. Heart weight/body weight ratios were significantly elevated in the dogs with volume overload. In addition, clinical signs of pulmonary and peripheral congestion were seen in all dogs. In these respects, this model is similar to that which is seen in low output failure.

The mechanism(s) responsible for the alteration in left atrial receptor discharge in heart failure are not completely understood; however, there are several aspects of this abnormality which are clear. In all of our dogs with chronic heart failure, the endings were either absent or grossly altered histologically [15]. In the sham dogs all endings examined were normal in appearance with clear myelinated fibers and encapsulated endings. This finding had not been described before; however, there have been observations made on arterial baroreceptor morphology in animals with long-standing hypertension in which the endings appeared anatomically abnormal [20].

Another possible mechanism considered was a reduction in atrial compliance. If dogs with chronically distended atria exhibit a reduction in atrial diastolic compliance, a decrease in atrial receptor discharge sensitivity may imply increased atrial stiffness. Left atrial diastolic compliance was measured using sonomicrometer techniques (two sham and two AV fistula dogs). The relationship between left atrial diameter and the change in left atrial diastolic pressure was plotted. The slope of this relationship was significantly steeper for dogs with chronic AVFs compared to sham dogs. In addition, the control atrial diameter was significantly increased in AVF dogs, suggesting that dogs with chronic AVFs have a reduced atrial compliance and are probably at the top of their length-tension curve. Therefore, atrial stretch receptor discharge would be attenuated. After closing the AVF and allowing a subgroup of dogs to recover for 8–10 weeks, heart size and discharge sensitivity returned to normal. It was found that in this subgroup of dogs, a large number of the receptor endings still appeared abnormal [21].

In dogs with chronic mitral stenosis, Zehr et al. [22] showed a failure of vasopressin levels to rise in response to a nonhypotensive hemorrhage. Histological examination of the left atrium in these dogs indicated hypertrophy and fibrosis, thus making the atrium stiffer, indicating that the most likely explanation for the reduction in atrial receptor discharge sensitivity in heart failure is a reduction in atrial compliance.

Investigations into the reflex effects of left atrial receptor stimulation in heart failure have shown a substantial attenuation, if not a complete loss of atrial receptor-mediated reflexes. Since atrial receptors have been implicated in the control of fluid balance, the failure of patients or animals with heart failure to exhibit a diuresis in the face of markedly elevated left atrial pressure may be due, in part, to the attenuation of left atrial reflex mechanisms [2]. Left atrial pressure was elevated in anesthetized dogs that were either sham operated or were in heart failure. Pressure was elevated by inflation of a balloon in the left atrium. Balloon inflation raised left atrial pressure in the sham dogs from 11.7 ± 1.2 to 23.5 ± 1.9 mmHg and in the heart failure dogs from 17.5 ± 2.6 to 28.2 ± 3.0 mmHg. There were no significant changes in arterial pressure during the balloon inflation in either group. Although a prompt diuresis and increase in free water clearance was seen in the sham group during balloon inflation, there was no change in these parameters in the heart failure dogs. Glomerular filtration rate (GFR) and renal blood flow were unchanged during balloon inflation in both groups. Arginine vasopressin (AVP) levels were measured in both groups of dogs before, during, and after balloon distension. AVP levels were significantly elevated in heart failure dogs. During balloon distension there was a reduction in AVP levels in both groups of dogs; however, the level to which AVP fell in the heart failure dogs (10.2 ± 3.3 μU/ml) was still considerably above the level at which a diuresis and increase in free water clearance would be seen. These data are consistent with those of others who have seen elevated plasma vasopressin levels in patients and in animals with heart failure [3,22,23]. These data strongly suggest that abnormal atrial receptor mechanisms may contribute to the elevated plasma AVP, which exacerbates and contributes to the elevation in extracellular fluid volume in patients with heart failure.

Atrial receptor modulation of renal sympathetic nerve activity (RSNA) has been demonstrated in dogs and nonhuman primates [24,25]. Since changes in RSNA can potentially influence such renal parameters are renal blood flow, renin release, and sodium reabsorption, we investigated the extent to which this modulation was altered in dogs with heart failure [26]. In normal dogs, left atrial balloon distension significantly reduced RSNA. In dogs with chronic AVFs, increases in left atrial pressure caused an increase in RSNA. This increase was due to a concomitant fall in arterial pressure and an unloading of the arterial baroreceptors.

The increase in RSNA per mmHg change in left atrial pressure in dogs with AVFs was completely abolished after carotid sinus denervation (Fig 1), but was actually potentiated in normal dogs. Vagotomy plus sinoaortic denervation abolished all reflex activity. The administration of norepinephrine and nitroprusside to elicit the arterial baroreflex showed that the dogs with chronic volume overload had a normal baroreflex control of renal nerve activity at the time that these studies were carried out. These data are consistent with the altered discharge characteristics of atrial receptors seen in heart failure and with the depressed diuretic reflex. In summary, atrial receptor-mediated reflex control of the circulation is likely to be substantially attenuated in heart failure, and this may contribute to some of the problems of fluid balance that patients in heart failure exhibit.

Ventricular receptor function in heart failure has not been extensively investigated. Both chemically sensitive and mechanically sensitive receptors exist in the ventricles. The reflex effects of left ventricular receptor stimulation have been described in normal, conscious, and anesthetized animals since the original work of von Bezold and Hirt [27]. The Bezold-Jarisch reflex is elicited by the chemical stimulation of left ventricular receptors with one of the veratrum alkaloids and results in hypotension and bradycardia as a result of vagal efferent activation and peripheral sympathetic withdrawal. These receptors can also be activated by mechanical stimuli such as ventricular distension.

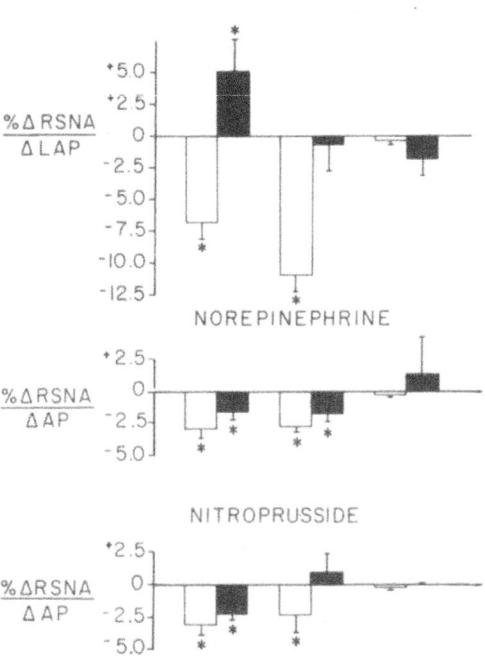

Fig. 1. The mean data on renal sympathetic nerve activity changes derived from normal and AV fistula dogs in response to left atrial balloon inflation, norepinephrine injection, and nitroprusside infusion. *Open bars*, data from normal dogs; *closed bar* data from AV fistula dogs; *asterisk*, significantly different from zero. *RSNA*, renal sympathetic nerve activity; *LAP*, left atrial pressure; *AP*, arterial pressure; *CSD*, carotid sinus denervation; *Vx + SAD*, vagotony plus sino-aortic denervation. (From [26])

In patients with aortic stenosis, leg exercise results in forearm vasodilation, while in normal patients or in patients with mitral stenosis vasoconstriction results [28]. Presumably, increases in stroke volume against a fixed outflow resistance caused extensive left ventricular distension, thus activating left ventricular receptors and causing a withdrawal of sympathetic tone to nonexercising muscle. It has been shown that the discharge rate of ventricular receptors will increase and evoke bradycardia when severely unloaded, as occurs during severe hemorrhage [29]. A similar response was noted by LeWinter et al. [30] in conscious dogs with chronic AVFs. In this study, a progressive hemorrhage was performed while heart rate and blood pressure were continuously monitored. Before the AVF was produced, a tachycardia was observed in response to the decrease in blood volume. However, several weeks after the fistula, hemorrhage resulted in little change in heart rate (albeit from a higher resting level) until approximately 800 ml had been withdrawn, at which time bradycardia was seen. This bradycardia could be completely abolished by atropine but not by propranolol. Similar results have been observed in our laboratory. Figure 2 shows recordings from a dog instrumented with balloon occluders on the descending thoracic aorta and on the thoracic inferior vena cava in order to change arterial blood pressure. Lowering of arterial pressure by inflation of the vena caval occluder resulted in a stimulus-related increase in heart rate (top tracings). Increasing arterial pressure by inflation of the aortic occluder resulted in bradycardia. Two weeks after construction of an AVF similar vena caval occlusion resulted in a bradycardia (bottom tracing). Although the arterial baroreflex is attenuated in heart failure, this could not explain reversal of the heart rate response (Fig. 2) or in the study of LeWinter et al. [30].

A more plausible explanation might be that the sensitivity and/or activity of ventricular mechanoreceptors is altered in states in which heart size is chronically increased. In the dogs with chronic AVF, unloading of the ventricles by hemorrhage or by vena caval occlusion may have stimulated ventricular afferents, which in turn caused a reflex bradycardia. This is similar to the observation of Oberg and Thoren following severe hemorrhage in the cat [29]. The mechanism by which ventricular receptors inhibit the baroreflex and reverse the heart rate response is not completely understood; however, it seems clear from the reflex and electrophysiological studies that, in heart failure, the ability of these receptors to increase their discharge is enhanced. A central mechanism is most likely responsible for suppressing the normal baroreflex [31,32].

Arterial Baroreceptors

Several studies have confirmed that the arterial baroreflex is depressed in humans and in animals with heart failure, at least as far as the control of heart rate is concerned [6-8]. Most data suggest that a major mechanism involved in this attenuation of the baroreflex is a failure of the efferent vagus to modulate heart rate during increases in arterial pressure, and, to some degree, poor sympathetic

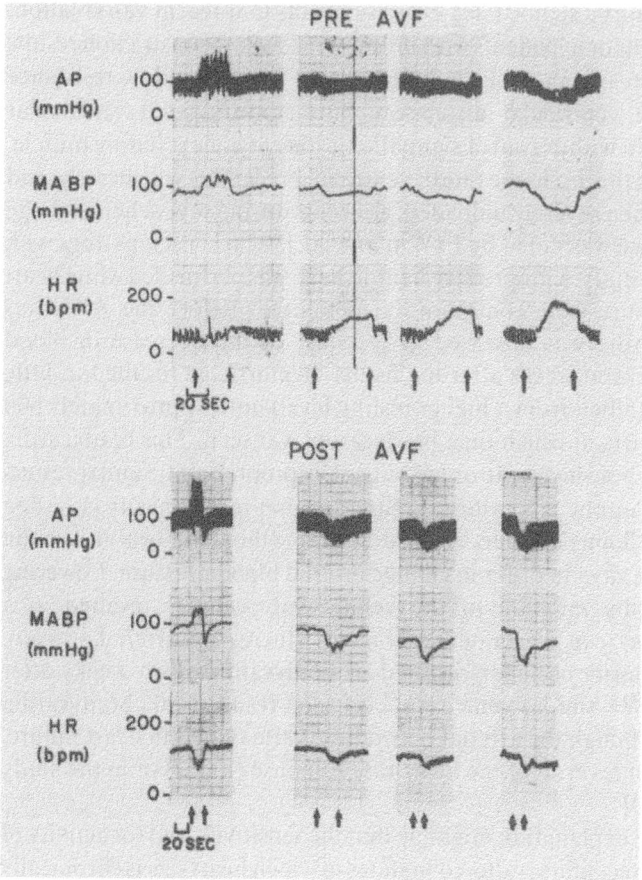

Fig. 2. The heart rate response of a conscious dog to changes in arterial pressure (using vena caval and aortic hydraulic occluders) before (*PRE A VF*) and 2 weeks following (*POST A VF*) the construction of an infrarenal aortocaval fistula. Note that in the post-AVF state, bradycardia is evoked in response to hypotension as well as to hypertension. *A P*, aortic pressure;. *MA BP*, mean arterial blood pressure; *HR*, heart rate

control of heart rate is also involved. Although efferent autonomic control of heart rate is certainly abnormal in heart failure, the possibility that afferent mechanisms may also contribute to the poor baroreflex sensitivity in heart failure has largely been ignored.

Two of our studies have examined the effects of high-output heart failure on baroreceptor afferent activity. In the first study, afferent discharge from aortic baroreceptors was recorded in open-chest anesthetized dogs which were either sham operated or had chronic AVFs [33]. Aortic diameter was measured and wall strain was calculated at the point where aortic pressure was measured. Systolic baroreceptor discharge-systolic pressure curves were generated using appropriately placed vascular occluders. The curves were characterized by determining threshold pressure, saturation pressure, midpoint pressure, and the normalized maximal gain.

The data from heart failure dogs indicated a reduced baroreceptor sensitivity and a resetting of the operating point to a higher pressure. The mechanism of this finding is unclear; however, the dogs with AVFs showed a significant elevation in the aortic diameter at the midpoint pressure and the saturation pressure, whereas the midwall strain at these points was increased. The only aortic hemodynamic parameter that was altered was pulse pressure, being 45.7 ± 2.4 and 24.4 ± 2.0 mmHg in the AVF and normal dogs, respectively ($p < 0.001$). Systolic arterial pressure was elevated in the AVF dogs (136.6 ± 8.7 mmHg) compared to the normal dogs (118.0 ± 5.5 mmHg), but this difference failed to reach statistical significance. These data suggest that, in this model of heart failure, there is a decrease in baroreceptor discharge sensitivity which is unrelated to wall strain but which may be conditioned by the increased aortic pulse pressure seen in dogs with AVFs.

A similar experiment used the isolated perfused carotid sinus in normal and heart failure dogs [34]. The left carotid sinus was perfused with a Krebs-Henseleit solution at a constant pressure of 100 mmHg until a baroreceptor discharge-carotid sinus pressure curve was generated. Piezoelectric crystals were placed across the carotid sinus so that an estimate of diameter could be recorded. Recordings of single-unit baroreceptor discharge were made from filaments of the carotid sinus nerve. Two types of curves were generated using this technique. First, carotid sinus pressure was increased in discrete steps from a carotid sinus pressure of about 50 mmHg to over 300 mmHg. The steady-state discharge rate was plotted against carotid sinus pressure. Secondly, carotid sinus pressure was increased by ramps at pressure rates ranging between 20 and 200 mmHg/s. In this way, both static and dynamic characteristics of the baroreceptor could be evaluated. Each curve was fitted with a second-order polynomial regression and characterized by determining: (a) the threshold pressure; (b) the saturation pressure; and (c) the maximal gain. Dogs with chronic AVFs had increased baroreceptor threshold pressures for the step pressure curve and the three lowest ramp rates; the saturation pressures were significantly higher in the AVF group for the step and the lowest ramp rate. A significantly lower gain was observed for the steps and for the lowest ramp rate (4.7 ± 0.22 mmHg/s) in the AVF group compared to the normal group. This decrease in static gain could not be attributed to differences in compliance of the carotid sinus or to differences in sodium, potassium, or water content (using the contralateral, blood-perfused sinus) of the carotid sinuses of the two groups of dogs.

The results of the above two studies suggest that the arterial baroreceptors become less sensitive in this model of heart failure. The mechanism for this abnormality remains to be elucidated; however, some possibilities may include alterations in sympathetic tone to the carotid sinus [35] or to changes in ionic flux across the receptor membrane. Part of the depressed baroreflex sensitivity in heart failure may be due to a depression at the afferent arm of the baroreflex. This could contribute to changes in systemic sympathetic tone which in turn may alter peripheral vascular resistance and organ function.

Finally, it is possible that some of the therapeutic benefits of the cardiac glycosides are related to their neuroexcitatory and neurosensitizing effects [36,37]. Therapeutic doses of glycosides administered to experimental animals have clearly been shown to increase the discharge sensitivity of atrial[37], arterial [36], and ventricular receptors[38]. In addition, cardiovascular reflexes have been shown to be potentiated in the presence of a variety of different glycosides[39,40]. In preliminary studies, we have recorded from single units in the carotid sinus nerves from normal dogs and from dogs with chronic heart failure due to rapid and continuous ventricular pacing (250 bpm for about 4 weeks). After constructing control, static pressure-discharge curves, we repeated the experiment during the perfusion of the isolated carotid sinus with a solution containing 0.01 $\mu g/ml$ of ouabain for 10 min. Figure 3 shows that ouabain did not alter the threshold pressure or the peak discharge at the saturation pressure in the normal dogs; however, this dose of ouabain (which did not alter carotid sinus diameter in either group) in the dogs with heart failure restored the sensitivity of the receptor in that the threshold was lowered and the peak discharge at saturation was increased. This would suggest that there may be an enhancement of a neural Na-K ATPase pump in chronic heart failure, which contributes to the reduction in discharge sensitivity of these endings. More extensive work in this area of heart failure therapy is needed to elucidate the mechanism(s) involved.

Summary

Neurohumoral events may play a major role in the compensatory adjustments which take place in heart failure, albeit at the expense of a deterioration in organ function. Many neurohumoral control mechanisms are abnormal in heart failure. These come about from changes in both efferent and afferent components of the reflex arcs.

The fact that sensory endings in the heart and blood vessels may play an important role in the abnormal reflex control of the circulation in heart failure has not been generally appreciated. Clinical and animal studies suggest that mechanoreceptor function in the atria, ventricles, aorta, and carotid sinus is abnormal in heart failure. In most cases, these receptors function at a depressed sensitivity, with the possible exception of left ventricular receptors. The mechanism(s) responsible for the receptor abnormalities in heart failure are not completely understood; however, both structural and compliance changes may cause the abnormalities observed for atrial receptors. The cause of the decrease in arterial baroreceptor discharge sensitivity is not known; however, it is not due to a change in compliance of the carotid sinus or aortic arch. Evidence suggests that the depressed carotid baroreceptor sensitivity in heart failure may be due to increases in the activity of a Na-K ATPase pump. The mechanism of the enhanced reflexes from ventricular receptor stimulation is not known.

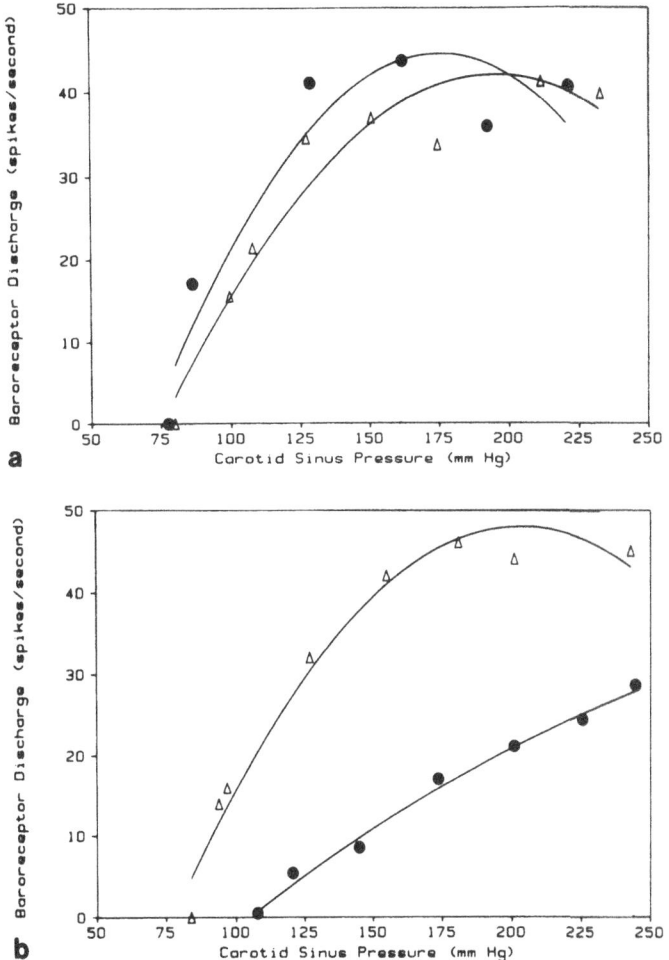

Fig. 3a,b. Pressure discharge curves from a normal dog (**a**) and from a dog with pacing-induced heart failure (**b**). The carotid sinus was perfused with 0.01 μg/ml of ouabain (*triangles*) after the control curves (*circles*) were constructed. Ouabain normalized the pressure-discharge relationship in the heart failure dog

Acknowledgements. The author would like to acknowledge the expert technical assistance of Ms. Johnnie F. Hackley and Mrs. Kay Bliss. I also wish to thank Mrs. Glennora Flanagan for her secretarial support.

References

1. Rutenberg HL, Spann JF Jr (1966) Alterations of cardiac sympathetic neurotransmitter activity in congestive heart failure. In: Mason DT (ed) Congestive heart failure: mechanisms, evaluation and treatment. York Medical Books. Dun-Donnelly, New York, pp 85-95
2. Zucker IH, Share L, Gilmore JP (1979) Renal effects of left atrial distension in dogs with chronic congestive heart failure. Am J Physiol 236:H554-560

3. Goldsmith SR, Francis GS, Cowley AW Jr, Levine TB, Cohn JN (1983) Increased plasma arginine vasopressin levels in patients with congestive heart failure. Am J Coll Cardiol 1:1385–1390
4. Watkins L, Burton JA, Haber E, Cant JR, Smith FW, Barger AC (1976) Renin in the pathogenesis of congestive heart failure. J Clin Invest 57:1606–1617
5. Newman WH, Frankis MB, Halashka PV (1983) Increased myocardial release of prostacyclin in dogs with heart failure. J Cardiovasc Pharmacol 5:194–201
6. Eckberg DL, Drabinsky M, Braunwald E (1971) Defective cardiac parasympathetic control in patients with heart disease. N Engl J Med 385:877–883
7. White CW (1981) Abnormalities in baroreflex control of heart rates in canine heart failure. Am J Physiol 240:H793–H799
8. Vatner SF, Higgins CB, Braunwald E (1974) Sympathetic and parasympathetic components of reflex tachycardia induced by hypotension in conscious dogs with and without heart failure. Cardiovasc Res 8:153–161
9. Chidsey CA, Harrison DC, Braunwald E (1962) Augmentation of plasma norepinephrine response to exercise in patients with congestive heart failure. N Engl J Med 267:650–654
10. Pool PE, Covell JW, Levitt M, Gibb J, Braunwald E (1967) Reduction of cardiac tyrosine hydroxylase activity in experimental heart failure: its role in depletion of cardiac norepinephrine stores. Circ Res 20:249–353
11. Newman WH (1977) A depressed response of left ventricular contractile force to isoproterenol and norepinephrine in dogs with congestive heart failure. Am Heart J 93:216–221
12. Zucker IH, Waltke E, Gilmore JP (1980) Cardiac responses to beta-adrenergic stimulation on anesthetized dogs with chronic congestive heart failure. Basic Res Cardiol 75:697–711
13. Goldstein RE, Beiser GD, Stampfer M, Epstein SE (1975) Impairment of autonomically mediated heart rate control in patients with cardiac dysfunction. Circ Res 36:571–578
14. Greenberg TT, Richmond WH, Stocking RA, Gupta PD, Meehan JP, Henry JP (1973) Impaired atrial receptor responses in dogs with heart failure due to tricuspid insufficiency and pulmonary artery stenosis. Circ Res 32:424–433
15. Zucker IH, Earle AM, Gilmore JP (1977) The mechanism of adaptation of left atrial stretch receptors in dogs with chronic congestive heart failure. J Clin Invest 60:323–331
16. Zelis R, Nellis SH, Longhurst J, Lee G, Mason DT (1975) Abnormalities in the regional circulations accompanying congestive heart failure. Prog Cardiovasc Dis 18:181–199
17. Bainbridge FA (1915) The influence of venous filling upon the rate of the heart. J Physiol (Lond) 50:65–84
18. Henry JP, Gauer OH, Reeves JS (1956) Evidence of the atrial location of receptors in influencing urine flow. Circ Res 4:85–90
19. Gilmore JP (1983) Neural control of extracellular volume in the human and nonhuman primate. In: Shephard JJ, Abhoad FM (eds) Handbook of physiology – the cardiovascular system III. American Physiological Society, Bethesda, pp 885–915
20. Angell-James JE (1973) Characteristics of single aortic and right subclavian baroreceptor fiber activity in rabbits with chronic renal hypertension. Circ Res 32:149–161
21. Zucker IH, Earle AM, Gilmore JP (1979) Changes in the sensitivity of left atrial receptors following reversal of heart failure. Am J Physiol 237:H555–H559
22. Zehr JE, Howe A, Tsakiris G, Rastelli GC, McGoon DC, Segar WE (1971) ADH levels following nonhypotensive hemorrhage in dogs with chronic mitral stenosis. Am J Physiol 221:312–337
23. Goldsmith SR, Dodge D (1985) Response of plasma vasopressin to ethanol in congestive heart failure. Am J Cardiol 55:1354–1357
24. Karim F, Kidd C, Malpus CM, Penna PE (1972) The effects of stimulation of the left atrial receptors on sympathetic efferent nerve activity. J Physiol (Lond) 227:243–260
25. Echtenkamp SF, Zucker IH, Gilmore JP (1980) Characterization of high and low pressure baroreceptor influences on renal nerve activity in the primate Macaca fascicularis. Circ Res 46:726–730
26. Zucker IH, Gorman AJ, Cornish KG, Lang M (1985) Impaired atrial receptor modulation of renal nerve activity in dogs with chronic volume overload. Cardiovasc Res 19:411–418
27. Bezold A von, Hirt L (1867) Über die physiologischen Wirkungen des essigsauren Veratrins. Unters Physiol Lab Würzburg 1:75–156

28. Mark AL, Kioschos JM, Abboud FM, Heistad DD, Schmid P (1973) Abnormal vascular responses to exercise in patients with aortic stenosis. J Clin Invest 52:1138-1146

29. Oberg B, Thoren P (1972) Increased activity in left ventricular receptors during hemorrhage or occlusion of caval veins in the cat. A possible cause of vasovagal reaction. Acta Physiol Scand 85:164-173

30. LeWinter MM, Karliner JS, Covell JW (1978) Alteration in heart rate response to hemorrhage in conscious dogs with volume overload. Am J Physiol 235:H422-H428

31. Holmberg MJ, Gorman AJ, Cornish KG, Zucker IH (1983) Attenuation of arterial baroreflex control of heart rate by ventricular receptor stimulation in the conscious dog. Circ Res 52:597-607

32. Holmberg MJ, Gorman AJ, Cornish KG, Zucker IH (1984) Intracoronary epinephrine attenuates baroreflex control of heart rate in the conscious dog. Am J Physiol 247:R237-R245

33. Niebauer MJ, Holmberg MJ, Zucker IH (1986) Aortic baroreceptor discharge characteristics in dogs with chronic volume overload. Basic Res Cardiol 81:111-122

34. Niebauer MJ, Zucker IH (1985) Static and dynamic responses of carotid sinus baroreceptors in dogs with chronic volume overload. J Physiol (Lond) 369:295-310

35. Tomomatsu E, Nishi K (1981) Increased activity of carotid sinus baroreceptors by sympathetic stimulation and norepinephrine. Am J Physiol 240:H650-H658

36. Gillis RA, Quest JA (1980) The role of the nervous system in the cardiovascular effects of digitalis. Pharmacol Rev 31:19-97

37. Zucker IH, Peterson TV, Gilmore JP (1980) Ouabain increases left atrial stretch receptor discharge in the dog. J Pharmacol Exp Ther 212:320-324

38. Thames MD, Waickman L, Abboud F (1980) Sensitization of cardiac receptor (vagal efferents) by intracoronary acetylstrophanthidin. Am J Physiol 239:H628-H635

39. Sleight P, Lall A, Muers M (1969) Reflex cardiovascular effects of epicardial stimulation by acetylstrophanthidin in dogs. Circ Res 25:705-711

40. Thames MD, Miller BD, Abboud FM (1982) Sensitization of vagal cardiopulmonary baroreflex by chronic digoxin. Am J Physiol 243:H815-H818

Ventricular Function in Heart Failure

Matching of Ventricular Properties with Arterial Load Under Normal and Variably Depressed Cardiac States

S. SASAYAMA

Cardiovascular Interaction

The regulation of cardiac output and venous return was diagramed classically by Guyton et al. [1] within the framework of venoventricular coupling, in which ventricular pump function was depicted by a cardiac output curve and properties of the vascular system and blood volume by the venous return curve. The equilibrium cardiac output can be obtained at the intersection between the two curves. Nearly 1 decade after, Sunagawa et al. [2] advanced Guyton's concept further to analysis of ventriculoarterial coupling by modeling both the ventricular pump and the arterial conducting system in terms of the relationship between ventricular or arterial end-systolic pressures and stroke volume. The ventricular system is characterized by the end-systolic pressure-volume relationship. This relationship is approximately linear over a physiologic range with slope of Ees and constant volume axis intercept of Vo. The former varies in response to changes in contractility. According to this relationship, the end-systolic pressure (Pes) varies inversely with stroke volume (SV) for a given end-diastolic volume (Ved) as follows:

$$Pes = Ees\,(Ved - SV - Vo) \tag{1}$$
$$= Ees\,(Ves - Vo) \tag{2}$$

where Ves is the end-systolic volume.

The arterial system is also characterized in terms of the Pes-SV relationship. In this framework, the slopes of both relationships are represented by the dimension of volume elastance (mmHg/ml), and hence both arterial and ventricular systems are similarly treated like an elastic chamber with a volume elastance Ea and Ees, respectively. The equilibrium SV can be obtained analytically as follows:

$$SV = (Ves - Vo)/(1 + Ea/Ees) \tag{3}$$
$$Pes = Ea \cdot SV \tag{4}$$

Sunagawa et al. [2] proposed the method of practical graphic analysis in the pressure (P) volume (V) diagram of the ventricle in which arterial system is characterized by arterial Pes-V relationship with the slope of Ea and the volume axis intercept of Ved. The SV that the ventricle can eject from a given Ved is

B.S. Lewis, A. Kimchi (Eds.)
Heart Failure Mechanisms and Management
© Springer-Verlag Berlin Heidelberg 1991

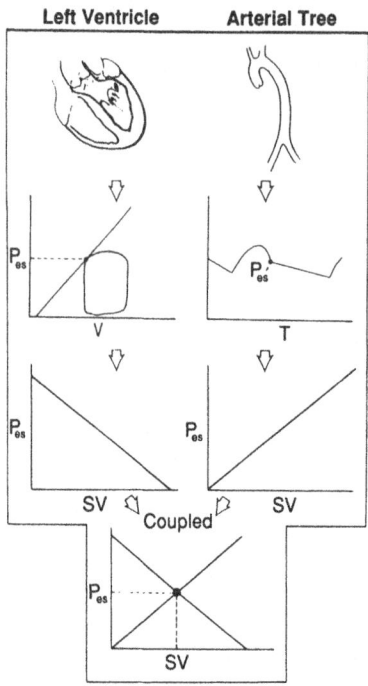

Fig. 1. Framework for coupling of the ventricle with the arterial load. The mechanical characteristics of both the ventricle (*left middle panel*) and the arterial system (*right middle panel*) are expressed by the Pes-SV relationship. Within this coupling framework, stroke volume (*SV*) is obtained as the intersection between these two Pes-SV relationships (*bottom panel*). (From [2])

represented as the intersection of these two lines (Fig. 1). Within this coupling framework, Sunagawa et al. [3] demonstrated that the external work of the ventricle becomes maximal, providing maximal transfer of mechanical energy of contraction to the arterial system, when the slopes of the ventricular (Ees) and arterial (Ea) Pes-V relationship are identical.

On the other hand, from the point of view on economical fuel consumption or mechanical efficiency defined as the ratio of stroke work (*SW*) to ventricular oxygen consumption, the coupling between an energy source and its load has been considered the another criterion for optimal coupling. Burkhoff and Sagawa [4] derived an analytical model that relates the properties of the vascular system and the left ventricle as expressed in terms of an effective elastance (Ees and Ea) to the mechanical work done by the heart and the amount of chemical energy consumed by the heart to perform that work. They estimated oxygen consumption by ventricular pressure-volume area, which has been shown to be linearly related to oxygen consumption [5], and theoretically analyzed the arterial load that would maximize SW and mechanical efficiency of ventricular contraction. Then, they showed that the coupling condition for maximal SW is $Ea = Ees$, whereas that for maximal efficiency is $Ea = Ees/2$, concluding the latter is the case under physiologic conditions.

Ventriculoarterial Coupling in Normal and Failing Human Hearts

Using the above-mentioned matching principles, we recently investigated resting humans' matching of the ventricular properties with arterial load properties under normal and variably depressed cardiac conditions [6]. We determined both the slope of the left ventricular end-systolic pressure-volume relationship (ventricular elastance) and the slope of the arterial end-systolic pressure-stroke volume relationship (effective arterial elastance) in three groups of subjects: group A, 12 subjects with ejection fraction of 60% or more; group B, seven patients with ejection fraction of 40%–59%; and group C, nine patients with ejection fraction of less than 40%. We also determined the left ventricular SW, end-systolic potential energy and the ventricular work efficiency defined as SW/pressure-volume area (PVA; SW + potential energy). In group A, ventricular elastance was nearly twice as large as arterial elastance. In group B, ventricular elastance was almost equal to arterial elastance. In group C, ventricular elastance was less than one-half of arterial elastance, resulting in increased potential energy and decreased work efficiency (Fig. 2).

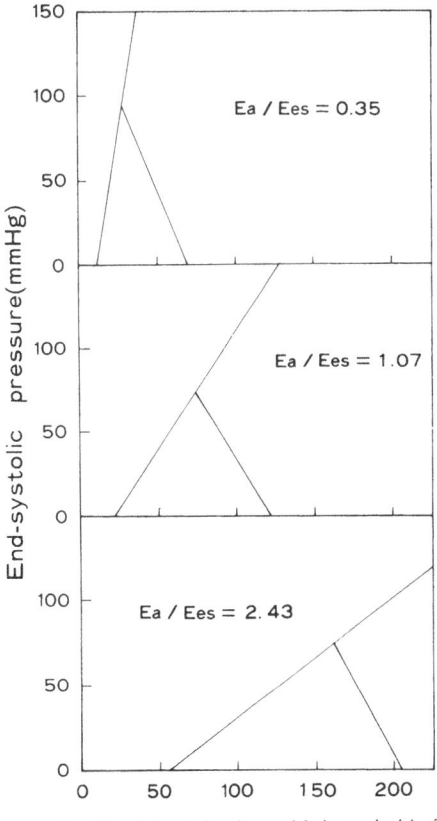

Fig. 2. Representative Pes-V relationship and Pes-SV relationship in subjects with ejection fraction of 60% or more (group A), those with ejection fraction of 40%–59% (group B), and those with ejection fraction of less than 40% (group C). In group A, Ees is nearly twice as high as Ea. In group B, Ees is almost equal to Ea. In group C, Ees is less than one-half of Ea. (Modified from [6])

Thus, the normal coupling condition in group A is surprisingly similar to the data of Burkhoff and Sagawa [4], and cardiovascular interaction in normal subjects appears to be set to optimize left ventricular work efficiency in the resting state. The moderately depressed hearts maximize SW but generate a greater potential energy with resultant reduction in work efficiency. Severely depressed hearts are no longer capable of maintaining SW or work efficiency properly.

Ventriculoarterial Coupling in Exercise

The coupling concept also provides a useful framework to understand the exercise response in the normal and failing heart. Patients with heart failure exhibit excessive sympathetic activity as evidenced by a progressive increase in plasma norepinephrine along with the increased severity in heart failure. The resting levels of plasma norepinephrine inversely correlate with exercise capacity expressed in terms of peak oxygen consumption and anaerobic threshold [7,8], and this rise in norepinephrine in patients with congestive heart failure is assumed to be related to the inability of the heart to provide adequate peripheral perfusion during exercise [9]. In patients with moderate heart failure, SV and Pes can be maintained normally over the wide range of plasma norepinephrine levels, whereas ventricular-load coupling variables (Ea/Ees, Ved, or Ved-Vo) as determinants of SV show substantial correlation with the resting plasma norepinephrine levels (Fig. 3). From Eq. 3 it is apparent that an increase in the Ea/Ees ratio directly reduces SV. However, early use of the Frank-Starling mechanism provides a fundamental compensation for the maintenenace of normal SV in these hearts.

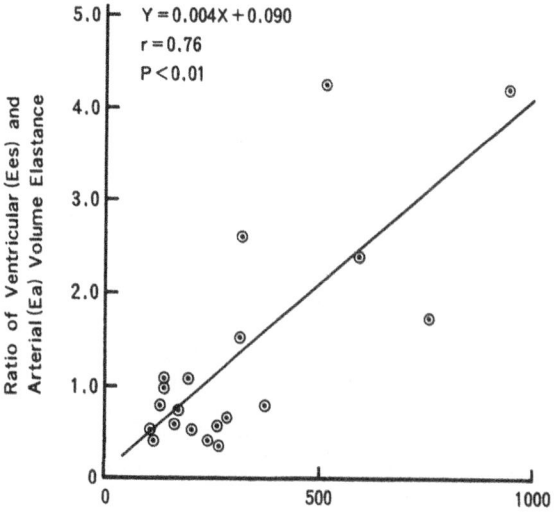

Fig. 3. Relation between the Ea/Ees ratio and plasma norepinephrine. Increased severity in heart failure is characterized by an increase in plasma norepinephrine levels together with a parallel increase in Ea/Ees ratio. (From [7])

The cardiovascular system can adjust to a moderate degree of exercise sufficient to supply oxygen to working muscle. When oxygen availability to the tissue becomes inadequate with more streneous exercise, an anaerobic threshold is reached. At this point, energy is generated by anaerobic metabolism through production of lactate, which leads to carbon dioxide production. In normal subjects and patients with chronic congestive heart failure (ejection fraction averaged 36 ± 12%), the anaerobic threshold was determined during graded exercise as the point at which the linear relationship between ventilation and oxygen uptake was lost, and ventricular-load coupling was analyzed at workloads 30% above and 30% below anaerobic threshold.

In normal subjects, SV increases during exercise due either to an increase in preload or an increase in the contractile state. Though the preload effect is more responsible during low levels of exercise, the contractility change comes into play leading to a reduction in the left ventricular end-systolic dimension at high levels of exercise. This response is represented by an increased in Ees and a decrease in Ea, mechanical efficiency therefore being markedly augmented (Fig. 4, left panel).

In patients with severe cardiac dysfunction, SV is generally augmented during anaerobic exercise by an increase in end-diastolic volume rather than a decrease in end-systolic volume. Hereby, Ees and Ea remained unchanged both during aerobic and anaerobic exercise (Fig. 4, right panel). The failure of Ees to rise during anaerobic exercise despite an excessive sympathetic stimulation is a result of reduced contractile reserve in these hearts. Thus, in advanced heart

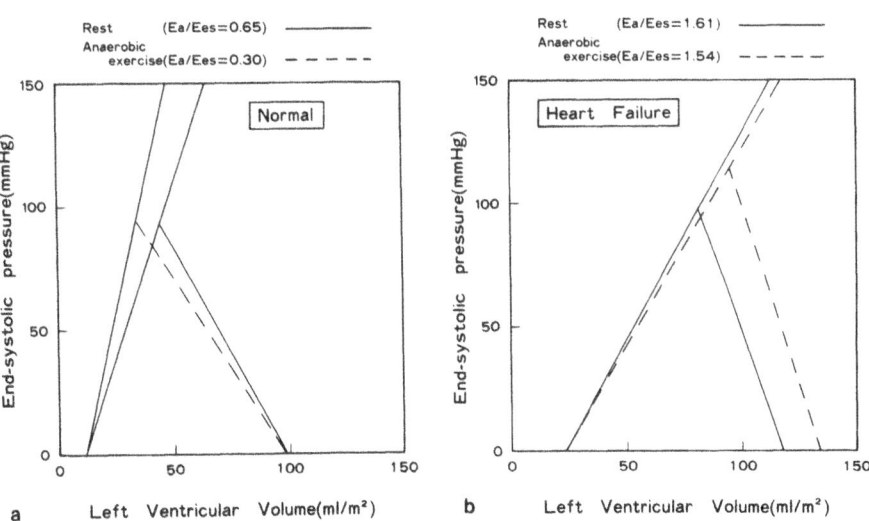

Fig. 4a,b. Changes in ventricular system properties and in arterial system properties during exercise. Ventriculoarterial coupling at rest (*solid line*) and during exercise (*dashed line*). **a** In the normal heart, SV is augmented from the essentially unchanged end-diastolic volume by enhanced contractility with a resultant increase in Ees and a decrease in Ea. **b** In the failing heart, an increase in SV during anaerobic exercise is mediated by an increase in preload without detectable changes in Ees and Ea

failure, the regulation of SV during exercise shifts from a catecholamine-mediated reduction in end-systolic volume to a greater reliance on the Frank-Starling mechanism [7].

Effect of Vasodilator Therapy

There is ample evidence that vasodilator therapy corrects afterload mismatch and augments SV in the failing heart. Most afterload-reducing agents have little or no direct effect on the cardiac contractility. If a mixed venous and arteriolar dilator is employed, there is usually an accompanying reduction in mean circulatory pressure and venous return. Thus, the resultant decrease in Ved attenuates the magnitude of augmentation of cardiac output along with the decrease in adjustment through the Frank-Starling mechanism [10]. The proposed coupling concept provides a convenient framework to evaluate the specific roles of the preload and afterload in determining the SV during infusion of nitroprusside.

In 11 patients with moderate congestive heart failure, infusion of nitroprusside produced a 9% reduction in Ved with unaltered SV and a 19% fall in Pes. In order to separate the pure preload effect from this balanced action of the drug on the arteriolar and venous beds, we applied a negative pressure chamber on the lower half of the body which enabled us to produce the desired amount of decrease in Ved by regulating venous return [11]. With the lower body negative pressure (LBNP), an equivalent reduction in Ved (-8%) was produced in the same patients. Hereby, Pes was maintained unchanged but SV was substantially decreased (-15%). Changes in Ved or Pes did not alter the end-systolic pressure-volume relationship (Ees), while the arterial elastance value (Ea) achieved considerable changes (being decreased by a decreasing afterload, and being increased by a decreasing preload) to meet the SV. The ratio of Ea to Ees (Ea/Ees) fell with nitroprusside and rose with LBNP. Both nitroprusside and LBNP decreased SW (-16% and -12%, respectively) mediated primarily by a decrease in Pes with the former and by a decrease in SV with the latter. Accordingly, work efficiency of the ventricle, expressed as the ratio of EW to PVA, was significantly augmented (by 11%) with nitroprusside and slightly decreased with LBNP (Fig. 5). Thus, we concluded that vasodilator thereby restored the more optimal ventriculoarterial coupling in patients with congestive heart failure. This response was mediated largely by the reduction in afterload rather than preload [12].

Effect of Inotropic Agents

A failing heart is unable to meet the demands for blood flow, and its treatment is directed to recruiting the energetic reserve of the heart most efficiently and economically to restore normal circulation.

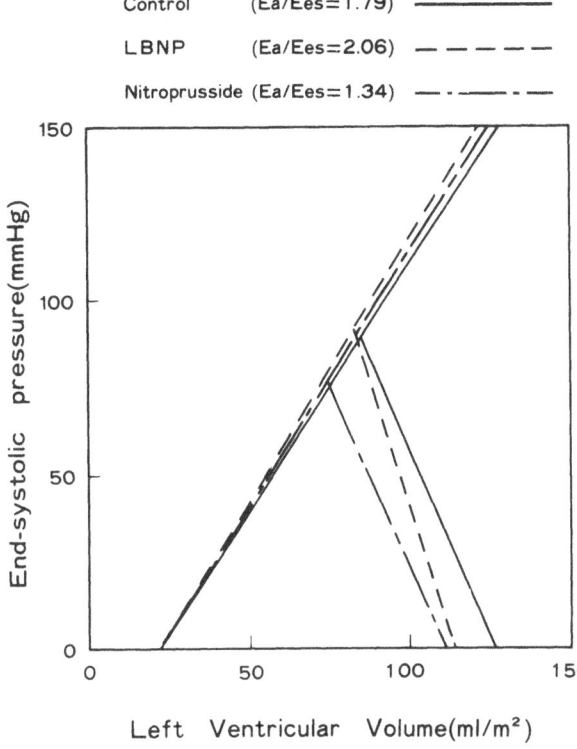

Control   (Ea/Ees=1.79) ——————

LBNP   (Ea/Ees=2.06) — — — — —

Nitroprusside (Ea/Ees=1.34) —·——·——·—

Fig. 5. Effects of changes in end-diastolic volume by LBNP and similar changes in end-diastolic volume together with afterload reduction by nitroprusside on ventriculoarterial coupling. The slope of the ventricular Pes-SV relation (Ees) is unchanged by both procedures. The slope of the arterial Pes-SV relation (Ea) decreased with augmented SV by nitroprusside. while it increased with reduced SV by LBNP. Consequently, the Ea/Ees ratio decreased with nitroprusside and increased with LBNP

With the proposed coupling concept, we also evaluated the specific roles of contractility change in determining the SV in nine patients with heart failure [13]. To determine the end-systolic pressure-volume relationship, linear regression analysis was applied to several data points collected under varying afterloads induced by phenylephrine or nitroprusside. With dobutamine, both Ved and Ves decreased significantly, and the slope of this Pes-Ves relationship (Ees) increased by 41% without a change in its volume intercept (Vo). If ejection precedes at a constant pressure, the slope of arterial Pes-volume relationship (Ea) decreases as long as the changes in the Ved are minimal (Fig. 6). Thus, the ratio of Ea/Ees was reduced by less than one, indicating that the heart would come to achieve a higher work efficiency by generating less potential energy relative to the external work. The mechanical efficiency is the product of work efficiency (SW/PVA) and PVA/myocardial oxygen consumption (MVO_2). Inotropic intervention shifts up the linear relationship between PVA and MVO_2 without changing the slope [14]. This non-zero positive intercept for $PVA = O$ is assumed to represent the oxygen consumption for basal metabolism and for activation of the contractile machinery. Consequently, with the enhanced contractile state PVA/MVO_2 is reduced for a given PVA, which renders an increase in mechanical efficiency less relative to the extent of an increase in SW/PVA.

Though there is still considerable dispute as to what extent muscle energetics can be estimated from the graphic analysis based on these simplifying assump-

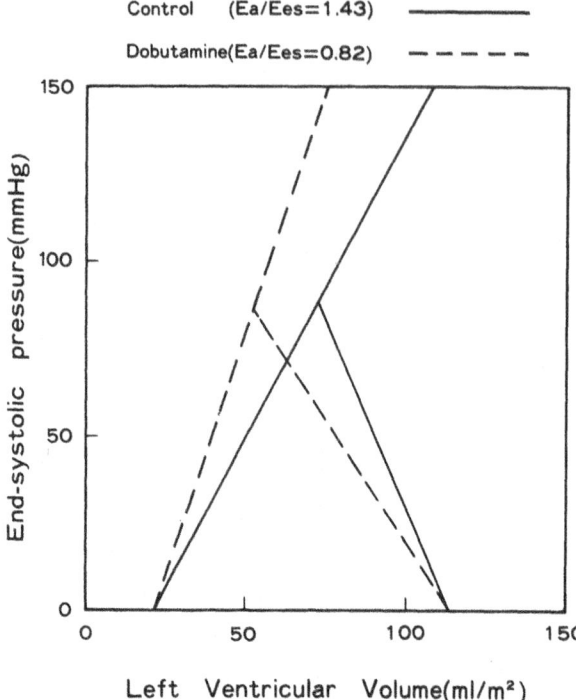

Control   (Ea/Ees=1.43)

Dobutamine(Ea/Ees=0.82)

Fig. 6. Changes in ventricular system properties (Ees) and in arterial system properties (Ea) via changes in contractility with dobutamine. Ventriculoarterial coupling framework at rest (*solid line*) and during infusion of dobutamine (*dashed line*). Augmented contractility is indicated by an increase in Ees and a decrease in Ea, resulting in an augmented work efficiency. (From [13])

tions, the PVA can be used practically to calculate the efficiency of energy utilization, defined as the ratio of mechanical energy to total liberated energy. Thus, we concluded that an enhancement of the inotropic state adjusts the ventriculoarterial coupling toward optimizing ventricular work efficiency.

Summary

These analyses delineated the distinctive aspect between normal and variably failing hearts, responses to exercise, or effects of pharmacologic interventions with vasodilators and inotropic agents in terms of the matching concept and were considered to have great potential in gaining insight into the relevance of adaptational changes and therapeutic responses in congestive heart failure.

References

1. Guyton AC, Jones CE, Coleman TG (1973) Circulatory physiology: cardiac output and its regulation, 2nd edn. Saunders, Philadelphia, pp 147–157
2. Sunagawa K, Maughan WL, Burkhoff D, Sagawa K (1983) Left ventricular interaction with arterial load studied in isolated canine ventricle. Am J Physiol 245:H773–H780
3. Sunagawa K, Maughan WL, Sagawa K (1985) Optimal arterial resistance for the maximal stroke work studied in isolated canine left ventricle. Circ Res 56:586–595
4. Burkhoff D, Sagawa K (1986) Ventricular efficiency predicted by an analytical model. Am J Physiol 250:R1021–R1027
5. Suga H, Hayashi T, Shirahata M (1981) Ventricular systolic pressure-volume area as predictor of cardiac oxygen consumption. Am J Physiol 240:H39–H44
6. Asanoi H, Sasayama S, Kameyama T (1989) Ventriculo-arterial coupling in normal and failing heart in man. Circ Res 65:483–493
7. Asanoi H, Sasayama S (1989) Relationship of plasma norepinephrine to ventricular-load coupling in patients with heart failure. Jpn Circ J 53:131–140
8. Francis GS, Goldsmith SR, Cohn JN (1982) Relationship of exercise capacity to resting left ventricular performance and basal plasma norepinephrine levels in patients with congestive heart failure. Am Heart J 104:725–731
9. Wilson JR, Martin JL, Schwartz D, Ferraro N (1984) Exercise intolerance in patients with chronic heart failure: role of impaired nutritive flow to skeletal muscle. Circulation 69:1079–1087
10. Sasayama S, Ohyagi A, Lee JD, Nonogi H, Sakurai T, Wakabayashi A, Fujita M, Kawai C (1982) Effect of the vasodilator therapy in regurgitant valvular disease. Jpn Circ J 46:433–441
11. Asanoi H, Sasayama S, Iuchi K, Kameyama T (1987) Acute hemodynamic effects of a new inotropic agent (OPC-8212) in patients with congestive heart failure. J Am Coll Cardiol 9:865–871
12. Kameyama T, Asanoi H, Ishizaka S, Sasayama S (1987) Modulation of ventriculo-arterial coupling by unloading therapy in patients with cardiac dysfunction. Circulation 76:IV–162
13. Ishizaka S, Asanoi H, Kameyama T, Sasayama S (1988) Effect of dobutamine on ventriculo-arterial coupling and ventricular work efficiency in patients with cardiac failure. J Cardiol 18:457–465
14. Suga H, Hayashi T, Shirahata M et al. (1981) Regression of cardiac oxygen consumption on ventricular pressure-volume area in dog. Am J Physiol 240:H320–H325

Targeting Evaluation and Treatment of Heart Failure by Pressure-Volume Relations

D.A. KASS and W.L. MAUGHAN

Introduction

The framework of pressure-volume relations provides a means to separately assess ventricular systolic and diastolic pump properties, ventriculo-vascular interactions, and myocardial energetics, *all* using common physiologic variable terms. While previously the domain of isolated heart and intact animal studies, recent technologic developments now make this approach practical and applicable to the clinical assessment of heart failure. There clearly are inherent limitations in studying conscious man (as opposed to isolated animal hearts), thus aspects of these relations in situ require careful reexamination. In the following sections, we will describe several such studies and provide an integrated approach for cardiac-vascular function assessment.

Obtaining Pressure-Volume Relations in Patients

Pressure-volume analysis has generally been difficult to apply in humans owing to the requirement for multiple pressure-volume loops obtained over a loading range. Calculation of volume from ventriculography or echocardiography is cumbersome, geometric model dependent, and not performed in real time. Alteration of loads by vasodilators or constrictors is time consuming and may alter the cardiac muscle under study. This situation has changed with development of a catheter system that provides continuous measurements of ventricular volume simultaneously with pressure [1,2]. By combining this technique with transient occlusion of the inferior vena cava by a large balloon catheter, reproducible left ventricular pressure-volume relations can be easily obtained in humans [3].

The procedure is performed using routine left heart cardiac catheterization techniques. Introducer sheaths are placed in a femoral vein and artery (9F and 8F, respectively). A 12-electrode conductance (volume) catheter is advanced through the femoral artery and placed in the ascending aorta. A 3F micromanometer catheter is placed within the lumen of the volume catheter, and then the assembly is advanced retrograde across the aortic value and positioned at the LV apex. The catheter is used in conjunction with a stimulator-microprocessor unit (VCU, Cardiac Pacemakers Inc., St Paul, Minn.) which generates an AC current field

B.S. Lewis, A. Kimchi (Eds.)
Heart Failure Mechanisms and Management
© Springer-Verlag Berlin Heidelberg 1991

between electrodes positioned at the apex and above the aortic valve. Voltage differences measured between multiple intervening electrode pairs are related to a segmental volume of blood within the ventricular chamber. The net signal is the sum of the segments and provides an on-line continuous volume signal synchronized with pressure.

While the raw volume signal appears linear with absolute volume, it requires calibration. This is achieved using two simple techniques. A thermodilution catheter is placed in the pulmonary artery to determine cardiac output. The relation between this measurement and the cardiac output obtained by the catheter (stroke volume × heart rate) provides the slope of the calibration line. The calibration offset is largely due to muscle wall conductance and that of other surrounding intrathoracic structures. This is estimated by injecting a small volume (10 ml) of hypertonic saline (7.6 g/100 ml) into the pulmonary artery. Mixed with blood, this bolus arrives in the LV a few beats later and alters the conductivity (not volume) of the blood within the chamber. As the conductivity (σ) increases slightly with each beat, a relation can be obtained that displays apparent volume (from the catheter signal) as a function of the altered conductivity. Extrapolated to a theoretically measured volume at zero σ, this gives an estimate of the component of the volume signal only due to conductance of structures surrounding the blood chamber, and thus the offset of the linear calibration. In a set of 15 patients [3], the average offset was 146 ± 32 ml, with a mean difference between multiple determinations of 4.7%. Comparison of calibrated end-diastolic volumes determined by this technique to those obtained by ventriculography ($n = 25$) revealed a good correlation ($r = 0.89, p < 0.001$) with a slope of 0.92 and offset not significantly different from zero.

To obtain pressure-volume relations, a large occlusion balloon (Cordis, FL) is advanced to the right atrium. Rapid inflation with 20–30 ml of CO_2, pulling back on the balloon to assure occlusion of the inferior vena cava (IVC), typically produces a 25–40 mmHg drop in systolic pressure over seven to ten consecutive cardiac cycles. Heart rate is little altered during this period, and thus these beats can be used to construct pressure-volume relations (Fig. 1). The balloon is rapidly deflated (an advantage to CO_2 over saline or contrast), and status returned to baseline. Pressure-volume relation determinations can be made repeatedly with excellent reproducibility. They can also be repeated following pacing, pharmacologic, or other interventions without altering the system under study.

Critical to a meaningful interpretation of such data is that the pressure-volume loops can be obtained without initiating significant reflex stimulation. In an animal study [4], data collected within the first 6–8 s of preload reduction was found to be minimally influenced by reflex change. In patients we have found that, despite reduction of systolic pressure by 26 mmHg during IVC occlusion, heart rate does not significantly change (3.2 ± 1.8 variation, p = NS). This also suggests little reflex activation for the first approximately eight beats of preload reduction.

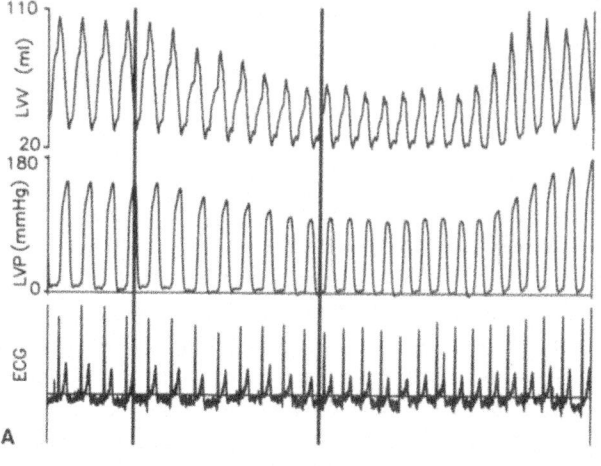

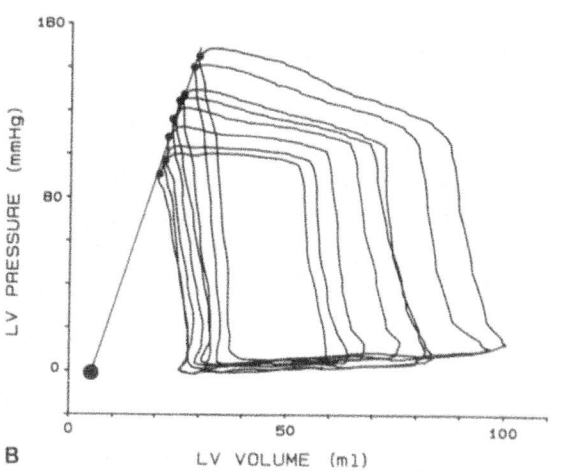

Fig. 1A,B. A Time plots of ECG, LV pressure (*LVP*), and LV volume (*LVV*) obtained in a patient before, during, and after transient IVC occlusion. The *vertical lines* identify the period of decreasing LV preload, and there is little heart rate change during this period (i.e. little change in RR interval). Some reflex activation (heart rate increase) is evident after this period. **B** Pressure-volume loop display of the data between cursors from **A**. Points of maximal P/(V-Vo) are identified, and the resulting relation can be described by linear regression (*r* = 0.99) with slope (Ees = 6.0 mmHg/ml) and volume intercept (Vo = 5.1 ml). (Reproduced with permission from Kass et al. [3])

Systolic Function Assessment

Critical to an index of chamber systolic function is that it sensitively reflect changes in chamber properties yet be minimally influenced by alterations in chamber or vascular loading conditions [5]. A substantial added benefit would be if the index could be easily coupled to measures of ventricular diastolic properties and vascular function so that overall cardiovascular performance could be described and predicted. While there are several indices that satisfy the first requirement, it is the addition of the second attribute that makes the end-systolic pressure-volume relation (ESPVR) so useful.

Figure 2 displays example data from a normal patient in whom six successive cardiac cycles were obtained during transient IVC occlusion. The points of

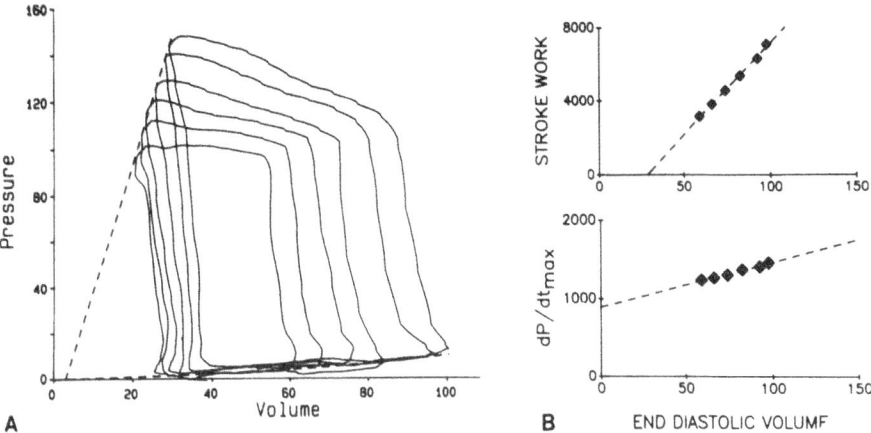

Fig. 2A,B. Assessment of systolic function by pressure-volume relations. **A** Six sequential pressure-volume loops obtained during IVC occlusion by conductance catheter technique. The *dashed line* (ESPVR) provides one index. Other measures **B** can be obtained by regressing either stroke work or dP/dt_{max} against end-diastolic volume. The slopes of both relations have also been found to be relatively load insensitive measures of contractile state. (Reproduced with permission from Kass et al. [8])

maximal $P/(V-Vo)$ for each beat are determined by an iterative technique (assuming $Vo = O$ to start), and the locus of such points defines the ESPVR, with a slope (Ees) providing a measure of contractile function. A variety of other measures are just as easily derived from the same data. The two right hand panels display stroke work – end-diastolic volume (Ved) [6] and dP/dt_{max}-Ved [7] relations. Both stroke work and dP/dt_{max} have preload sensitivity which is quite linear within a physiologic range, but has only small afterload sensitivities in this same range. Thus, by regressing either variable against a range of preloads, the resulting slope is both pre- and afterload independent and provides a measure of contractile function.

There are advantages and disadvantages to each of these indices. The stroke work relation has units of mmHg (work/volume) and is thus essentially chamber size independent. This is an advantage in comparing hearts in patients with markedly different wall geometries. By integrating pressure-volume data over the cardiac cycle, it is also less sensitive to small signal noise in either measurement, which can be problematic for dP/dt_{max} relations. While both indices can provide valuable measurements, a major disadvantage is that they cannot be as easily integrated with other cardiovascular properties.

The end-systolic elastance (Ees) has its own limitations which we have recently reviewed [8]. ESPVRs in intact hearts frequently display an apparent negative extrapolated volume axis intercept (Vo), which clearly has no physiologic meaning. However, we found this behavior to be likely explained by ESPVR nonlinearity [9,10], with linear fits to data obtained in higher loading ranges often displaying flatter slopes and negative intercepts compared to fits over a lower load range from the same ESPVR. Changes in contractile state both influenced the nonlinear shape of ESPVRs and the extrapolated Vo value [9]. In patients, the limited range of altered loading produced by IVC occlusion generally prevents demonstration of significant nonlinearity; however, the derived relations with "negative" extrapolated intercepts strongly suggest a similar phenomena. Comparisons between patient ESPVRs need to consider this potential effect, particularly if very disparate ranges of loads are examined in contrasting two relations.

ESPVRs demonstrate some load [11,12] and contraction history [13] sensitivity. The extent to which these effects interfere with more simplistic interpretations of the relations or their changes following pharmacologic interventions is not completely clear, but does not appear large [8]. Studies in intact animal models have shown the greatest effects when afterload resistance is markedly altered beat-to-beat to construct the ESPVR [14], a load sequence that can amplify contraction history influences.

Despite these and other limitations, such as influences from chamber geometry [15], the ESPVR provides a useful measure of systolic function for several reasons. It defines an operating upper limit of systolic chamber performance under steady-state contractile conditions. Changes in ESPVR due to loading history appear smaller than the easily discerned alterations with pharmacologic agents (Ees typically falling by 45% with 300 μg kg^{-1} min^{-1} esmolol, or rising by more than 100% with 10 μg kg^{-1} min^{-1} dobutamine). Finally, unlike other measures, it is easily coupled with ventricular diastolic and vascular property measurements.

Diastolic Function

Diastolic dysfunction often accompanies systolic pump failure and can, in some instances, constitute the principal cause of clinical symptoms. While frequently assessed by early relaxation indices such as peak negative dP/dt or time constant of pressure fall, and early and late peak filling rates, it is the diastolic pressure-volume relation that comes closest to providing a measure of chamber "passive" properties. While preload change alone will significantly alter $-$dP/dt$_{max}$ and various filling rates and ratios, the diastolic pressure-volume relation derives from data obtained over a range of chamber volumes.

The majority of clinical studies reporting on pressure-volume relations in humans have analyzed single steady-state beats, using much of the filling portions of diastole to provide data. However, this approach is not ideal and can lead to erroneous conclusions about diastolic properties as much as attempts to derive measures of systolic function from steady-state beats [16]. Early diastolic pressure-volume relations can be influenced by incomplete relaxation, and viscoelastic properties manifest during rapid filling. Furthermore, studies have demonstrated an important role of pericardial constraint in mediating RV-LV interaction and its effect on diastolic pressure-volume relations. For example, seemingly beneficial effects of vasodilating agents on diastolic compliance are mostly due to such interactions coupled through an intact pericardium rather than alterations in muscle properties [16].

By obtaining multiple pressure-volume loops and using the IVC occlusion technique, while simultaneously measuring right atrial pressure, these effects can be minimized. IVC occlusion markedly unloads the right heart prior to any LV preload reduction, thereby lowering potential RV-LV crosstalk. Secondly, using only the end-diastolic points from multiple pressure-volume relations enables pressure-volume relations (end-diastolic pressure-volume relations, EDPVR) to be constructed over a range of volumes that are unlikely to be influenced by delayed relaxation or viscoelastic properties. Determination of the EDPVR is shown in Fig. 3. The end-diastolic points are identified from each beat obtained during IVC occlusion, and the locus of points fit to a monoexponential relation. The early diastolic pressure-volume curve often lies slightly above the EDPVR, with small parallel downward shifts as preload is reduced. However, considering the large change in preload volume (nearly 50% reduction in this example) this shift is quite small owing to substantial unloading of the right heart by the IVC balloon several beats *prior* to any left heart volume changes.

The disparity between single beat (steady-state) diastolic data and data obtained from multiple beats is more apparent in the setting of acute ischemia. Figure 4 shows steady-state data before and after 60 s of acute coronary occlusion via percutaneous transluminal coronary angioplasty (PTCA) balloon. With ischemia, the diastolic pressure-volume relation was markedly shifted upward, with an increased pressure at any matched volume. However, when the EDPVRs were obtained by IVC occlusion during both control and ischemic periods, the diastolic relations were superimposable. Thus, by unloading the right heart and

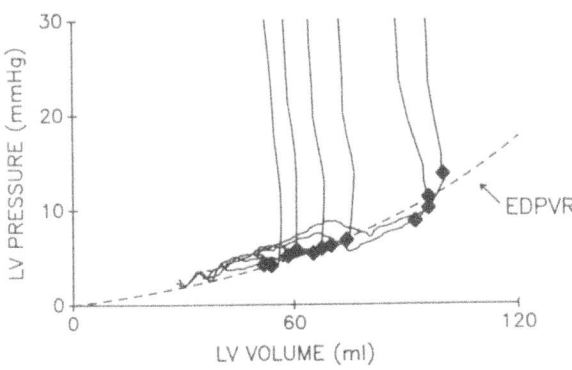

Fig. 3. Measurement of diastolic pressure-volume relation during transient IVC occlusion. There are only small parallel downward shifts in the diastolic pressure-volume relations with each sequential beat despite the large preload reduction (nearly 50% in this example). This is due to right heart unloading by IVC occlusion prior to any fall in LV preload. By selecting only end-diastolic points from each loop, an end-diastolic pressure-volume relation (*EDPVR*) can be assessed which is less influenced by loading, relaxation, or filling effects. This relation is slightly different that what would be obtained from any one steady-state beat

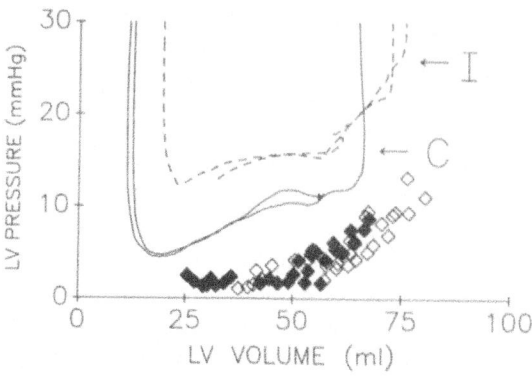

Fig. 4. Effect of loading interaction on diastolic pressure-volume relations during acute coronary occlusion by PTCA balloon in humans. After 60 s of ischemia (*I*), the steady-state pressure-volume relation is significantly elevated in parallel compared to the baseline control (*C*). However, when EDPVRs (see Fig. 3) are determined during IVC occlusion, the load effects are effectively eliminated, and the control (*solid symbols*) and ischemia (*open symbols*) data are virtually superimposable

reducing pericardial constraint and by using only end-diastolic data to avoid relaxation abnormalities, seemingly large diastolic changes during acute coronary occlusion are effectively eliminated [17].

Ventricular-Vascular Coupling

Characterization of ventricular systolic and diastolic properties by elastance can also be applied to the peripheral vasculature [18,19]. The larger the stroke volume (*SV*) introduced into the arterial system, the higher the developed arterial pressure at end-systole (*Pes*). The slope of the linear *SV-Pes* relation, which has elastance units, provides a measure of the arterial load and is called the "effective" arterial elastance (*Ea*) [18]. The term "effective" is used as *Ea* does not represent the property of a specific anatomic component of the vascular system, but rather lumps several properties of the arterial input impedance together. The major determinants of *Ea* are arterial resistance and heart rate, and *Ea* can be approximated by the product of these variables.

A potential advantage of *Ea* is that it defines ventricular load in a manner that is minimally influenced by preload volume, in contrast to estimated wall stress of arterial pressure. This has been found to be the case in humans, for when *Ea* (*Pes/SV*) is calculated for each beat during IVC occlusion, there is no significant change in *Ea* despite the fall in arterial pressure. In a group of 12 patients, the average coefficient of variation (SD/mean·100) *Ea* during preload reduction was only 8.3%, with no significant correlation between *Ea* and reducing preload. Thus,

Ea can provide a measure of ventricular afterload that is reasonably independent of preload change.

The *Ea* description of vascular properties can be easily coupled with the pressure-volume characterization of ventricular properties, enabling prediction of stroke volume [18], stroke work [20], ejection fraction [21], systolic pressure, and other variables. This is particularly valuable in assessing the potential value of specific pharmacologic interventions. Using the data obtained from a set of pressure-volume loops, a series of cardiac function curves can be derived which, unlike traditional relations, embody the relative load independence of the pressure-volume relations from which they originate. Pressure-volume loops are used to define systolic and diastolic pressure-volume relations. These are fit by the following equations: SYSTOLE $[Ees = Pes/(Ves-Vo)]$, and DIASTOLE $[Ped = Po + A(e^{B \cdot Ved} - 1)]$. Lastly, *Ea* is calculated by the ratio of *Pes/SV*. By manipulation of a simple coupling equation [5], it can be shown that stroke work (*SW*) is approximately equal to:

$$SW = \frac{Ea \cdot Ees^2}{(Ea + Ees)^2} \cdot (Ved - Vo)^2$$

$$\text{where } Ved = \frac{\ln[(Ped - Po)/A + 1]}{B}$$

These equations enable stroke work (or stroke volume) to be predicted as a consequence of varying only one parameter (preload, afterload resistance, or contractile state) at a time. In addition, the patient's current status can be superimposed on these relations to define the range of potential functional reserve through manipulation of each respective variable.

An example of this analysis is shown in Fig. 5. Panel A displays the measured pressure-volume data from which systolic, diastolic, and arterial property variables are obtained. The three lower panels (B-D) display the theoretical function curves produced by selective alterations in preload (plotted as filling pressure), afterload resistance (*Ea*), and contractile state (*Ees*). The solid circle indicates the position of steady-state beats for this patient. For a normal heart, there remains a great amount of functional reserve from enhancing contractile state, while preload change can only modestly further increase stroke work, and alterations in afterload in either direction tend to reduce it. Similar function curves from patients with cardiomyopathy can predict which form of therapy is most likely to be successful. In patients with very steep *Ees* (often accompanying hypertrophy), afterload resistance reduction will only minimally increase stroke volume [18]. Likewise, little is achieved by further increasing *Ees*. In contrast, patients with very shallow ESPVRs are more sensitive to afterload and contractile change. Diastolic pressure-volume relation abnormalities can markedly inhibit the preload reserve relation. Heterogeneity of each factor's influence in a given patient may be a major source of variability in heart failure studies. The ability to improve the specificity of our diagnostic assessment of heart failure patients by use of pressure-volume relations should help in this regard.

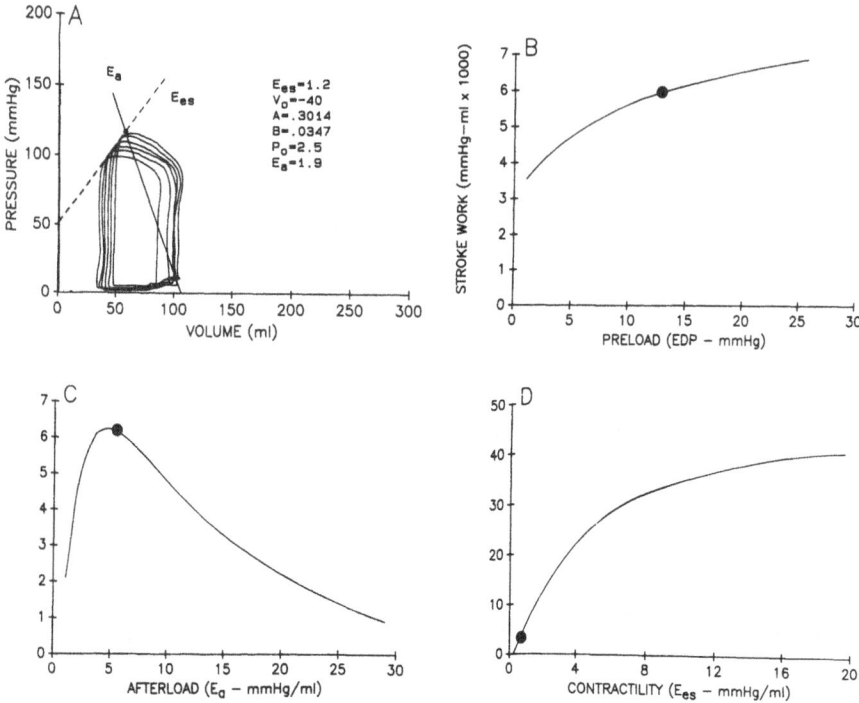

Fig. 5A-D. Generations of LV function curve sets from pressure-volume data. Pressure-volume relations are used to define systolic, diastolic, and vascular coupling parameters (see text for details). From these parameters, theoretical function curves can be determined which display cardiac reserve capacity for changes purely in preload, afterload resistance, or contractility, respectively. The status of the patient at rest (*solid circle*) identifies the relative placement along these function curves and can suggest more successful modes of therapy

Separation of Vascular Unloading from Inotropic Change

For the clinical assessment of heart function and evaluation of drug therapy, it is valuable to quantitatively separate improvements in pump output due to lowered afterload resistance from those secondary to enhanced contractile performance. While ejection fraction is almost equally influenced by changes in either variable, separation of *Ees* and *Ea* using pressure-volume relations provides a means to quantify these effects.

An example is provided by the cardiovascular response to the bipyridine derivative amrinone which has both inotropic and vasodilator effects [21]. The relative influence of both can be quantified as shown in Fig. 6. An anesthetized dog with blocked autonomic reflexes (hexamethonium/vagotomy) received an acute i.v. infusion of 2 mg/kg amrinone. The steady-state control loop shifted leftward after infusion with a 16% fall in end-diastolic volume. Mean arterial resistance also fell by 30% leading to flatter wider pressure-volume loops. Using the coupling relations to predict ejection fraction (a variation of the one above for

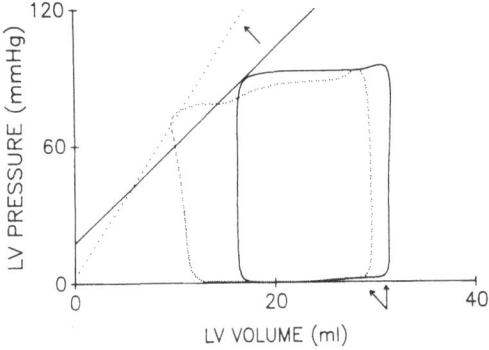

Fig. 6. Separation of afterload versus contractile change produced by intravenous amrinone injection. Steady state loops at control (*solid lines*) and after amrinone (*dotted lines*) are shown, along with their respective ESPVRs. In addition to the increase in contractile state, loops also became flatter and squatter, with a lower ratio of end-systolic pressure to stroke volume [Pes/SV ≃ effective arterial elastance (Ea)]. This is consistent with lowered afterload resistance and can be quantified independently from Ees change

stroke work), one could predict that ejection fraction would increase by only 18% from these loading changes alone. In fact, ejection fraction rose by 35%, thus nearly half of the net increase stemmed from alterations in peripheral loading, while the other half was due to an increase in inotropic state (*Ees*). The inotropic change was easily assessed by the ESPVR slope which rose from 4.4 to 6.4 mmHg/ml. By separate identification of ventricular preload, afterload resistance, and contractile function, the specific sources of a drugs influence on chamber pump function can be quantified.

Summary

The application of pressure-volume analysis to the study of cardiac and vascular physiology in various animal models has a long and distinguished history, yet the clinical application of this approach for assessment of human cardiac disease and therapy remains at an early stage. The power of the approach for quantifying mechanisms of drug action, better defining individual patient pathophysiology, and helping target therapy seems evident. It is hoped that future studies will lead us to a new level of definition, understanding, and treatment of human cardiac disease.

References

1. Baan J, van der Velde ET, Bruin HG, Smeenk GJ, Koops J, van Duk AD, Temmerman D, Senden J, Buis B (1984) Continuous measurement of left ventricular volume in animals and humans by conductance catheter. Circulation 70:812
2. McKay R, Spears JR, Aroesty J, Baim D, Royal H, Heller G, Lincoln W, Salo R, Braunwald E, Grossman W (1984) Instantaneous measurement of left and right ventricular stroke volume and pressure-volume relationships with an impedance catheter. Circulation 69:703
3. Kass DA, Midei M, Graves W, Brinker JA, Maughan WL (1988) Use of a conductance (volume) catheter and transient inferior vena caval occlusion for rapid determination of pressure-volume relationships in man. Cathet Cardiovasc Diagn 15:192–202
4. Kass DA, Yamazaki T, Burkhoff D, Maughan WL, Sagawa K (1986) Detemination of left ventricular end-systolic pressure-volume relationships by the conductance (volume) catheter technique. Circulation 73:586
5. Kass DA, Maughan WL, Guo AM, Kono A, Sunagawa K, Sagawa K (1987) Comparative influence of load versus inotropic states on indexes of ventricular contractility: experimental and theoretical analysis based on pressure-volume relationships. Circulation 76:1422
6. Glower DD, Spratt JA, Snow ND, Kabas JS, Davis JW, Olsen CO, Tyson GS, Sabiston DC Jr, Rankin JS (1985) Linearity of the Frank-Starling relationship in the intact heart: the concept of preload recruitable stroke work. Circulation 71:994
7. Little WC (1985) The left ventricular dP/dt_{max}-end diastolic volume relation in closed-chest dogs. Circ Res 56:808
8. Kass DA, Maughan WL (1988) From E_{max} to pressure-volume relations: a broader view. Circulation 77:1203
9. Kass DA, Beyar R, Lankford E, Heard M, Maughan WL, Sagawa K (1989) Influence of contractile state on curvilinearity of In Situ end-systolic pressure-volume relations. Circulation 79:167
10. Burkhoff D, Sugiura S, Yue DT, Sagawa KL (1987) Contractility-dependent curvilinearity of end-systolic pressure-volume relations. Am J Physiol 252: (Heart Circ Physiol 21) H1218
11. Freeman GL, Little WC, O'Rourke RA (1986) The effect of vasoactive agents on the left ventricular end-systolic pressure-volume relations in closed-chest dogs. Circulation 74:1107
12. Maughan WL, Sunagawa K, Burkhoff D, Sagawa K (1984) Effect of arterial impedance changes on the end-systolic pressure-volume relation. Circ Res 54:595
13. Hunter WC (1989) End-systolic pressure as a balance between opposing effects of ejection. Circ Res 64:265
14. Baan J, van der Velde E (1988) Sensitivity of left ventricular end-systolic pressure-volume relation to type of loading intervention in dogs. Circ Res 62:1247
15. Suga H, Hisano R, Goto Y, Hamada O (1984) Normalization of end-systolic pressure-volume relation and E_{max} in different sized hearts. Jpn Circ J 48:136
16. Gilbert JC, Glantz SA (1989) Determinants of left ventricular filling and of the diastolic pressure-volume relation. Circ Res 64:827
17. Kass DA, Midei M, Brinker J, Maughan WL (1990) Influence of coronary occlusion during PTCA on end-systolic and end-diastolic pressure-volume relations in man. Circulation 81:447–460
18. Sunagawa K, Maughan WL, Burkhoff D, Sagawa K (1983) Left ventricular interaction with arterial load studied in isolated canine ventricle. Am J Physiol 215: (Heart Circ Physiol 14) H773
19. Sunagawa K, Maughan WL, Sagawa K (1985) Optimal arterial resistance for the maximal stroke work studied in isolated canine left ventricle. Circ Res 56:586
20. Maughan WL, Kass DA, Sagawa K (1988) Accurate prediction of stroke work from systolic and diastolic pressure-volume relations in the isolated canine heart. Phys Med Biol 33 [Suppl 1]:179
21. Kass DA, Grayson R, Marino P (1990) Pressure-volume analysis as a method for quantifying simultaneous drug (Amrinone) effects on arterial load and contractile state in vivo. J Am Coll Cardiol 16:726–732

Importance of the Pericardium in Relation to Normal and Abnormal Ventricular Diastolic Function

R. Shabetai

Heart failure can be defined as symptomatic ventricular dysfunction. In some types of heart failure, systolic or pump dysfunction predominates; whereas in others, such as that which may follow hypertension and left ventricular hypertrophy, diastolic dysfunction predominates or may even occur when indices of systolic left ventricular function are normal. Nevertheless, it is important to emphasize that, in the vast majority of instances of heart failure of every variety, there is usually an element of diastolic dysfunction.

It is well known that cardiac tamponade and constrictive pericarditis are largely disorders of diastolic filling of the heart. While the older literature tended to emphasize the extremes of these two compressive disorders of the heart, it is now increasingly appreciated that it is important to recognize milder and atypical forms of tamponade and constrictive pericarditis in which, although the patient is not dramatically ill, it is clear that the pericardium is exerting a major abnormal influence on hemodynamics. It is not surprising that this thinking has been logically extended to inquire into the extent to which the pericardium influences the heart in the absence of disease of either the heart or the pericardium.

The unstressed pericardium is slightly larger in volume (perhaps in the order of 10%) than the volume of the contents that it encloses under the conditions of euvolemia. This reserve of volume permits changes in heart size to occur in response to such physiological variables as the respiratory cycle, changes in posture or heart rate, and state of hydration. Another factor facilitating the occurrence of these dimensional changes without inducing secondary changes in cardiac pressure is that the unstressed pericardium is compliant and can increase in volume with little, if any, pressure change to accommodate small changes in cardiac volume. However, thereafter the pericardium rapidly becomes stiffer and eventually inextensible. The shape of the pericardial pressure-volume curve illustrating this physiology is shown in Fig. 1 obtained during aspiration of a large pericardial effusion. The pericardium was prestretched by the effusion; therefore the pericardium was not as stiff as normal, and the early part of the curve is correspondingly less steep.

The implication to be derived from the foregoing paragraphs is that the pericardium and the heart may exert considerable contact pressure on each other when cardiac volume is relatively large, but that this influence is less at smaller cardiac volumes. Ventricular diastolic chamber compliance is derived from the change of ventricular volume during diastole relative to the change in ventricular pressure. Myocardial fiber compliance is calculated from the changes in diastolic

B.S. Lewis, A. Kimchi (Eds.)
Heart Failure Mechanisms and Management
© Springer-Verlag Berlin Heidelberg 1991

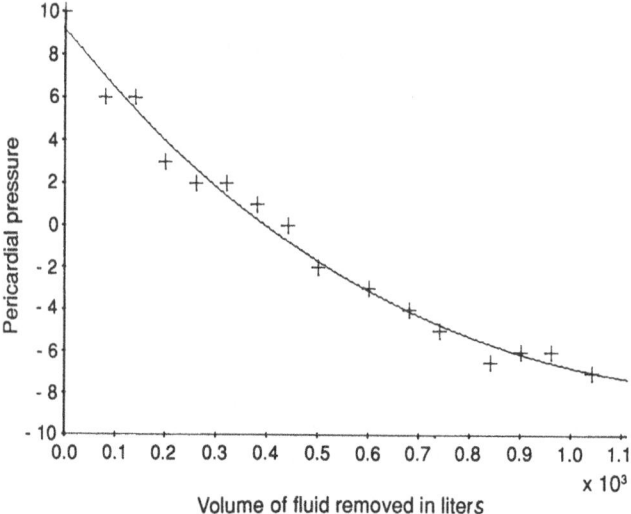

Fig. 1. Pericardial pressure-volume curve. The data were obtained during pericardiocentesis for moderately severe cardiac tamponade. One litre of fluid was obtained. Aspiration of the first 200 ml dropped the pericardial pressure from 6 mmHg to 2 mmHg. The curve is exponential

stress and strain. Ventricular diastolic pressure is a component of both these compliance calculations and should be factored not as the instantaneous diastolic pressure within the ventricle, but as the ventricular diastolic transmural pressure. To calculate transmural pressure, it is necessary to know pericardial pressure. When pericardial pressure is close to atmospheric, the error introduced into compliance calculations by using luminal rather than transmural pressure is negligible, but at high pericardial pressure becomes appreciable.

Unfortunately, the pericardial space is not easily accessible for pressure measurement. When catheters are placed in the pleural and pericardial spaces, and attached to pressure transducers, the recorded pressure from the two cavities is essentially equal throughout the respiratory cycle. Thus, until relatively recently, it was assumed that one could substitute pleural pressure for pericardial pressure to calculate ventricular transmural pressure. Thus, for quiet respiration, it was assumed that pericardial pressure was close to ambient, and that during inspiration pericardial pressure would be a few millimeters of mercury subambient. However, recently it has been posited that, since the pericardial space is potential rather than actual, measurement of pressure within it using conventional means of catheter and transducer grossly underestimates the true pericardial surface contact pressure, i.e., the force exerted by the pericardium and heart against each other [1]. The nearest approximation to pericardial surface contact pressure is the pressure exerted on a flat air- or liquid-filled balloon placed between the heart and pericardium. Pressure measured by this technique is usually close to right atrial pressure and right ventricular diastolic pressure. This close approximation of the three pressures has several important physiological consequences [2], the most important of which are (a) that the right ventricle would operate at close to zero transmural pressure over a large range of diastolic volumes; and (b) that in calculations of left ventricular compliance using transmural pressure, it would be necessary only to subtract right atrial pressure from measured left ventricular diastolic pressure. The difference is transmural ventricular diastolic pressure, comparing conventional to surface pressure measurements, can be appreciated if one considers the case in which right atrial pressure is 12 mmHg and ventricular diastolic pressure is 15 mmHg. Using conventional liquid pressure measurement in the pericardium, pericardial pressure can be assumed to be zero during expiration and –5 at peak inspiration. The ventricular diastolic pressure would then be 15 mmHg during expiration and 20 mmHg at the peak of inspiration. Using right atrial pressure as a surrogate for pericardial pressure, however, transmural ventricular diastolic pressure would be only 5 mmHg. Another physiological consequence stemming from the concept of surface contact pressure is that pericardial pressure is not uniform around the ventricle but subject to regional variation which may change depending upon the volume of individual cardiac chambers.

Acute Cardiac Dilatation

When cardiac volume is rapidly expanded by intravenous infusion, right atrial and left atrial pressure rise rapidly. However, if pericardial pressure is measured at the same time, a substantial increase in intrapericardial pressure is found to have occurred simultaneously with the rise in atrial pressure. Thus, the rise in transmural atrial and ventricular diastolic pressures is much less than the change in absolute diastolic pressures (Fig. 2).

Equalization of left and right ventricular diastolic pressures is a hemodynamic hallmark of compression of the heart by the pericardium in either constrictive pericarditis or cardiac tamponade. From this observation, it has been postulated that equalization of left and right ventricular diastolic pressures, in the face of a normal pericardium, is an expression of restriction caused not by disease of the pericardium, but by an enlarged heart which has engaged the pericardium and stretched it to the point of low compliance. Abundant experimental and clinical evidence supports this concept. Thus, in animals and in humans, the entire left ventricular diastolic pressure-volume relationship can be displaced along the pressure axis by infusion of volume, angiotensin or nitroprusside [3]. In many cases of acute heart failure or acute exacerbations of chronic heart failure, left and right ventricular diastolic pressures are found to be equal. Furthermore, infusion of nitroprusside not only lowers both diastolic pressures, but lowers right ventricular diastolic pressure to a lower level than left. Relatively acute severe tricuspid regurgitation caused by carcinoid can produce a hemodynamic picture difficult to distinguish from constrictive pericarditis. Ruptured chordae tendineae of the mitral valve creates severe mitral regurgitation, manifest not only by giant peaked systolic waves of left atrial and pulmonary wedge pressure, but also by the

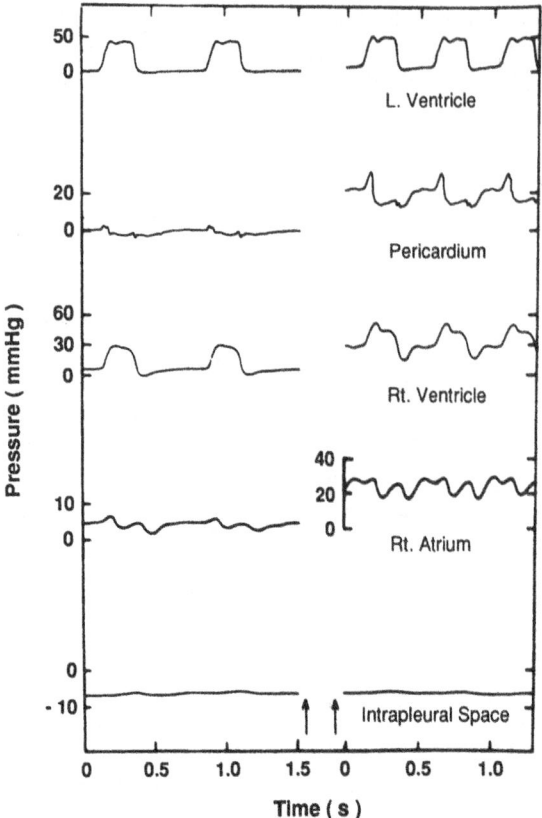

Fig. 2. Effect of rapid intravenous volume expansion in a dog. Note increase in ventricular diastolic pressures and atrial pressure is accompanied by a significant increase in pericardial pressure. Infusion caused a relatively small increase in transmural cardiac pressures. (From [10])

development of equal pressure in the left atrium, right atrium, and both the ventricles during diastole. Another well-known example of this phenomenon occurs in right ventricular infarction. Here, the relatively acute dilatation of the right ventricle fills the pericardial reserve volume, so that the pericardium engages the heart, once more generating hemodynamics that simulate constrictive pericarditis. Acute aortic regurgitation occurring in such conditions as infectious endocarditis or rupture of the sinus Valsalva may produce similar effects. Finally, experimental evidence suggests that the well-known upward shift of the left ventricular diastolic pressure-volume relation in myocardial ischemia, while due in considerable measure to reduced compliance of the left ventricular myocardium, is accentuated by engagement with the pericardium when cardiac volume increases.

Chronic Volume Overload and Chronic Heart Failure

Evidence that when cardiac volume is acutely expanded, pericardial pressure rises because the heart engages the pericardium and stretches it to the limit of its compliance (Fig. 1 and 2) is highly convincing. It is then appropriate to examine to what extent the same phenomenon can be documented in the case of chronic cardiac enlargement. In the animal laboratory, inferarenal aorta-caval fistula has been used as a model to create chronic cardiac enlargement and hypertrophy. When dogs were studied 7-10 days after the creation of such a shunt, the restraining effect of the pericardium was still evident, but when the dogs were studied at 45 days, evidence of pericardial restraint could no longer be demonstrated [4] (Fig. 3). Subsequent studies showed that the pericardium had undergone both hypertrophy and an increase in compliance [5]. Opportunities to study this phenomenon in human subjects have been relatively few, but, in some instances, evidence of pericardial restraint has been presented in cases with cardiomegaly secondary to chronic congestive heart failure [6]. Since cardiac catheterization in patients with chronic heart failure is frequently indicated because of worsening symptoms, it is possible that pericardial restraint is present because of an acute further enlargement of the heart. Preload reduction, for instance by infusion of nitroprusside, shrinks the volume of the heart until it no

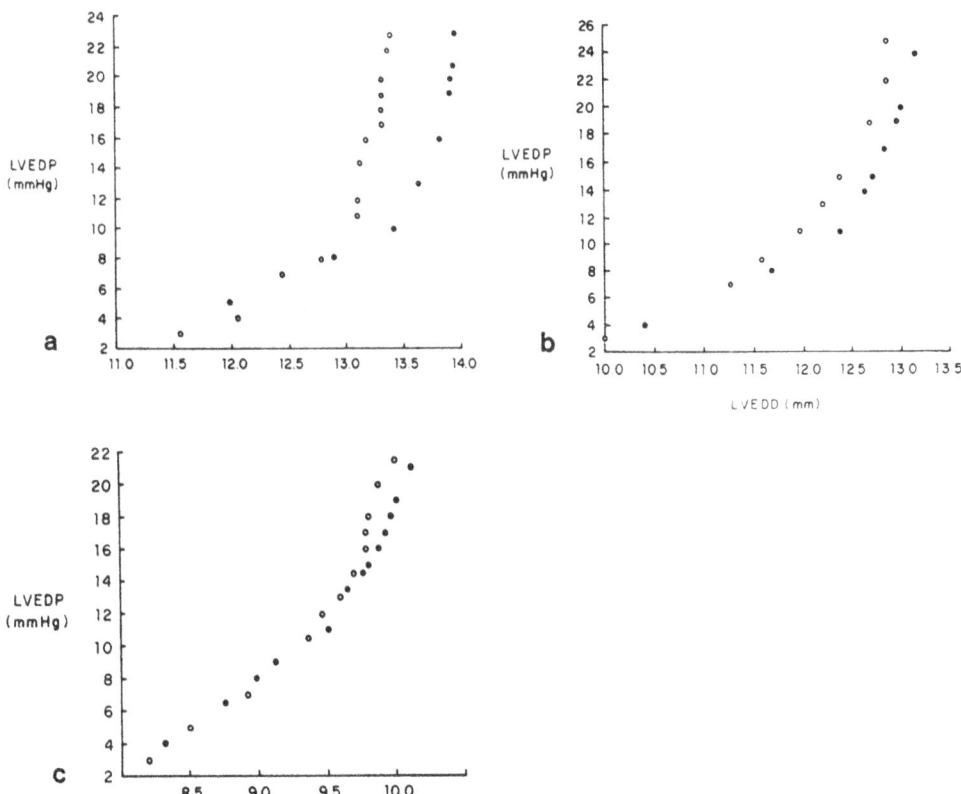

Fig. 3a-c. Left ventricular end diastolic pressure-volume curve. Nine (**a**) and eight (**b**) days after creation of a chronic volume overload. Pericardial restraint is evident at higher ventricular volumes. (**c**) After 36 days. The pericardium has adapted and its restraining effect can no longer be demonstrated. *Open circles,* before pericardiectomy; *closed circles,* after pericardiectomy

longer engages the pericardium. When this occurs, diastolic pressure falls in both the ventricles, but right ventricular diastolic pressure becomes lower than left. These results indicate that the mechanism by which preload-reducing agents improves cardiac status in heart failure depends in part on their ability to disengage the heart from the pericardium by reducing cardiac volume.

Diastolic Heart Failure

Some cases of heart failure are manifest by predominantly, and in some cases only, by diastolic dysfunction. The most common cause of this syndrome is left ventricular hypertrophy secondary to hypertension, but predominantly diastolic heart failure occurs in some cases of ischemic heart disease. Diastolic heart failure is sometimes of unknown etiology, and in some of these there may be myocardial fibrosis. Although the hemodynamics resemble those of constrictive pericarditis, so far as is known at present, the pericardium plays no role in the pathophysiology of such cases.

Recording Doppler velocity patterns of left ventricular filling is a common means of assessing diastolic heart failure and other abnormalities of diastolic function. Thus, in constrictive pericarditis, and in some case of restrictive cardiomyopathy, early rapid filling is predominant and characterized by an early and steep early filling peak. On the other hand, many cases of diastolic heart failure, other than restrictive cardiomyopathy, are characterized by slower early rapid filling and predominance of late over early filling. However, caution should be exercised in interpreting phenomena such as alteration of the ratio of early to late filling peaks as evidence of myocardial dysfunction. This caution is necessary because a number of factors other than myocardial compliance strongly influence the pattern of left ventricular filling. These include heart rate, age, ventricular volume, and, of particular relevance to this communication, the pericardium [7]. Thus, with tachycardia, the early and late filling waves merge and the pattern becomes monophasic. Late diastolic filling of the left ventricle is seen in infancy and again in old age, whereas in young adults the early rapid filling wave is often predominant. The pericardium influences the ventricular filling pattern; thus, pericardiectomy converts predominance of the early rapid filling wave to dominance by the late filling wave [7]. Also, we have observed alterations in the early to late filling ratio and in deceleration times in response to mental stressors administered during Doppler study.

After cardiac transplantation some patients develop a picture of restrictive cardiomyopathy [8] with hemodynamics indistinguishable from constrictive pericarditis, but sometimes this syndrome is related, at least in part, to scarring of the pericardium or mediastinum. Rarely, acute myocarditis presents with predominant diastolic dysfunction, the clinician should evaluate the patient for constrictive pericarditis, because acute pericardial constriction can occur early in the course of some cases of myocarditis.

Ventricular Interaction

The pericardium can influence ventricular diastolic function via chamber interaction as well as by the direct mechanisms discussed thus far. Right ventricular enlargement as a result of tricuspid regurgitation bulges the intraventricular septum toward the left ventricle, often creating paradoxical motion of the septum. Left ventricular volume is then compressed by the right heart as well as by the pericardium. The short axis of the left ventricle is selectively reduced and the resulting shape change of the chamber tends to reduce ventricular diastolic compliance. Numerous studies have made it clear that interaction among the cardiac chambers is greatly strengthened by the presence of the pericardium [9].

Summary

The pericardium, by virtue of its strategic position around the heart, exerts a restraining influence on cardiac volume. This influence tends to be small or negligible at low cardiac volume, but is quite marked when cardiac volume is increased. Many investigators measure pericardial contact pressure via balloons placed between the heart and pericardium rather than by using conventional liquid pressure measurements when there is no pericardial effusion. With pericardial effusion, pressures measured by balloons and catheters are identical because the pericardium no longer contacts the heart. Pericardial contact pressure is considerably higher than conventionally measured pressure and approaches right atrial pressure. Unlike liquid pressure, regional variations occur in contact pressure. These aspects of pericardial pressure are relevant to the measurement of ventricular transmural pressure and hence the estimation of ventricular diastolic compliance. Exactly how pericardial pressure should be estimated is still a subject for investigation. In acute volume load secondary to infusion, acute subacute valve dysfunction or heart failure, the heart enlarges more rapidly than the pericardium can stretch. The pericardium therefore bears a considerable proportion of the resulting increase in ventricular diastolic pressure. This phenomenon should be borne in mind when considering the benefits of preload reduction in acute heart failure. The role of the pericardium in the response to preload reduction for chronic heart failure is less certain; although the pericardium probably plays a part when acute exacerbations of heart failure further enlarge the heart. The pericardium modulates the pattern of ventricular filling, and this should be borne in mind when using Doppler parameters to assess ventricular diastolic function.

References

1. Tyberg JV, Taichman GC, Smith ER et al. (1986) The relation between pericardial pressure and right atrial pressure. An intraoperative study. Circulation 73:428
2. Shabetai R (1988) Pericardial and cardiac pressure. Circulation 77:1
3. Shirato K, Shabetai R, Bhargava V et al. (1978) Alteration of the left ventricular diastolic pressure-segment length relation produced by the pericardium. Circulation 57:1191
4. LeWinter MM, Pavelec RS (1978) Influence of the pericardium on left ventricular end-diastolic pressure-segment length relations during early and later stages of experimental chronic volume overload in dogs. Circ Res 42:433
5. Freeman G, LeWinter MM (1984) Pericardial adaptations during chronic cardiac dilatation. Circ Res 54:294
6. Boltwood CM, Tei C, Wong M et al. (1983) Inspiratory tracking of diastolic pressures; a hemodynamic sign of ubiquitous pericardial restraint. Circulation 68 [Suppl 3]:3–340
7. Hoit BD, Bhargava V, Shabetai R (1989) Influence of the pericardium or dynamic right and left ventricular filling. J Am Coll Cardiol 13:207A
8. Appleton CP, Hatle LK, Popp RL (1987) Central venous flow velocity patterns can differentiate constrictive pericarditis from restrictive cardiomyopathy. J Am Coll Cardiol 9:119A
9. Hess OM, Bhargava V, Ross J Jr et al. (1983) The role of the pericardium in interactions between the cardiac chambers. Am Heart J 106:377
10. Holt JP (1970) The normal pericardium. Am J Cardiol 26:455–465

Non-Invasive Imaging Techniques in the Assessment of Patients with Heart Failure

Radionuclide Evaluation of Ventricular Performance in Congestive Heart Failure: An Overview

B.L. ZARET and R. SOUFER

Introduction

The radionuclide assessment of ventricular performance provides relevant data concerning global and regional systolic and diastolic function, and right as well as left ventricular function. In addition, assessment may be made under varying conditions such as exercise or pharmacologic intervention, and technology has been miniaturized such that ambulatory patients can be evaluated during routine activity. This review will address radionuclide cardiologic techniques for evaluating ventricular performance and focus specifically on their applicability to the clinical and investigative study of congestive heart failure.

Left Ventricular Ejection Fraction

Left ventricular ejection fraction is a well-standardized measure of global systolic performance [1], it is objective, reproducible, and operator independent. From a physiologic standpoint, it must be recognized that the measure is influenced significantly by loading conditions as well as intrinsic contractility. Nevertheless, the clinical utility of this measure as a meaningful approximation of global systolic performance and as a prognostic index in patients with coronary artery disease are well established [2,3]. In addition, ejection fraction can be used to identify patients with stable coronary disease who might benefit from surgical as opposed to medical therapy [4]. Left ventricular ejection fraction is also a potent predictor of survival in patients who have been resuscitated from out-of-hospital ventricular tachycardia and fibrillation [5]. However, there is controversy concerning the relative contribution of left ventricular ejection fraction as a major independent determinant of survival in congestive heart failure [6]. This is probably owing to the fact that the impact of the measurement may also in part be dependent on the etiology of congestive heart failure.

Serial measures of ejection fraction can be of significant value in following patients receiving potentially cardiotoxic agents. The largest clinical experience has been is cancer patients receiving the antinaoplastic drug doxorubicin [7]. Based on the study of over 1000 patients, guidelines have been developed for the utilization of resting left ventricular ejection fraction as a means of guiding therapy in patients receiving doxorubicin. Prior to the institution of

B.S. Lewis, A. Kimchi (Eds.)
Heart Failure Mechanisms and Management
© Springer-Verlag Berlin Heidelberg 1991

such guidelines, monitoring resided primarily with endomyocardial biopsy, a procedure not without risk, discomfort, and expense [8]. In the absence of some form of effective monitoring, congestive heart failure will not be an uncommon endpoint in patients receiving doxorubicin therapy [9].

The following therapeutic guidelines have been proposed based upon serial radionuclide resting left ventricular ejection fraction [7]. A baseline radionuclide angiocardiogram should be performed prior to the administration of drug or at a level of less than 100 mg/m^2. Subsequent studies should be performed prior to subsequent dose increments according to the following scheme. In patients with normal baseline left ventricular ejection fraction ($\leqslant 50\%$), a second study should be performed after 250–300 mg/m^2. A repeat study should be obtained after 400 mg/m^2 in patients with known heart disease, radiation exposure, abnormal electrocardiograms, or cyclophosphamide therapy. In the absence of these risk factors, a second study should be performed after 450 mg/m^2. Thereafter, sequential studies should be performed prior to each dose. Doxorubicin therapy should be discontinued once ejection fraction evidence of cardiotoxicity develops: that is, an absolute decrease in LVEF of $\geqslant 10\%$ (ejection fraction units) associated with a decline to a level less than 50% (ejection fraction units). In patients with abnormal baseline LVEF ($< 50\%$), doxorubicin therapy should not be initiated if the baseline level is less than 30%. In individuals with ejection fractions between 30% and 50%, sequential studies should be done prior to each dose. Therapy should be discontinued for an absolute fall of LVEF of $\geqslant 10\%$ and/or a final LVEF value of $< 30\%$. Implementation of these management guidelines led to a significant improvement in survival without evidence of congestive heart failure [7]. In this series, death due to heart failure did not occur when appropriate ejection fraction guidelines were followed. The total incidence of heart failure in this series of high-risk patients was only 16% [7]. In addition, when congestive heart failure did develop, it was generally mild and responded to routine anti-heart-failure medication.

Ventricular Volumes

Within the spectrum of heart failure, the majority of patients will present with substantial depression of ejection fraction and overall systolic performance. Ejection fraction in this instance may not be sufficiently discriminatory to distinguish subpopulations or to show major interventional changes. However, more meaningful changes may be demonstrable with the use of absolute ventricular volume measurements. Nuclear techniques offer the ability to measure ventricular volume in a nongeometric manner, based upon calibration of measured activity with actual blood samples [10]. Volume measurements also can be integrated with catheterization laboratory-derived intraventricular pressure measurements such that pressure-volume relations can be evaluated [11]. This can also be done noninvasively if one uses peak systolic pressure measured peripherally as the pressure parameter [12]. Pressure-volume data provide more load-independent measures of ventricular function and contractility [13].

Serial pressure-volume measures have been obtained in the intensive care unit in a group of patients with unstable angina and varying degrees of ventricular dysfunction and have been used to evaluate the impact of graded intravenous nitroglycerin infusions on ventricular performance [14]. Using the radionuclide technique, it can be demonstrated that, despite major drug-induced changes in ejection fraction (usually increments), overall contractility as assessed by systolic pressure-volume relation does not change [14]. Similar approaches can be used for the detailed assessment of therapeutic interventions in heart failure.

Finally, ventricular volume measurements may provide important data for defining the phenomenon of remodeling of ventricular architecture in acute coronary artery disease. Recent studies have emphasized the importance of this particular phenomenon as it relates to survival and congestive heart failure [15]. Recent studies in this sphere have involved development of appropriate processing techniques for quantitatively defining abnormalities in systolic and diastolic shape. Specific measures relating to curvature as well as bending energy have been proposed and are currently under active investigation [16].

Regional Function

In the setting of coronary artery disease, regional abnormalities in ventricular performance may play a major role in defining both risk and prognosis. The most dramatic regional wall motion abnormality involves the postinfarction development of a left ventricular aneurysm. This can be readily defined from multiview radionuclide studies. In a series of patients presenting with an initial anterior wall myocardial infarction, those individuals developing a left ventricular aneurysm had a substantial increase in mortality compared to those without aneurysms [17]. This occurred despite the fact that both groups had comparable ejection fractions. The definition of left ventricular aneurysm should include three specific criteria: the presence of akinesis or dyskinesis, a distinct diastolic deformity, and the presence of normally adjacent contracting myocardium. All three criteria must be met for an aneurysm to be considered present [17] (Fig. 1.).

It is clear that visual assessment of regional wall motion abnormality is insufficient for a complete evaluation. Quantitative approaches are mandatory. One technique, perhaps used most widely, involves measurement of regional ejection fraction [1]. With this approach, the left ventricular region of interest in the left anterior oblique view is divided into four to six specific regions (Fig. 2). The same count-based volume curve analysis employed for global function is utilized for analysis of regional function. The method is relatively independent of ventricular geometry. With this technique, post-thrombolysis differences in regional performance were noted in the initial phase of the TIMI study (TIMI)

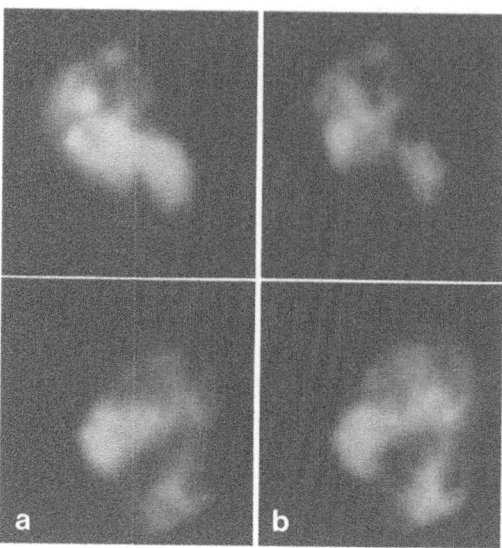

Fig. 1a,b. A radionuclide ventriculogram of a patient with a recent anterior myocardial infarction in the anterior (*upper*) and left lateral (*lower*)
views. **a** End-diastolic (ED) and **b**
end-systolic (ES) frames are shown.
Note the aneurysm of the anteroapical segment

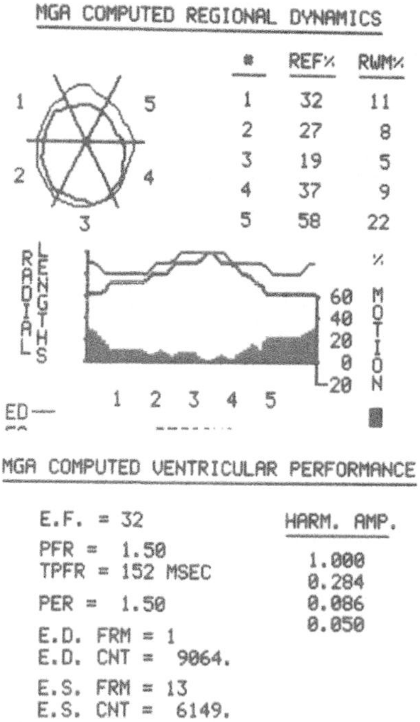

MGA COMPUTED REGIONAL DYNAMICS

#	REF%	RWM%
1	32	11
2	27	8
3	19	5
4	37	9
5	58	22

MGA COMPUTED VENTRICULAR PERFORMANCE

E.F. = 32

PFR = 1.50
TPFR = 152 MSEC

PER = 1.50

E.D. FRM = 1
E.D. CNT = 9064.

E.S. FRM = 13
E.S. CNT = 6149.

HARM. AMP.

1.000
0.284
0.086
0.050

Fig. 2. Regional ejection fraction data. The *upper panel* shows the division of the left ventricle in the
LAO (left anterior oblique) view into five regions. Regions 1 and 2 represent the upper and lower
septal zones, region 3 the inferoapical zone, region 4 the inferolateral zone, and region 5 the
posterolateral zone. The greatest abnormality in regional ejection fraction is in regions 3 and 4. In the
lower panel the patients global *LVEF* (left ventricular ejection fraction) is shown at 27%

between streptokinase and rt-PA therapy patients [18]. These differences were not apparent from analysis of global function alone. This represents the first data involving direct comparisons between two thrombolytic therapies that correlate enhanced vessel patency to improved ventricular performance.

A second regional approach is geometry dependent and involves adaptation of the center line method (initially developed for contrast angiography) for radionuclide studies [19]. These are performed in lateral-view equilibrium studies, which are comparable mirror images of the left ventricular contrast angiographic right anterior oblique projection [20]. Using artificial intelligence-based edge detection algorithms, the outline of the left ventricle in these lateral views is defined from the radionuclide studies [21]. End-diastolic and end-systolic contours are then superimposed and evaluated with the centerline approach. With this technique, a series of 100 chords are derived perpendicular to a centerline which is midway between the end-diastolic and end-systolic outlines. The length of each chord is a measure of the degree of contraction in that particular region. Based upon the length of the chord, shortening is defined as a value normalized to the end-diastolic perimeter and expressed as "shortening fraction." This can then be related to a normal database, in comparison to which deviation can be derived. This technique has also been applied in the TIMI trial [22].

Finally, it may be possible to assess regional performance using the technetium-99m-labeled perfusion agents, the isonitriles. These particular radionuclides remain within the myocardium following an initial flow-related distribution. Appropriate gating of these perfusion images allows definition of regional performance on a count-based basis. This allows for simultaneous measurement of perfusion and function from the same radionuclide study. Preliminary work with this approach in our laboratory has yielded encouraging results [22a].

Diastolic Performance

Diastolic function can be readily evaluated from the equilibrium radionuclide angiocardiogram by assessment of ventricular filling. The two measurements used most widely for this are peak filling rate, generally normalized to end-diastolic volume, and time to peak filling [23] (Fig. 3). These volumetric indices represent an approximation of true diastolic function which is a pressure-volume phenomenon. The preference of our own laboratory has been to utilize peak filling rate since this can be determined in a more reproducible and objective operator-independent manner. Preliminary studies from our laboratory suggest that diastolic function may be the major determinant of exercise performance in patients with congestive heart failure [24]. This was noted in a group of 19 patients with congestive heart failure recently evaluated in our laboratory, in whom resting radionuclide measures of ventricular performance were compared to upright bicycle exercise performance and total body oxygen consumption [24].

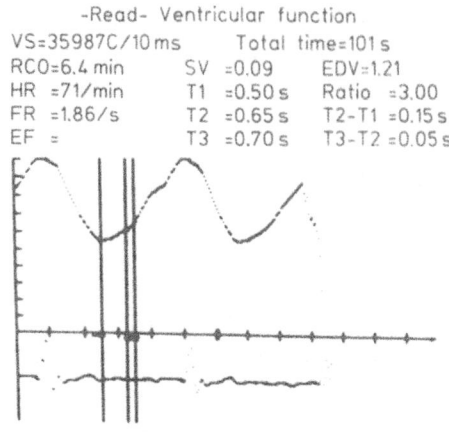

-Read- Ventricular function
VS=35987C/10 ms   Total time=101 s
RCO=6.4 min   SV =0.09   EDV=1.21
HR =71/min   T1 =0.50 s   Ratio =3.00
FR =1.86/s   T2 =0.65 s   T2-T1 =0.15 s
EF =   T3 =0.70 s   T3-T2 =0.05 s

Fig. 3. A radionuclide ventricular volume curve. The two cursors on the right-hand portion of the diastolic filling phase of the volume curve are separated by 60 ms. It is within this time frame that the most rapid change in counts, i.e., the peak filling rate, is measured. This is 1.86 *EDV/s* (end-diastolic volumes per second) in this patient. The single cursor is at end systole. The time between the single cursor and the mid-portion of the peak filling rate is the time to peak filling

Seven baseline variables (right and left ventricular ejection fraction, cardiac output, stroke volume, end-diastolic and end-systolic volumes, peak filling rate) were compared to maximal total oxygen consumption using multivariate and stepwise discriminate analysis. The single most important determinant of exercise performance in this study was peak filling rate; all other parameters appeared to play a lesser role.

Over the past 5 years there has been increasing recognition of the importance in congestive heart failure patients of diastolic dysfunction in the absence of systolic performance abnormalities. Over a 1-year period we were able to define a group of 58 patients presenting with heart failure and intact systolic function [25]. Within this subgroup, radionuclide peak filling rate was abnormal in 38%. An additional 24% of patients had borderline abnormalities in diastolic function. The most characteristic clinical correlates of diastolic dysfunction heart failure in these patients were the antecedent presence of hypertension and coronary artery disease, either alone or in combination. Of note, clinical phenomena were not helpful in distinguishing these patients from other more routine systolic dys-function heart failure patients. These results have been corroborated by other investigators [26,27]. To assess the relative frequency of this phenomenon, we evaluated patients referred to the noninvasive laboratoy with a clinical diagnosis of heart failure over a 3-month period. Forty-two percent of these patients were found to have intact systolic function [25]. Thus diastolic dysfunction is not an uncommon occurrence, and it must be thought of in the evaluation of indi-viduals presenting with heart failure and no apparent etiology, particularly in the elderly.

Those presenting with heart failure, diastolic dysfunction, and intact systolic performance do not necessarily have a benign outcome. This was initially demonstrated in individuals presenting with pulmonary edema in the course of myocardial infarction [28]. We have now followed our initial study group for an average of 7 years. In this group, a cardiovascular mortality of 46% and an additional cardiovascular morbidity of 29% were noted. Combined morbidity and mortality from cardiovascular causes was 75%. Thus, patients with congestive heart failure who have preserved systolic function but diastolic dysfunction do not have a comparatively favorable long-term prognosis. The risk of future cardiovascular events is substantial.

Therapy for this particular condition is not well defined. However, based upon experience in hypertrophic cardiomyopathy, it would seem reasonable to consider calcium channel-blocking agents as a therapeutic possibility [29]. We have recently completed a trial evaluating this possibility. The study involved 20 patients with heart failure who had intact left ventricular function as measured by ejection fraction, and abnormal diastolic filling as measured by peak filling rate. No patient had active coronary or valvular disease. Patients were treated in a double-blind crossover trial involving verapamil. Verapamil significantly improved an objective clinicoradiographic heart failure score, exercise capacity, and peak filling rate as compared to placebo. In contrast, there was no change in ejection fraction during this study. Thus, there are meaningful therapeutic options for individuals with diastolic abnormality and intact systolic performance. Radionuclide approaches allow definition of such patients. Whether application of therapy will result in improved survival remains to be defined.

Right Ventricular Ejection Fraction

Nuclear cardiology techniques have been employed for measurement of right ventricular ejection fraction for over a decade. Because of the complex geometry of this chamber, the use of count-based nongeometric techniques has been the key for obtaining this measurement [30]. Right ventricular ejection fraction is best measured by the first pass as opposed to the equilibrium technique. This arises from the fact that there is considerable overlap of right atrium and right ventricle that cannot be avoided using the equilibrium technique. The right atrial contamination will substantially alter right ventricular measurements [30]. Right ventricular ejection fraction was initially thought to be an important determinant of exercise performance in patients with congestive heart failure [31]. This has not been corroborated by subsequent studies [24,32]. Nevertheless, right ventricular ejection fraction provides important information concerning both the diffuse nature of ventricular involvement in heart failure and the presence of pulmonary hypertension. Because the right ventricle is afterload dependent, abnormal right ventricular ejection fraction can be used as a potential index of pulmonary hypertension. In the absence of intrinsic disease, abnormal right ventricular ejection fraction is clearly associated with pulmonary hypertension [33]. Right ventricular ejection fraction is of significant value in defining the extent of abnormality in specific subsets of patients with heart failure including those with significant pulmonary disease, congenital heart disease, or valvular disease. Using the gated first pass technique, right ventricular ejection fraction measurement can be easily combined with the widely used equilibrium radionuclide angiocardiogram.

Ambulatory Left Ventricular Function

Recently, a radionuclide technique has been developed for monitoring ventricular function in ambulatory patients [34]. This particular approach utilizes principles of equilibrium imaging. With the aid of a conventional scintillation camera, a miniaturized detector is placed over the left ventricular region of interest. Employing miniaturized electronics and a tape-recording system comparable to that used for Holter arrhythmia monitoring, ECG and nuclear data are recorded simultaneously for several hours during routine activity. Off-line analysis provides trended data of left ventricular ejection fraction, relative ventricular volumes, heart rate, and ECG ST segment changes. Ejection fraction measured in this manner has been correlated with conventional gamma camera measurements under conditions of rest and exercise [35]. In addition, the technique has been shown to be sensitive to immediate detection of ventricular dysfunction during coronary artery balloon occlusion in the course of coronary angioplasty. In a recent study involving patients following thrombolysis, ambulatory ventricular functional abnormalities were noted in individuals who did not manifest similar degrees of dysfunction during exercise radionuclide angiocardiography. Furthermore, abnormalities in ambulatory ventricular function were associated with poor clinical outcome and subsequent clinical events. Abnormalities detected during routine ambulatory activities were generally not associated with either chest pain or ECG changes. In addition, they did not occur in the presence of substantial increments in heart rate. These observations suggest that the ambulatory ventricular function approach may provide important insights into silent myocardial ischemia, and that the mechanism of such abnormalities may be based more upon alterations in myocardial oxygen supply than on demand. This new approach to ventricular function may offer new opportunities for the assessment of cardiac performance in man.

Summary

Nuclear cardiologic approaches to ventricular function clearly offer substantial opportunity for evaluating the heart failure patient under a variety of conditions. Parameters of global, regional, systolic, and diastolic performance may be measured. They give insight into etiology and prognosis as well as providing therapeutic algorithms in appropriate clinical situations. The next decade should continue to see further application of these approaches to patient categorization as well as in therapeutic and functional assessment.

References

1. Zaret BL, Berger HJ (1986) Nuclear cardiology. In: Hurst JW (ed) The heart. McGraw Hill, New York, pp 1809-1857
2. Multicenter postinfarction research group (1983) Risk stratification and survival after myocardial infarction. N Engl J Med 309:331-336
3. van der Wall EE, Res JCJ, van Eenige MJ, Verheugt FWA, Wijns W, Braat S, de Zwaan C, Reeme WJ, Vermeer F, Reber JHC, Simoons ML (1986) Effects of intracoronary thrombolysis on global left ventricular function assessed by an automated edge detection technique. J Nucl Med 27:478-484
4. Passamani E, Davis KB, Gillespie MJ, Killip T (1985) A randomized trial of coronary artery bypass surgery: survival of patients with a low ejection fraction. N Engl J Med 312:1665-1671
5. Ritchie JL, Hallstrom AP, Troubaugh CB et al. (1985) Out-of-hospital sudden coronary death: rest and exercise left ventricular function in survivors. Am J Cardiol 55:654-651
6. Franciosa JA (1987) Why patients with heart failure die: hemodynamic and functional determinants of survival. Circulation 75:IV-20-IV-27
7. Schwartz RG, McKenzie WB, Alexander J, Sager P, D'Souza A, Manatunga A, Schwartz PE, Berger HJ, Setaro J, Surkin L, Wackers FJ, Zaret BL (1987) Congestive heart failure and left ventricular dysfunction complicating doxorubicin therapy. Am J Med 82:1109-1118
8. Bristow MR, Mason JW, Billingham ME, Daniels JR (1981) Dose-effect and structure-function relationships in doxorubicin cardiomyopathy. Am Heart J 102:709-718
9. Minow RA, Benjamin RS, Lee ET, Gottlieb JA (1977) Adriamycin cardiomyopathy-risk factors. Cancer 39:1397-1402
10. Links JM, Becker LC, Shindledecker JG et al. (1982) Measurement of absolute ventricular volume from gated blood pool studies. Circulation 65:82-89
11. Kronenberg MW, Parrish MD, Jenkins DW Jr et al. (1985) Accuracy of radionuclide ventriculography for estimating left ventricular volume changes and end-systolic pressure-volume relationships. J Am Coll Cardiol 6:1064-1072
12. Borow KM, Neumann A, Wynne J (1982) Sensitivity of end-systolic pressure dimension end pressure-volume relations to the inotropic state in humans. Circulation 65:988-997
13. Mehmel HC, Stochins B, Ruffmann K, Olshauser K, Schuler G, Kubler W (1981) The linearity of the end-systolic pressure-volume relationship in man and its sensitivity for assessment of left ventricular function. Circulation 63:1216-1222
14. Breisblatt WM, Vita NA, Armuchastegui, Cohen LS, Zaret BL (1988) Usefulness of serial radionuclide monitoring during graded nitroglycerin infusion for unstable angina pectoris for determining left ventricular function and individualized therapeutic dose. Am J Cardiol 161:685-690
15. Pfeffer MA, Pfeffer JM (1987) Ventricular enlargement and reduced survival after myocardial infarction. Circulation 75:IV-93-IV-97
16. Duncan JS, Smeulders A, Lee F, Zaret BL (1988) Measurement of end diastolic shape deformity using bending energy. Computers in cardiology. IEEE Press, Washington DC
17. Meizlich JL, Berger HJ, Plankey M, Errico D, Levy W, Zaret BL (1984) Functional left ventricular aneurysm formation with acute myocardial infarction: incidence natural history and prognostic implications. N Engl J Med 311:1001-1006
18. Wackers FJ, Terrin ML, Kayden D, Knatterud G, Forman S, Braunwald E, Zaret BL (1989) Quantitative radionuclide assessment of regional ventricular function after thrombolytic therapy for acute myocardial infarction: results of Phase I TIMI trial. J Am Coll Cardiol 13:998-1005
19. Sheehan FH, Stewart DK, Dodge HT, Mitten S, Bolsen EL, Brown BG (1983) Variability in the measurement of regional wall motion from contract angiograms. Circulation 68:550-558
20. McKenzie W, Duncan J, Kayden D, Fetterman R, Green R, Sheehan F, Bolson E, Dodge H, Canner P, Wackers FJ, Zaret BL (1985) A new method for quantifying regional wall motion on radionuclide angiocardiography (abstract). Circulation 72:III-480
21. Duncan J (1984) Intelligent determination of left ventricular wall motion from multiple view nuclear medicine image sequences. In: Proceedings of the 1984 joint international symposium on medical images and icons (ISMII) Arlington Va, July 1984. IEEE Computer Society, Silver Springs, pp 265-269

22. McKenzie W, Duncan J, Greene R, Fetterman R, Kayden D, Wackers FJ, Zaret BL (1985) Hyperkinesis in myocardial infarction: quantificative assessment on multiple view equilibrium radionuclide angiocardiography (abstract). Circulation 72:111-481

22a. Maniawski PJ, Allan AH, Wackers FJ, Zaret BL (1990) A new non-geometric technique for simultaneous evaluation of regional function and myocardial perfusion from gated planar isonitrile images. (Submitted for publication)

23. Bonow RO, Bacharach SL, Green MV, Kent KM, Lipson LC, Leon MB, Epstein SE (1981) Impaired left ventricular diastolic filling in patients with coronary artery disease: assessment with radionuclide angiography. Circulation 64:315-323

24. Soufer R, Lindo C, Kanakis J, Gradman A, Zaret BL (1986) The relationship of baseline peak filling rate to exercise capacity in congestive heart failure (abstract). Circulation 74:II-138

25. Soufer R, Wohlgelernter D, Vita NA, Amuchestegui M, Sostman HD, Berger HJ, Zaret BL (1985) Intact systolic left ventricular function in clinical congestive heart failure. Am J Cardiol 55:1032-1036

26. Dougherty AH, Maccarelli GV, Gray EL, Hicks CH, Goldstein RA (1984) Congestive heart failure with normal systolic function. Am J Cardiol 54:778-782

27. Echeverria HH, Blisker MS, Myerburg RJ, Kessler KM (1983) Congestive heart failure: echocardiographic insights. Am J Med 75:750-755

28. Warnowicz MA, Parker H, Cheitlin MD (1983) Prognosis of patients with acute pulmonary edema and normal ejection fraction after acute myocardial infarction. Circulation 67:330-334

29. Bonow RO, Rosing DR, Bacharch SL, Green MV, Kent FM, Lipson LC, Maron BJ, Leon MB, Epstein SE (1981) Effects of verapamil on left ventricular systolic function and diastolic filling in patients with hypertrophic cardiomyopathy. Circulation 64:787-795

30. Berger HJ, Matthay RH, Loke J, Marshall RC, Gottschalk A, Zaret BL (1978) Assessment of cardiac performance with quantitative radionuclide angiocardiography: right ventricular ejection fraction with reference to findings in chronic obstructive pulmonary disease. Am J Cardiol 41:897-905

31. Baker BJ, Wilen MM, Boyd CM, Dinh H, Fronciosa JA (1984) Relation of right ventricular ejection fraction to exercise capacity in chronic left ventricular failure. Am J Cardiol 54:596-601

32. Zaret BL, Wackers FJ (1987) Measurement of right ventricular function. In: Gerson M (ed) Cardiac nuclear medicine. McGraw Hill, New York, pp 161-172

33. Brent BN, Mahler D, Matthay RA, Berger HJ, Zaret BL (1984) Noninvasive diagnosis of pulmonary hypertension in chronic obstructive pulmonary disease: right ventricular ejection fraction at rest. Am J Cardiol 53:1349-1353

34. Wilson RA, Sullivan PJ, Moore RH, Boucher CA, Hutter AM, Strauss HW (1983) An ambulatory ventricular function monitor: validation and preliminary clinical results. Am J Cardiol 52:601-606

35. Tamaki N, Yasuda T, Moore RH, Gill JB, Boucher CA, Hutter AM, Gold HK, Strauss HW (1988) Continuous monitoring of left ventricular function by an ambulatory radionuclide detector in patients with coronary artery disease. J Am Coll Cardol 12:669-679

New Method for the Assessment of Right Ventricular Systolic and Diastolic Function Using Digital Subtraction Right Ventriculography

F.P. Chappuis, P.A. Dorsaz, and W. Rutishauser

Introduction

Evaluation of the right ventricle with conventional methodologies is fraught with difficulty. The chamber has an unusual geometric shape, namely, that of a truncated pyramid, that does not conform readily to geometric analysis or modeling. Furthermore, the right ventricular wall is thin and heavily trabeculated, which makes outlining of the endocardial contour on contrast angiograms quite difficult, particularly at end-systole.

To obviate these difficulties, we developed a new approach based on densitometric analysis of digital subtraction right ventriculograms [1]. This method is based on the Lambert-Beer law which states that radiographic density is directly proportional to the amount of contrast medium traversed by the X-ray beam. If mixing of the contrast medium is homogeneous (and this is the case in the right ventricle following intravenous injection), the radiographic density is directly proportional to the volume occupied by the contrast medium. Using this technique, a time-volume curve of the right ventricle can be generated, which describes volume changes of the right ventricle throughout the cardiac cycle without any geometric assumption. Since digital subtraction right ventriculograms are acquired with high spatial and temporal resolution (as compared with radionuclide ventriculograms), this time-volume curve can be reconstructed without any mathematical fitting procedure. From this curve, quantitative parameters of systolic and diastolic right ventricular functions can be derived.

This study was undertaken to (a) assess systolic and diastolic right ventricular function using this new method at baseline and after nitroglycerin; and (b) to determine which systolic and diastolic parameters most sensitively reflected small nitroglycerin-induced changes in loading conditions.

Method

Patients

Eight patients with a normal right ventricle were studied. The right ventricle was considered normal if (a) the right ventricular pressure was normal; (b) there was no previous inferior myocardial infarction; and (c) there were no right ventricular wall motion abnormalities. Mean age ($\pm$SD) was 56 ($\pm$9) years. There were six men and two women. Six patients had coronary artery disease, one had Prinzmetall angina, and one had atypical chest pain.

Image Acquisition

Digital subtraction right ventriculography was performed by injecting 30 cc iopamidol (Iopamiro) at 20 cc/s in the femoral vein. Images were acquired directly in the digital format with a temporal and spatial resolution of 50 frames per second and 256 $\times$ 256 $\times$ 10 bits (Digitron, Siemens), respectively, with fixed kilovolts, milliamperes, and pulse width. The digital subtraction right ventriculogram was repeated with the same settings 3 min after 0.5 mg sublingual nitroglycerin.

Image Processing and Analysis

The cycle with peak opacification was chosen for analysis. End-diastole was assigned to the image corresponding to the ECG R-wave. Logarithmic transformation and mask mode subtraction were performed. Reregistration of the mask image was performed if necessary to correct for motion artifact. Care was taken to prevent over- and underflow. The subtracted digital images were then transferred to our imaging system (Vax 11–750 and Gould Denaza IP8500) for further analysis.

An end-diastolic region of interest was manually outlined around the right ventricle with a trackball. Background density was determined using a U-shaped region of interest drawn around the right ventricle at end-systole and calculating a mean pixel density for this region over three frames, beginning one frame before and ending one frame after end-systole. Right ventricular ejection fraction was determined from the background-corrected time-density curve (end-diastolic minus end-systolic divided by end-diastolic density). Peak ejection rate (PER; maximum negative first derivative), peak filling rate (PFR; maximum negative first derivative), and time to PER (TPER) and to PFR (TPFR) were also determined.

Right Ventricular Pressure

Right ventricular pressure was simultaneously recorded using a 7-F micromanometer (Millar). Systolic and end-diastolic pressures were measured.

Statistical Analysis

Differences between baseline and post-nitroglycerin measurements were analyzed with paired t tests. The level of statistical significance was defined at $p < 0.05$. Data are reported as means $\pm$ SEM.

Results

Hemodynamic Findings

After nitroglycerin, both systolic and end-diastolic right ventricular pressures decreased slightly, but significantly (from 28.7 ± 2.6 to 24.0 ± 3.3 mmHg and from 7.5 ± 1.5 to 5.3 ± 2.0 mmHg, respectively; both $p < 0.05$), indicating a decrease in preload and afterload (Fig. 1).

Systolic Function

Following nitroglycerin, right ventricular ejection fraction increased slightly, but significantly, while PER and TPER remained unchanged (Table 1; Fig. 2).

Diastolic Function

Following nitroglycerin, PFR decreased significantly, whereas TPFR did not change significantly (Table 1; Fig. 3).

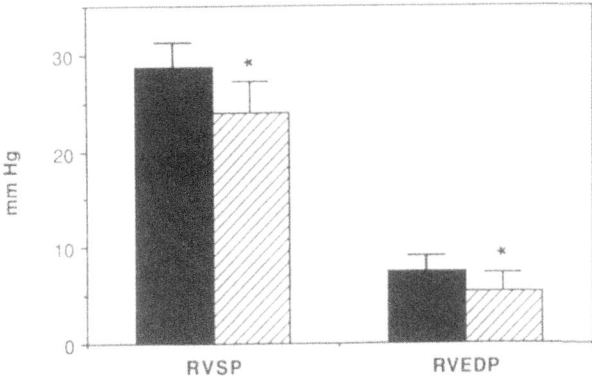

Fig. 1. After nitroglycerin there is a slight, but significant decrease in both systolic and end-diastolic right ventricular pressure. *Shaded columns*, baseline; *hatched columns*, after nitroglycerin; *asterisk*, $p < 0.01$

Table 1. Parameters of systolic and diastolic right ventricular function at baseline and after nitroglycerin

	Baseline	After nitroglycerin
Ejection fraction (%)	44.0 ± 3.3	46.4 ± 2.6[a]
Peak ejection rate (EDV/s)	2.6 ± 0.6	2.5 ± 0.4
Time to peak ejection rate (ms)	138 ± 31	138 ± 10
Peak filling rate (PFR; EDV/s)	2.2 ± 0.2	1.8 ± 0.2[a]
Time to peak filling rate (ms)	162 ± 10	155 ± 7

[a]$p < 0.05$.
EDV, end-diastolic volume; *PFR*, peak filling rate. Mean ± SEM.

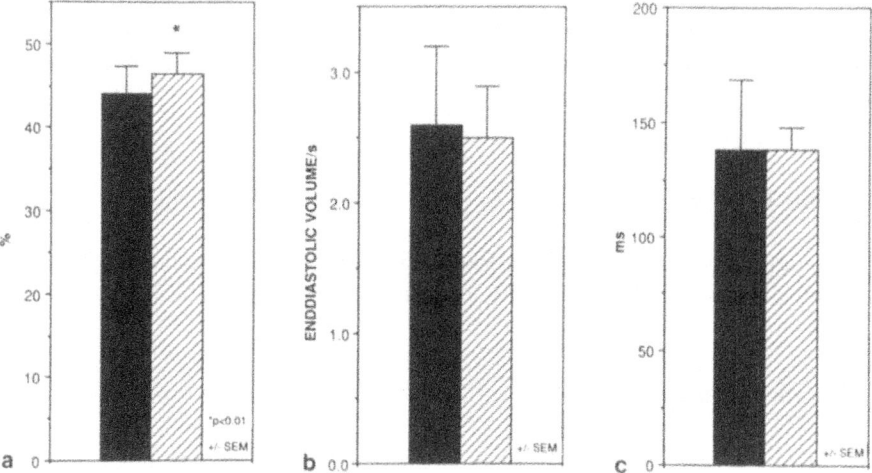

Fig. 2a-c. Systolic right ventricular function; **a** RV ejection fraction; **b** RV peak ejection rate; **c** time to peak ejection. After nitroglycerin there is a slight increase in right ventricular ejection fraction, but no change in PER or TPER. *Shaded columns*, baseline; *hatched columns* after nitroglycerin; *asterisk*, $p < 0.01$

Discussion

Digital Subtraction Right Ventriculography

We have developed a new method based on densitometric analysis of digital subtraction angiography. This new approach has previously been used for the assessment of global and regional left ventricular function both in humans and animals [2,3]. We have now extended this technique to the assessment of right ventricular systolic and diastolic function. Using this method, several parameters of systolic and diastolic function can be quantified. Among these parameters, right ventricular ejection fraction and PFR appeared most sensitive in reflecting

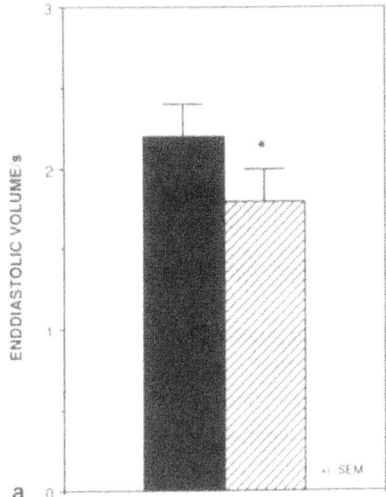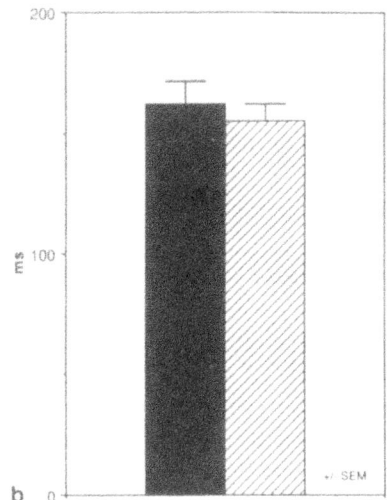

Fig. 3a,b. Diastolic right ventricular function; **a** RV peak filling rate; **b** time to peak filling rate. After nitroglycerin there is a decrease in PFR, but no change in TPFR. *Shaded columns,* baseline; *hatched columns,* after nitroglycerin; *asterisk,* $p < 0.01$

small, nitroglycerin-induced changes in loading conditions. In contrast, PER, TPER, and TPFR were unaffected by the discrete changes in loading conditions.

Following nitroglycerin, ejection fraction increased slightly, while PFR decreased. Nitroglycerin decreased both preload and afterload slightly, but significantly. A decrease in preload tends to decrease ejection fraction, while a decrease in afterload will increase it. The net result of these two opposing effects was a small increase in ejection fraction. The decreased preload alone probably accounts for the reduction in PFR.

Detrano et al. [4] employed a method similar to ours for the determination of right ventricular ejection fraction. However, other parameters of systolic and diastolic function were not determined. Similar time-volume curves can be obtained by radionuclide ventriculography. However, the suboptimal spatial and temporal resolution of this method limits its usefulness. High resolution is particularly important for the assessment of peak ejection and filling rate since the first derivative augments the noise level.

Advantages

This technique has several advantages. First, it provides three-dimensional assessment of right ventricular function without any geometric assumption. Second, it not only provides isolated measurements of end-diastolic and end-systolic volumes, but also a continuous time-volume curve reflecting right volume changes throughout the cardiac cycle. Third, the digital subtraction right ventriculogram is obtained by intravenous injection and does not require heart catheterization. Finally, it does not require delineation of the end-systolic contour; this may be of value because the right ventricular wall is heavily trabeculated, particularly at end-systole. Also, operator interaction is reduced, making the technique faster and more reproducible than conventional geometric methods.

Limitations

Several limitations must also be addressed. First, motion artifacts may degrade the quality of digital subtraction images. However, this can be at least partly corrected by mask reregistration. Second, the relation between the amount of contrast medium traversed by the X-ray beam and the digital gray scale level may be nonlinear because of beam hardening, X-ray scatter, and veiling glare. These potential problems, however, contribute little to the errors in assessing density changes. Lastly, background correction may affect the accuracy of the method. However, most of the bone and soft tissue was subtracted using a preinjection mask. In addition, the analyzed cycle was chosen at peak opacification, before significant opacification of the pulmonary vasculature has taken place.

Conclusion

This new method allows (a) to assess volume changes of the RV during the entire cardiac cycle, with high spatial and temporal resolution, and without any geometric assumption; and (b) to determine systolic and diastolic parameters of RV function. Among these parameters, PFR and EF appear most sensitive to nitroglycerin-induced decrease in preload and afterload.

References

1. Mancini GBJ, Higgins CB (1985) Digital subtraction angiography: a review of cardiac application. Prog Cardiovasc Dis 28:111–131
2. Chappuis F, Widmann T, Nicod P, Peterson KL (1988) Densitometric regional ejection fraction: a new three-dimensional index of regional left ventricular function. Comparison with geometric methods. J Am Coll Cardiol 11:72–82
3. Chappuis F, Widmann T, Guth B, Nicod P, Peterson KL (1988) Quantitative assessment of regional left ventricular function by densitometric analysis of intravenous digital subtraction ventriculograms. Correlation with myocardial systolic shortening in dogs. Circulation 77:457–467
4. Detrano R, MacIntyre W, Salcedo EE, O'Donnell J, Underwood DA, Simpfendorfer C, Go RT, Butters RK, Withrow S (1985) Videodensitometric ejection fraction from intravenous digital subtraction right ventriculograms: correlation with first pass radionuclide ejection fraction. J Am Coll Cardiol 5:1377–1383

Heart Failure in Acute Ischemic Syndromes and Acute Myocardial Infarction

Left Ventricular Systolic and Diastolic Function Immediately After Acute Coronary Artery Occlusion

M.E. Bertrand, J.M. Lablanche, J.L. Fourrier, A. Gommeaux, and I. Mirsky

Introduction

The acute changes in left ventricular (LV) function after coronary artery ligation have mostly been studied in animals [1-6], where differences in coronary and collateral circulation [7] may influence the results.

The detection of ischemia-induced wall motion changes in humans has until recently been limited to observations recorded after atrial pacing [8-10], exercise [11], or during the early stage of acute myocardial infarction [12-14]. Percutaneous transluminal coronary angioplasty offers the opportunity to study sequential changes of LV function during the transient occlusion of the vessel. Several reports have described modifications of myocardial relaxation [15], coronary blood flow [16,17], and acute wall motion changes during coronary angioplasty [18,19]. However, few studies have included the simultaneous recording of LV pressure and LV cineangiograms. Abnormalities of relaxation and segmental wall motion [20], the time course of changes during the transient interruption of coronary flow by balloon occlusion [21], and the effect of acute occlusion on left ventricular chamber stiffness [22] have recently been reported.

The aim of this study was to examine the possible changes in LV diastolic and systolic function induced by coronary balloon occlusion in patients with single left anterior descending coronary artery disease without angiographic evidence of collateral circulation. If dysfunction occurs, is LV function restored to normal levels following coronary angioplasty?

Methods

Patients

This study included 16 patients (15 males and one female) who underwent percutaneous transluminal coronary angioplasty of a proximal left anterior descending coronary artery narrowing. All patients experienced angina pain on effort and had no history of a previous myocardial infarction. All had single significant ($>75\%$) vessel disease and normal left ventricular segmental wall motion. The diagnostic angiography showed no collateral circulation filling the distal left anterior descending artery.

B.S. Lewis, A. Kimchi (Eds.)
Heart Failure Mechanisms and Management
© Springer-Verlag Berlin Heidelberg 1991

Informed consent was given by all patients, and the day before the procedure, the patients received nifedipine 30 mg and aspirin 1 g. No drugs were given on the day of the procedure except heparin IV (10 000 IU i.v.).

Study Protocol

An 8F pigtail Millar micromanometer was introduced into the left ventricle from the left femoral route. The guiding catheter for the angioplasty was introduced from a right femoral approach. LV and aortic pressures were simultaneously recorded. A first LV cineangiogram was performed in the 30° RAO projection and was obtained by injection of 0.5 ml/kg of sodium and meglumine amidotrizoate (Radioselectan). LV pressures and a frame-marker signal were recorded during cineangiography. Fifteen minutes later, the narrowing of the left anterior descending artery was dilated with a 3-mm or 3.5-mm balloon. LV and aortic pressures were recorded and a second LV cineangiogram was performed during the first coronary balloon inflation. To examine time-related abnormalities, patients were divided into two groups. Data were collected at 30 s after coronary occlusion in eight patients (group A). In a second group, balloon inflation was continued for 50 s, and LV cineangiography and pressure measurements were obtained at that time (Group B). All patients had ST segment elevation during the coronary occlusion and all had successful coronary angioplasty. In group B patients, a third LV cineangiogram was performed, and LV and aortic pressures were recorded 15 min after completion of the procedure.

Data Analysis

Pressures were measured with a computer system (Syscomoran). Frame-by-frame left ventricular volumes and corresponding pressures were obtained simultaneously from early to end diastole. LV contours were detected and volumes calculated according to the area-length method [23]. Segmental wall motion was obtained by the radial method [24] using a center located at 69% of a line joining the upper edge of the aorta to the left ventricular apex in end-systole. Nine radii were obtained in end-diastole (ED) and end-systole (ES), and for each, the segmental wall shortening (SWS) was calculated as $SWS = 100. (ED - ES)/ED$. Segments 1–4 were related to the anterior wall. Segments 6–9 corresponded to the inferior wall and segment 5 was related to the apex.

Assessment of Chamber and Myocardial Stiffness Constants

Since chamber stiffness (dP/dV) depends on several factors including chamber size (V), myocardial stiffness (E), cavity volume/wall volume ratio (V/Vw), and external constraints, appropriate normalizations must be employed if comparisons between ventricles are to be made.

A rationale is provided in Appendix A that normalization to wall volume Vw yields an index of chamber stiffness, whereas normalization to cavity volume V provides an index of myocardial stiffness.

Specifically, by curve-fitting the diastolic pressure-volume points from minimal pressure to end-diastole in the

forms $P = A \, e^{\alpha(V/Vw)}; P = B \, V^{\beta}$; we obtain

$$dP/(dV/Vw) = \alpha A \, e^{\alpha(V/Vw)} = \alpha P$$

and $dP/(dV/V) = \beta B \, V^{\beta} = \beta P.$

Therefore, α (the slope of the $dP/(dV/Vw)$ vs. P relation) and β (the slope of the $dP/(dV/V)$ vs. P relation) may be employed as indices of chamber and myocardial stiffness respectively.

In Appendix B, alternative methods are presented for the quantitation of global myocardial stiffness (E) and regional myocardial stiffness (Er) with the results

$$E = K \, Dm \, (d \, \sigma/d \, Dm) = k \, \sigma$$

and $Er = - dP/(dh/h) = \delta P$

where K is a geometric factor, h is the LV wall thickness, and κ, β, δ are indices of myocardial stiffness. It should be emphasized here that comparisons of chamber stiffness must be made at common levels of pressure, and myocardial stiffness must be compared at common stress levels.

Assessment of Time Constants of Relaxation

The LV pressure tracings were digitized from the point of peak negative dP/dt to the time at which pressure decreased to 5 mmHg above end-diastolic pressure. The pressure-time data (P-t) were then curve-fitted in the

forms $P = C \, e^{-1/\tau w}; P = a + b \, e^{-\gamma t}$

where τ_w is the time constant as evaluated by the Weiss method [25], and $\tau_M = (1/\gamma) \log [e \, b/(a + b - a \, e)]$ is the time constant evaluated on the basis of a three-constant curve-fit ([26] and Appendix C).

Statistical Analysis

All data were expressed as mean $\pm$ standard deviation. Paired t tests were employed for patients in group A who were studied before and after 30 s of coronary balloon occlusion. An analysis of variance was conducted in group B patients where three sequential measurements were made and the results obtained by the Bonferroni correction [27].

Results

Left Ventricular Pressures

LV end-diastolic pressures (Tables 1, 2) were significantly increased ($p < .01$) at 30 s of occlusion (group A) and in patients studied at 50 s of occlusion (group B). The magnitudes of these increases were similar in both groups. However, little or no change was observed in peak LV pressures.

Segmental Wall Motion

The visual analysis of the LV cineangiogram clearly demonstrated a marked dyskinesia of the anterior and apical wall in all cases. Figure 1 shows the important modifications occurring during total occlusion of the left anterior descending coronary artery: occlusion for only 30 s resulted in a marked decrease of the anterior and anteroapical wall shortening with the appearance of a systolic outward displacement.

Table 1. Hemodynamic data in group A patients

Patient		LVEDP (mmHg)	LVEDVI (ml/m²)	LVESVI (ml/m²)	SVI (ml/m²)	EF (%)	Vw (ml)
1	Pre	21	83	24	58	70	211
	30 s	27	91	47	44	48	
2	Pre	19	100	25	75	75	162
	30 s	34	94	56	38	40	
3	Pre	25	93	24	69	74	287
	30 s	32	99	56	33	33	
4	Pre	18	111	32	79	71	189
	30 s	32	100	49	51	51	
5	Pre	34	93	23	70	75	173
	30 s	46	116	78	38	32	
6	Pre	14	140	34	106	76	239
	30 s	20	115	42	73	63	
7	Pre	6	72	13	58	81	111
	30 s	34	93	50	43	45	
8	Pre	7	98	33	65	66	243
	30 s	44	112	57	55	49	
Mean ± SD							
	Pre	18 ± 9	98 ± 20	26 ± 7	72 ± 15	73 ± 4	202 ± 55
	30 s	33 ± 8[a]	102 ± 10	54 ± 11[b]	46 ± 12[b]	45 ± 10[b]	

[a] $p < 0.01$.
[b] $p < 0.001$.
EF, ejection fraction; *LVEDP*, left ventricular end-diastolic pressure; *LVEDVI*, left ventricular end-diastolic volume index; *LVESVI*, left ventricular end-systolic volume index; *SVI*, stroke index; *Vw*, left ventricular wall volume.

Table 2. Hemodynamic data in group B patients

Patient		LVEDP (mmHg)	LVEDVI (ml/m²)	LVESVI (ml/m²)	SVI (ml/m²)	EF (%)	Vw (ml)
1	Pre	18	98	26	72	73	234
	50 s	22	105	55	50	48	
	Post	19	111	20	91	82	
2	Pre	33	90	37	53	58	184
	50 s	43	103	67	36	34	
	Post	27	93	37	56	60	
3	Pre	15	82	14	68	82	170
	50 s	22	88	39	48	55	
	Post	19	85	13	72	84	
4	Pre	32	130	47	83	63	278
	50 s	41	143	97	46	31	
	Post	24	130	63	67	51	
5	Pre	24	92	28	64	68	209
	50 s	31	103	48	55	52	
	Post	26	115	27	88	76	
6[a]	Pre	18	92	20	70	77	205
	50 s	36	102	50	52	50	
	Post	19	88	22	66	74	
7	Pre	20	100	25	75	75	204
	50 s	36	109	46	63	57	
	Post	28	98	18	80	81	
8[a]	Pre	14	90	28	62	69	200
	50 s	39	90	53	37	41	
	Post	8	79	23	56	71	
Mean ± SD							
	Pre	22 ± 7	97 ± 14	28 ± 10	68 ± 9	70 ± 7	211 ± 33
	50 s	34 ± 7[b]	105 ± 16	56 ± 18[c]	48 ± 9[c]	46 ± 9[c]	
	Post	21 ± 6	99 ± 17	29 ± 15	72 ± 13	72 ± 11	

[a] Omitted from the analysis.
[b] $p < 0.01$ (pre vs. 50 s).
[c] $p < 0.001$ (pre vs. 50 s).
Abbreviations as in Table 1.

Left Ventricular Volumes and Ejection Fraction

Complete occlusion of the left anterior descending coronary artery resulted in a significant increase ($p < .001$) in end-systolic volume index (ESVI) from 26 ± 7 to 54 ± 11 ml/m² at 30 s in group A (Table 1) and from 28 ± 10 to 56 ± 18 ml/m² in group B (Table 2). LV end-diastolic volume index (EDVI) was slightly but insignificantly increased at 30 s and 50 s of occlusion. In both groups, a dramatic and significant decrease of stroke index and ejection fraction was noted ($p < .001$). Thus occlusion of the left anterior descending coronary artery for 30–50 s resulted in a marked depression of LV systolic function.

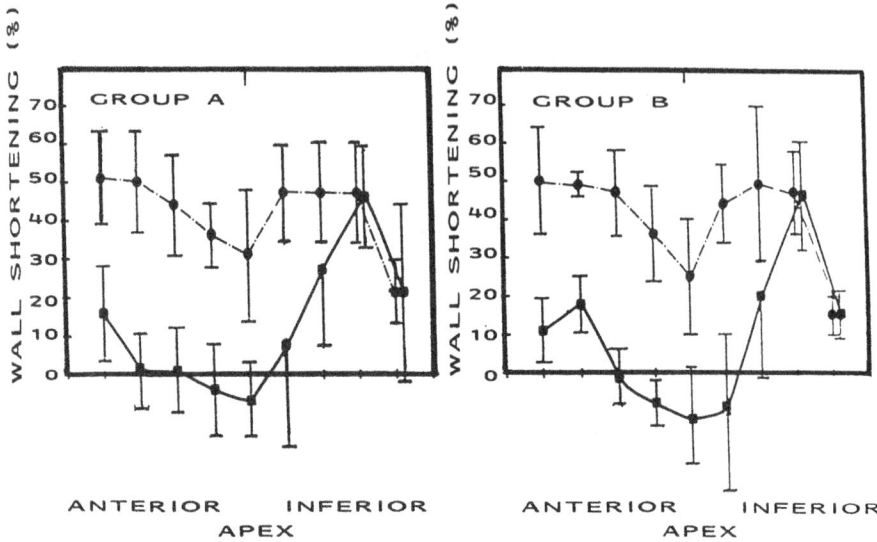

Fig. 1. Radial wall motion in group A and in group B. *Dashed lines*, before occlusion; *solid lines*, during coronary occlusion

Time Constants of Relaxation (τ_W, τ_M)

The changes in time constants of relaxation are shown in Tables 3 and 4. The occlusion of the left anterior descending coronary artery for 30 s resulted in important and significant increases in τ_W from 48.5 $\pm$ 9.4 to 63.7 $\pm$ 13.3 ($p <$ .01) and in τ_M from 48.9 $\pm$ 7.6 to 62.0 $\pm$ 11.2 ($p <$ .025). In patients studied 50 s after the onset of occlusion, significant increases were also observed. The time constant τ_W increased from 43.3 $\pm$ 5.4 to 57.7 $\pm$ 10.4 ($p <$ .005) and τ_M increased from 46.1 $\pm$ 7.5 to 59.2 $\pm$ 13.2 ($p <$ .03). Both time constants returned to preocclusion levels 15 min after the procedure.

Chamber Stiffness Constant (α)

Since chamber stiffness must be compared at common levels of pressure, two patients from each group were excluded from the statistical analyses. No significant alterations were observed in the chamber stiffness constant following coronary occlusion at 30 and 50 s although there was a tendency for an increase in the group A patients. In group A, the constant α increased from 2.08 $\pm$ 1.00 to 2.87 $\pm$ 2.26 after 30 s and in group B after 50 s there was no change (pre: 2.28 $\pm$ 1.00; 50 s: 1.94 $\pm$ 0.66). Fifteen minutes after the procedure in group B patients, α remained within the preocclusion levels (2.19 $\pm$ 0.96).

Table 3. Diastolic function parameters in group A patients

Patient		Myocardial stiffness constants			Chamber stiffness constant	Time constants of relaxation (ms)	
		κ	δ	β	α	τ_W	τ_M
1	Pre	8.46	2.83	1.33	2.19	46.1	46.9
	30 s	6.91	5.09	2.08	2.48	70.0	68.8
2	Pre	4.88	4.43	1.92	2.07	52.9	53.4
	30 s	4.90	4.68	1.99	1.37	65.1	64.7
3	Pre	7.18	5.30	1.99	3.96	36.9	37.5
	30 s	6.75	5.55	2.30	4.02	57.4	56.7
4	Pre	4.93	2.36	1.16	1.18	52.5	50.5
	30 s	4.51	3.76	1.70	1.57	66.0	63.6
5	Pre	5.41	2.51	1.14	1.52	62.5	59.9
	30 s	3.27	2.00	0.95	0.87	81.8	75.2
6	Pre	4.66	2.56	1.10	1.54	40.3	45.4
	30 s	12.22	10.63	4.44	6.88	42.0	42.7
7[a]	Pre	6.05	2.62	3.06	1.62	43.6	49.0
	30 s	6.17	3.43	2.05	1.73	92.7	88.8
8[a]	Pre	–	–	–	–		–
	30 s	–	–	–	–	–	–
Mean ± SD							
	Pre	5.92	3.33	1.44	2.08	48.5	48.9
		± 1.55	± 1.23	± 0.41	± 1.00	± 9.4	± 7.6
	30 s	6.43	5.29	2.24	2.87	63.7[b]	62.0[c]
		± 3.16	± 2.90	± 1.17	± 2.26	± 13.3	± 11.2

[a] Omitted from analysis.
[b] $p < .01$.
[c] $p < .025$.
β, δ, κ, myocardial stiffness constants obtained from pressure-volume, pressure-thickness, and stress-diameter relationships respectively; α, chamber stiffness constant obtained from pressure – V/Vw relation; τ_W, τ_M, time constants of relaxation obtained from two- and three-constant curve-fits, respectively.

Myocardial Stiffness Constants (κ, β, δ)

The myocardial stiffness constants were evaluated by three different methods, and each yielded the same qualitative results for each group. Again there were no significant alterations following coronary occlusion for 30 and 50 s; however, the increases were more pronounced in group A (30 s) than in group B (50 s). Preocclusion levels were maintained 15 min following the procedure. The values for these constants are shown in Table 5.

M.E. Bertrand et al.

Table 4. Diastolic function parameters for group B patients

Patient		Myocardial stiffness constants			Chamber stiffness constant	Time constants of relaxation (ms)	
		κ	δ	β	α	τ_W	τ_M
1	Pre	5.37	2.91	1.21	1.89	36.2	36.0
	50 s	5.24	4.27	1.76	2.71	47.4	47.2
	Post	4.57	3.33	1.49	1.75	34.5	35.0
2	Pre	4.70	3.52	1.67	2.13	41.1	44.0
	50 s	2.18	1.45	0.72	0.76	57.6	55.6
	Post	4.96	4.10	1.69	2.45	38.3	39.7
3	Pre	7.49	4.63	1.88	3.09	39.9	41.4
	50 s	5.62	4.21	1.76	2.40	42.5	40.3
	Post	4.72	3.47	2.26	2.60	40.3	41.0
4	Pre	4.60	2.72	1.16	1.73	46.4	52.7
	50 s	5.75	3.76	1.77	2.13	60.4	57.1
	Post	6.98	6.94	2.99	3.78	49.8	50.0
5	Pre	4.26	3.59	1.50	2.19	39.2	39.3
	50 s	6.28	4.60	1.82	2.32	57.6	77.0
	Post	3.80	1.77	0.82	1.19	41.6	39.7
6[a]	Pre	3.63	3.18	1.26	1.92	46.1	46.2
	50 s	8.59	5.85	2.69	3.36	54.7	54.2
	Post	–	–	–	–	39.9	42.0
7	Pre	2.46	1.35	0.52	0.92	53.2	58.3
	50 s	3.83	2.53	1.05	1.52	76.9	77.3
	Post	2.35	1.55	0.59	1.00	54.1	58.5
8	Pre	6.36	6.60	2.70	4.02	45.4	50.9
	50 s	4.42	2.86	1.28	1.77	64.4	65.1
	Post	3.82	3.67	1.30	2.54	41.1	44.1
Mean ± SD							
	Pre	5.03	3.62	1.52	2.28	43.4	46.1
		± 1.60	± 1.65	±0.68	± 1.00	± 5.4	± 7.5
	50 s	4.76	3.38	1.45	1.94	57.7[b]	59.2[c]
		± 1.41	± 1.14	± 0.44	± 0.66	± 10.5	± 13.2
	Post	4.46	3.55	1.59	2.19	42.5	43.8
		± 1.41	± 1.78	± 0.83	±0.96	± 6.4	± 7.3

[a] Omitted from statistical analysis of chamber and myocardial stiffness constant.
[b] $p < .005$ (pre vs. 50 s)
[c] $p < .03$ (pre vs. 50 s).

Table 5. Values for myocardial stiffness constants

		κ	δ	β
Group A				
	Pre	5.92 ± 1.55	3.33 ± 1.23	1.44 ± 0.41
	30 s	6.43 ± 3.16	5.29 ± 2.90	2.24 ± 1.17
Group B				
	Pre	5.03 ± 1.60	3.62 ± 1.65	1.52 ± 0.68
	50 s	4.76 ± 1.41	3.38 ± 1.14	1.45 ± 0.44
	Post	4.46 ± 1.41	3.55 ± 1.78	1.59 ± 0.83

Discussion

LV systolic and diastolic function were markedly affected shortly after occlusion of the left anterior descending coronary artery. Stroke volume and ejection fraction decreased, LV end-diastolic pressure increased, and LV relaxation was delayed. There was a tendency for both chamber and myocardial stiffness to increase indicating a reduction in compliance; however, these changes were not statistically significant, and the changes appeared to be more pronounced in the group A patients. Generally, the results were similar to those in animal studies [1-4]; however, in coronary artery occlusion experiments, the pressure-segment length relationship has repeatedly been shown to move to the right. The present study involved patients with single vessel disease and significant narrowing of the proximal left anterior descending artery. Thus, interruption of coronary flow induced by transient balloon inflation during percutaneous transluminal coronary angioplasty is a situation that completely mimics the experimental coronary artery ligation performed during animal studies.

The results of the present study agree in part with those described by Serruys et al. [21] and Wijns et al. [22], namely (a) there were upward shifts in the diastolic pressure-volume relations immediately following the angioplasty procedure; and (b) systolic function and the time constants of relaxation returned to near preocclusion levels 12-15 min after completion of the procedure. On the other hand, these investigators [22] showed that abnormalities in the chamber stiffness persisted 12 min after the procedure, a result not observed in the present study. In previous studies [22], pressure and angiographic measurements were obtained 20 s during the second dilation and 50 s during the fourth dilation. The interval between two sequential angiograms was at least 10 min, and one cannot exclude the possible influence of contrast medium in these consecutive examinations. Moreover, immediate collateral circulation may occur after a first coronary occlusion. In the present study, all measurements at 30 and 50 s were done during the first balloon inflation. Another possible explanation for the differences may reside in the different methods employed for the assessment of chamber stiffness. Global stiffness was analyzed in this study and not regional chamber stiffness. However, earlier studies [22] considered parameters of chamber stiffness which were size dependent, and comparisons were not always conducted over common pressure ranges.

After 30 or 50 s of coronary occlusion, LV systolic function was depressed with a marked decrease of the ejection fraction due to an increase in end-systolic volume. This is clearly related to the large ischemic area as demonstrated by the depression of wall motion shortening which affected specifically the anterior and apical segments. In both groups, a systolic outward displacement of the ischemic segment was observed. Serruys et al. [21] showed that the moment of maximal wall displacement for the anterior wall shifted from end-systole to early diastole. This late systolic outward displacement of the ischemic segment is probably passive and could be due to the increased inward displacement of the non-ischemic segments. This is similar to the results obtained by Tyberg et al. [28] who described the relationship between transient asynergy, myocardial ischemia, and alteration in the course of relaxation, and observed that prolongation of this parameter was seen only upon reoxygenation. In humans, prolongation of the time constant of the early relaxation phase is the earliest hemodynamic marker of myocardial ischemia. In both series of patients, marked increases were observed in the time constants of relaxation τ_W, τ_M. By careful analysis of the LV cineangiogram, Serruys et al. [21] showed that these changes accompanied a biphasic wall displacement of the ischemic area after aortic valve closure. The deformation occurring in the ascending limb of the negative dP/dt tracing occurred simultaneously with the beginning of the second wave of inward displacement. After 50 s of occlusion (group B), the deformation of peak negative dP/dt generally disappeared.

Although three approaches were employed here for the assessment of myocardial stiffness, these indices also have their limitations. The stiffness constants κ and β describe global stiffness and may not be valid in cases of segmental disease as considered in the present study. On the other hand, the radial stiffness constant δ does more closely represent a regional stiffness parameter. The possibility exists that pericardial pressure may have been elevated during these procedures and was not accounted for in these or the earlier studies [21,22]. Future studies should include measurements of right atrial pressures [29] enabling one to consider these pericardial effects in a semiquantitative manner.

The results of the present studies and those of Serruys et al. [21,22] have important clinical implications since changes in LV systolic and diastolic function were observed as early as 30 or 50 s after coronary occlusion. Generally, diastolic parameters returned to preocclusion values; however, there may be a subset of patients in whom dysfunction persists after completion of the angioplasty procedure. More sophisticated methods for analyzing chamber and myocardial stiffness need to be developed along the lines described by Pasipoularides et al. [30].

Appendix A

Rationale for the Development of Simple Indices of Chamber and Myocardial Stiffness

Employing the theory of elasticity and assuming a spherical geometry for the left ventricle [31], chamber stiffness may be expressed in the form

$$dP/dV = [(4/9) Es - P(V/Vw)]/V (1 + V/Vw)$$

where Es = myocardial stiffness, Vw = LV wall volume, P = LV diastolic cavity pressure, and V = LV cavity volume.

Normalizing chamber stiffness to Vw, we obtain

$$dP/(dV/Vw) = [(4/9) Es - P (V/Vw)]/(1 + V/Vw) (V/Vw).$$

This parameter is predominantly a function of pressure and the V/Vw ratio and suggests that the $dP/(dV/Vw)$ vs. P relation may provide an appropriate index for chamber stiffness.

Normalizing chamber stiffness to the volume V yields

$$dP/(dV/V) = [(4/9) Es - P(V/Vw)]/(1 + V/Vw).$$

This parameter is dominated by myocardial stiffness Es, and the $dP/(dV/V)$ vs. P relation may yield an index of myocardial stiffness.

In particular, curve-fitting the pressure-volume data in the forms

$P = A e^{\alpha(V/Vw)}; P = B V^\beta$, we obtain
$dP/(dV/Vw) = \alpha A e^{\alpha(V/Vw)} = \alpha P$ and
$dP/(dV/V) = \beta B V^\beta = \beta P.$

Thus α and β may be employed as indices of chamber and myocardial stiffness respectively.

Appendix B

Alternative Evaluation of Myocardial Stiffness Constants

Two additional methods for assessing myocardial stiffness are outlined here:

Method 1: Incremental Modulus — Stress Relation

From earlier studies [32], the incremental modulus is given by

$Einc = (3/2) Dm (d\sigma/d Dm)/(2 + Dm^2/Lm^2)ave$
where $\sigma = \sigma_o - \tau_r$
$= P[1 + DL/H(L + D + 2H)]$

is the difference in circumferential and radial global average stress.

The quantities D and L are, respectively, the short and long axes of an ellipsoid of revolution, which is the assumed geometry for the left ventricle.

If the stress — diameter $(\sigma - Dm)$ data are curve-fit in the form $\sigma = A_d Dm^c$ one obtains

$Einc = (3/2) c Dm (A_d Dm^{c-1})/(2 + Dm^2/Lm^2)ave$
$= (3/2) c (A_d Dm^c)/(2 + Dm^2/Lm^2)ave$
$= K c (A_d Dm^c) = Kc \sigma = \kappa \sigma$
where $\kappa = (3/2) c/(2 + Dm^2/Lm^2)ave.$

The parameter κ is the slope of the stiffness vs. stress relation and represents an index of circumferential myocardial stiffness.

This method has been employed with moderate success in studies on pacing-induced angina in humans [33]. Radial myocardial stiffness Er is defined by $Er = -h \, (dP/dh)$ where P is the diastolic LV pressure, and h is LV wall thickness. Curve-fitting the pressure-thickness data $(P - h)$ in the form $P = A_h \, h^{-\delta}$ one obtains $Er = -h \, (-\delta \, A_h \, h^{-\delta-1}) = (A_h \, h^{-\delta}) \, \delta = \delta \, P$. Hence δ (the slope of the radial stiffness-pressure relation) may be employed as an index of radial myocardial stiffness.

Appendix C

Evaluation of the Time Constant (τ_M)

The pressure-time data from peak negative dP/dt to the time at which pressure decreased to 5 mmHg above end-diastolic pressure were curved-fitted in the form

$$P = a + b \, e^{-\gamma t} \qquad\qquad [1]$$

where a, b, and γ are regression coefficients.

At time $t = 0$ (time of peak negative dP/dt), the pressure P_o is given by

$$P_o = a + b \qquad\qquad [2]$$

Now τ_M is defined as the time required for P_o to be reduced by the factor $1/e$ where e is the base of the natural logarithm. Hence τ_M is represented by the relation

$$
\begin{aligned}
P_o/e &= a + b \, e^{-\gamma \tau_M} && \text{(using Eq. 1)}\\
&= (a + b)/e && \text{(employing Eq. 2)}\\
\text{i.e., } e^{-\gamma \tau_M} &= [(a + b)/e - a]/b\\
&= (a + b - ae)/eb
\end{aligned}
$$

Taking the logarithm of both sides, this yields

$$
\begin{aligned}
-\gamma \tau_M &= \log [(a + b - ae)/eb]\\
\text{or } \tau_M &= (1/\gamma) \log [eb/(a + b - ae)]
\end{aligned}
$$

which is the desired result.

References

1. Theroux P, Ross J Jr, Franklin D, Kemper WS, Sasayama S (1976) Regional myocardial function in the conscious dog during acute coronary occlusion and response to morphine, propranolol, nitroglycerine and lidocaine. Circulation 53:302-314
2. Heyndrickx GR, Millard RW, Mc Ritchie RJ, Maroko PR, Vatner SF (1975) Regional myocardial function and electrophysiological alterations after brief coronary artery occlusion in conscious dogs. J Clin Invest 56:978-986
3. Pagani M, Vatner SF, Baig H, Braunwald E (1978) Adjustments to brief periods of ischemia and reperfusion in the conscious dog. Circ Res 43:83-91
4. Kumada T, Karliner JS, Pouleur H, Gallagher KP, Shirato K, Ross J Jr (1979) Effects of coronary occlusion on early ventricular diastolic events in conscious dogs. Am J Physiol 237:H542-549
5. Gaasch WH, Bernard SA (1977) The effects of acute changes in coronary blood flow on left ventricular diastolic wall thickness. An echocardiographic study. Circulation 56:593-977
6. Forrester JS, Wyatt HL, Da Luz PL, Tyberg JV, Diamond GA, Swan HJC (1976) Functional significance of regional ischemic contraction abnormalities. Circulation 54:64-70
7. Gensini GG, Da Costa BCG (1969) The coronary collateral circulation in living man. Am J Cardiol 24:393-400
8. Dwyer EM Jr (1970) Left ventricular pressure. Volume alterations and regional disorders of contraction during myocardial ischemia induced by atrial pacing. Circulation 42:1111-1122
9. Mc Laurin LP, Rolett EL, Grossman (1973) Impaired left ventricular relaxation during pacing-induced ischemia. Am J Cardiol 32:751-757
10. Barry WH, Brooker JZ, Alderman EL, Harrison DC (1974) Changes in diastolic stiffness and tone of the left ventricle during angina pectoris. Circulation 49:255-263
11. Carroll JD, Hess OM, Hirzel HO, Krayenbuehl HP (1983) Exercise induced ischemia: the influence of altered relaxation on early diastolic pressures. Circulation 67:521-527
12. Bleifeld W, Mathey D, Hanrath P (1974) Acute myocardial infarction. VI Left ventricular wall thickness in the acute phase and in the convalescent phase. Eur J Cardiol 2:191-198
13. Bertrand ME, Rousseau MF, Lefebvre JM, Lablanche JM, Asseman PH, Carre AG, Lekieffre JP (1978) Left ventricular compliance in acute transmural myocardial infarction. Eur J Cardiol 7:179-193
14. Bertrand ME, Rousseau MF, Lablanche JM, Carre AG, Lekieffre JP (1979) Cineangiographic assessment of left ventricular function in the acute phase of transmural myocardial infarction. Am J Cardiol 43:472-480
15. Bertrand ME, Lablanche JM, Thieuleux FA (1983) Changes in left Ventricular relaxation during transient coronary occlusion in man. Eur Heart J 4 [Suppl E]:49
16. Feldman RL, Conti R, Pepine CJ (1983) Regional coronary venous flow responses to transient coronary artery occlusion in human beings. J Am Coll Cardiol 2:1-10
17. Rothman MT, Baim DS, Simpson JB, Harrison DC (1982) Coronary hemodynamics during percutaneous transluminal coronary angioplasty. Am J Cardiol 49:1615-1622
18. Hauser AM, Vellappilil G, Ramos RG, Gordon S, Timmis GC (1985) Sequence of mechanical electrocardiographic and clinical effects of repeated coronary artery occlusion in human beings. J Am Coll Cardiol 5:193-197
19. Das SK, Serruys PW, Van Den Brand M, Domenicucci S, Vletter WB, Roelandt J (1983) Acute echocardiographic changes during percutaneous coronary angioplasty and their relationship to coronary blood flow. J Cardiovasc Ultrasonogr 2:269-271
20. Sigwart V, Orbic M, Essinger A, Fischer A, Morin D, Sadeghi H (1982) Myocardial function in man during acute coronary balloon occlusion (abstract). Circulation 66 [Suppl II]:86
21. Serruys PW, Wijns W, Van Der Brand M et al. (1984) Left ventricular performance, regional blood flow, wall motion and lactate metabolism during transluminal angioplasty. Circulation 70:25-36
22. Wijns W, Serruys PW, Slager C et al. (1986) Effect of coronary occlusion during percutaneous transluminal angioplasty in humans on left ventricular chamber stiffness and regional diastolic pressure-radius relations. J Am Coll Cardiol 7:455-463

23. Kennedy JW, Trendholme SE, Kasser IS (1970) Left ventricular volume and mass from single plane cineangiogram. A comparison of anteroposterior and right anterior oblique methods. Am Heart J 80:343–350
24. Ingels N, Daughters G, Stinson E, Alderman E (1980) Evaluation of methods for quantitating left ventricular segmental wall motion in man using myocardial markers as a standard Circulation 61:966–972
25. Weiss JL, Fredericksen JW, Weisfeldt ML (1978) Hemodynamic determinants of the time course of fall in canine left ventricular pressure. J Clin Invest 58:751–760
26. Mirsky I (1984) Assessment of diastolic function: suggested methods and future considerations. Circulation 69:836–841
27. Gill JL (1978) Design and analysis of experiments in the animal and medical sciences, vol 3. Iowa State Univ Press, Ames, pp 72–75
28. Tyberg JV, Parmley WW, Sonnenblick EH (1969) In vitro studies of myocardial asynchrony and regional hypoxia. Circ Res 25:569–579
29. Tyberg JV, Taichman GC, Smith ER, Douglas NWS, Smiseth OA, Keon WJ (1986) The relationship between pericardial pressure and right atrial pressure: an intraoperative study. Circulation 73:428–432
30. Pasipoularides A, Mirsky I, Hess OM, Grimm J, Krayenbuehl HP (1986) Myocardial relaxation and passive diastolic properties in man. Circulation 74:991–1001
31. Mirsky I, Pfeffer JM, Pfeffer MA, Braunwald E (1983) The contractile state as the major determinant in the evolution of left ventricular dysfunction in the spontaneously hypertensive rat. Circ Res 53:767–778
32. Mirsky I, Rankin JS (1979) The effects of geometry, elasticity and external pressures on the diastolic pressure-volume and stiffness-stress relations. How important is the pericardium? Circ Res 44:601–612
33. Bourdillon PD, Lorell BH, Mirsky I, Paulus WJ, Wynne J, Grossman W (1983) Increased regional myocardial stiffness of the left ventricle during pacing-induced angina in man. Circulation 67:316–323

Can Thrombolysis Prevent Ischemic Heart Failure?

P.G. HUGENHOLTZ

Introduction

Pump failure, whether early and severe such as in acute cardiogenic shock, or insidious and late by congestion of upstream organs, is now the leading cause of cardiac death. Efforts at temporary mechanical or pharmacologic support of the heart have been largely unsuccessful so that attention is now more and more directed toward *prevention* of ventricular failure. When ischemic heart disease as a consequence of coronary artery obstruction(s) is the cause, limitation of the initial myocardial infarct size or even outright prevention of infarction itself appears to be the best approach now that early reperfusion efforts with thrombolytic agents have proven to be very successful in this regard.

The dramatic effects of early thrombolysis in acute myocardial infarction (AMI) on enzymatic infarct size, left ventricular function, and early mortality have been demonstrated in relatively few patients in comparison with the many large-scale trials with late β-blockade. Although experimental data with a variety of these pharmacologic agents seemed promising, in recent large-scale clinical trials in which early administration of β-adrenergic blockers was part of the procedure, such as the MIAMI trial [1] and also the ISIS-1 trial [2], neither these agents nor the various calcium antagonists [3–6] have shown a reduction in mortality even approaching that achieved by early thrombolysis. Thus the efficacy of early reperfusion by thrombolysis is now generally being recognized and implemented.

The randomized trial by the Netherlands Interuniversity Cardiology Institute is a good example of these observations [7]. It demonstrated that early (i.e., within 4 h) thrombolytic therapy with intracoronary streptokinase (152 patients) or with intracoronary streptokinase preceded by still earlier intravenous streptokinase (117 patients) achieved patency of the infarct-related artery in 85% of patients when compared to conventional treatment in 264 patients (consisting of bed rest, sedatives, antiarrhythmics and/or antihypertensive drugs whenever the hemodynamic state of the patient required this). Enzymatic infarct size, measured from cumulative α-hydroxybutyrate dehydrogenase (α-HBDH) release, was a median of 760 units in patients allocated to thrombolytic therapy versus 1179 units per liter in control subjects, $p = 0.0001$. This reflected a limitation of infarct size of approximately 30%. Left ventricular ejection fraction measured by radionuclide angiography before discharge was higher after thrombolytic therapy (median 50% versus 43% in control subjects, $p = 0.0001$). In later evaluations

B.S. Lewis, A. Kimchi (Eds.)
Heart Failure Mechanisms and Management
© Springer-Verlag Berlin Heidelberg 1991

with contrast angiography at 4–6 weeks after AMI, these differences were even more striking. While there was a statistically insignificant reduction in terms of early cardiac failure in favor of lytic therapy early on, 1-year follow up showed a highly significant reduction of 37 versus 53 deaths in patients conventionally treated, $p < 0.05$ (Table 1–5). For all of these reasons, 12-month mortality at 8% was much lower in patients allocated to thrombolytic therapy versus 16% in the control group ($p < 0.01$; at 3 months $p < 0.03$). Recently it was shown [8] that treatment beginning within < 60 min after onset of symptoms in a mobile coronary care system results in even better preservation of cardiac function.

In the last 2 decades, coronary care units have made it possible to recognize and treat in time previously fatal arrhythmias during the acute stage of myocardial infarction. This has reduced, at least the in-hospital, mortality from $\pm 30\%$ to $< 15\%$. Now the emphasis is on early reperfusion which can restore potentially jeopardized tissue to a "life sustainable" level. This in turn results in a reduction of later congestive heart failure. Indeed, all our attention must now be directed toward limitation of myocardial infarct size or even outright prevention of the infarction itself in order to reach a further significant reduction in hospital mortality to less than 5%.

Role of Coronary Thrombosis in Myocardial Infarction

The causal role of thrombosis in acute myocardial infarction has for a long time been a matter for debate. Although since Herrick's days it had been assumed that thrombosis was always the cause of an infarction, careful postmortem studies in the 1960s cast doubt on this theory because many patients showed infarction without complete coronary obstruction. Some researchers postulated, therefore, that thrombosis was the sequel of infarction. Such theories, based on postmortem examinations, were corrected through the detailed anatomic studies of Fulton et al. [9] and corroborated by DeWood et al. [10], whose coronary arteriographic studies in the first few hours after myocardial infarction showed that thrombosis was present in 86% of 517 patients within 4 h after onset of symptoms. These data were similar to those from the Netherlands Interuniversity Cardiological Institute [7] which indicated complete obstruction in 84% of the patients who were randomized to early angiography and intracoronary thrombolysis (Table 1). Thus, provided patients are studied early enough, most authors confirm that in acute infarction thrombotic obstruction is the most frequent cause.

Recently, Falk [11] identified a ruptured atheromatous plaque to be the cause of 40 of 51 recent coronary artery thromboses. This points to the significance of a sudden rupture of an atherosclerotic plaque in the genesis of coronary artery obstruction, either by hemorrhage into an expanding plaque or by serving as a nidus for rapid intraluminal platelet aggregation. Davies and Thomas [12] found that the same mechanism was operative regardless whether the ultimate clinical outcome was unstable angina, myocardial infarction, or sudden death.

Table 1. Clinical course in hospital. (Data modified from [7])

	Controls (n)	Thrombolysis (n)	p^a
Patients	264	269	
Hospital mortality (14 days)	26	14	0.05
Recurrent infarction (14 days)	9	12	
Angina pectoris	55	57	
Heart failure in coronary care unit:			
Mild	55	54	
Severe	12	10	
Shock	24	13	
Dopamine/dobutamine treatment	42	26	0.03
Respiratory support	11	6	
Intraaortic balloon pump	10	16	
Heart failure reconvalescence	53	37	0.05
Ventricular fibrillation	61	38	0.01
Pericarditis	46	19	0.0004
Bleeding	7	53	0.0001
Percutaneous transluminal coronary angioplasty	9	59^b	
Bypass surgery	16	29	

[a] Only p values < 0.05 are reported.
[b] PTCA was performed more frequently in the thrombolysis group, when the 46 PTCA immediately after thrombolysis are included.

These observations therefore bring several fundamental concepts into focus: (a) angiography can be carried out in acute myocardial infarction without major risks to establish whether obstruction is the cause of ischemia; (b) thrombosis is present in the majority of cases when studied within the first few hours after symptoms; (c) such an obstructing thrombus can be resolved in the majority of cases by immediate thrombolytic therapy for which a multitude of agents now present themselves; (d) although the prevalence of complete obstruction declines as the time after the onset of symptoms lengthens, myocardial loss is permanent after the first few hours; (e) while residual obstruction in and around the plaque remains a major problem even after successful lysis, efforts at early reperfusion will salvage tissue and preserve myocardial function particularly when followed by more permanent revascularization efforts such as percutaneous transluminal coronary angioplasty (PTCA) or coronary artery bypass graft (CABG) on a semi-urgent but elective basis.

It is therefore likely that limitation of infarct size and avoidance of later congestive heart failure will be successful only in those patients who present themselves for therapy within hours after onset of symptoms of AMI. This is evident from the data in Tables 2, 3, and 5. Indeed, the experimental evidence of

Table 2. Mortality by hours from onset of symptoms

Hours	Streptokinase (n)	(%)	Controls (n)	(%)	p	Risk ratio	95% (CI)	Total (n)	(%)
< 3*	278/3016	9.2	369/3078	12.0	0.0005	0.74	0.63–0.87	647/6094	10.6
> 3–6	217/1849	11.7	254/1800	14.1	0.03	0.80	0.66–0.98	471/3649	12.9
> 6–9	87/693	12.6	93/659	14.1	NS	0.87	0.64–1.19	180/1352	13.3
> 9–12	46/292	15.8	41/302	13.6	NS	1.19	0.75–1.87	87/594	14.6
< 1*	52/635	8.2	99/642	15.4	0.0001	0.49	0.34–0.69	151/1277	11.8

NS, not significant; *CI*, confidence interval.

Table 3

		Streptokinase, i.v. (0-3 h) GISSI + ISAM		Streptokinase, i.v. (0-4 h) NL − ICI		Streptokinase, i.v. (0-4 h) W. Washington	
		Control (%)	Lysis (%)	Control (%)	Lysis (%)	Control (%)	Lysis (%)
Patency		±20	±50	±20	85		
Infarct size			−15		−30		−10.3
LVEF		54	57	48	54	47	51
Mortality (3-4 weeks)	ISAM	7	5	12	6		
	GISSI	12	9				
Mortality (1 year)				18	9	30	17

GISSI, Gruppo Italiano per lo studio della streptochinas; nell' infarcto myocardico [14]; *ISAM*, intravenous streptokinase in acute myocardial infarction study group [35]; *NL-ICI*, Netherlands Interuniversity Cardiology Institute [7]; *W. Washington*, Western Washington trial [15].

Sobel et al. [13] demonstrated that only reperfusion within 4 h will limit the ultimate infarct size and achieve return toward normal cardiac function and metabolism. By now, overwhelming clinical evidence [7,8,14–16] has accrued, which confirms the efficacy of reperfusion in the first 0–4 h, with the greatest reductions in mortality and limitation of infarct size being achieved in those patients in whom lysis could be achieved within 2 h or less.

In an editorial in 1982 [17], in which the published data up to that year were reviewed, Rentrop and Hugenholtz voiced various notes of caution against excessive early enthusiasm for thrombolytic therapy. They pointed to the many factors which could positively or negatively influence the ultimate outcome. These included the need to know the time interval between the onset of symptoms and reperfusion, the extent of restoration of myocardial function in the region perfused by the infarct-related artery, the functional availability of collateral flow, the best route and optimal dose of the thrombolytic agents, the best agent and its side effects, and the degree to which the usual sequelae of myocardial infarction, such as subsequent angina, reinfarction, *congestive heart failure*, and death, could be reduced in the treatment group when compared to a control group randomly assigned to conventional treatment. That evidence is now available, and it can be stated without ambiguity that the most effective manner to reduce the incidence of (or avoid altogether) subsequent congestive heart failure in ischemic heart disease is early restoration of bloodflow to the area affected by obstruction to coronary flow.

What Proof is Available?
Intravenous and Intracoronary Studies in Humans

Early Reperfusion Studies

The feasibility of rapid dissolution of intracoronary thrombi by systemic or selective infusion of thrombolytic substances was convincingly demonstrated in experimental series and in clinical pilot studies as long as 30 years ago. However, because of lack of proper study design, the older experience should be eliminated from current considerations, although Yusuf et al. [18] concluded from a pooled analysis of some 6000 patients in 24 randomized trials with intravenous streptokinase between 1950 and 1980 that a reduction in the odds of death by 22% ± 5% could be deduced, this despite the fact that nonsignificant results were achieved in most individual studies.

Systematic efforts at restoration of anterograde flow after intracoronary administration were not introduced into clinical practice until 1979 by Rentrop et al. [19,20] in the Federal Republic of Germany. Since then we have witnessed a dramatic increase in the number of patients with acute ischemic cardiac disorders who have been treated by intracoronary streptokinase infusion [21–23]. The advantages of early intravenous administration combined with intracoronary lysis and aggressive follow-up treatment of residual coronary artery obstruction with coronary angioplasty or bypass surgery to optimize coronary bloodflow have recently been adequately investigated [17,24,25]. These striking benefits are entirely consistent with experimental evidence. Thus, most advanced cardiac centers now favor immediate and optimal reperfusion. An example of its significant influence on ventricular fibrillation is given in Table 4.

Table 4

Ventricular fibrillation	Controls (n = 264)		Thrombolysis (n = 269)	
	(n)	(%)	(n)	(%)
Total VF	60	23	36	13
Primary VF (< 48 h)[a]	24	9	13	5
Catheter-induced VF	9	3	15	5
Late VF (> 48 h)	10	4	2	1
Shock + VF	17	7	6	2

[a] Median delay after symptoms: 3 h   2 h

More Recent Studies in Thrombolysis

Returning to the question posed in our editorial [17]: what *have* we learned from the experience in the years since 1980? Most importantly, early recanalization, whether by guidewire alone [19] or by clot lysis with urokinase [27] or recombinant tissue plasminogen activator (rt-PA) [28–30], with or without PTCA [31], have all been shown to limit infarct size [7,8,32], preserve cardiac function [7,8,33], and reduce early as well as late mortality [7,8,14,15]. Thus the earlier requirements to demonstrate efficacy have largely been met, and it is now more a matter of implementation of this strategy than of finding the optimal agent or technique.

Which Patients Should We Select?

Here I cite from a recent study from our institute [34]:

In the present study the beneficial effects of streptokinase in patients admitted between 2 and 4 hours after onset of chest pain were observed only in those with extensive myocardial ischemia, as reflected by a high ΣST^1, and in patients in Killip class III or IV at admission. Although recanalization was also observed in a high percentage (68%) of patients with low ΣST, this did not lead to limitation of enzymatic infarct size, improvement in LVEF, or reduction in mortality (Table 5).

In the Western Washington trial [15], mean time to initiation of streptokinase infusion was 276 min, and patients with newly formed Q waves or receiving maintenance therapy for congestive heart failure were excluded. A significant reduction in early mortality was reported, although no beneficial effect on infarct size by thallium imaging or on left ventricular function was observed. Apparently this study included many patients who could not benefit from thrombolytic therapy according to our analysis, while patients with extensive ischemia leading to left ventricular failure, who might have benefitted from thrombolytic therapy, were excluded. In two other studies, the infusion of strepto-kinase started on average more than 5 hours after the onset of symptoms and patients with signs of cardiogenic shock were excluded. No improvement in left ventricular function or reduction in mortality was observed, which is consistent with our observations. Among three relatively small

Table 5. The effect of intracoronary thrombolytic therapy on enzyme infarct size, global left ventricular function, and 3-month mortality in patients. (Data from [7])

Interval between symptoms and admission (h) Sum ST elevation (mV)	< 2 > 1.2		2–4 > 1.2		< 2 > 1.2		2–4 < 1.2	
	C	SK	C	SK	C	SK	C	SK
Number of patients	112	92	35	372	72	81	24	35
HBDH release (U/l)	1440[a]	820	1640[b]	1180	800[b]	500	680	660
LVEF (%)	40[a]	48	44	46	44[a]	57	52	47
Mortality (%)	16[b]	7	17	8	10	4	8	9

[a] C vs. SK, $p < 0.0005$.
[b] C vs. SK, $p < 0.05$.
C, conventional treatment; SK, intracoronary streptokinase.

---

[1] ΣST, sum of ST segment elevation in precordial leads.

studies beneficial effects of thrombolytic therapy were observed in only one, in which the mean time between onset of symptoms and admission was 160 min [23]. In most of these studies patients with newly formed Q waves or signs of cardiogenic shock were excluded, and these groups of patients were shown to benefit greatly from thrombolytic therapy in the present trial [7,34].

This underlines once more that the interval of symptoms to onset of therapy may not exceed 4 h except when obvious signs of cardiac ischemia are still present.

Which Patients Benefit Most from Thrombolytic Therapy by Streptokinase?

Thrombolytic therapy with intracoronary streptokinase led to significant limitation of infarct size, improvement in left ventricular function, and reduction in mortality in patients with extensive myocardial ischemia, that is in those patients with a high ΣST, in whom thrombolytic therapy was started in the first few hours after onset of symptoms. Data from the GISSI trial [14] and the ISAM study [35] also indicate that beneficial effects from intravenous streptokinase dominate in patients admitted within 3 hours after onset of symptoms. Thus, it can now be recommended that thrombolytic therapy be offered to patients admitted within the first few hours after the onset of symptoms, and only to those patients who show extensive ST segment elevation on the ECG.

Recent publications such as ISIS-II [43], although involving much larger numbers and thus gaining power, have tended to confirm these recommendations, while also suggesting that a smaller benefit may be achieved in those treated for acute ischemia entering beyond the 6th h.

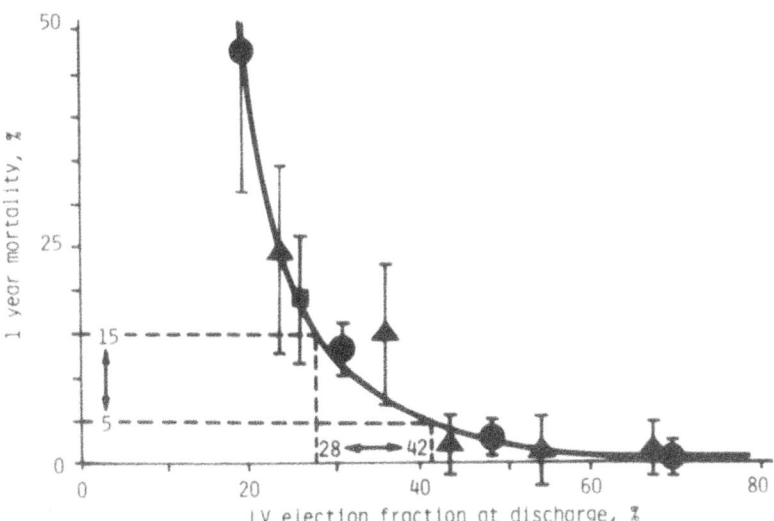

Fig. 1. There is a curvilinear relationship between the resting left ventricular ejection fraction at discharge and 1st year mortality. This relationship has been found by many authors [38–40]. If one could move the immediate postinfarct ejection fraction from say, 45% to 60%, the gains in 1-year survival (85%–95%) appear to be impressive. *LV*, left ventricle. *Circles*, n = 799 [38]; *squares*, n = 179 [39]; *triangles*, n = 214 [40]

Quality of Life after Thrombolysis

In the cost-benefit analysis of the randomized trial conducted by the Netherlands Interuniversity Cardiology Institute [34,44], we observed the following:

All hospital admissions were recorded and functional class was defined for each patient at regular intervals during the first year after entry. The method proposed by Olsson et al. [36], allows the analysis of differences in the quality of life, morbidity and mortality between the two treatment groups. While the symptoms of angina pectoris or heart failure are dependent on the patient's opinion, quality of life can be measured in an objective manner from the ability to carry on normal activity [37], as estimated by the Karnofsky Performance Status Scale. As shown earlier in patients with anterior infarction, thrombolytic therapy improved life expectancy, while the analysis depicted in Figs. 2 and 3 also demonstrates a striking effect on quality of life. However, the salutary effects of thrombolytic therapy in inferior infarction remained small, while costs for intervening episodes and procedures were in fact higher. Although total duration of hospital stay appeared to be equal in both treatment groups, admissions in the thrombolysis group were more often related to ischemia (reinfarction and additional revascularisation procedures as coronary angioplasty or bypass surgery). In the control group more admissions were due to symptoms and signs of *heart failure*. This confirms the more severe impairment of left ventricular function in conventionally treated patients over the first year of follow up.

The true "costs" of thrombolytic therapy include the acute intervention as well as the higher incidence of reinfarction and additional revascularisation procedures. It should be noted that the number of days "in hospital" was based on a weekly assessment of functional status. It was 21 days in both treatment groups.

Recently some have advocated even earlier release from hospital after successful lysis. Our calculation of total costs was based on actual hospital stay, catheterizations, coronary angioplasty, and bypass surgery during follow up. The increased workload due to the administration of thrombolytic therapy was balanced by the lower incidence of complications in the coronary care unit as thrombolytic therapy reduced the occurrence of ventricular fibrillation (Table 4), cardiogenic shock, and heart failure, workload on the coronary care unit was not affected [41]. Therefore the average costs for stay at the coronary care unit were used. Medication was not taken into account since this did not differ between the two treatment groups.

Total costs per patient during the 1 year of follow-up were higher after thrombolytic therapy. This was mainly owing to the costs of acute angiography and subsequent coronary angioplasty or bypass surgery. Even so, the cost-benefit analysis of intracoronary thrombolytic therapy with streptokinase is very favorable when compared with other established medical therapies. For example, while costs for 1 year increase in quality-adjusted life expectancy after bypass surgery as calculated by Weinstein varied from Dfl 20 000 to Dfl 75 000 [42], treatment of moderate diastolic hypertension requires Dfl 30 000–Dfl 90 000 per year of life gained. The excellent cost-benefit ratio for thrombolytic therapy is related to the fact that it requires but a single intervention at the time of hospital admission, with considerable salutary effects in a well-defined and easily recognized group of patients, while hypertension therapy must be given to large numbers of patients over a long period of time in order to prevent or delay a relatively small number of cardiovascular events.

Having engaged upon the strategy of reperfusion, a disadvantage of thrombolytic therapy remains the frequent need for preferably elective, but still

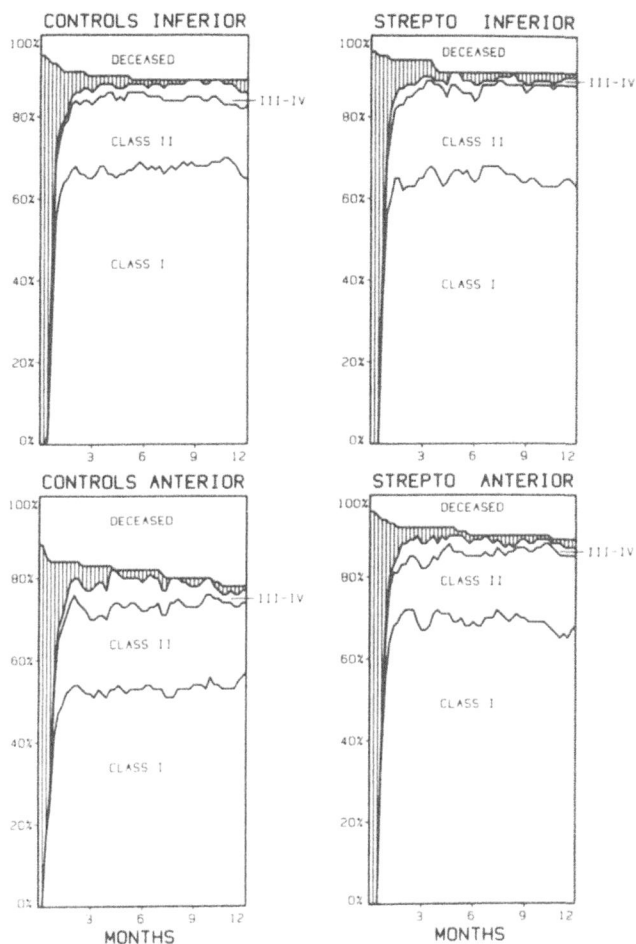

Fig. 2. A schematic overview of the symptomatic state during the first 12 months after onset of thrombolysis (*strepto*) or start of conventional therapy (*controls*). Class I reflects an asymptomatic course, class II occasional visits to the clinic for minor complications, classes III, IV congestive heart failure or other signs of dysfunction or need for interventions. The *hatched areas* indicate hospitalization days. *Horizontal axis*, duration of observation in months; *vertical axis*, percentage of all patients in each subgroup divided over the various classes. It is evident that patients with anterior wall infarction treated by streptokinase show the greatest improvement in the quality of life. (Data from [44])

(sub)acute angiography. It should be noted, however, that the costs of equipment and personnel for 24-h angiography service were included within our analysis. It is as yet unknown how the cost-benefit ratio of intracoronary thrombolysis relates to intravenous thrombolysis only. Intravenous administration of streptokinase is initially less expensive, but also considerably less effective than intracoronary treatment both in achieving patency, in terms of salvage of myocardial function,

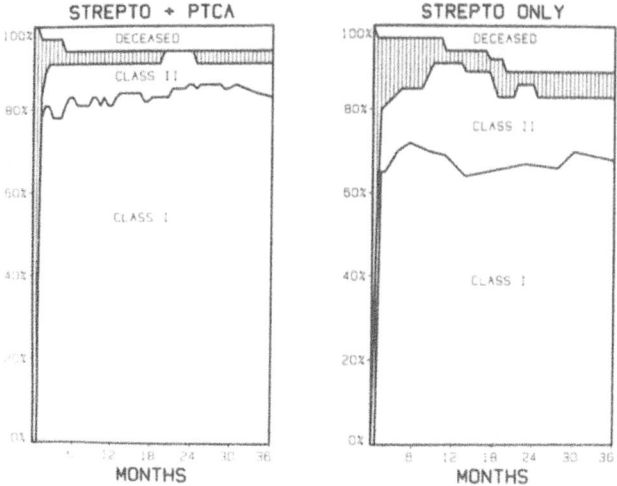

Fig. 3. As Fig. 2. It is evident that the group treated with streptokinase and percutaneous transluminal coronary angioplasty (*PTCA*) experiences the greatest benefit

and mortality reduction. Careful analysis of follow-up data of ongoing trials with intravenous streptokinase, intravenous tissue plasminogen activator, and intracoronary treatment with or without immediate coronary angioplasty should enable physicians and health authorities eventually to decide upon the most cost-effective method for a reperfusion/recanalization strategy. From presently available data, thrombolysis (preferably begun as intravenous lytic therapy) can be recommended as a cost-effective therapy in patients with extensive anterior myocardial ischemia, provided such therapy begins early after the onset of symptoms of myocardial infarction (i.e., 0–5 h). The result will be better residual ventricular function and reduced incidence of congestive heart failure, not to speak of a host of other benefits among which is improved quality of life.

Summary

In the present era of thrombolysis, congestive heart failure secondary to (sub)acute coronary artery obstruction can be reduced to a considerable extent or even avoided altogether, provided reperfusion is carried out within hours of occlusion.

References

1. The MIAMI Trial Research Group (1985) Metoprolol in acute myocardial infarction. Eur Heart J 6:199-226
2. ISIS-I (first international study of infarct survival) collaborative group (1986) Randomised trial of intravenous atenolol among 16 027 cases of suspected acute myocardial infarction. Lancet II:57-65
3. The Danish Study Group on Verapamil in Myocardial Infarction (1984) Verapamil in acute myocardial infarction. Eur Heart J 5:516-528
4. Muller JE, Morrison J, Stone PH, Rude RE, Rosner B, Roberts R, Pearle DL, Turi ZG, Schneider JF, Serfas DH, Tate C, Scheiner E, Sobel BE, Hennekens CH, Braunwald E (1984) Nifedipine therapy for patients with threatened and acute myocardial infarction: a randomized double blind, placebo controlled comparison. Circulation 69:740-747
5. Muller JE, NAMIS Study Group (1985) Nifedipine therapy for unstable angina and myocardial infarction: randomized double blind evaluations. In: Hugenholtz PG, Goldstein B (eds) Unstable angina. Schattauer, Stuttgart, pp 199-210
6. Sirnes PA, Overskeid K, Pederson TR, Bathen J, Drivenes A, Froland GS, Kjekshus JK, Laudmark K, Rokseth R, Sirnes KE, Sundoy A, Torjussen BR, Westlund KM, Wik BA (1984) Evolution of infarct size during the early use of nifedipine in patients with acute myocardial infarction: the Norwegian nifedipine multicenter trial. Circulation 70:638-644
7. Simoons ML, van den Brand M, de Zwaan C, Verheught FWA, Remme WJ, Serruys PW, Bar F, Res J, Krauss XH, Vermeer F, Lubsen J (1985) Improved survival after early thrombolysis in acute myocardial infarction. Lancet I:578-582
8. Gotsman MS, Weiss AT (1986) Immediate reperfusion in acute myocardial infarctions. Bibl Cardiol 40:30-51
9. Fulton W, Lutz W, Donald KW (1972) Natural history of unstable angina. Lancet I:860-870
10. DeWood MA, Spores J, Notske R, Mouser LT, Borroughs R, Golden MS, Lang HT (1980) Prevalence of total coronary occlusion during the early hours of transmural myocardial infarction. N Engl J Med 303:897-902
11. Falk E (1983) Plaque rupture with severe pre-existing stenosis precipitating coronary thrombosis. Br Heart J 50:127-134
12. Davies MJ, Thomas A (1984) Thrombosis and acute coronary artery lesions in sudden cardiac ischemic death. N Engl J Med 310:1137-1150
13. Sobel BE, Geltman EM, Tiefenbrunn AJ, Jaffe AS, Spadaro JJ, Ter-Pogossian MM, Collen D, Ludbrook PA (1984) Improvement of regional myocardial metabolism after coronary thrombolysis induced with tissue type plasminogen activator or streptokinase. Circulation 69:983-990
14. GISSI (Gruppo Italiano per lo studio della streptochinasi nell'infarcto myocardico) Tognoni F, Rovelli F et al. (1986) Effectiveness of intravenous thrombolytic therapy in acute myocardial infarction. Lancet I:397-402
15. Kennedy JW, Ritchie JL, Davis KB, Stadius L, Maynard C, Fritz JK (1985) The Western Washington randomized trial of intracoronary streptokinase in acute myocardial infarction. N Engl J Med 312:1073-1078
16. Koren G, Weiss AT, Hasin Y, Appelbaum D, Welber S, Rozenman Y, Lotau C, Mosseri M, Sapoznikov D, Luria MH, Gotsman M (1985) Prevention of myocardial damage in acute myocardial ischemia by early treatment with intravenous streptokinase. N Engl J Med 313:1384-1389
17. Hugenholtz PG, Rentrop P (1982) Thrombolytic therapy for acute myocardial infarction: quo vadis? Eur Heart J 3:395-403
18. Yusuf S, Collins R, Peto R, Furberg C, Stampfer MJ, Goldhaber SZ, Hennekes CH (1985) Intravenous and intracoronary fibrinolytic therapy in acute myocardial infarction: overview of results on mortality, reinfarction and side effects from 33 randomized controlled trials. Eur Heart J 6:556-585
19. Rentrop P, De Vivie ER, Karsch KR et al. (1978) Acute coronary occlusion with impending infarction as an angiographic complication relieved by a guide wire recanalization. Clin Cardiol 1:101-107

20. Rentrop P, De Vivie ER, Karsch KR et al. (1979) Acute myocardial infarction: intracoronary application of nitroglycerin and streptokinase in combination with transluminal recanalization. Clin Cardiol 5:354–356

21. Serruys PW, van den Brand M, Hooghoudt TEH, Simoons ML, Rioretti P, Ruiter J, Fels PW, Hugenholtz PG (1982) Coronary recanalization in acute myocardial infarction: immediate results and potential risks. Eur Heart J 3:404–415

22. Schwarz F, Hofmann M, Schuler G, von Olshausen K, Zimmermann R, Kubler W (1984) Thrombolysis in acute myocardial infarction: effect of intravenous followed by intracoronary streptokinase application on estimates of infarct size. Am J Cardiol 53:1505–1510

23. Khaja F, Walton JA, Brymer JF, Lo E, Osterberger L, O'Neill WW, Colfer HT, Weiss R, Lee T, Kurian T, Goldberg AD, Pitt B, Goldstein S (1983) Intracoronary fibrinolytic therapy in acute myocardial infarction: report of a prospective randomized trial. N Engl J Med 308:1305–1311

24. Merx W, Dorr R, Rentrop P, Blanke H, Karsch KR, Mathey DG, Kriemer P, Rutsch W, Schmutzler H (1981) Evaluation of the effectiveness of intracoronary streptokinase infusion in acute myocardial infarction: postprocedure management and hospital course in 204 patients. Am Heart J 102:1181–1187

25. Meyer J, Merx W, Schmitz H, Erbel R, Kiesslich T, Dörr R, Lambertz H, Bethge C, Krebs W, Bardos P, Minale C, Messmer BJ, Effert S (1982) Percutaneous transluminal coronary angioplasty immediately after intracoronary streptolysis of transmural myocardial infarction. Circulation 66:905–913

26. Kambara M, Kawai C, Kammatsuse K, Sato H, Nobuyoshi M, Chino M, Miwa H, Uchida Y, Kodama K, Mitsudo K, Hayashi T, Kajiwara N, Sekiguchi M, Yasue H (1985) Coronary thrombolysis in urokinase infusion in acute myocardial infarction. A multicenter study in Japan. Cathet Cardiovasc Diagn 11:349–360

27. Van der Werf F, Bergmann SR, Fox KAA, De Geest H, Hoyng CF, Sobel BE, Collen D (1984) Coronary thrombolysis with intravenously administered human tissue type plasminogen activator produced by recombinant DNA technology. Circulation 69:605–610

28. TIMI Study Group (1985) The thrombolysis in myocardial infarction (TIMI) trial: phase I findings. N Engl J Med 310:932–946

29. Verstraete M, Bory M, Collen D et al. (1985) Randomized trial of intravenous recombinant tissue-type plasminogen activator versus intravenous streptokinase in acute myocardial infarction, II. Lancet I:842–847

30. Topol EJ, Eha JE, Brin KP et al. (1985) Applicability of percutaneous transluminal angioplasty to patients with recombinant tissue type plasminogen activator mediated thrombolysis. Cathet Cardiovasc Diagn 2:337–348

31. Simoons ML, Serruys PW, Van den Brand M et al. (1986) Early thrombolysis in acute myocardial infarction: limitation of infarct size and improved survival. J Am Coll Cardiol 7:717–728

32. Serruys PW, Simoons ML, Suryapranata M et al. (1986) Preservation of global and regional left ventricular function after early thrombolysis in acute myocardial infarction. J Am Coll Cardiol 7:729–742

33. Vermeer F, Simoons ML, Bar FW, Tijssen JGP, Van Domburg RT, Serruys PW, Verheugt FWA, Res JCJ, De Zwaan C, Van der Laarse A, Drauss XH, Lubsen J, Hugenholtz PG (1986) Which patients benefit most from early thrombolytic therapy with intracoronary streptokinase? Circulation 74:1379–1389

34. The ISAM study group (1986) A prospective trial of intravenous streptokinase in acute myocardial infarction (ISAM). Mortality, morbidity, and infarct size at 21 days. N Engl J Med 314:1465–1471

35. Olsson G, Lubsen J, van Es GA, Rehnqvist N (1986) Quality of life after myocardial infarction: effect of chronic etoprolol treatment on mortality and morbidity. Br Med J 292:1491–1493

36. Yates JW, Chalmer B, McKegney FP (1980) Evaluation of patients with advanced cancer using the Karnofsky performance status. Cancer 45:2220–2224

37. The Multicenter Postinfarction Research Group (1983) Risk stratification after myocardial infarction. N Engl J Med 50:266–272

38. De Feyter PJ, Van Eenige MG, Dighton DH et al. (1982) Prognostic value of exercise testing, coronary angiography and left ventriculography 6–8 weeks after myocardial infarction. Circulation 66:527–536

39. Fioretti P, Brower RW, Simoons ML et al. (1984) Prediction of mortality in hospital survivors of myocardial infarction. Br Heart J 52:292–298
40. Kint PP, Simoons ML, Vermeer F, de Graaf S (1986) Early thrombolysis in acute myocardial infarction does not increase CCU workload (abstract). Circulation 74 II:129
41. Weinstein MC, Stason WB (1982) Cost effectiveness of coronary artery bypass surgery. Circulation 66 III:56–65
42. ISIS-II (Second International Study of Infarct Survival) (1988) Randomised trial of intravenous streptokinase, oral aspirin, both, or neither among 17,187 cases of suspected acute myocardial infarction: ISIS-II. Lancet II:349–360
43. Vermeer F (1987) Thesis: Thrombolysis in acute myocardial infarction. Van Gorkum, Assen Maastricht

Acute Right Ventricular Infarction: Pathogenesis of Low Systemic Output and Therapeutic Implications

K. Chatterjee

Introduction

Right ventricular necrosis frequently accompanies left ventricular infarction. Isolated right ventricular infarction is rare, only observed in approximately 3% of hearts in autopsy studies [1]. Clinically, inferoposterior myocardial infarction is the most frequent association; but in patients who succumb due to cardiogenic shock, left ventricular anterior wall myocardial infarction occurs with higher frequency. Although right ventricular infarction is relatively common, a severe low-output state with or without clinical features of cardiogenic shock occurs only in about 10% of patients. In this brief review, the diagnosis, pathogenesis, and pharmacologic management of low-output state will be described.

Diagnosis of Right Ventricular Infarction

Table 1 shows the steps to be taken in the diagnosis of acute right ventricular infarction. As right ventricular infarction occurs almost exclusively in the presence of inferoposterior left ventricular infarction, findings suggestive of right ventricular infarction should always be sought in these patients. Initially hypotension in the absence of pulmonary congestion was regarded as the hallmark for the diagnosis of right ventricular infarction [2]; however, it is now recognized that such constellations of signs may occur in the absence of right ventricular infarction and do not occur in all patients with right ventricular infarction.

Clinical diagnosis depends on the recognition of the findings indicative of right ventricular failure in the absence of obvious left heart failure and pulmonary arterial hypertension. Elevated jugular venous pressure, right ventricular S3 gallop in the absence of accentuated pulmonary component of the second heart sound, and overt pulmonary congestion in a patient with inferior myocardial infarction is strong clinical evidence for right ventricular myocardial infarction. Lack of inspiratory collapse or inspiratory rise of jugular venous pressure (Kussmaul's sign), although only seen in 10%–15% of patients, is almost always diagnostic of right ventricular infarction [3]. Occasionally, a prominent "y" descent along with elevated mean jugular venous pressure is observed. It should be emphasized the abnormal physical findings are not present in all patients with right ventricular infarction, and their absence does not exclude the diagnosis.

B.S. Lewis, A. Kimchi (Eds.)
Heart Failure Mechanisms and Management
© Springer-Verlag Berlin Heidelberg 1991

Table 1. Diagnosis of acute right ventricular infarction

---

1. *Clinical.* Elevated jugular venous pressure with or without prominent 'y' descent, Kussmaul's sign, right ventricular S3 gallop, lack of pulmonary congestion
2. *Electrocardiogram.* Inferior or inferoposterior myocardial infarction and ST elevation in leads V_1 and V_1R
3. *Radionuclide Scintigraphy.* (a) Positive uptake of Tc99m pyrophosphate by the free walls of the right ventricle; (b) dilated, poorly contracting right ventricular and regional wall motion abnormalities by gated blood pool scintigraphy
4. *Two-dimensional Echocardiography.* Dilated, poorly contracting right ventricle, right ventricular wall motion abnormalities
5. *Hemodynamics.* Disproportionate elevation of right atrial pressure compared to pulmonary capillary wedge pressure (RAP/PCWP > 0.86); equalization – right and left ventricular diastolic pressures

---

"Volume loading," although it unmasks some of these findings, is rarely necessary for establishing the diagnosis of right ventricular infarction.

Careful analysis of the early electrocardiogram provides diagnostic clues in the vast majority of patients [4]. An elevation of ST segment by 0.1 mv or more in leads V1 and V4R, with or without Q waves, in the presence of electrocardiographic evidence of inferior wall myocardial infarction is highly suggestive of right ventricular infarction. In some patients, ST segment elevation may extend from lead V1 to V5, simulating acute anterior myocardial injury. Lack of significant reciprocal ST segment depression in leads V1 and V2, i.e., less than 50% of the magnitude of ST segment elevation in leads II, III, and AVF has been reported to be indicative of right ventricular dysfunction.

Other noninvasive investigations also aid in diagnosis. Chest X-ray is usually not helpful except that frank pulmonary edema is usually absent. Tc99m pyrophosphate imaging reveals "hotspots" in the areas of necrosis of right ventricle [5], but the value of Tc99m pyrophosphate imaging is considerably diminished in clinical practice as it is not usually positive before 12–24 h after the onset of infarction.

Blood pool scintigraphy and echocardiography provide assessment of right and left ventricular function. Right ventricular global ejection fraction declines significantly when left ventricular ejection fraction may be reasonably preserved [5]. Right ventricular ejection fraction of 40% or less associated with akinesis or dyskinesis of right ventricular walls provides a high degree of diagnostic accuracy, and the sensitivity of these scintigraphic criteria exceeds 80% [6]. Echocardiography provides similar information and is more easily performed and practical. Right ventricular dilatation and its impaired systolic function with its wall motion abnormalities are easily detected. Furthermore, echocardiography excludes the presence of pericardial effusion and signs of cardiac tamponade with which the diagnosis of right ventricular infarction can be confused. Thus, two-dimensional echocardiography, for practical purposes, is the noninvasive investigation of choice in the diagnosis of right ventricular infarction.

Determination of hemodynamics is rarely required for the diagnosis of right ventricular infarction. Hemodynamic monitoring, however, is useful, if not essential, during the management of low-output state complicating right ventricular infarction. The hemodynamic abnormalities of right ventricular infarction are a disproportionate elevation of right atrial pressure compared to pulmonary capillary wedge pressure. Right atrial pressure is frequently elevated and exceeds 10 mmHg, and the ratio of right atrial to pulmonary capillary wedge pressure is usually higher than 0.86 [7]. The sensitivity of these hemodynamic criteria for the diagnosis of right ventricular infarction is high and exceeds 80%. In patients with significant right ventricular dilatation, hemodynamic abnormalities similar to cardiac tamponade, i.e., equalization of right atrial and pulmonary capillary wedge pressures, are frequently observed [8].

Complications of Right Ventricular Infarction

Bradyarrhythmias are the most frequent complications of acute right ventricular infarction. Sinus bradycardia, sinus arrest, and second degree atrioventricular block are quite frequent and occur in approximately 40% of patients. The incidence of complete atrioventricular block is also high: about 20%. This relatively high incidence of sinoatrial and atrioventricular nodal dysfunction can be explained by the coronary artery lesions associated with right ventricular infarction, usually total occlusion of the right coronary artery, proximal to the right ventricular branches and atrioventricular nodal artery.

Complete atrioventricular block may precipitate hypotension and low-output state. Slower heart rate and lack of timed atrial systole appear to be poorly tolerated by patients with right ventricular infarction. Ventricular pacing and atrioventricular pacing at identical pacing rates indicates that cardiac output during atrioventricular sequential pacing is considerably higher than during ventricular pacing [9]. The therapeutic implication of this finding is that atrioventricular sequential pacing should be considered in preference to ventricular pacing if atrioventricular block is associated with low-output state.

Hypotension and decreased systemic output in the absence of bradyarrhythmias occur in approximately 10% of patients with acute right ventricular infarction. Severe acute tricuspid regurgitation resulting from right ventricular papillary muscle infarction is an infrequent but potentially life-threatening complication. Rarely, rupture of the right ventricular free wall without rupture of the interventricular septum, a catastrophic complication, may occur in right ventricular infarction. A reduction in arterial PO_2 and saturation, resulting from right to left shunt through a stretched open foramen ovale, has been reported in some patients. Pulmonary embolism associated with right ventricular mural thrombi may cause hemodynamic deterioration; however, such complications are rarely diagnosed clinically.

Pathogenesis of Low Output in Right Ventricular Infarction

Decrease in systemic output due to acute right ventricular infarction results from a number of interacting mechanisms which lead to a significant reduction in left ventricular preload. In experimental isolated right ventricular infarction in animals [10], left ventricular diastolic chamber size and transmural pressure decrease, indicating reduced left ventricular preload and filling pressures, respectively. Right ventricular diastolic volume and transmural pressure, however, increase. Both right and left ventricular stroke volume and stroke work indices decrease; decrease in right ventricular stroke volume results from impaired right ventricular pump function primarily owing to its reduced contractile function, whereas decreased left ventricular stroke volume is related to its decreased preload.

As right ventricular stroke volume contributes to left ventricular preload, the more severe the reduction of right ventricular stroke volume, the smaller the left ventricular preload. There is experimental evidence to suggest that volume expansion with the administration of intravenous fluids may increase right and left ventricular preloads, and right and left ventricular stroke volumes [11]. Thus, improvement in right ventricular function by augmenting the Frank-Starling mechanism enhances systemic output by increasing left ventricular preload. The degree of impairment of right ventricular systolic function is directly related to the extent of right ventricular infarction. In type I right ventricular infarction, 50% or less of the inferior wall of the right ventricle is involved, in addition to the infarction of the inferior part of the interventricular septum and part of the inferior wall of the left ventricle. In type II right ventricular infarction, more than 50% of the inferior wall of the right ventricle is infarcted, but the anterior wall of the right ventricle is spared. In types I and II right ventricular infarction, residual Frank-Starling function can be used to augment right ventricular stroke volume. In type III, 50% or less, and in type IV, more than 50% of the right ventricular anterior wall is infarcted in addition to its interior wall, part of the interventricular septum, and the inferior wall of the left ventricle. Types III and IV infarction are likely to be associated with marked right ventricular dilatation, and thus a further increase in right ventricular volume with "volume expansion" is unlikely to produce a significant increase in stroke volume.

Constraining effects of pericardium also contribute to decreased left ventricular preload. Pericardium, being a stiffer structure than atria and ventricles, does not stretch acutely and proportionately to right ventricular dilatation, causing increased intrapericardial pressure which impairs left ventricular filling. Increased intrapericardial pressure following right ventricular dilatation is also the hemodynamic mechanism for equalization of the diastolic pressure. In experimental isolated right ventricular infarction in dogs, right and left ventricular diastolic pressures and intrapericardial pressure increase concurrently, and all pressures are equal. Following pericardiectomy, equalization of the diastolic pressures is no longer observed. That decrease in left ventricular preload results partly from the constraining effect of pericardium is evident from the fact that, after pericardiectomy, left ventricular diastolic volume and transmural pressure increase along with an increase in systemic arterial pressure, stroke volume, and cardiac output. Although the role of pericardium in restricting left ventricular filling can be easily demonstrated in experimental isolated right ventricular infarction in dogs, its role in patients with right ventricular infarction has not been investigated.

Intact pericardium and increased intrapericardial and right ventricular diastolic pressure determine the transseptal pressure and the orientation of interventricular septum. Normally, left ventricular diastolic pressure exceeds right ventricular pressure causing a rightward shift of the interventricular septum. With a marked increase in intrapericardial pressure, right and left ventricular diastolic pressures may be equal, preventing diastolic rightward shift of the interventricular septum and thus causing a relative decrease in left ventricular preload. When right ventricular diastolic pressure exceeds that of the left ventricle, a leftward shift of the interventricular septum may occur, causing a further reduction of left ventricular preload. Although detailed analysis of changes in septal orientation in right ventricular infarction still needs to be performed, it is very likely that an abnormal septal shift contributes to decreased left ventricular volume [12].

An increase in pulmonary artery pressure improves increased resistance to right ventricular ejection which causes a further reduction in right ventricular forward stroke volume. When left ventricular diastolic pressure is already elevated due to associated left ventricular dysfunction, or when left ventricular diastolic pressure increases due to increased intrapericardial pressure, there is an obligatory increase in left atrial, pulmonary venous and pulmonary arterial pressures. Thus, secondary pulmonary arterial hypertension further impairs right ventricular systolic function. Right ventricular dilatation, which raises right ventricular afterload, also causes further reduction in right ventricular stroke volume. It is apparent that several interacting hemodynamic mechanisms impair right ventricular systolic function and decrease left ventricular preload, which, however, appears to be the principal mechanism for low-output state in right ventricular infarction.

Management of Low Output in Right Ventricular Infarction

Hemodynamic monitoring is frequently required to determine response to therapy during the management of low-output state. The major objectives are to improve right ventricular systolic function and increase left ventricular preload. In experimental isolated right ventricular infarction in dogs, volume expansion with the administration of intravenous fluids results in an improvement in right ventricular systolic function, an increase in left ventricular diastolic volume and transmural pressure, and a significant increase in systemic output and arterial pressure [11]. Right ventricular transmural pressure and chamber size also increase, suggesting that an augmented Frank-Starling function is the mechanism for improved right ventricular systolic performance during volume expansion. The magnitude of improvement, however, depends on right ventricular residual "Frank-Starling reserve." If the right ventricle is already markedly dilated, limited or no improvement in right ventricular function and systemic output is expected during volume expansion. Clinically, volume expansion is usually not associated with any significant increase in cardiac output when initial right atrial and pulmonary capillary wedge pressure are higher than 10–15 mmHg [13, 14]. Although intravenous fluid therapy causes a further increase in right atrial and pulmonary capillary wedge pressure, essentially there is no increase in systemic output. The precise explanation for this lack of response remains unclear; however, it is unlikely that significant improvement in right ventricular systolic function, or an increase in left ventricular preload results from volume expansion therapy in these patients.

Vasodilators such as sodium nitroprusside or nitroglycerin have been shown to be beneficial in correcting low-output state in some patients with right ventricular infarction [2]. The mechanisms of improvement in systemic hemodynamics with vasodilators, however, have not been clarified. It is likely that a reduction of both right and left ventricular ejection impedance contributes to improved systemic hemodynamics during vasodilator therapy. Maintenance of adequate right and left ventricular preloads is necessary, and thus concomitant intravenous fluid therapy is frequently required.

Inotropic therapy improves right ventricular systolic function and systemic hemodynamics in patients with right ventricular infarction. Dobutamine and dopamine are the two most frequently used inotropic agents, and both improve cardiac output. However, there are some differences between the hemodynamic effects of dobutamine and dopamine which should be considered for their use in individual patients. Pulmonary capillary wedge, pulmonary artery pressure, and total pulmonary arterial resistance may increase with dopamine, particularly when larger doses (exceeding 8–10 g kg^{-1} min^{-1}) are used. Thus, the potential exists for increased right ventricular ejection impedance with dopamine. Pulmonary capillary wedge and pulmonary artery pressure tend to decrease with dobutamine, which is thus preferable to dopamine in the management of low-output state complicating right ventricular infarction. Dobutamine, however, usually does not correct hypotension; thus, in the presence of hypotension, dopamine is preferable to dobutamine. Occasionally, the combination of dobutamine and dopamine is required to optimize hemodynamic improvement. It should be emphasized that inotropic and vasopressor therapy may enhance myocardial ischemia and induce ventricular arrhythmias, and such therapy should be employed only when vasodilators and fluid therapy fail to produce adequate hemodynamic response or when they are contraindicated. It is apparent that hemodynamic monitoring is required to assess the therapeutic response during various pharmacologic interventions for correction of hemodynamic abnormalities and low-output state complicating acute right ventricular infarction. Most patients with low-output and hypotension recover within 3–4 days with aggressive supportive therapy as outlined.

Summary

Acute right ventricular infarction is relatively common in patients with inferior myocardial infarction. Diagnosis can be made in most patients based on clinical and electrocardiographic findings. Radionuclide scintigraphy and echocardiography are helpful for the assessment of right and left ventricular function. Hemodynamic monitoring is recommended during the managemnt of low-output state complicating right ventricular infarction. Decreased left ventricular preload is the principal mechanism for decreased systemic output. Depressed right ventricular systolic function, constraining effects of pericardium, and the leftward shift of the interventricular septum cause impaired left ventricular filling. Aggressive supportive therapy with the administration of intravenous fluids, vasodilators, and inotropic agents is usually effective in increasing cardiac output and correcting other hemodynamic abnormalities resulting from acute right ventricular infarction.

References

1. Isner J, Roberts WC (1978) Right ventricular infarction complicating left ventricular infarction secondary to coronary heart disease. Am J Cardiol 42:885–894
2. Cohn JN, Guiha NH, Broder MI et al. (1974) Right ventricular infarction. Am J Cardiol 33:209–214
3. Dell'Italia LJ, Starling MR, O'Rourke RA (1983) Physical examination for exclusion of hemodynamically important right ventricular infarction. Ann Intern Med 99:608–611
4. Lopez-Sendon J, Coma-Cannella I, Alcasena S et al. (1985) Electrocardiographic findings in acute right ventricular infarction: sensitivity and specificity of electrocardiographic alterations in right precordial leads V4R, V3R, V1, V2 and V3. J Am Coll Cardiol 6:1273–1979
5. Sharpe DN, Botvinick EH, Shames DM et al. (1978) The noninvasive diagnosis of right ventricular infarction. Circulation 57:483–490
6. Rigo P, Murray M, Taylor DR (1978) Right ventricular dysfunction detected by gated scintiphotography in patients with acute inferior myocardial infarction. Circulation 52:268–274
7. Dell'Italia LJ, Starling MMR, Crawford MH et al. (1984) Right ventricular infarction: identification by hemodynamic measurements before and after volume loading and correlation with noninvasive techniques. J Am Coll Cardiol 4:931–939
8. Lorell B, Leinbach RC, Pohost GM et al. (1979) Right ventricular infarction. Clinical diagnosis and differentiation from cardiac tamponade and pericardial constriction. Am J Cardiol 43:465–471
9. Topol EJ, Goldschlager N, Ports TA, DiCarlo LA Jr, Schiller NB, Botvinick EH, Chatterjee K Hemodynamic benefit of atrial pacing in right ventricular myocardial infarction. Ann Intern Med 96:594–597
10. Goldstein JA, Vlahakes GJ, Verrier ED et al. (1982) The role of right ventricular systolic dysfunction and elevated intrapericardial pressure in the genesis of low output in experimental right ventricular infarction. Circulation 65:513–522
11. Goldstein JA, Vlahakes GJ, Verrier ED et al. (1983) Volume loading improves low cardiac output in experimental right ventricular infarction. J Am Coll Cardiol 2:270–278

12. Mikell FL, Asinger RW, Hodges M (1983) Functional consequences of interventricular septal involvement in right ventricular infarction: echocardiographic, clinical, and hemodynamic observations. Am Heart J 105:393-401
13. Dell'Italia LJ, Starling MR, Blumhardt R et al. (1985) Comparative effects of volume loading, dobutamine and nitroprusside in patients with predominant right ventricular infarction. Annu Rev Med 34:377-390
14. Shah PK, Maddahi J, Berman DS et al. (1985) Scintigraphically detected predominant right ventricular dysfunction in acute myocardial infarction: clinical and hemodynamic correlates and implications for therapy and prognosis. J Am Coll Cardiol 6:1264-1272

Rheumatic Heart Disease and Valvular Heart Disease

Mechanisms and Management of Heart Failure in Active Rheumatic Carditis

J.B. Barlow, R.H. Marcus, W.A. Pocock, C.W. Barlow, R. Essop, and P. Sareli

There is almost universal agreement that rheumatic fever and rheumatic heart disease are always preceded by infection with group A beta-hemolytic streptococcus. In most developed countries, the reported incidence of both rheumatic fever and rheumatic heart disease has declined drastically. The fact that the onset of this decline preceded the advent of antibiotics indicates that factors other than streptococcal infection must play a role in the pathogenesis of this condition. Despite worldwide research, the factors causing a high prevalence of rheumatic heart disease in any community remain uncertain. It is favored that socioeconomic factors are important; hence, the continued high prevalence of rheumatic heart disease in Third World countries. In 1978, Padmavati [1] concluded that "prophylaxis was hardly worthwhile" in patients encountered for the first time with a late stage of rheumatic heart disease. Such cases comprised 75% of those considered for a secondary prophylaxis program in India between 1968 and 1974. While it is now rare to encounter White patients under the age of 20 years with rheumatic heart disease, the clinical experience of those involved with the diagnosis and treatment of Black South African patients is that rheumatic heart disease remains prevalent and continues to affect young children. In 1972 a survey of 12 050 Black schoolchildren in the Johannesburg area [2] detected an overall prevalence rate for rheumatic heart disease of 6.9/1000, with a peak rate of 19.2/1000 in children aged about 15–18 years.

The exact nature of the relevant "co-factor(s)" that predispose to rheumatic fever or rheumatic heart disease remains uncertain. In 1930, Glover [3] stated that "no disease has a clearer-cut 'social incidence' than acute rheumatism which falls perhaps thirty times as frequently upon the poorer children of the industrial town as upon the children of the well-to-do ... the incidence of acute rheumatism increases directly with poverty, malnutrition, overcrowding and bad housing." Since Glover's comments, the socioeconomic factors that have received the most attention are poor nutrition and overcrowding. Hereditary, racial, geographical, and blood group factors have also been studied but are probably of minor or no importance. From the data obtained in our survey, we concluded that overcrowding was of importance, but that it alone was not the sole factor. All schools are "overcrowded" in that the pupils are in close contact with one another, and this will facilitate spread of the beta-hemolytic streptococcus. As many as 9% of pupils at an exclusive Johannesburg preparatory school in 1975 [4] had throat swabs that tested positive for the beta-hemolytic streptococcus, yet rheumatic fever or rheumatic heart disease has not, to our knowledge, been encountered in

B.S. Lewis, A. Kimchi (Eds.)
Heart Failure Mechanisms and Management
© Springer-Verlag Berlin Heidelberg 1991

a pupil at that school during the last 3 decades. A more recent survey [5], in which the throats of Coloured and of Indian schoolchildren were swab-tested revealed group A beta-hemolytic streptococci in 24% and 21%, respectively, during the summer months. The total number of 226 children examined was relatively small, but none had rheumatic heart disease. We did not detect significant malnutrition in the Black schoolchildren whom we examined in 1972, but it is possible that poor nutrition during the 1st year of life renders a child susceptible to rheumatic fever and rheumatic heart disease [6].

Elucidation of factors predisposing to acute rheumatic fever and rheumatic carditis has not been assisted by the recent apparent resurgence of these entities in the United States [7,8]. In many of the reported cases, the preceding pharyngitis was mild, the incidence of carditis high, and the rheumatic fever occurred in middle class families with ready access to medical care. In their recent excellent review on the pathogenesis of rheumatic fever, Kaplan and Markowitz [8] concluded that, just as the marked decline in incidence of rheumatic fever in Western countries remains "unexplained," so does the recent resurgence. More over, they stated that "unless and until the pathogenesis of rheumatic fever is fully understood, methods of control will not be optimal."

Active, Severe Rheumatic Carditis

A fulminating form of active rheumatic carditis continues to be encountered by us and has been observed by one of us (JBB) for more than 3 decades. It is difficult to assess the incidence, but there is no evidence to suggest that it is decreasing [9]. During 1986, for example, a total of 339 patients was subjected to mitral valve surgery in our institution (Fig. 1), and almost all of these cases had a rheumatic etiology.

Clinical Features

On the basis of an analysis of 80 patients subjected to valve replacement or repair while in the active phase of rheumatic carditis, the clinical presentation can be outlined [9] (Table 1). All but four of the 80 patients were under the age of 21 years. Eighteen patients (23%) were less than 10 years, and the youngest was 5 years. The children or their parents commonly claimed that symptoms such as tiredness, breathlessness, cough, and arthralgia had been present for a few weeks only. Tachycardia of more than 100 beats per minute and pyrexia greater than 38°C were present in 96% of patients. The clinical picture was often compatible with infective endocarditis, but the differentiation could usually be made. Relevant distinguishing features are negative blood cultures, absence of splinter hemorrhages or other evidence of systemic embolism, no vegetations on echocardiography, and lack of response to a trial of antibiotic therapy. There was definite clubbing of the fingers in about 15%. This is a little-recognized feature of

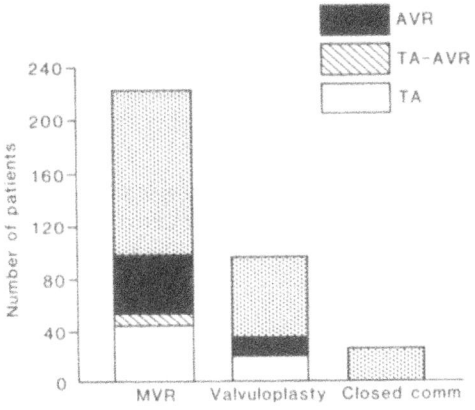

Fig. 1. Analysis of 339 patients who had mitral valve surgery at the Baragwanath and Johannesburg Hospitals during 1986. Additional aortic valve replacement (*AVR*) and tricuspid anuloplasty (*TA*), either alone or in combination, were required in about a third of the patients. *Closed comm,* closed commissurotomy; *MVR,* mitral valve replacement

Table 1. Clinical features of active severe rheumatic carditis in 80 patients subjected to valve surgery

		n	%
Age (years)			
< 10		18	23
10–20		58	72
> 20		4	5
Tachycardia (> 100/min)		77	96
Pyrexia		77	96
Chest pain		31	39
Arthralgia		13	16
Epistaxis		10	13
Cardiothoracic ratio			
(57 patients)	≥0.6	53	93
	< 0.6	4	7
PR interval (second)			
(55 patients)	> 0.20	30	55
	< 0.20	25	45
Cachexia		34	49
Emergency operation		52	65

active rheumatic carditis and may mislead clinicians into diagnosing infective endocarditis. Splenomegaly was detected in about 15% of patients. It is uncertain whether this is causally related to the rheumatic activity or a coincidental feature in a population with a high prevalence of parasitic infestation. A notable symptom was severe anterior chest pain (31 patients), which was typically aggravated by pressure of the palm of the examiner's hand on the sternum. A pericardial rub may be heard, and acute fibrinous pericarditis was confirmed at surgery in 24 of these patients. Hemodynamically significant pericardial effusion has seldom been encountered in our experience of acute rheumatic carditis and was not detected in any of these 80 patients. Cachexia was present in 34, and this may be extremely marked in some instances. Arthralgia or arthritis is infrequent and occurred in only 16%. Rheumatic nodules and erythema marginatum were rarely encountered. Considerable cardiomegaly was readily apparent on clinical examination and was confirmed by a cardiothoracic ratio on chest roentgenogram of 60% or more in most cases.

Regurgitation was invariably the predominant valvular lesion and almost always involved the mitral valve. Of the 80 patients, 72 had pure or predominant mitral regurgitation. A left atrial lift is an easily elicited and highly contributory physical sign, especially if the apical systolic murmur is only grade 2 or less in intensity[9]. Concomitant aortic regurgitation was present in 47 of our 80 patients, but marked aortic regurgitation as an isolated lesion (that is, without detectable associated mitral valve involvement) was encountered in only six subjects. Dominant mitral stenosis occurred in only one instance in this series, and there was no case of significant aortic stenosis. Associated tricuspid regurgitation is common and is usually due to dilatation of the tricuspid anulus. This was confirmed at operation in 22 patients. The systolic murmur of tricuspid regurgitation is often unimpressive or absent, but the entity may be clinically recognized by prominent systolic waves in the jugular venous pressure and systolic pulsation of the enlarged liver. Tricuspid regurgitation with anular dilatation in the absence of tricuspid leaflet disease is generally described as "functional," but we consider that rheumatic anular disease is a crucial factor in initiating or aggravating the tricuspid anular dilatation [10]. This is analogous to the functional anatomy of rheumatic mitral regurgitation which will be discussed below.

Pathogenesis and Functional Pathology of Severe Mitral Regurgitation in Active Rheumatic Carditis

Our recent analysis [11] of 73 patients, aged 7–27 years, with severe mitral regurgitation and active rheumatic carditis who were subjected to surgery over a 2-year period has confirmed and clarified our concepts of the functional anatomy [9,12]. Relevant clinical, hemodynamic, and other data are summarized in Table 2.

Table 2. Clinical, radiologic, and hemodynamic data and operative procedure in 73 patients with severe mitral regurgitation and acute rheumatic carditis

Age (years)	Sex M/F	NYHA III/IV	Rhythm SR/AF	CTR (%)	Pressures[a] LA mean (mmHg)	LA "V" (mmHg)	LVED (mmHg)	Procedure MVR/repair
13 ± 3	25/48	47/26	69/4	65 ± 7	25 ± 8	48 ± 17	16 ± 8	39(16)[b]/34(2)[b]

[a] Recorded at operation.
[b] Concomitant aortic valve replacement for significant aortic regurgitation.
Values are mean ± SD. *AF*, atrial fibrillation; *CTR*, cardiothoracic ratio; *LA*, left atrial; *LVED*, left ventricular end diastolic; *MVR*, mitral valve replacement; *SR*, sinus rhythm.

The predominant features of pure rheumatic mitral regurgitation comprise marked anular dilatation, chordal lengthening, and prolapse of the anterior leaflet. It is essential to emphasize that we define mitral valve prolapse as failure of leaflet coaptation resulting in displacement of an involved leaflet's *edge* toward the left atrium [11,13,14]. This definition of mitral valve prolapse is in accord with the morphologic observations of the pathologists Becker and De Wit [15] as well as those during operation of Carpentier et al. [16] and Antunes et al. [17], which are crucial in assessment for a reconstructive procedure. The terms "billowing," "floppy," and "flail" also require definition in the context of correlating the clinical evaluation with mitral valve functional anatomy [13,14]. "Billowing," and in its more advanced form "floppy," are *anatomic* terms that describe the leaflet *bodies*. There is a gradation of mild billowing of the normal leaflet bodies toward the left atrium during ventricular systole to marked displacement when the leaflets are voluminous and the chordae elongated. A floppy mitral valve may remain functionally competent throughout systole. Prolapse, and its more advanced form flail, reflect failure of leaflet *edge* apposition and therefore essentially describe valve *function*. Although two-dimensional echocardiography is contributory in the evaluation of both the rheumatic and degenerative processes that may involve the complex mitral valve mechanism and result in functional prolapse, the echocardiographic appearances are essentially different (Fig. 2).

Of the 73 patients, 69 (94%) showed varying degrees of anterior mitral leaflet prolapse on two-dimensional echocardiography, and this finding was confirmed at surgery. Dilatation of the mitral anulus was noted at operation in 70 patients, all but two of whom had demonstrable prolapse of the anterior mitral leaflet. Moreover, the external diameters of prosthetic valves ($n = 39$) and Carpentier rings ($n = 34$) inserted at the time of surgery were 28 ± 2.0 mm and 32 ± 2 mm (mean $\pm$ SD), respectively, disproportionately large for the young age (mean 13 years) of the patients studied [9,18]. The maximal diameter of the mitral anulus was measured on echocardiography in 12 patients and was significantly greater ($p < 0.0001$) than that obtained for ten control subjects matched for age, mass, and body surface area (37 ± 4 mm vs. 23 ± 1.9 mm). In six patients, in whom precise measurements of anular circumferences were made at surgery, the derived mean anular diameter of 36 ± 3 mm was similar to that independently evaluated on two-dimensional echocardiography.

Marked elongation of the marginal ('strut') chordae tendineae attaching to the anterior mitral leaflet, associated with prolapse of the leaflet, was observed at operation in 66 of the 73 patients. Of the 34 patients who underwent mitral valve repair, 33 required shortening of chordae to the anterior mitral leaflet. Posterior leaflet chordal elongation was uncommon and was present in only three patients. Anterior leaflet chordal rupture was detected in five patients and was invariably associated with elongation of intact chordae to that leaflet, dilatation of the anulus, and mitral valve prolapse. The mean maximal systolic chordal length measured by preoperative two-dimensional echocardiography in six patients was significantly greater ($p < 0.01$) than that of five age-matched control subjects (23 ± 4 mm vs. 17 ± 1 mm). The mean intraoperative value for chordal length in these

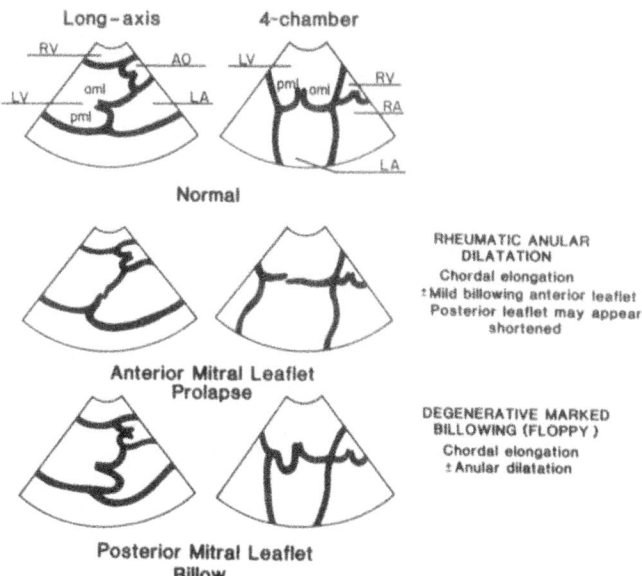

Fig. 2. Schematic two-dimensional echocardiographic appearance during systole of normal, prolapsed (rheumatic) and markedly billowing or floppy (degenerative) mitral valves in the parasternal long axis and apical 4-chamber views. In the normal valve the coaptation of the leaflets is readily apparent. In rheumatic mitral prolapse, the anulus is significantly dilated, and the free edge of the prolapsing anterior leaflet is displaced beyond the line of valve closure. In degenerative mitral billow, the body of the posterior leaflet bulges into the left atrium (*LA*), but the leaflet margins usually appear coapted. Principal functional anatomic features are listed on the *right. AO*, aorta; *LV*, left ventricle; *pml*, posterior mitral leaflet; *RA*, right atrium; *RV*, right ventricle; *aml*, anterior mitral leaflet

six patients was 23 ± 3 mm, similar to that measured by two-dimensional echocardiography.

Chordal elongation may result from primary involvement by the rheumatic inflammatory process or secondary exposure of the chordae to increased tensile stresses during ventricular systole, but it is probable that both primary and secondary factors play an important role. The rise in chordal tension in the normal mitral valve during ventricular systole is attenuated by the "keystone mechanism" whereby the pressure generated by left ventricular contraction is applied against opposite sides of the apposing mitral leaflets, forming a competent seal [19,20]. A normal valve leaflet:anular area ratio is essential for this mechanism to operate optimally [21]. Following anular dilatation, the area of apposition of the valve leaflets during ventricular systole is reduced, diminishing the keystone effect with resultant increase in chordal tension.

Scarring of the valve leaflets and commissural fusion were uncommon (16 of 73 patients) and mild. Although the leaflets are involved in active rheumatic carditis, the acute inflammatory change apparently has no important hemodynamic consequences during the active phase of the disease. The major structural changes in young patients with severe rheumatic mitral regurgitation and ongoing rheumatic activity involve the anulus and chordae. The functional consequence of these structural changes is mitral valve prolapse. Our recent data confirm that the majority (94%) of patients with severe mitral regurgitation due to active rheumatic carditis have readily demonstrable prolapse of the anterior leaflet. In the four patients in whom no obvious prolapse was demonstrated, mitral anular dilatation per se was probably the principal cause of the regurgitation [16], but some functional prolapse was presumably present (Fig. 3).

Figure 4 summarizes our concept of the evolution of severe pure mitral regurgitation in active rheumatic carditis. Acute rheumatic carditis causes inflammation of the connective tissue of the mitral apparatus, including the anulus, valve leaflets, and chordae tendineae (Fig. 4B). The inflamed anulus dilates, first diminishing (Fig. 4C) and later abolishing (Fig. 4D) the "keystone effect." Systolic tension along the length of the inflamed chordae rises, resulting in their elongation. Anular dilatation, chordal elongation, and possibly the leaflet inflammation act together to produce mitral valve prolapse and hemodynamically significant regurgitation (Fig. 4D). Because of the mitral regurgitation, the left atrium enlarges, dilating the anulus further (Fig. 4E) and perpetuating a vicious cycle [9,22]. The devastating clinical consequences of this cascade of events continue to manifest themselves in underdeveloped countries where rheumatic fever remains a major cause of morbidity and mortality [2,9,23]. Reasons for this accelerated or "malignant" form of rheumatic heart disease in Third World populations are unclear. The fact that such patients invariably show

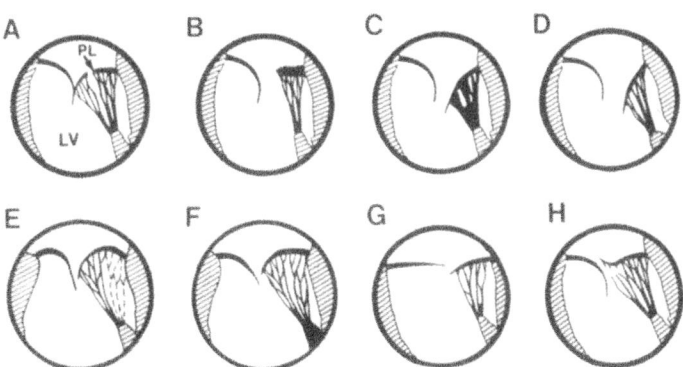

Fig. 3A-H. Mechanisms by which the mitral valve becomes incompetent. Some possible causes are: **A** perforation or cleft in a leaflet; **B** a scarred and shortened leaflet due to chronic rheumatic carditis or mitral anular calcification; **C** a retracted and tethered leaflet, the result of shortened chordae tendineae in chronic rheumatic carditis; **D** a leaflet that does not appose because the papillary muscle is retracted by a left ventricular aneurysm; **E** primary "degeneration" of mitral valve mechanism resulting in leaflet billowing, lengthened chordae tendineae, anular dilatation, and failure of leaflet edge apposition (prolapse); **F** failure of leaflet apposition due to papillary muscle dysfunction secondary to occlusive coronary artery disease; **G** marked anular dilatation causing anterior leaflet prolapse in acute rheumatic carditis; **H** flail leaflet with ruptured chordae – causes include infective endocarditis, "idiopathic rupture," and trauma. *PL*, posterior leaflet

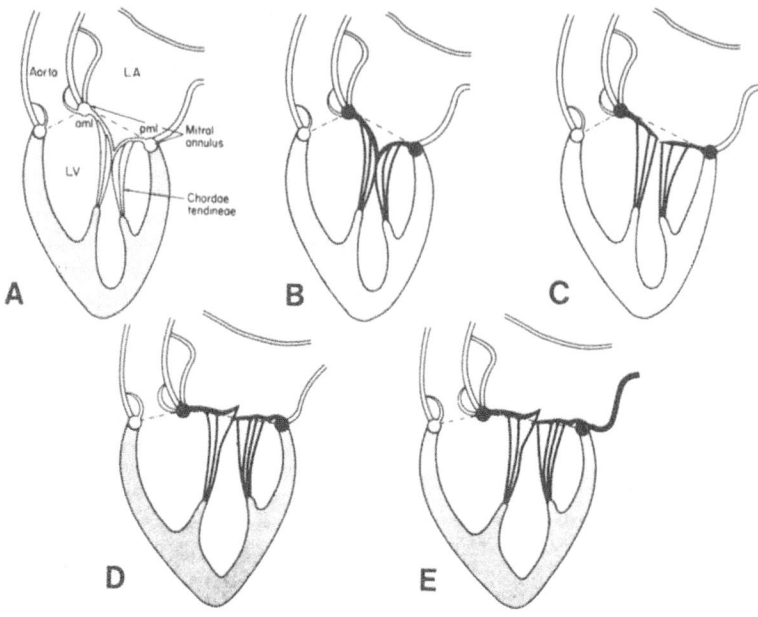

Fig. 4. A-E Evolution of pure mitral regurgitation in severe active rheumatic carditis. **A** Normal mitral valve; **B** components of the mitral apparatus principally affected. For full description, see text

histologic evidence of chronic rheumatic activity in addition to active carditis suggests that the severe hemodynamic lesion is seldom or never the result of a single attack, but rather of repeated episodes [11]. Reasons for such recurrences are environmental but include the potentially avoidable contributory factors of inadequate penicillin prophylaxis [24] and ongoing physical activity [9,11], both of which are discussed later.

Heart Failure and Severe Active Rheumatic Carditis

It is important to emphasize that left or right ventricular failure never results from active rheumatic carditis in the *absence* of a hemodynamically severe valvular lesion. We are uncertain of the cause or the role of the myocardial component referred to by Stollerman [25] as "toxic rheumatic myocarditis" but reiterate that, unlike viral myocarditis, it never by itself causes ventricular dilatation or heart failure. By far the most prevalent valve lesion encountered in patients in heart failure with active rheumatic carditis is mitral regurgitation. When depressed left ventricular function is associated [9], we are uncertain whether this is due to "rheumatic myocarditis" or is the consequence of work overload produced by the severe regurgitation. Evaluation of the "myocardial factor" in active rheumatic carditis requires clarification and is the subject of an ongoing study in our department.

Because "heart failure" associated with fulminant active rheumatic carditis principally results from a hemodynamically severe valve lesion, usually mitral regurgitation, the term is difficult to define in this context. An appropriate definition would be "an inadequate circulation at rest together with a raised pulmonary venous pressure, with or without high systemic venous pressure, in the absence of hemodynamically significant tricuspid valve disease or pericardial effusion." Although this definition does not clarify "inadequate circulation," a raised left ventricular end diastolic pressure has been encountered in most cases in which pressures were recorded, whether at cardiac catheterization or during operation (Table 2). Medical management of such cases is of limited value but requires brief consideration:

1. Antibiotic Therapy. This is mandatory and we use intramuscular benzathine penicillin G in a dose of 1 200 000 units (600 000 for children weighing < 30 kg) administered at 3–4-week intervals, or oral penicillin in a dose of at least 250 mg twice daily.

2. Salicylate, Steroid, and Other Medical Therapy. Salicylates are used by us for symptomatic relief of arthralgia, arthritis, or severe pericardial pain. Contrary to the conclusions of Czoniczer et al. [26], and which became accepted doctrine [27,28], steroids are never a "life-saving" measure in patients who have severe active rheumatic carditis with heart failure and are therefore in danger of dying. Steroids may make the tissues more friable and the task of the surgeon more difficult. We have encountered a number of patients with fulminating rheumatic carditis and severe regurgitant valve lesions who have been treated with steroids [9] but have yet to observe improvement of the heart failure on such therapy!

We seldom use digitalis unless atrial fibrillation is present (5% of patients) [11]. Diuretic and vasodilator therapy, including angiotensin-converting enzyme inhibitors, cause temporary symptomatic improvement, mainly by decreasing pulmonary venous pressure, but clinical evidence of rheumatic activity and of heart failure invariably persist.

Pathogenesis, Prevention, and Management of Fulminant Rheumatic Carditis with Severe Mitral Regurgitation and Heart Failure

It is relevant to discuss the early course of active rheumatic carditis and our concept of its progression with inappropriate management (Fig. 5). A first or early attack of active rheumatic carditis may cause mild mitral regurgitation which is probably due to the failure of normal anular contraction [29], and which we originally called "anular dysfunction" [30]. If the patient remains sedentary at this stage and penicillin is administered, the rheumatic activity abates, and the mitral regurgitation diminishes or disappears [9,31,32]. Should the patient continue to exercise and not receive or not comply with penicillin therapy, rheumatic activity

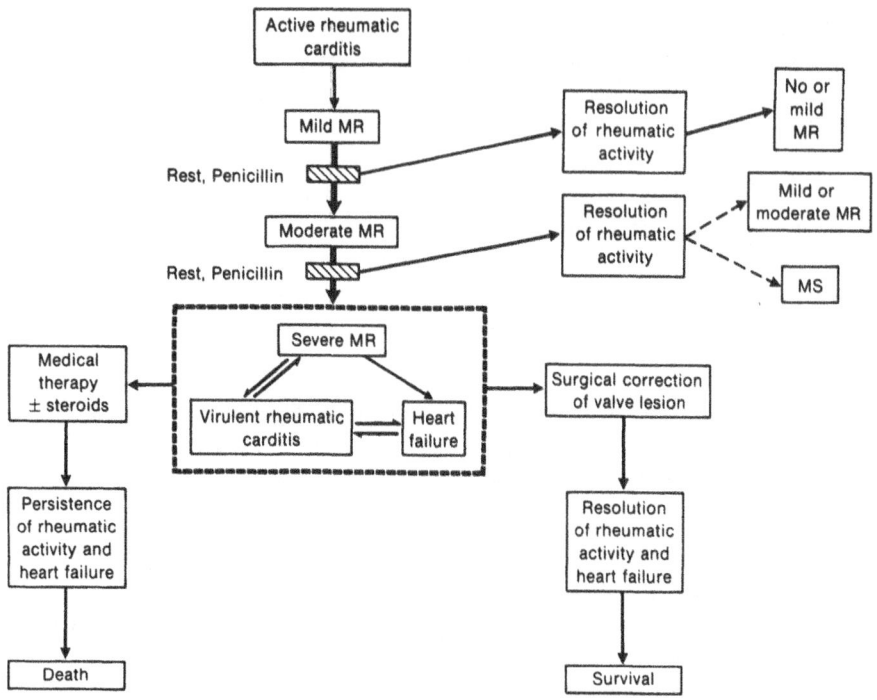

Fig. 5. Progression of untreated mild rheumatic mitral regurgitation to virulent carditis, severe regurgitation, and heart failure. Alternate pathways to death (medical therapy) or survival with resolution of rheumatic activity (surgical correction of valve lesion) are illustrated. Appropriate treatment with penicillin and rest at an early stage, together with long-term penicillin prophylaxis, avoid this disastrous sequence. *MR*, mitral regurgitation; *MS*, mitral stenosis. For details, see text

continues and moderate mitral regurgitation ensues. Even at this stage, rest and penicillin therapy will usually eliminate the rheumatic activity and reduce the mitral regurgitation. While it is possible that steroid therapy may contribute at that time to improvement of rheumatic activity, this has not been well substantiated. It is almost certain, however, that many of these patients subsequently have scarring of leaflets and commissures with resultant mitral stenosis. When patients with moderate mitral regurgitation and active carditis are still not treated with penicillin, the rheumatic process continues and severe mitral regurgitation supervenes. There is then a formidable hemodynamic overload which sometimes aggravates the rheumatic activity and may initiate virulent rheumatic carditis[9]. A vicious cycle is now established, and heart failure results. The sole effective management of patients with cardiac failure and active rheumatic carditis is surgical. Neither the rheumatic activity nor the cardiac failure will respond satisfactorily to steroid or other medical therapy. Surgery should not be delayed [33] and, in our experience [9,18,34], at least 90% of patients survive surgery. The rheumatic activity abates dramatically during the first few weeks of the postoperative period. We conclude that a principal factor predisposing to postoperative resolution of rheumatic activity is the removal of the cardiac workload by correction of the valve lesion. This concept is in accord with observations [35,36] prior to the antibiotic era that manifestations of acute rheumatic fever receded more rapidly with bed-rest. The excessive workload on the heart of a patient with severe rheumatic mitral regurgitation produces an analogous situation to that of a patient with active carditis and a mild valve lesion being forced to exercise continuously.

Finally, it cannot be too strongly emphasized that in active rheumatic carditis and heart failure, death is due to the heart failure. Whether or not rheumatic myocarditis is a contributory factor, the heart failure is predominantly or entirely a sequel of the severe mitral regurgitation or other hemodynamically significant valve lesion! Treatment is surgical correction of the valve lesion and medical therapy should not be unduly prolonged.

References

1. Padmavati S (1978) Rheumatic fever and rheumatic heart disease in developing countries. Bull WHO 56(4):543-550
2. McLaren MJ, Hawkins DM, Koornhof HJ, Bloom KR, Bramwell-Jones DM, Cohen E, Gale GE, Kanarek K, Lachman AS, Lakier JB, Pocock WA, Barlow JB (1975) Epidemiology of rheumatic heart disease in black school children of Soweto, Johannesburg. Br Med J 3:474-478
3. Glover JA (1930) Incidence of rheumatic diseases. Lancet 1:499-505
4. Devaux P (1979) Some aspects of rheumatic fever in Soweto. The Leech 49:67-68
5. Ransome OJ, Roode H, Spector I, Reinach SG (1983) Pharyngeal carriage of group A beta-haemolytic streptococci in Coloured and Indian schoolchildren. S Afr Med J 64:779-781
6. Aryanpur-Kashani I (1980) On rheumatic fever in children (letter to editor). Am Heart J 100:942-943
7. Veasy LG, Wiedmeier SE, Orsmond GS, Ruttenberg HD, Boucek MM, Roth SJ, Tait VF, Thompson JA, Daly JA, Kaplan EL, Hill HR (1987) Resurgence of acute rheumatic fever in the intermountain area of the United States. N Engl J Med 316:421-427
8. Kaplan EL, Markowitz M (1988) The fall and rise of rheumatic fever in the United States: a commentary. Int J Cardiol 21:3-10
9. Barlow JB, Kinsley RH, Pocock WA (1987) Rheumatic fever and rheumatic heart disease. In: Barlow JB Perspectives on the mitral valve. Davis, Philadelphia, pp 227-245
10. Barlow JB, Pocock WA, Antunes MJ, Sareli P, Meyer TE (1987) Surgical aspects of mitral valve disease. In: Barlow JB Perspectives on the mitral valve. Davis, Philadelphia, pp 281-282
11. Marcus RH, Sareli P, Pocock WA, Meyer TE, Magalhaes MP, Grieve T, Antunes MJ, Barlow JB (1989) Functional anatomy of severe mitral regurgitation in active rheumatic carditis. Am J Cardiol 63:577-584
12. Marcus R, Sareli P, Antunes M, Magalhaes M, Meyer T, Grieve T, Barlow J (1986) Functional pathology of mitral regurgitation in active rheumatic carditis – surgical and echocardiographic observations (abstract). J Am Coll Cardiol 7:8A
13. Barlow JB, Pocock WA (1985) Billowing, floppy, prolapsed or flail mitral valves? Am J Cardiol 55:501-502
14. Barlow JB, Pocock WA (1988) Mitral valve billowing and prolapse: perspective at 25 years. Herz 13:227-234
15. Becker AE, De Wit APM (1979) Mitral valve apparatus. A spectrum of normality relevant to mitral valve prolapse. Br Heart J 42:680-689
16. Carpentier A, Lessana A, D'Allaines C, Blondeau P, Piwnica A, Dubost C (1980) Reconstructive surgery of mitral valve incompetence. J Thorac Cardiovasc Surg 79:338-348
17. Antunes MJ, Magalhaes MP, Colsen PR, Kinsley RH (1987) Valvuloplasty for rheumatic mitral valve disease. A surgical challenge. J Thorac Cardiovasc Surg 94:44-56

18. Kinsley RH, Girdwood RW, Milner S (1981) Surgical treatment during the acute phase of rheumatic carditis. In: Nyhus LM (ed) Surgery annual, vol 13. Appleton Century Crofts, East Norwalk, pp 299–323
19. Salisbury PF, Cross CE, Rieben P (1963) Chorda tendineae tension. Am J Physiol 205:385–392
20. Cobbs BW (1974) Clinical recognition and medical management of rheumatic heart disease and other acquired valvular disease. In: Hurst JW, Logue RB, Schlant RC, Wenger NK (eds) The heart. McGraw-Hill, New York, p 862
21. Brock RC (1952) The surgical and pathologic anatomy of the mitral valve. Br Heart J 14:489–513
22. Levy MJ, Edwards JE (1962) Anatomy of mitral insufficiency. Prog Cardiovasc Dis 5:119–144
23. Agarwal BL (1981) Rheumatic heart disease unabated in developing countries. Lancet I:910–911
24. Dajani AS, Bisno AL, Chung KJ, Durack DT, Gerber MA, Kaplan EL, Millard HD, Randolph MF, Shulman ST, Watanakunakorn C (1988) Prevention of rheumatic fever. A statement for health professionals by the Committee on Rheumatic Fever, Endocarditis, and Kawasaki Disease of the Council on Cardiovascular Disease in the Young, the American Heart Association. Circulation 78:1082–1086
25. Stollerman GH (1975) The pathology of rheumatic fever. In: Rheumatic fever and streptococcal infection. Grune and Stratton, New York, pp 127–131
26. Czoniczer G, Amezcua F, Pelargonio S, Massell BF (1964) Therapy of severe rheumatic carditis. Comparison of adrenocortical steroids and aspirin. Circulation 29:813–819
27. Sukumar IP (1987) Acute and chronic rheumatic heart disease. In: Anderson RH, Macartney FJ, Shinebourne EA, Tynan M (eds) Paediatric cardiology. Churchill Livingstone, London, p 1193
28. Bland EF (1987) Rheumatic fever: the way it was. Circulation 76:1190–1195
29. Barlow JB, Antunes MJ (1987) Functional anatomy of the mitral valve. In: Barlow JB Perspectives on the mitral valve. Davis, Philadelphia, pp 11–12
30. Barlow JB, Pocock WA (1975) The problem of nonejection systolic clicks and associated mitral systolic murmurs: emphasis on the billowing mitral leaflet syndrome. Am Heart J 90:636–655
31. Tompkins DG, Boxerbaum B, Liebman J (1972) Long-term prognosis of rheumatic fever patients receiving regular intramuscular benzathine penicillin. Circulation 45:543–551
32. Sanyal SK, Berry AM, Duggal S, Hooja V, Ghosh S (1982) Sequelae of the initial attack of acute rheumatic fever in children from North India. A prospective 5-year follow-up study. Circulation 65:375–379
33. Lewis BS, Geft IL, Milo S, Gotsman MS (1979) Echocardiography and valve replacement in the critically ill patient with acute rheumatic carditis. Ann Thorac Surg 27:529–535
34. Magalhaes M, Antunes M, Marcus R, Sareli P, Meyer T, Grieve T, Barlow J (1986) The role of surgery in acute rheumatic valvulitis – a 2 year experience of 70 cases. Abstract of the X World Congress of Cardiology, Washington 1986, 115
35. Miller R (1937) Rheumatic heart disease in children. In: Rolleston H (ed) The British encylopaedia of medical practice, vol 6. Butterworth, London, p 250
36. Bywaters EGL (1950) The general management of rheumatic fever. Proc R Soc Med 43:199–206

Morphometric Structure
of the Failing Left Ventricular Myocardium
in Aortic Valve Disease
Before and After Valve Replacement*

H.P. Krayenbühl, O.M. Hess, E.S. Monrad, J. Schneider, G. Mall, and M. Turina

Chronic pressure and/or volume overload in aortic valve disease is associated with marked left ventricular angiographic [1-3] as well as cellular hypertrophy [4,5]. This process of secondary hypertrophy is accompanied by an increase in interstitial tissue. Are the microscopic alterations different in patients with preserved and depressed left ventricular function? Comparing intraoperative transmural biopsies from patients with compensated and decompensated aortic stenosis, Schwarz et al. [6] found a reduced volume fraction of myofibrils in those with depressed left ventricular function. In patients with aortic insufficiency and a massively impaired left ventricular ejection fraction of 32%, volume fraction of myofibrils was smaller and muscle fiber diameter larger than in patients with aortic insufficiency and only a moderately depressed ejection fraction of 48% [7]. The purpose of the present study was to evaluate left ventricular morphometric structure from endomyocardial biopsies in patients with aortic valve disease with compensated and failing left ventricles and to report changes of morphometric variables at an intermediate time after aortic valve replacement.

Patients and Methods

A total of 49 patients with pure or predominant aortic stenosis (AS) and 35 patients with aortic insufficiency (AI) were studied hemodynamically prior to surgery. Left ventricular cineangiography and endomyocardial biopsies using a transseptal technique were performed [5]. Coronary arteriography was carried out in all patients with aortic stenosis and in those with aortic insufficiency who were older than 37 years. In none of these patients was coronary artery narrowing of more than wall irregularities present. The patients were divided into two groups. In group 1 with left ventricular failure there were 15 patients with AS and 17 with AI. Left ventricular failure was said to be present when ejection fraction (EF) was < 57% and either cardiac index (CI) was < 2.5 L/min/m² and/or left ventricular end-diastolic pressure (LVEDP) was > 20 mmHg. In the nonfailing group (group 2) there were 34 patients with AS and 18 with AI. In these patients EF was ⩾ 57%, CI ⩾ 2.5 L/min/m² and LVEDP ⩽ 20 mmHg. Eleven patients in group 1

*This work was supported by a grant from the Swiss National Science Foundation.

B.S. Lewis, A. Kimchi (Eds.)
Heart Failure Mechanisms and Management
© Springer-Verlag Berlin Heidelberg 1991

and 19 in group 2 were recatheterized 22.5 and 24.0 months, respectively, after successful aortic valve replacement.

Left ventricular quantitative angiography and assessment of angiographic muscle mass was carried out as reported previously [5]. Morphometric evaluation of left ventricular endomyocardial biopsies included the determination of muscle fiber diameter (MFD), percentage interstitial fibrosis (IF), volume fraction of myofibrils (VFM), and the calculation of left ventricular fibrous content (FC) [5].

Results

Because left ventricular morphometric structure was not different between patients with aortic stenosis and aortic insufficiency in both the failing and the nonfailing group, only the pooled data of group 1 and group 2 are reported. Patients in group 1 were older than patients in group 2 (55.7 versus 48.2 years, $P < 0.02$). Figure 1 shows EF, CI, and LVEDP in groups 1 and 2. Left ventricular muscle mass index (LMMI) was 234 g/m² in group 1 and 161 g/m² in group 2 ($P < 0.001$, Fig. 1). MFD amounted to 32.4 μ in group 1 and 29.6 μ in group 2 ($P < 0.02$). IF and VFM did not differ in the two groups (Fig. 2). FC was 49.9 g/m² in group 1 and 30.6 g/m² in group 2 ($P < 0.001$). The increased FC in group 1 was due to the larger LMMI in group 1 as compared to that in group 2.

After valve replacement in group 1, EF increased from 44% to 59% ($P < 0.005$), and LVEDP decreased from 26.3 to 11.0 mmHg ($P < 0.001$) (Fig. 3). CI increased slightly but not significantly. LMMI decreased markedly from 236 to 146 g/m² ($P < 0.001$). MFD decreased in group 1 from 34.4 to 29.6 μ ($P < 0.001$), whereas IF, VFM, and FC did not change significantly after valve replacement (Fig. 4).

In the patients with a nonfailing left ventricle prior to surgery (group 2), EF and CI did not change postoperatively (Fig. 5). LVEDP decreased from 13.7 to 9.2 mmHg ($P < 0.001$) and LMMI from 162 to 103 g/m² ($P < 0.001$) (Fig. 5). MFD decreased from 29.4 to 26.9 μ ($P < 0.025$), and IF increased from 19.7% to 23.5% ($P < 0.05$) (Fig. 6). VPM did not change, whereas there was a decrease of fibrous content from 32.6 to 24.7 g/m² ($P < 0.05$).

Figure 7 depicts the hemodynamics in the two groups at postoperative catheterization. EF, CI, and LVEDP did not differ. LMMI was, however, still significantly larger in group 1 than in group 2 ($P < 0.01$). Similarly, cellular hypertrophy as evaluated from MFD was greater ($P < 0.05$) in group 1 than in group 2 (Fig. 8). At the postoperative study there was no difference between group 1 and group 2 with respect to EF, VFM, IF, and FC.

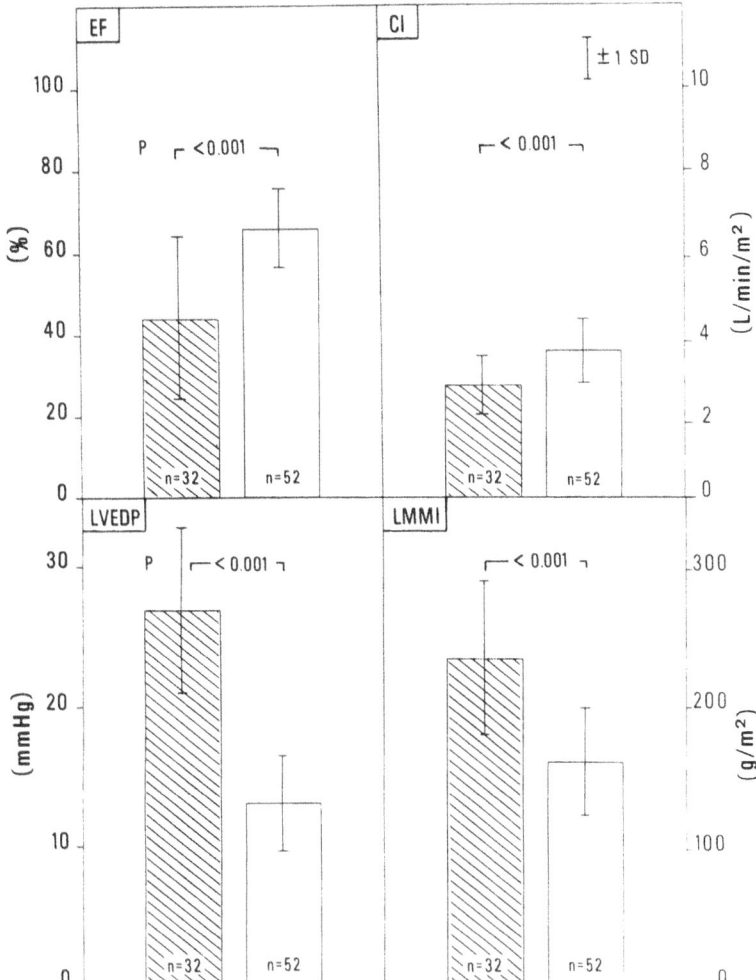

Fig. 1. Preoperative hemodynamic data in aortic valve disease. *Hatched columns*, group 1: failing left ventricle; *open columns*, group 2: nonfailing left ventricle. *EF*, left ventricular ejection fraction; *CI*, cardiac index; *LVEDP*, left ventricular end-diastolic pressure; *LMMI*, left ventricular muscle mass index. *P* values were obtained by the unpaired Student's *t* test

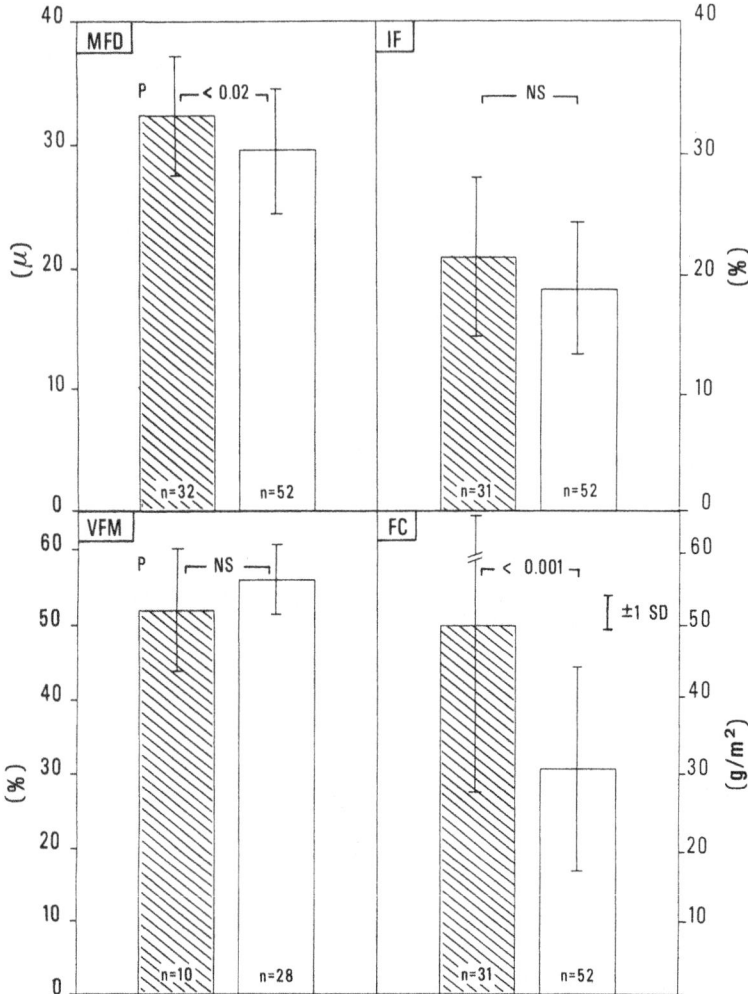

Fig. 2. Preoperative morphometric data in patients with aortic valve disease. *Hatched columns*, group 1: failing left ventricle; *open columns*, group 2: nonfailing left ventricle. *MFD*, muscle fiber diameter; *IF*, percentage interstitial fibrosis; *VFM*, volume fraction of myofibrils; *FC* left ventricular fibrous content (LMMI × IF/100). The P values were obtained by the unpaired Student's *t* test

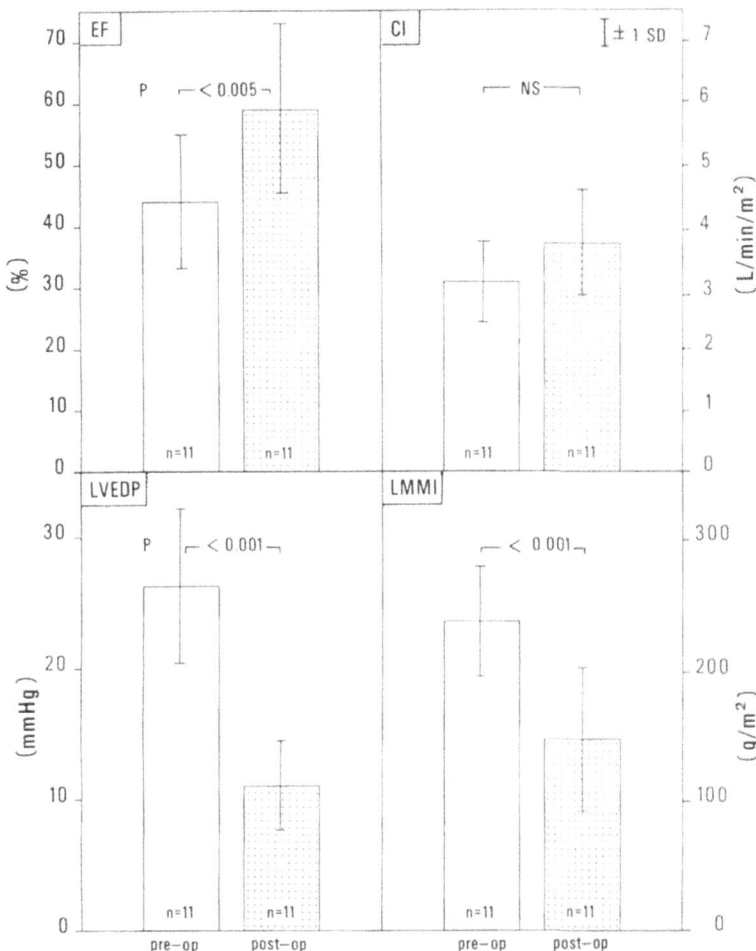

Fig. 3. Pre- (*open columns*) and 22.5-month postoperative (*dotted columns*) hemodynamic data in a subset of patients with aortic valve disease who had preoperative left ventricular failure. Abbreviations as in Fig. 1. The P values were obtained by the paired Student's *t* test

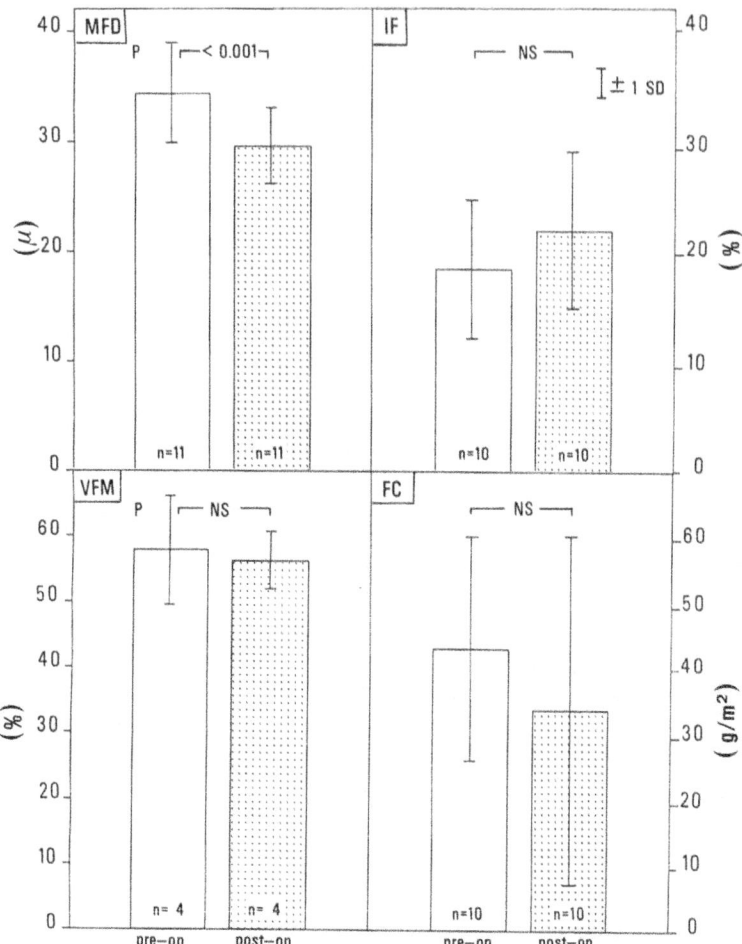

Fig. 4. Pre- (*open columns*) and 22.5-month postoperative (*dotted columns*) morphometric data in a subset of patients with aortic valve disease who had preoperative left ventricular failure. The abbreviations are the same as in Fig. 2. The *P* values were obtained by the paired Student's *t* test

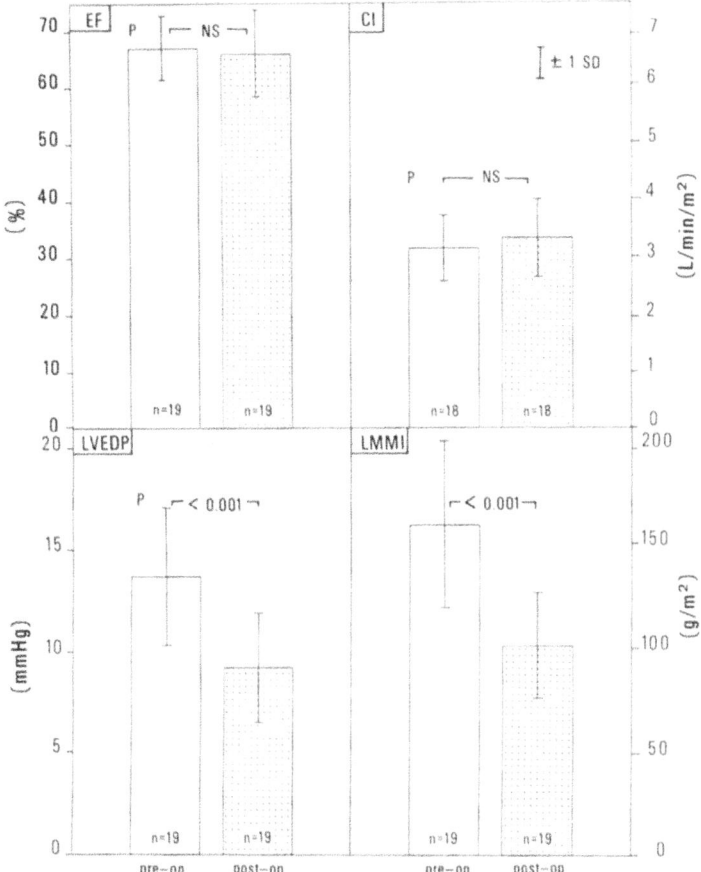

Fig. 5. Pre- (*open columns*) and 24-month postoperative (*dotted columns*) hemodynamic data in a subset of patients with aortic valve disease and preoperative nonfailing left ventricle. The abbreviations are the same as in Fig. 1. The *P* values were obtained by the paired Student's *t* test

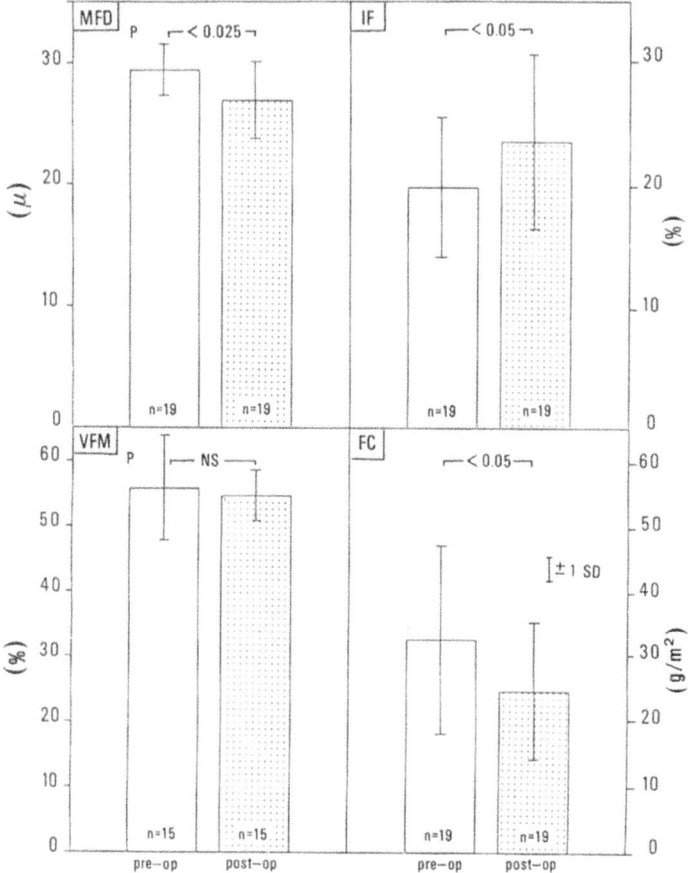

Fig. 6. Pre- (*open columns*) and 24-month postoperative (*dotted columns*) morphometric data in a subset of patients with aortic valve disease and preoperative nonfailing left ventricle. The abbreviations are the same as in Fig. 2. The *P* values were obtained by the paired Student's *t* test

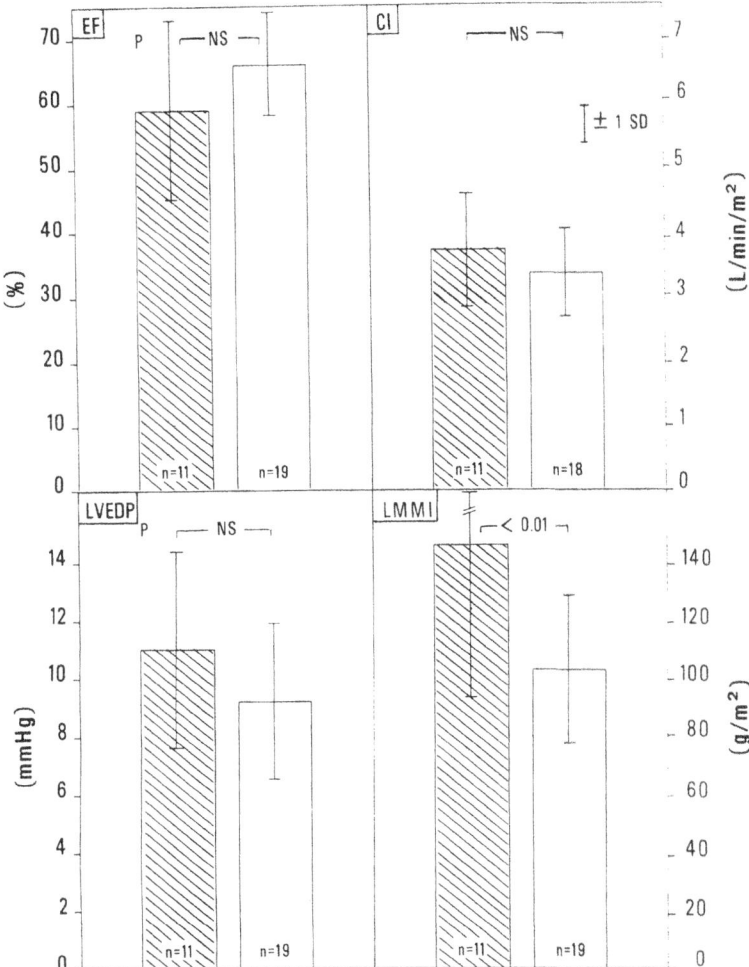

Fig. 7. Hemodynamic data at postoperative (22.5 and 24 months) catheterization in patients with aortic valve disease who had a failing (group 1. *hatched columns*) or a nonfailing (group 2. *open columns*) left ventricle at the preoperative study. Abbreviations as in Fig. 1. The *P* values were obtained by the unpaired Student's *t* test

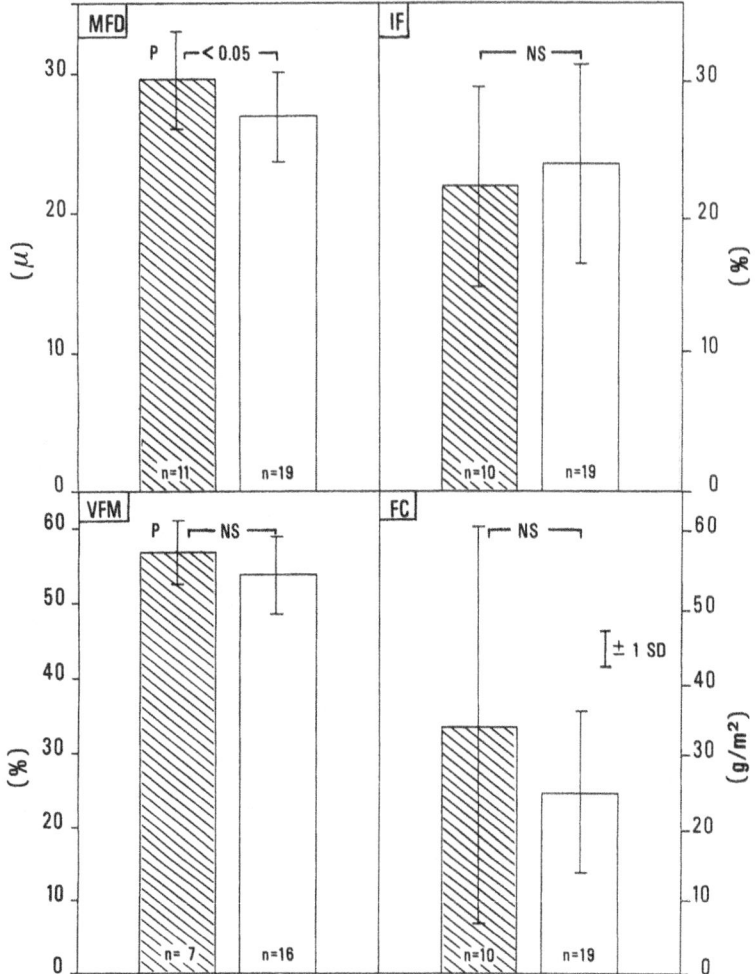

Fig. 8. Postoperative (22.5 and 24 months) morphometric data in patients with aortic valve disease who had a failing (group 1, *hatched columns*) or a nonfailing (group 2, *open columns*) left ventricle at the preoperative study. Abbreviations as in Fig. 2. The *P* values were obtained by the unpaired Student's *t* test

Discussion

In patients with aortic valve disease and hemodynamically defined left ventricular failure, macroscopic and microscopic hypertrophy is more marked than in patients with compensated left ventricular function. Left ventricular pump function was not related to percentage interstitial fibrosis. This observation is in agreement with the findings of others in aortic stenosis [6] and aortic insufficiency [7]. In contrast to these authors [6,7], volume fraction of myofibrils was not depressed in our patients with left ventricular failure. The reason for this discrepancy is not clear but might be related to patient selection. It should be noted that the patients of Perennec et al. [7] who had aortic insufficiency and an unfavorable postoperative outcome were in a more advanced stage of left ventricular dysfunction, their ejection fraction being only 32%. Because in our patients with preoperatively depressed left ventricular function but no intracellular depletion of myofibrils there was postoperative restoration of ejection fraction in contrast to those of Perennec et al. [7], one might speculate whether the reduction of volume fraction of myofibrils represents a stage of no recuperable contractile dysfunction. On the other hand, it is evident from our study that reduction of volume fraction of myofibrils is not a prerequisite for some milder form of hemodynamic left ventricular failure. In these instances a functional rather than an anatomical derangement of the myofibrils is likely to be the origin of left ventricular dysfunction. Finally, this investigation emphasizes that there is residual macroscopic and microscopic left ventricular hypertrophy 2 years after aortic valve replacement. This residual hypertrophy is more marked in patients who have preoperative left ventricular failure.

References

1. Gould KL, Kennedy JW, Frimer M, Pollack GH, Dodge HT (1976) Analysis of wall dynamics and directional components of left ventricular contraction in man. Am J Cardiol 38:322-331
2. Gunther S, Grossman W (1979) Determinants of ventricular function in pressure-overload hypertrophy in man. Circulation 59:679-688
3. Herreman F, Ameur A, De Vernejoul F, Bourgin JG, Gueret P, Guerin F, Degeorges M (1979) Pre- and post-operative hemodynamic and cineangiographic assessment of left ventricular function in patients with aortic regurgitation. Am Heart J 98:63-72
4. Schaper J, Schwarz F, Hehrlein F (1981) Ultrastructural changes in human myocardium with hypertrophy due to aortic valve disease and their relationship to left ventricular mass and ejection fraction. Herz 6:217-225
5. Hess OM, Ritter M, Schneider J, Grimm J, Turina M, Krayenbuehl HP (1984) Diastolic stiffness and myocardial structure in aortic valve disease before and after valve replacement. Circulation 69:855-865
6. Schwarz F, Schaper J, Kittstein D, Flameng W, Walter P, Schaper W (1981) Reduced volume fraction of myofibrils in myocardium of patients with decompensated pressure overload. Circulation 63:1299-1304
7. Perennec J, Herreman F, Cosma H, Ilers F, Djigouadi Z, Degeorges M, Hatt PY (1988) Relationship of myocardial morphometry in aortic valve regurgitation to myocardial function and post-operative results. Basic Res Cardiol 83:10-23

Heart Failure in Patients with Valve Disease: The Timing of Valve Replacement

J.S. Alpert, J.R. Benotti, and I.S. Ockene

Timing of valve replacement has traditionally been linked with the development of heart failure or symptoms resulting from pathophysiologic sequences resembling heart failure [1,2]. Almost 30 years after the first valve replacement, patients with aortic, mitral, or tricuspid valve *stenosis* receive prosthetic valves primarily to relieve symptoms associated with pulmonary and/or systemic venous congestion. Only patients with aortic stenosis have actual left ventricular dysfunction as the cause of these symptoms. Individuals with mitral and tricuspid stenosis usually develop pulmonary and systemic venous congestion, respectively, despite normal left and right ventricular function.

Thus, the end-points for recommending mitral, aortic, or tricuspid valve stenosis are usually straightforward and clearcut; these indications often involve symptoms of pulmonary or systemic venous congestions. Unfortunately, indications for valve replacement are often not as obvious in patients with valvular regurgitation.

Aortic Regurgitation

Two dinstinct clinical syndromes of aortic regurgitation exist, i.e., acute and chronic. Acute aortic regurgitation (AAR) is often the result of endocarditis, dissection, or traumatic injury to the valve itself. Patients with AAR often present with symptoms of severe left ventricular failure: marked dyspnea and even pulmonary edema. These symptoms develop rapidly over hours or days. The diagnosis may not be suspected initially because of the absence of the usual peripheral manifestations of chronic aortic regurgitation (CAR), i.e., bounding arterial pulses with rapid upstroke and fall-off. Often the murmur of AAR is short and early diastolic in location. It may be overlooked if the patient is tachypneic or suffering from pulmonary edema. Echocardiography with Doppler often characterizes the lesion with considerable accuracy.

Management of these patients usually occurs in an intensive care unit since they are often quite unstable. Initially, individuals are managed medically with diuretics, supplemental inspiratory oxygen, vasodilation, and positive inotropes, e.g., nitroprusside and dobutamine or amrinone [3-5]. Hemodynamic monitoring may be required. If the patient is exceedingly unstable, urgent aortic valve replacement may be necessary [6,7]. A minority of patients become stable during

B.S. Lewis, A. Kimchi (Eds.)
Heart Failure Mechanisms and Management
© Springer-Verlag Berlin Heidelberg 1991

intravenous vasodilator and positive inotropic therapy. A trial of oral medications is warranted in these individuals, e.g., an ACE inhibitor such as captopril or enalapril combined with digoxin. Patients with AAR who respond to oral medication should be followed closely with careful attention to clinical and echocardiographic signs of left ventricular decompensation. Elective but urgent aortic valve replacement may be required in these individuals [8].

Patients with CAR present a different challenge for the clinician compared with the hectic, often stormy course of AAR. Individuals with CAR remain stable for decades without developing signs and symptoms of left ventricular failure. The diagnosis is usually made quite easily even by inexperienced clinicians who recognize the bounding peripheral pulses, the enlarged left ventricle, and the easily audible diastolic murmur. The difficulty in managing patients with CAR involves the decision concerning aortic valve replacement. Indeed, the appropriate timing of aortic valve replacement in patients with CAR is one of the most difficult clinical problems of modern cardiology [9].

Objective manifestations of left ventricular failure can often be demonstrated at cardiac catheterization in patients who are asymptomatic. Indeed, such patients may remain clinically stable for years despite having a severe hemodynamic abnormality [10]. This paradoxical situation has resulted in controversy among cardiologists concerning the timing of surgical therapy (aortic valve replacement) in patients with aortic regurgitation. On the one hand, irreversible left ventricular dysfunction can develop that persists despite successful aortic valve replacement [11]. Indeed, patients whose heart size, measured by roentgenography, fails to decrease during the first 6 months after operation face a 57% 6-year mortality, as opposed to a 15% 6-year mortality in those whose heart size decreases [12]. This implies that irreversible left ventricular dysfunction adversely affects survival after successful aortic valve replacement. On the other hand, recent results of aortic valve replacement in patients with aortic regurgitation and severe left ventricular dysfunction are not as discouraging as they once were [13,14]. Prosthetic heart valves and cardiac surgery with cardiopulmonary bypass can, however, entail significant complications, mortality, or both.

The long-term prognosis is poor in patients with aortic regurgitation and electrocardiographic evidence of left ventricular hypertrophy with ST-T changes. Long-term prognosis is similarly impaired in patients with markedly dilated, hypocontractile left ventricles secondary to long-standing aortic regurgitation [15–20]. These individuals have left ventricles with markedly increased end-diastolic and end-systolic volumes, reduced regurgitant volume to end-diastolic volume ratios, and inappropriately elevated mean and end-systolic wall stress [16–20].

These findings have led a number of investigators to advise cardiac catheterization in these patients, with aortic valve replacement to follow for patients demonstrating left ventricular dysfunction even in the absence of symptoms [15–20]. Prospective studies to support such arguments are lacking although the reasoning and conclusions that have led to these recommendations seem quite reasonable. On the other side of this debate are a number of reports confirming excellent long-term results in patients who undergo aortic valve replacement

even after severe, symptomatic, left ventricular dysfunction has developed
[21–23].

Medical therapy can lead to markedly improved ventricular function in
patients with CAR. For example, afterload reduction therapy with intravenous
nitroprusside can result in improvement in left ventricular function with reduced
aortic regurgitant fraction in patients with CAR. This had led some authorities to
advocate the long-term use of afterload-reducing agents in patients with early
evidence of left ventricular dysfunction secondary to aortic incompetence.

Clearly, there is no consensus among cardiologists concerning the optimal
timing of aortic valve replacement in patients with severe aortic regurgitation. If
valve replacement carried little or no short- or long-term morbidity or mortality,
the decision for aortic valve replacement would be straightforward: any person
with severe aortic incompetence, regardless of symptoms or the state of left
ventricular function, would undergo aortic valve replacement. Unfortunately,
valve prostheses are not perfect, and aortic valve replacement carries a surgical
mortality of approximately 5%.

The following protocol is suggested as one approach to the management of
patients with aortic insufficiency:

1. Patients with mild or moderate insufficiency should be followed at 6–12-
    month intervals, and an ECG and chest roentgenogram should be obtained
    every 1–2 years. Echocardiographic or radionuclear determination of left
    ventricular function are not absolutely necessary but may be obtained at
    intervals of approximately 5 years. If deterioration occurs in left ventricular
    function, catheterization should be performed to assess the severity and
    consequences of aortic regurgitation.
2. Asymptomatic persons with moderately severe or severe aortic insufficiency
    should be followed at 3–6-month intervals with an ECG, chest roentgeno-
    gram, and echocardiographic or radionuclear determination of left ven-
    tricular function performed each year. Patients with the electrocardiographic
    pattern of "diastolic overload" left ventricular hypertrophy (no ST-T
    changes) should be observed closely. Patients with the electrocardiographic
    pattern of "systolic overload" left ventricular hypertrophy (ST-T changes
    present) should undergo cardiac catheterization for assessment of the
    severity and consequences of aortic regurgitation. Patients in whom symp-
    toms develop (chest discomfort suggestive of angina pectoris, left ventricular
    failure) or patients who demonstrate deterioration of left ventricular function
    by echocardiography or radionuclear ventriculography should also be
    referred for cardiac catheterization.
3. Cardiac catheterization should confirm the presence of moderately severe to
    severe aortic regurgitation, determine the state of left ventricular function,
    and ascertain the presence of associated lesions (mitral valve disease, co-
    ronary artery disease). Patients with markedly abnormal left ventricular
    function (biplane ejection fraction < 40%) should be advised to undergo
    aortic valve replacement regardless of symptoms. Patients with marginally
    abnormal left ventricular function (biplane ejection fraction 40%–55%) may

be treated medically and followed closely, or aortic valve replacement may be advised.

4. Patients who are awaiting operation or who have symptoms of left ventricular failure should be digitalized. Diuretics may also be employed in patients who remain symptomatic. Afterload reduction therapy is used in patients with marginally abnormal left ventricular function in whom medical therapy is elected. Such patients should also be digitalized. Afterload reduction therapy may also be used with success in patients with severe left ventricular dysfunction who are awaiting valve replacement. An effective regimen for afterload reduction therapy consists of isosorbide dinitrate (20–40 mg orally every 4–6 h and hydralazine (50 mg orally every 6 h), or captopril (25–50 mg orally three times a day), or enalapril (5–10 mg orally twice a day).

5. Patients who undergo successful aortic valve replacement but continue to manifest signs or symptoms (or both) of left ventricular failure may require therapy with digitalis and diuretics. Afterload reduction therapy may also be beneficial in such patients.

Mitral Regurgitation

Acute mitral regurgitation (AMR) resembles AAR with respect to the rapidity of presentation and the severity of the patient's unstable hemodynamic status. These individuals may have endocarditis, myxomatous degeneration, or myocardial infarction as the cause of the AMR. Often, such patients require urgent intensive care and mitral valve replacement [24]. Echocardiography with Doppler is usually quite accurate in delineating the presence and severity of AMR as well as the state of left ventricular function [11].

The mainstays of medical therapy for AMR are vasodilating drugs and the intraaortic balloon pump (IABP) [25]. Hemodynamic improvement in AMR following administration of vasodilating agents such as nitroprusside, captopril, or hydralazine occurs by several mechanisms. First, lowered systemic vascular resistance favors increased forward cardiac output and diminished regurgitant volume. Secondly, as left ventricular volume decreases, the size of the regurgitant orifice also declines. The use of intravenous diuretics such as furosemide may further reduce left ventricular size as well as relieve pulmonary congestion.

Intravenous nitroprusside is the vasodilating agent of choice for the initial treatment of patients with AMR [26]. Pulmonary artery pressure should be monitored with a balloon-tipped pulmonary artery catheter, and intraarterial pressures are monitored with an indwelling cannula. The nitroprusside infusion should be titrated to maintain the systemic systolic pressure in the 90–100-mmHg range and the pulmonary capillary wedge pressure in the 15–18-mmHg range.

It is not uncommon for patients with severe AMR to require support of the systemic arterial pressure as well as afterload reduction. Urgent insertion of the IABP should be done; however, combination of nitroprusside and dobutamine may provide enough hemodynamic stability to improve the safety of IABP insertion. If the major problem is systemic hypotension, the combination of nitroprusside and dopamine may be preferable, while the combination of nitroprusside and dobutamine is more efficacious if the primary hemodynamic problem is pulmonary congestion with mild hypotension. Dopamine may carry the disadvantage of elevating systemic vascular resistance and exacerbating AMR.

In relatively mild cases of AMR, it may be possible to stabilize the patient with intravenous nitroprusside and then switch to an oral vasodilator. This may be particularly appropriate when AMR accompanies acute myocardial infarction and the clinician hopes to postpone surgical correction of the AMR until some time has passed after the acute ischemic event. Therapy with captopril usually begins with a dosage of 6.25 mg orally three times a day. If hypotension does not ensue, the dosage is progressively increased to 25 or 50 mg orally three times a day or until systemic hypotension results. Hydralazine has also been used for this purpose. Oral inotropic therapy with digoxin is also usually employed.

While these measures to enhance hemodynamic stability are being instituted, a plan for definitive treatment should be formulated. Urgent cardiac catheterization is generally required. In the absence of cardiogenic shock, cardiac catheterization should be performed within 24 h of the onset of AMR. If cardiogenic shock is present (even if hemodynamic improvement occurs with the IABP), emergency catheterization should be performed. The cardiac surgical team should be placed on standby as soon as the decision to proceed to cardiac catheterization has been made. Urgent or emergent mitral valve replacement is often required.

The patient with chronic mitral regurgitation (CMR) presents the clinician with the same therapeutic dilemma as noted earlier for the patient with CAR. Individuals with CMR may also remain asymptomatic for decades while insidious left ventricular dysfunction develops [27].

The current operative mortality of 5%–10% associated with mitral valve repair or replacement, the lack of a perfect valve substitute, and the persistence of symptoms of low cardiac output following surgery argue against earlier mitral valve surgery. The benefits of surgery, however, both in terms of functional improvement and a probable decrease in mortality, are obtained if mitral valve surgery is instituted before irreversible left ventricular dysfunction has supervened. A recent report indicates better surgical results in terms of regression of left ventricular hypertrophy and decrease in left ventricular size without worsening of ejection fraction up to 15 months following mitral valve surgery in patients in whom there was only moderate left ventricular dilatation, normal ejection fraction, and minimal elevation of the PC wedge pressure prior to surgery [28].

Mitral valve surgery entails either valve replacement or reconstruction of the patient's own mitral value apparatus. Previously, it was felt that only congenitally abnormal mitral valves were suitable for primary repair; however, in experienced hands, reconstruction of the mitral valve (valvuloplasty) is the operation of choice for all forms mitral valve disease. A valve that is pliable, minimally damaged, or moderately fibrosed without calcification is ideal for repair rather than replacement. Suture and plication techniques with or without the incorporation of a rigid or flexible annuloplasty ring (such as the Carpentier ring) constitute the majority of valvuloplasty techniques. The most favorable candidates for valvuloplasty are patients with mitral regurgitation caused by mitral valve prolapse, ruptured chordae tendineae (congenital, prolapse, or ischemic), and rheumatic heart disease without calcification.

Currently, mitral valve replacement carries an overall mortality of 5%-10%; however, the risks of surgery vary and may be as high as 25% in patients in NYHA class IV. The risk of prosthetic mitral valve replacement depends on left atrial size and NYHA class. The surgical risk is greater in patients over the age of 50, with reduced cardiac index, elevated pulmonary capillary wedge pressure (greater than 16 mmHg), and reduced left ventricular ejection fraction.

Unfortunately, patients with preoperative left ventricular dysfunction often continue to manifest signs and symptoms of left ventricular failure despite successful mitral valve replacement or repair. This is particularly true if the preoperative left ventricular ejection fraction is less than 40%.

Despite these difficulties, the following protocol is advised for the management of patients with CMR:

1. Patients with asymptomatic CMR should have a clinical evaluation (physical examination, ECG, and chest roentgenogram) at yearly intervals. Observe patients for the development of symptoms, ECG evidence of increasing left ventricular hypertrophy, changes in cardiac rhythm, and increasing heart size by chest roentgenogram. An echocardiogram/Doppler study should be performed every 1-2 years to detect changes in left ventricular contractility and to determine left ventricular dimensions, left atrial size, and severity of mitral regurgitation. No treatment is required unless a significant change occurs in the preceding studies. Antibiotic prophylaxis for dental work or potentially septic surgical procedures is important.

2. Patients with mild to moderate CMR should have a clinical evaluation (physical examination, ECG, and chest roentgenogram) at 6-month intervals. An echocardiogram, or radioisotope ventriculogram, or both should be obtained every 1-2 years. If the patient is stable, antibiotic prophylaxis for dental and surgical procedures is all that is required. If marked electrocardiographic LVH with ST-T changes or deterioration in echocardiographic indices of left ventricular function or size develop, cardiac catheterization should be performed. It should also be done, even in the absence of symptoms, if there is an increase in cardiac size greater than 2 cm, with evidence of upper lobe pulmonary venous redistribution on the chest roentgenogram. At catheterization, hemodynamic measurements should be obtained at rest and during exercise if they are normal at rest. Patients with abnormal left ventricular function should be strongly considered for mitral valve repair or replacement.

3. The decision for surgical intervention should be based on the foregoing data. Medical treatment consists of digitalization for left ventricular failure or atrial fibrillation, diuretics, a low-salt diet, and vasodilators (hydralazine, ACE inhibitors) for left ventricular failure, and anticoagulants for atrial

fibrillation. Antibiotic prophylaxis for dental work and potentially septic surgery is also indicated. Afterload reduction therapy with oral hydralazine (or ACE inhibitors) or long-acting nitrates or both is indicated for patients with symptomatic CMR, either before surgery or if the patient refuses surgery.

Conclusions

Aortic or mitral valve replacement is indicated in patients with stenotic valves and signs/symptoms of pulmonary congestion. Individuals with AMR or AAR usually require urgent valve replacement following a variable period of medical therapy aimed at hemodynamic stabilization of these individuals. Patients with CMR or CAR present the greatest dilemma. In general, valve replacement or repair should be offered to patients with CAR or CMR who demonstrate objective signs, symptoms, or laboratory evidence of deteriorating left ventricular function.

References

1. Levinson GE (1987) Aortic stenosis. In: Dalen JE, Alpert JS (eds) Valvular heart disease, 2nd edn. Little, Brown, Boston
2. Dalen JE (1987) Mitral stenosis. In: Dalen JE, Alpert JS (eds) Valvular heart disease, 2nd edn. Little, Brown, Boston
3. Miller RR et al. (1976) Afterload reduction therapy with nitroprusside in severe aortic regurgitation: improved cardiac performance and reduced regurgitant volume. Am J Cardiol 38:564
4. Warner RA et al. (1977) Treatment of acute aortic insufficiency with sodium nitroferricyanide. Chest 72:375
5. Sonnenblick EM, Frishman WH, LeJemtel TH (1979) Dobutamine: a new synthetic cardioactive sympathetic amine. N Engl J Med 300:17
6. Prager RL et al. (1989) Early operative intervention in aortic bacterial endocarditis. Ann Thorac Surg 32:347
7. Hunter AM Jr et al. (1970) Aortic valve surgery as an emergency procedure. Circulation 41:623
8. Benotti JR (1987) Acute Aortic Insufficiency. In: Dalen JE, Alpert JS (eds) Valvular heart disease, 2nd edn. Little, Brown, Boston
9. Alpert JS (1987) Chronic aortic regurgitation. In: Dalen JE, Alpert JS (eds) Valvular heart disease, 2nd edn. Little, Brown, Boston
10. Goldschlager N et al. (1973) The natural history of aortic regurgitation: a clinical and hemodynamic study. Am J Med 54:577
11. Gault JH et al. (1970) Left ventricular performance following correction of free aortic regurgitation. Circulation 42:773
12. Hirshfield JW Jr et al. (1974) Indices predicting long-term survival after valve replacement in patients with aortic regurgitation and patients with aortic stenosis. Circulation 50:1190
13. Clark D, McAnulty JH, Rahimtoola S (1978) Results of valve replacement in aortic incompetence with left ventricular dysfunction. Circulation 58 [Suppl II]:22
14. Herreman F et al. (1979) Pre- and postoperative hemodynamic and cineangiographic assessment of left ventricular function in patients with aortic regurgitation. Am Heart J 98:63

15. Kumpuris AG et al. (1982) Importance of preoperative hypertrophy, wall stress, and end-systolic dimension as echocardiographic predictors of normalization of left ventricular dilatation after valve replacement in chronic aortic insufficiency. Am J Cardiol 49:1091

16. Carroll JD et al. (1983) Serial changes in left ventricular function after correction of chronic aortic regurgitation. Dependence on early changes in preload and subsequent regression of hypertrophy. Am J Cardiol 51:476

17. Gaasch WH et al. (1983) Chronic aortic regurgitation: Prognostic value of left ventricular end-systolic dimension and end-diastolic radius/thickness ratio. J Am Coll Cardiol 1:775

18. Levine HJ, Gaasch WH (1983) Ratio of regurgitant volume to end-diastolic volume: a major determinant of ventricular response to surgical correction of chronic volume overload. Am J Cardiol 52:406

19. Henry WL et al. (1980) Observations on the optimum time for operative intervention for aortic regurgitation. II. Serial echocardiographic evaluation of asymptomatic patients. Circulation 61:484

20. Bonow RO et al. (1982) Timing of operation for chronic aortic regurgitation. Am J Cardiol 50:325

21. Thompson R et al. (1979) Influence of preoperative left ventricular function on results of homograft replacement of the aortic valve for aortic regurgitation. J Thorac Cardiovasc Surg 77:411

22. Stone PH et al. (1984) Determinants of prognosis of patients with aortic regurgitation who undergo aortic valve replacement. J Am Coll Cardiol 3:1118

23. Clark DG, McAnulty JH, Rahimtoola SH (1980) Valve replacement in aortic insufficiency with left ventricular dysfunction. Circulation 61:411

24. Rippe JM, Howe JP (1987) Acute mitral regurgitation. In: Dalen JE, Alpert JS (eds) Valvular heart disease. 2nd edn. Little, Brown, Boston

25. Harshaw CW et al. (1975) Reduced systemic vascular resistance as therapy for severe mitral regurgitation of valvular origin. Ann Intern Med 83:312

26. Chatterjee K, Swan HJC (1974) Vasodilator therapy in acute myocardial infarction. Mod Concepts Cardiovasc Dis 43:119

27. Haffajee CI (1987) Chronic mitral regurgitation. In: Dalen JE, Alpert JS (eds) Valvular heart disease. 2nd edn. Little, Brown, Boston

28. Schuller G et al. (1979) Temporal response of left ventricular performance to mitral valve surgery. Circulation 59:1218

Cardiomyopathies

Cardiomyopathies: Morphological Aspects

E.G.J. Olsen

Cardiomyopathies[1] are defined as heart muscle diseases of unknown cause and subdivided into three major types: dilated cardiomyopathy, hypertrophic cardiomyopathy and restrictive cardiomyopathy.

Dilated Cardiomyopathy[1]

In the late stages of the disease, all cardiac chambers are dilated, often to a severe degree. Heart weights are, not infrequently, double normal values, yet despite the undoubted hypertrophy, measurements of the ventricular (and atrial) walls are normal or less than normal, due to dilatation masking the degree of hypertrophy. The myocardium is often pale and flabby, and occasionally naked eye inspection will show areas of fine fibrosis scattered throughout the ventricular walls, most noticeable in the inner third of the left ventricular wall. Endocardial thickening, randomly or uniformly distributed, particularly in the left ventricle, is typical [2] (Fig. 1). In over 50% of hearts, thrombus, particularly in the apical region, is found [3]. The coronary arteries are, with rare exceptions, normal [4], even if the patient is of advanced age, in whom atherosclerosis is not unexpected.

Histological Changes

The myocardial fibres are in normal alignment with evidence of hypertrophy of the nuclei, taking the form of pyknosis, vesicular change or unusual shapes resembling a horseshoe. The diameter of the fibres is, however, normal or less than normal, this being due to the stretching or attenuation of the fibres [5], particularly to the inner half of the myocardial walls. An increase of interstitial fibrous tissue of varying degrees or areas of fibrous replacement of myocardial fibres are not unusual, particularly in cases with long-standing heart failure [6]. The intramyocardial vessels are usually normal [7] despite suggestions to the contrary [8,9]. Occasional small vessels may show intimal thickening composed of fibroelastic tissue, rarely, however, obstructing the lumina. The abnormal

---

[1] The recommendations of the WHO/ISFC Task Force on nomenclature of cardiomyopathies and specific heart muscle diseases will be followed [1].

B.S. Lewis, A. Kimchi (Eds.)
Heart Failure Mechanisms and Management
© Springer-Verlag Berlin Heidelberg 1991

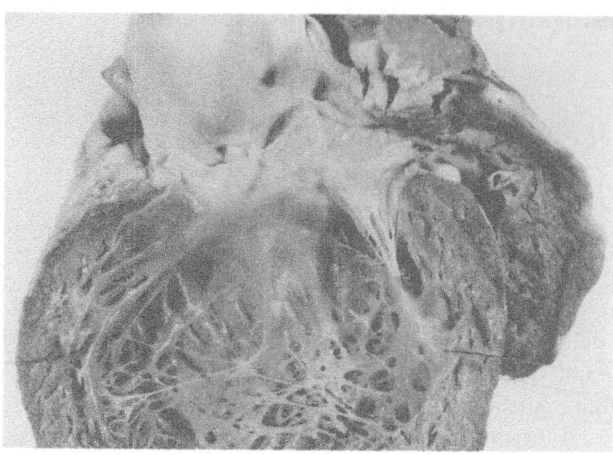

Fig. 1. The heart of a patient with dilated cardiomyopathy. The left ventricle has been displaced showing severe dilatation. Despite the hypertrophy, measurements of the left ventricular walls are normal

vessels are frequently found in areas of fibrosis and are therefore considered secondary change, rather than primary events. The endocardium is usually thickened to a mild to moderately severe degree (over 40 μm) and, if heart failure has been present for at least 6 weeks, shows varying degrees of prominence of the normally present smooth muscle component [10]. Pericardial changes are usually not evident.

Death may occur at any time during the natural history of dilated cardiomyopathy, and thus the morphological details described above may not necessarily be seen. The changes may therefore include hypertrophy only or hypertrophy and some dilatation.

From this description, it is evident that the morphological changes are non-specific, and a diagnosis can only be made if conditions that can give rise to a hypertrophied, dilated myocardium are excluded.

One further morphological change has been found. This concerns a decrease of neuronal cells. By serially sectioning right atrial strips between venae cavae, a significant decrease of these cells has been noted in patients with dilated cardiomyopathy, compared to normal controls [11].

Detailed examination of endomyocardial biopsies obtained by bioptome from nearly 2000 patients has permitted histochemical and ultrastructural evaluation of endomyocardial tissue to be undertaken.

Histochemical Changes

An increase, decrease, or normal amounts of substances such as glycogen or succinic dehydrogenase may be found. An increase is noted when hypertrophy dominates the picture, whilst a decrease is noted in those hearts which had been in failure for some time; in severe instances glycogen is almost or totally absent, and succinic dehydrogenase is severely decreased [12].

Electron-Microscopical Changes

The arrangement of myocardial fibrils is normal and regular in parallel alignment, but occasional irregular foci may be found, interpreted as an accompaniment of hypertrophy. An increase in the number of mitochondria to more than one per two sarcomeres reflects the presence of hypertrophy, together with crenellation of nuclear membranes. Glycogen, reflecting histochemical analysis, may either be focally increased, normal in distribution or decreased. The interstitium may show collagen bundles and occasional lymphocytes. Capillaries are usually normal, but occasional artefactual oedema of the walls may be encountered. Varying degrees of degenerative changes have, however, been observed, consisting of myelin figures, membrane-bound vesicles and focal or more widespread dissolution of actin and myosin [13,14].

Myocarditis

In a number of patients, clinically suspected of suffering from dilated cardiomyopathy, endomyocardial biopsy has shown evidence of myocarditis by many workers. Morphological – like clinical – diagnosis is difficult, and the reported incidence has varied between 2% and 63% [15]. This wide fluctuation has, in the past, been attributed, among other things, mainly to morphological interpretation. Among a group of pathologists [16], great variation has been reported, and it is for this reason that a group of cardiac pathologists met in Dallas [17] to define and establish criteria for myocarditis. The suggested criteria, based on previously reported definition and classification [18], has been adopted and expanded. Classification into acute or active, on-going, resolving (healing) and resolved (healed) phases is recommended, together with a category of borderline myocarditis.

In acute or active myocarditis, interstitial inflammatory cells, usually consisting of lymphocytes and other chronic inflammatory cells, are in close contact with adjacent myocardial fibres, which show areas of necrosis. In on-going myocarditis, the inflammatory infiltrate is at least as severe as the most recent biopsy, whilst in resolving (healing) myocarditis, the inflammation is less. In these cases, an increase in interstitial fibrous tissue can usually be found, as well as a very occasional focus of necrosis. Increasing degrees of fibrosis and progressive diminution of the cellular infiltrate heralds the resolved (healed) phase. Grading of myocarditis is important as it may have therapeutic implication and can only be achieved by sequential biopsy examination.

Virus has been implicated as being causally related, but until recently, such suggestions could only be confirmed by indirect virological techniques [19]. The adaptation of a hybridization probe has shown the presence of virus in over 50% of cases, not only in those with evidence of myocarditis, but also in instances where only the non-specific morphological changes of a hypertrophied, dilated myocardium were present [20,21]. It can therefore be concluded that, together with evidence of immunological idiosyncrasy, virus, especially Coxsackie B virus, is implicated in the pathogenesis of dilated cardiomyopathy, which finds morphological expression in the form of myocarditis or in specialized techniques of examination.

Hypertrophic Cardiomyopathy

In contrast to dilated cardiomyopathy, morphological characteristics exist in this type of cardiomyopathy. The hearts are overweight, globular in shape and firm to the touch. Macroscopically, asymmetric hypertrophy of the interventricular septum is typical and, if severe (i.e. twice or more the thickness of the already hypertrophied free left ventricular wall [22], permit categorisation of this condition at naked eye examination (Fig. 2). The maximal bulge of the asymmetry of the septum may be at the apex, in the mid-region or beneath the aortic valve [23]. Interference with the normal closure of the mitral valve is frequent, especially due to displacement of the papillary muscles, and may result in severe endocardial thickening, forming a mirror image of the anterior leaflet of the mitral valve onto the outflow tract of the left ventricle [24]. Elsewhere in the left ventricle endocardial thickening is usual. The coronary arteries are also normal, but infarct-like lesions have been described [25]. Sectioning of the asymmetric regions shows the myocardium to be arranged in a whorled fashion.

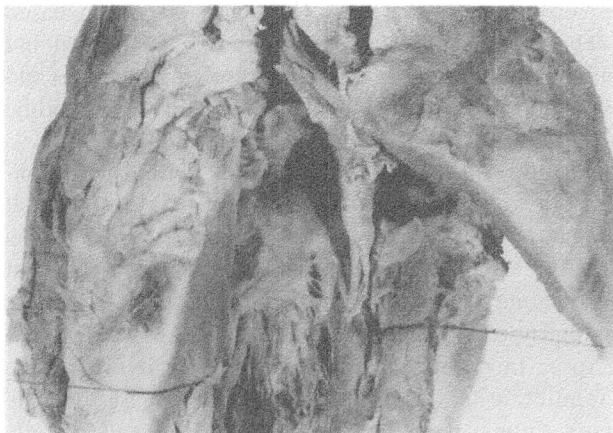

Fig. 2. Hypertrophic cardiomyopathy. Close-up view of the left ventricular outflow tract showing endocardial thickening representing a "mirror image" of the anterior leaflet of the mitral valve

Further experience has shown that milder forms of asymmetry of the interventricular septum can occur as an accompaniment of other disease processes, particularly of congenital heart disease affecting the right side, as well as in the neonate, and therefore great care has to be taken to attribute these changes to hypertrophic cardiomyopathy [26,27].

Asymmetry may not always be present, and echocardiographic analysis has shown that in up to 31% of cases symmetric hypertrophic cardiomyopathy does occur [28].

Histological Changes

Disarray of myocardial fibres dominates the histological picture and occupies at least 5% in 94% of 54 patients' heart tissue examined [29]. In addition, severe hypertrophy, short runs of myocardial fibres, bizarre nuclear shapes often surrounded by clear zone — the perinuclear halo — together with an increase in cellular connective tissue are found. These findings have been semi-quantitatively assessed and have resulted in the histological index of hypertrophic obstructive cardiomyopathy [30].

Intramyocardial vessels have, in my experience, been found to be normal, based on examination of hearts at post mortem in approximately 80 cases and on tissue obtained by bioptome in 160 cases. Occasionally, intimal thickening has, however, been observed, but, as in dilated cardiomyopathy, these vessels are usually located in fibrous tissue, not significantly narrowing the lumina. More extensive changes in the small vessels have been reported, and in 40 out of 48 patients medial thickening often accompanied by intimal thickening has been observed in vessels, particularly located in the septum and the anterior left ventricular wall [31]. These findings have been attributed to a congenital anomaly and would explain ischaemic symptoms and also perhaps the infarct-like lesions noted macroscopically, even if the extra-mural coronary arteries are not significantly abnormal.

The endocardium, where thickened, is composed of an increase in all the normal constituents. Smooth muscle hyperplasia is rare and only occurs in heart failure, which heralds a very poor prognosis. The epicardium is usually unremarkable.

Of the *histochemical* changes, an immense increase of glycogen is often found, resulting in pooling, particularly in the perinuclear areas. This serves as an additional diagnostic marker. Other parameters, such as succinic dehydrogenase, non-specific esterases, acid or alkaline phosphatases, may be increased, but these are interpreted as an accompaniment of the severe hypertrophy [32].

Ultrastructural Changes

Disarray of myocardial myofibrils may be striking with fibrils running in all directions. In addition, there is an increase of inter- and intra-fibrillar connections forming a basket weave [33,34]. The relevance of these findings is debateable, but they have been suggested as explaining the failure of diastolic compliance considered to be the underlying mechanism of symptoms of hypertrophic cardiomyopathy.

Aggregations of mitochondria, referred to as mitochondriosis, are frequent, together with extreme crenellation of nuclear membranes and severe focal accumulations of glycogen. Intercellular spaces frequently show an increase in collagen fibrils and occasional lymphocytes. Vessels are normal [34].

Restrictive Cardiomyopathy

Endomyocardial fibrosis [35] and Löffler's endocarditis parietalis fibroplastica [36] were considered to be separate entities, the former confined to tropical or sub-tropical zones, whilst the latter considered to be restricted to the temperate zones. Evidence has accumulated over the years that both these conditions are in fact a single entity [37,38]. Irrespective of the geographical distribution, in the late phase the striking lesions are found in the endocardium, taking the form of extreme thickening, not infrequently exceeding 5000 μm (10 μm is normal for the left ventricle inflow tract). The right, left or both ventricles (and atria) may be affected. Typically, when the left ventricle is involved, the inflow tract, the apex and part of the outflow tract are involved, ending abruptly in the thick rolled edge [39] (Fig. 3) as the region of the opened anterior mitral valve leaflet is approached. The papillary muscles and the posterior leaflet of the mitral valve are also frequently involved. Thrombus is often superimposed, particularly at the apex. From the thick endocardium, fibrous septa can be seen extending, occasionally

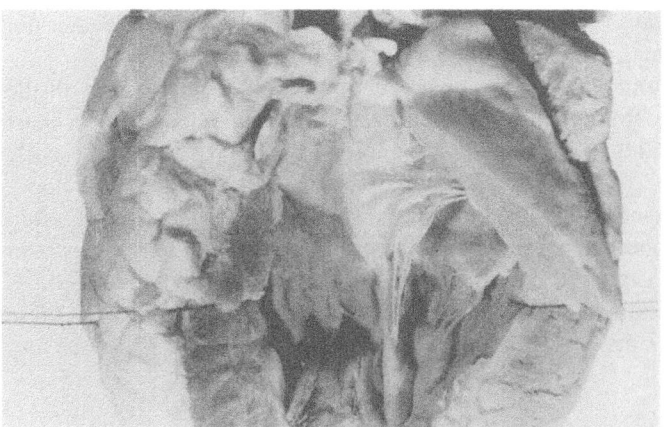

Fig. 3. The left ventricular outflow tract in the heart of a patient with endomyocardial fibrosis. The thick endocardium (overlaid by thrombus) ends abruptly (shadowed area) beneath the anterior leaflet of the mitral valve, which has been deflected

transmurally, into the underlying myocardium [40]. The coronary arteries are normal.

In right ventricular involvement, the apex and the area beneath the posterior leaflet of the tricuspid valve are affected with progressive obliteration of the apex and involvement of papillary muscles and the tricuspid valve.

In either event, the *microscopical findings* are identical. The thick endocardium is arranged in layers. Superficially, fibrin or thrombus is found, followed by a zone of dense collagen tissue in which elastic fibres may abound. Foci of calcification may form in this layer in previously degenerated collagen tissue. The deepest layer – the granulation tissue layer – is composed of loose connective tissue and dilated vascular channels, together with varying degrees of inflammatory cells, occasionally also eosinophils [37,40]. It is from this layer that the septa, noted by the naked eye, extend into the myocardium. Remnants of the original normal endocardium may occasionally be preserved.

In a retrospective study examining the morphology of 30 cases [37], three major stages have been identified, depending on the length of history. If the clinical symptomatology has lasted for an average of 5 weeks, the necrotic stage, exemplified by intense myocarditis rich in eosinophils and arteritis/arteriolitis is evident. The thrombotic stage is attained when the length of history has lasted, on average, for a period of 10 months, characterised by thrombus superimposition upon the already thickening endocardium which, in extreme cases, may totally occlude the ventricular cavities. The myocarditic process has at this stage largely abated, and small vessels may show thrombotic material within the lumina. The final, fibrotic stage, reached after an average length of history of 2.5 years, is exemplified by the changes that have already been described above.

Further studies have shown that the morphology of the eosinophils is abnormal. The abnormality consists of vacuolation of the cytoplasm and a decrease, or even absence, of the normal granular content [40]. It has been shown that, if 15% of circulating eosinophils are significantly degranulated, then endomyocardial fibrosis is present, even in the absence of clinical symptoms.

In view of the association of eosinophils with this disease, it is no longer tenable to include endomyocardial fibrosis under the heading of cardiomyopathy; it should be reclassified under specific heart muscle diseases [41].

There is, however, a group of patients emerging with signs and symptoms of restriction, but with inconsistent morphology. The endocardium in some instances may be severely thickened, whilst in others interstitial fibrous tissue may be held responsible for the restrictive symptomatology. But not infrequently, both endocardial thickening and fibrosis are absent, and a hypertrophied, dilated myocardium, similar to that found in dilated cardiomyopathy, is all that can be found. There is, thus, no consistent clinico-pathological correlation in this group of patients. The aetiology is totally unknown, and much research is needed to evaluate these patients. It is suggested that this group alone justifies inclusion under restrictive cardiomyopathy.

References

1. WHO/ISFC (1980) Task Force on the definition and classification of cardiomyopathies. Br Heart J 44:672-673
2. Olsen EGJ (1979) Pathology of cardiomyopathies – a critical analysis. Am Heart J 98:385-392
3. Olsen EGJ (1976) Pathologie der "primären" Kardiomyopathien. Muench Med Wochenschr 118:735-740
4. Gau GT, Goodwin JF, Oakley CM, Olsen EGJ, Rahimtoola SH, Raphael MJ, Steiner RE (1972) Q Qaves and coronary arteriography in cardiomyopathy. Br Heart J 34:1034-1041
5. Olsen EGJ (1975) Pathological recognition of cardiomyopathy. Postgrad Med J 51:277-281
6. Olsen EGJ (1981) Pathology of Congestive Cardiomyopathy. In: Goodwin JF, Hjalmarson A, Olsen EGJ (eds) Congestive cardiomyopathy. Hassle, Molndal, pp 66-74
7. Olsen EGJ (1983) What is the pathologic anatomy of cardiomyopathy? Controv Cardiol 3:240-243
8. James TN (1964) An etiologic concept concerning the obscure myocardiopathies. Progr Cardiovasc Dis 7:43
9. Factor SM, Cho S, Sonnenblick EH (1989) Verapamil treatment of cardiomyopathic Syrian hamsters: effects on the micro circulation and the extent of myocardial necrosis. Fed Proc 40:758
10. Olsen EGJ (1983) Endomyocardial biopsies. Int J Cardiol 3:240-243
11. Amorim DS, Olsen EGJ (1982) Assessment of heart neurons in dilated (congestive) cardiomyopathy. Br Heart J 47:11-18
12. Olsen EGJ (1978) Special investigations of COCM: endomyocardial biopsies (morphological analysis). Postgrad Med J 54:486-490
13. Olsen EGJ (1978) Endomyocardial biopsies. Invest Cell Pathol 1:139-157
14. Ferrans VJ (1978) Myocardial ultrastructure in the cardiomyopathies. In: Sekiguchi M, Olsen EGJ (eds) Cardiomyopathy. Univ Tokyo Press, Univ Park Press, pp 107-137
15. Fowles RE (1985) Treatment of myocarditis and cardiomyopathy in the USA. In: Sekiguchi M, Olsen EGJ, Goodwin JF (eds) Myocarditis and related disorders. Springer, Berlin Heidelberg New York Tokyo, pp 173-174
16. Shanes JG, Ghali J, Billingham ME, Ferrans VJ, Fenoglio JJ, Edwards WD, Tsai CC, Saffitz JE, Isner J, Furner S, Subramanian R (1987) Interobserver variability in the pathologic interpretation of endomyocardial biopsy results. Circulation 75:401-405
17. Aretz HT, Billingham Margaret E, Edwards WD, Factor SM, Fallon JT, Fenoglio JJ Jr, Olsen EGJ, Schoen FJ (1987) Myocarditis – a histopathologic definition and classification. Am J Cardiovasc Pathol 1:3-14
18. Olsen EGJ (1981) Panel discussion. In: Goodwin JF, Hjalmarson A, Olsen EGJ (eds) Congestive cardiomyopathy, Kiruna Sweden 1980. Hassle, Molndal, p 122
19. Olsen EGJ (1983) Myocarditis – a case of mistaken identity? Br Heart J 50:303-311
20. Bowles NE, Richardson PJ, Olsen EGJ, Archard LC (1986) Detection of Coxsackie B virus-specific RNA sequences in myocardial biopsy samples from patients with myocarditis and dilated cardiomyopathy. Lancet I:1120-1123
21. Archard LC, Bowles NE, Olsen EGJ, Richardson PJ (1987) Detection of persistent coxsackie B virus RNA in dilated cardiomyopathy and myocarditis. Eur Heart J 8 [Suppl J]:437-440
22. Olsen EGJ (1983) Anatomic and light microscopic characterization of hypertrophic obstructive cardiomyopathy and non-obstructive cardiomyopathy. Eur Heart J 4 [Suppl F]:1-8
23. Wigle ED, Silver MD (1978) Myocardial fiber disarray and ventricular septal hypertrophy in asymmetrical hypertrophy of the heart (editorial). Circulation 58:398-402
24. Davies MJ, Pomerance A, Teare RD (1974) Pathological features of hypertrophic obstructive cardiomyopathy. J Clin Pathol 27:529-535
25. Maron BJ, Epstein SE, Roberts WC (1979) Hypertrophic cardiomyopathy and transmural myocardial infarction without significant atherosclerosis of the extramural coronary arteries. Am J Cardiol 43:1086-1102
26. Maron BJ, Edwards JE, Moller JH, Epstein SE (1979) Prevalence and characteristics of disproportionate ventricular septal thickening in infants with congenital heart disease. Circulation 59:126-133

27. Bulkley BH, Weisfelt ML, Hutchins GM (1977) Asymmetric septal hypertrophy and myocardial fiber disarray. Features of normal, developing and malformed hearts. Circulation 56:292–298
28. Shapiro LM, McKenna WJ (1983) Distribution of left ventricular hypertrophy in hypertrophic cardiomyopathy: a two-dimensional echocardiographic study. J Am Coll Cardiol 2:437–444
29. Maron BJ, Roberts WC (1979) Quantitative analysis of cardiac muscle cell disorganization in the ventricular septum of patients with hypertrophic cardiomyopathy. Circulation 59:689–706
30. Van Noorden S, Olsen EGJ, Pearse AG (1971) Hypertrophic obstructive cardiomyopathy. A Histological histochemical and ultrastructural study of biopsy material. Cardiovasc Res 5:118–131
31. Maron BJ, Wolfson JK, Epstein SE, Roberts WC (1986) Intramural ("small vessel") coronary artery disease in hypertrophic cardiomyopathy. J Am Coll Cardiol 8:545–557
32. Van Noorden S, Pearse AGE (1971) Histochemistry and electron microscopy of the heart in hypertrophic obstructive cardiomyopathy. In: Wolstenholme GEW, O'Connor M (eds) Ciba Foundation Study Group N 37. Churchill, London, pp 92–121
33. Olsen EGJ (1978) In: Kaltenbach M, Loogen F, Olsen EGJ (eds) Cardiomyopathy and myocardial biopsy. Springer, Berlin Heidelberg New York, pp 52–61
34. Ferrans VJ, Morrow AG, Roberts WC (972) Myocardial ultrastructure in idiopathic hypertrophic subaortic stenosis. A study of operatively excised left ventricular outflow tract muscle in 14 patients. Circulation 45:769
35. Davies JNP (1948) Endocardial fibrosis in Africans. East Afr Med J 25:10–14
36. Loffler W (1936) Endocarditis parietalis fibroplastica mit Bluteosinophilie. ein eigenartiges Krankheitsbild. Schweiz Med Wochenschr 66:817–820
37. Brockington IF, Olsen EGJ (1973) Loffler's endocarditis and Davies' endomyocardial fibrosis. Am Heart J 85:308
38. Oakley CM, Olsen EGJ (1977) Eosinophilia and heart disease. Br Heart J 39:233–237
39. Davies JNP (1968) The ridge in endomyocardial fibrosis. Lancet I:631–632
40. Olsen EGJ, Spry CJF (1979) The pathogenesis of Loffler's endomyocardial disease. and its relationship to endomyocardial fibrosis. In: Yu PN, Goodwin JF (eds) Progress in cardiology. Lea and Febiger, Philadelphia, pp 281–303
41. Olsen EGJ (1990) Morphological overview and pathogenetic mechanism in Endomyocardial Filerosis associated with eosinophilia. In: Sekiguchi M, Olsen EGJ (eds) Cardiomyopathy. Tokyo Univ Press, pp 1–8

Morphological Correlates of Cardiac Failure in Patients with End-stage Cardiomyopathy

Jutta Schaper, S. Bernotat-Danielowski, R. Froede, S. Hein, and N. Bleese

In earlier studies, our group determined as the morphological correlate of reduced cardiac function: fibrosis, degenerative ultrastructural changes, and the lack of contractile material. These studies were carried out in patients with either coronary heart disease or left ventricular hypertrophy due to aortic valve disease using intraoperative needle biopsies for the histological and electron microscopical investigation [1]. Owing to the development of cardiac transplantation surgery and therefore the availability of greater amounts of tissue from the explanted hearts, these studies can now be extended by additional techniques such as immunofluorescence using various monoclonal antibodies.

The present study is concerned with histological investigations, i.e., light microscopy, electron microscopy, and immunofluorescence for components of the cytoskeleton as well as of the growth factor EGF and its receptor in myocardium from explanted hearts from patients with end-stage dilated cardiomyopathy. The purpose of the study was to determine the various structural changes and to try to identify the morphological correlates of reduced cardiac function.

Myocardial tissue was obtained from eight explanted hearts from patients undergoing transplantation surgery because of chronic cardiac failure (NYHA class IV, ejection fraction $< 15\%$) due to dilated cardiomyopathy. The tissue was immediately frozen in liquid nitrogen and stored at $-70°C$ for immunocytochemical studies or it was fixed in glutaraldehyde and embedded in Epon for light and electron microscopy.

The most prominent features in all tissues investigated were the varying cell size of the myocytes, many of them hypertrophied, others showing atrophy, as well as the presence of significant fibrosis. Fibrosis consisted of large amounts of collagen, elastic material, and extracellular ground substance as well as fibroblasts, fibrocytes, numerous macrophages, and cellular debris (Fig. 1).

Many myocardial cells, hypertrophied or atrophic, exhibited lack of contractile material by light microscopy which could be very prominent so that the cells appeared like bags filled with fluid but otherwise empty. This became even more obvious by electron microscopy: the myofilaments were present in varying amounts with great variations from one cell to the other, but in most cells they were reduced (Fig. 2). The apparently "empty" cells were mostly filled with unspecified cytoplasm as well as tubular structures resembling sarcoplasmic reticulum, small mitochondria, fat droplets, glycogen, and myelin bodies (Fig. 3). The nuclei were often enlarged and exhibited abnormal chromatin clumping,

B.S. Lewis, A. Kimchi (Eds.)
Heart Failure Mechanisms and Management
© Springer-Verlag Berlin Heidelberg 1991

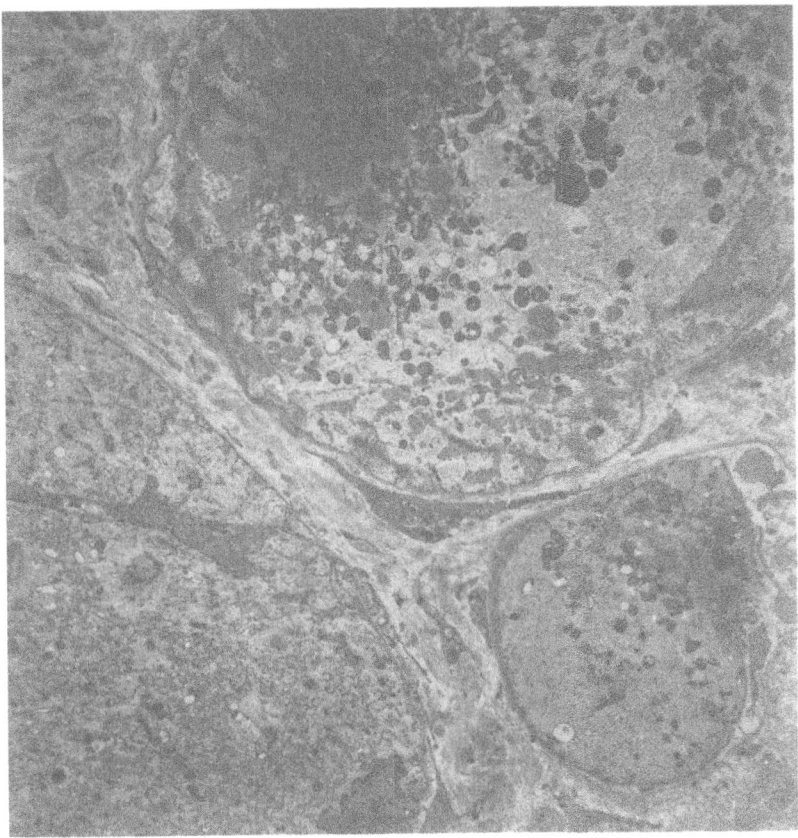

Fig. 1. Hypertrophic as well as atrophic cells in diseased human myocardium. The extracellular space contains collagen and cellular debris. × 6000

inclusions of cytoplasmic material as well as prominent nucleoli (Fig. 4). The T tubules were enlarged and more numerous than in normal tissue. These ultrastructural alterations are similar to those observed by our group in myocardium hypertrophied due to aortic valve disease or in coronary heart disease [1]. It appears that myocardium chronically overloaded or stressed reacts in only one way, i.e., by hypertrophy and degeneration, independent of the type of the cardiac disease. The nuclear changes, however, are indicative of compensatory synthetic processes possibly still occurring which is evident from our cytochemical studies.

For immunocytochemistry, monoclonal antibodies against desmin, tubulin, vinculin, vimentin as well as laminin and fibronectin were used, the second antibodies were labeled with FITC for fluorescence detection. Generally, these antibodies showed a stronger labeling of the various proteins in diseased human myocardium than in any normal control tissue. Tables 1 and 2 list the localization

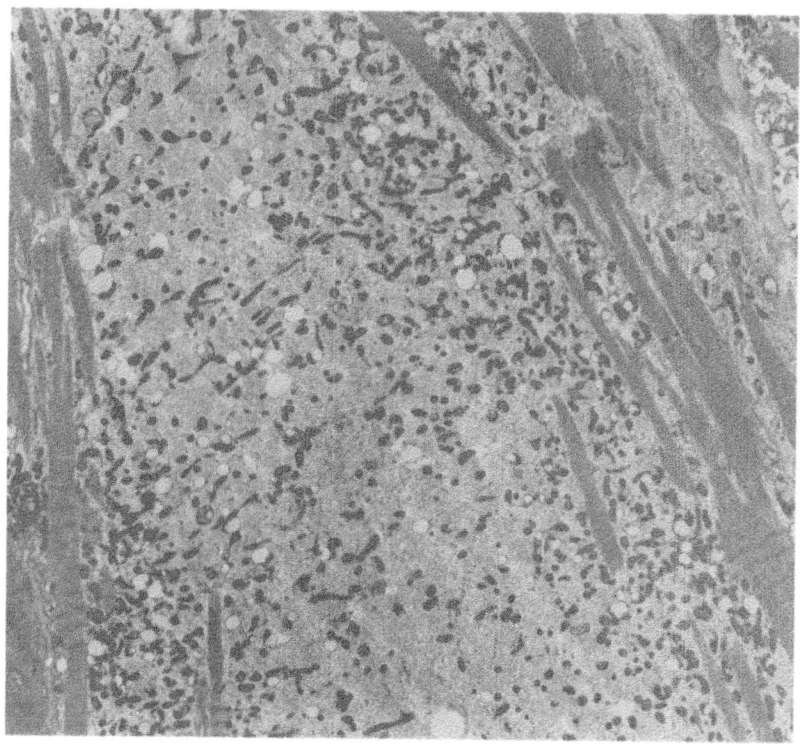

Fig. 2. Lack of contractile material in human myocardium. The cytoplasm contains many small irregular mitochondria. × 6000

of the various components of the cytoskeleton in normal and diseased tissue. It is evident that there is an increase in occurrence of the different proteins which may result in the functional disturbances listed in Table 2. It may well be that by augmenting the different components of the cytoskeleton and associated proteins like vinculin and laminin the total stability or even stiffness of the myocytes is increased, thereby contributing to the impairment of contractile function, which primarily seems to be disturbed because of the lack of myofilaments.

For the localization in myocardial tissue of the epidermal growth factor EGF and its receptor (EGF-R) commercially available monoclonal antibodies were used (Collab. Research, Lexington, Mass.; and Biomakor, Rehovot, Israel, respectively). In explanted cardiomyopathic hearts the receptor for EGF was strongly expressed in vascular cells and in fibroblasts of the interstitium. The myocardial cells were completely devoid of any fluorescent labeling for EGF-R. EGF itself could never be detected in any of the tissues tested, but it was found in cultured human endothelial cells providing proof that (a) this growth factor does occur in human cells; and (b) that the antibody is specific for EGF. The interpretation of these data is difficult. Since EGF has been shown to influence angiogenesis in tumors [2], it could be hypothesized that vascular adaptation to

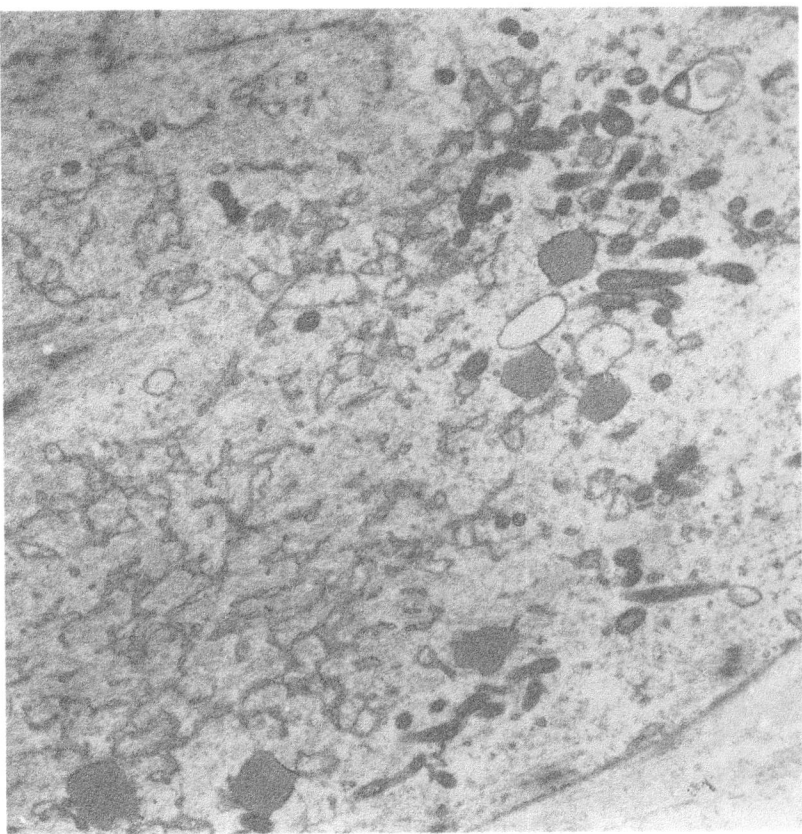

Fig. 3. The cytoplasm of a myocardial cell at higher magnification. Note the lipid inclusions, small mitochondria, and the prominent elements of the sarcoplasmic reticulum. Only remnants of myofilaments are present in the *upper left* and the *lower right corners*. × 18 000

the process of hypertrophy may be disturbed in late stages of dilated cardiomyopathy. Further studies need to be done to evaluate the importance of the absence or presence of growth factors in dilated cardiomyopathy.

Summary

The morphological correlates of chronic heart failure appear to include fibrosis, lack of myofilaments, degenerative subcellular changes, increased proliferation of the cytoskeleton and proteins associated with it, and possible abnormalities in the distribution of epidermal growth factor and its receptor. All these factors may contribute to the reduction of cardiac function in patients with chronic heart disease such as dilated cardiomyopathy.

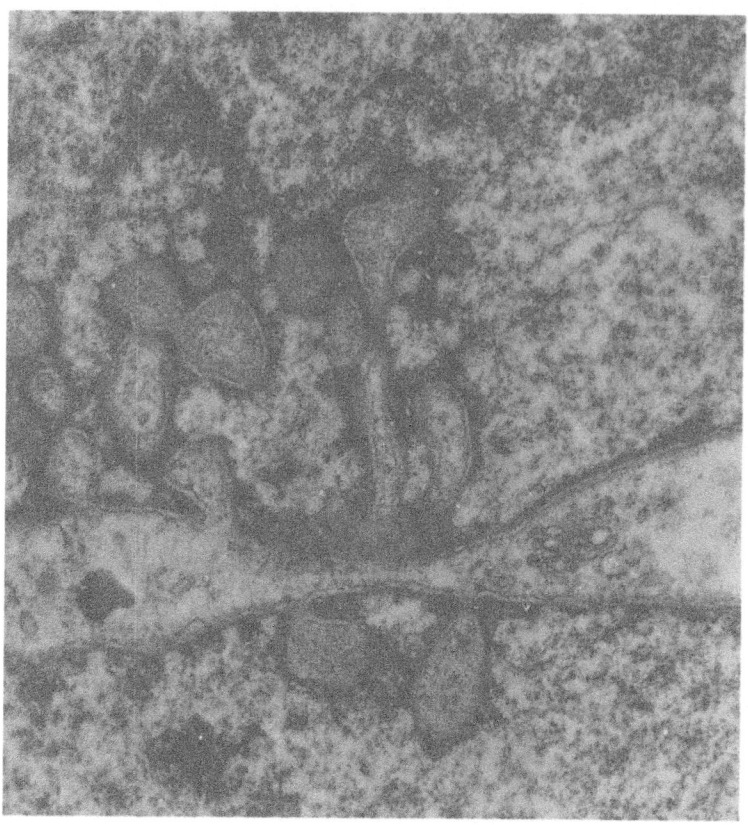

Fig. 4. Inclusions of cytoplasm in the nucleus of a myocardial cell. × 48 000

Table 1. Localization and supposed function of several intermediate filaments and proteins present in cardiac tissue

Protein	Localization	Function
Desmin	Z-line	Alignment of adjacent Z discs
Tubulin	Microtubules, mostly perinuclear	Longitudinal alignment of cell organelles, growth regulation (?)
Vinculin	Intercalated disc, sarcolemma	Binding of actin to membranes
Laminin	Basement membrane	Binds to collagen IV, continuous with cytoskeleton
Vimentin	Endothelial cells, fibroblasts	Cytoskeleton

Table 2. Localization of intermediate filaments and proteins in cardiomyopathic human hearts and the possible functional disturbances resulting from the altered distribution

Protein	Localization in cardiomyopathy	Disturbance of:
Desmin	Z-line, also diffuse irregular	Alignment of sarcomeres
Tubulin	Around nucleus, increased number of tubules	Cytoskeleton, growth regulation?
Vinculin	Also in cell center	Alignment of sarcomeres
Laminin	Irregular	Cytoskeleton, cell attachment
Vimentin	Localization normal but more structures labeled	Equivalent to fibrosis

References

1. Schaper J, Schaper W (1986) Morphological changes in myocardium from patients with coronary heart disease and cardiac hypertrophy. Adv Cardiol 34:16–24
2. Shiurba RA, Eng LF, Vogel H, Lee Y, Horonpian DS, Urich H (1988) Epidermal growth factor receptor in meningiomas is expressed predominantly on endothelial cells. Cancer 62:2139–2144

Influence of Ventricular Structure and Function on the Management of Heart Failure in Cardiomyopathies

J.F. GOODWIN

Congestive heart failure occurs in all forms of cardiomyopathy; it is invariable, except in the earliest stages, and uncommon, but well recognised in hypertrophic cardiomyopathy, and usual in the later stages of restrictive cardiomyopathy due to endomyocardial fibrosis [1].

Hypertrophic Cardiomyopathy

In hypertrophic cardiomyopathy there are striking disorders of structure and function that can predispose to congestive cardiac failure, but often do not do so. The main abnormalities are the massive ventricular hypertrophy, the rapid powerful contraction of the left ventricle and the severely abnormal diastolic function characterised mainly by delayed relaxation and reduced compliance. These changes can be either global or regional and are aggravated by the extensive fibrosis, myofibrillar disarray and the narrowing of the lumen of intra-myocardial arterioles and small arteries in many patients.

Pathology

This is largely confined to the ventricles – mainly the left ventricle and ventricular septum. There is impressive asymmetrical hypertrophy of the septum, mainly of the upper portion, but hypertrophy can involve any portion of the septum or be symmetrical throughout the septum. The ventricles are not dilated, except in rare cases with heart failure, and, indeed, the volume of the left ventricle appears to be reduced and is slit-like. The papillary muscles are hypertrophied and project into the cavity of the ventricle. The hypertrophied muscle is interlaced with pale areas of fibrous tissue. There is usually a plaque of fibrous tissue present on the upper surface of the anterior leaflet of the mitral valve and on the septum in direct apposition to the septum. The atria are commonly dilated but are not usually involved in the disease. Commonly, the right ventricle is not involved except for the septal portion. The extramural coronary arteries are normal, being of particularly wide bore and smooth. The intra-muscular arterioles or small arteries may be thickened and narrowed, particularly in the subendocardial zone. Typical obstructive atherosclerotic disease in the major coronary arteries

B.S. Lewis, A. Kimchi (Eds.)
Heart Failure Mechanisms and Management
© Springer-Verlag Berlin Heidelberg 1991

may be found in association with hypertrophic cardiomyopathy as a separate condition.

The characteristic histological features are short, thick, greatly hypertrophied degenerate muscle fibres interrupted by connective tissue and arranged in the circular "whorled" fashion. On electron microscopy, striking myofibrillar disarray may be found, mainly in the septum.

Haemodynamics

Contraction of the left ventricle is powerful and rapid, the contents being expelled in the first half to two-thirds of systole. End-systolic volume is less than normal, and emptying of the cavity is complete with an ejection fraction of well over 80%. In many, but not all patients, systolic gradients are found within the body of the left ventricle. The powerful rapid contraction of the left ventricle is in striking contrast to the severe pathological and histological abnormalities that are present. In patients with gradients, the anterior mitral valve apparatus impinges on the septum at the site of the fibrous plaque, which is presumably the result of the impaction. The mitral valve is crumpled in the reduced ventricular volume, and mid-systolic closure of the aortic valve may occur.

The abnormalities of diastolic function are probably even more important. Left ventricular end-diastolic pressure tends to be elevated at rest and particularly on effort. The isovolumic relaxation period is prolonged. Relaxation is slow, and the diastolic closure rate of the mitral valve is prolonged. These changes all suggest an increase in stiffness and reduction in compliance of the left ventricle [2].

Patterns of Heart Failure

The pathophysiology of hypertrophic cardiomyopathy discourages the development of congestive heart failure until an advanced stage of the pathology has been reached at an end stage of the disease after many years of only moderate symptoms. The most common causes of heart failure are progressive fibrosis, myofibrillar disarray and hypertrophy of the left ventricle which gradually impair systolic function to a stage when the combination of abnormal diastolic function and reduced pump function summate to produce heart failure. Congestive cardiac failure may be precipitated by:

1. The onset of atrial fibrillation, especially if the ventricular rate is rapid and the arrythmia persists.
2. Severe mitral regurgitation due to fibrosis and calcification of the mitral valve.
3. Infective endocarditis on aortic or mitral valves.
4. Myocardial infarction.
5. Associated severe hypertension.

The natural history of hypertrophic cardiomyopathy in most patients is one of mild or moderate symptoms of dyspnoea, anginal pain, palpitations or dizziness for many years. Patients with a poor prognosis are those with a family history of sudden death, severe signs or symptoms in youth, marked haemodynamic disturbance and ventricular arrythmia. Many such patients die suddenly without previous heart failure [2].

The onset of atrial fibrillation removes the atrial drive needed to fill the stiff ventricles and also reduces the time available for the ventricle to fill. Thus, cardiac output often falls precipitously. Pulmonary oedema may occur if ventricular rate is very rapid. Although usually a serious complication, atrial fibrillation may be surprisingly well tolerated if the ventricular rate is well controlled, but systemic embolism is a hazard. *Severe mitral regurgitation* is a complication of the disease which may precipitate pulmonary oedema and congestive heart failure because of the sudden intolerably high left atrial pressure. *Infective endocarditis* may cause congestive heart failure as a result of severe aortic or mitral valve damage. *Myocardial infarction* can occur in the absence of significant occlusive disease of the major coronary arteries [3], possibly as a result of ischaemia due to fibrosis, impaired relaxation, and small vessel disease. It can result both in serious disorder of systolic function and in further decrease in ventricular compliance due to scarring.

Ventricular arrhythmias, an important cause of sudden death, do not seem likely to induce congestive heart failure. Regular ECG ambulatory monitoring is needed.

How the Structural and Functional Disorders Influence Management

Management is directed towards improving compliance, relaxation and filling of the ventricles; diminishing the force of contraction of the ventricles, diminishing the incidence of arrythmias and controlling them when they occur; and controlling symptoms and reducing the risk of sudden death. At the present time there is no certain way of diminishing hypertrophy or slowing the progression of the disease.

From the haemodynamic aspect, the single most important group of drugs are the beta-adrenergic blocking agent which reduce the force of contraction of the ventricle, reduce gradients, improve diastolic function and allow better filling by slowing the heart rate. The best beta-adrenergic blocking agent is still propranolol, but other agents may be used with success.

Calcium-blocking agents are good second-line drugs, but verapamil carries dangers of sudden death and pulmonary oedema and should be used with care. Nifedipine has the disadvantage of producing peripheral dilatation, thus tending to diminish the volume of the left ventricle. The effects of diltiazem are probably midway between those of verapamil and nifedipine. Other calcium-blocking agents have not been sufficiently studied for comment.

An alternative drug for haemodynamic purposes is disopyramide which diminishes the force of the left ventricle and may reduce arrythmia. Its effect on diastolic function is uncertain.

Serious ventricular arrythmias may be significantly reduced and prognosis improved by the use of amiodarone, which is indicated in patients with repeated episodes of non-sustained ventricular arrythmia or multifocal, multiple ventricular ectopic beats, especially if there is a family history of sudden death. If amiodarone is not tolerated, sotolal, which has a similar anti-arrythmic action and a weak beta-adrenergic blocking action may be an alternative.

In patients who have significant symptoms and also arrythmias, the combination of propranolol and amiodarone is acceptable. The combination of a beta-blocking agent with nifedipine may be useful in reducing the reflex tachycardia produced by the nifedipine [2,4].

Other Methods of Treatment

Implanted triggered defibrillators and sequential atrioventricular pacing are under investigation for preventing ventricular fibrillation and improving ventricular function, respectively. Atrial fibrillation is an emergency and requires immediate control. Cardioversion should be carried out under anticoagulant cover and oral (or, if necessary, intravenous) amiodarone should be given. Amiodarone should be continued in routine oral maintenance doses to maintain the patient in sinus rhythm. It must be remembered that amiodarone potentiates the effect of factor VII anticoagulants and digitalis.

When congestive heart failure is established, the treatment regimen changes. Large doses of beta-adrenergic blocking agents are contraindicated, but small doses may be useful in slowing the heart rate. Diuretics will be needed, and amiodarone may be required to control ventricular rate if there is atrial fibrillation. If congestive heart failure develops and cannot readily be relieved by control of supraventricular arrhythmia, mitral valve replacement or treatment of infective endocarditis, then cardiac transplantation must urgently be considered. Finally, the tendency for sudden death to occur during or after violent exercise makes it necessary to advise against energetic competitive sports.

Dilated Cardiomyopathy

In many ways, dilated cardiomyopathy is the opposite of hypertrophic cardiomyopathy: systolic contraction is severely impaired, and ventricular dilatation is almost the rule. Hypertrophy is at most moderate, and diastolic faults do not develop until congestive heart failure is well established. While it is now possible to diagnose dilated cardiomyopathy before overt cardiac failure occurs, cardiac failure is an inevitable progression in practically all cases. It is due to a combination of reduced ventricular systolic power and ventricular dilatation. Dilatation initially helps to maintain systolic function, but eventually the increase in wall stress and oxygen demand add a further burden. Minute cardiac volume is maintained by tachycardia which also increases the oxygen demand of the failing myocardium. Accumulation of catecholamines in the heart muscle reduces beta adrenergic receptors, further compromising contractility.

Pathology

Grossly, the heart is dilated and overweight. The dilatation of the ventricles may conceal hypertrophy by stretching and thinning the walls. The heart is flabby and the myocardium pale. The valves are normal except for stretching of the atrioventricular valve ring. There may be ante-mortem intra-cardiac thrombus in the atria or ventricles. The atria are commonly dilated. The major coronary arteries are unobstructed and appear normal, though associated atherosclerotic coronary disease may coincide in a few patients with dilated cardiomyopathy [1].

Microscopical Findings

The appearances are usually non-specific. Cellular infiltration is often only slight. There may be little myocytolysis or fibrosis. In some cases there may be considerable cellular infiltration, and this, together with extensive fraying of myocardial fibres, suggests an acute virus infection. Extensive fibrosis due to replacement of diseased myocardial cells suggests a chronic inflammatory or infective process.

There seems little doubt that some patients with dilated cardiomyopathy have suffered a previous viral myocarditis [1].

Haemodynamics

The essential disturbances are those of impaired systolic pump function. Thus, cardiac output and cardiac index are reduced, left ventricular diastolic pressures are elevated, as are right ventricular pressures. Pulmonary hypertension is thus common, but rarely severe. In early cases, before overt congestive heart failure has developed, ejection fraction is reduced. Systolic and diastolic dimensions of the ventricles measured by echocardiography are increased, and radionuclide studies may show areas of impaired uptake indicating local damage, which also suggests previous viral myocarditis.

When atrial fibrillation occurs, as it does in around 20% of patients, cardiac output falls further, and congestive failure may be precipitated. Ventricular arrhythmias are common and, if persistent, may precipitate heart failure.

Atrioventricular valvar regurgitation is common as the result of ventricular dilatation rather than of organic damage to the valve apparatus. Valvar regurgitation is seldom sufficient to affect congestive heart failure significantly. If heart failure is severe, pericardial effusion may occur.

Right ventricular failure is usually the result of preceding left ventricular failure, but in certain cases (right ventricular dilated cardiomyopathy, right ventricular dysplasia) the right ventricle may be severely affected with little or no damage to the left ventricle. In this situation, congestive heart failure is common and serious ventricular arrhythmias almost the rule. Right ventricular failure may be aggravated or precipitated by repeated pulmonary embolism as the result of deep vein thrombosis in the lower extremities or thrombus in the right atrium or right ventricle.

Influence of Structural and Functional Abnormalities on Management

The basic principles of management of dilated cardiomyopathy are three in number: treatment of low-output cardiac pump failure, control of arrhythmias, and prevention and treatment of embolism.

The most satisfactory treatment of heart failure is the combination of diuretics with ACE inhibitors such as captopril or enalapril [5]. The early use of ACE inhibitors may improve prognosis. Digoxin may be used to control ventricular rate in atrial fibrillation but is probably better avoided in patients in sinus rhythm because of its tendency to produce ventricular arrhythmias and uncertainty as to its long-term benefit.

The most effective drug for repetitive ventricular arrhythmias is amiodarone because its negative inotropic action is only slight. It is important to avoid antiarrhythmic drugs with a definite negative inotropic effect, and to remember that almost all antiarrhythmic drugs have some potential to produce arrhythmia themselves.

Anticoagulants are indicated in patients with severe congestive heart failure who are immobilised or when there is a history of systemic or pulmonary embolism or when atrial fibrillation occurs. In view of the natural history of the disease, it may be reasonable, if there are no contraindications, to prescribe anticoagulants for every patient with an established diagnosis of dilated cardiomyopathy, but there is not yet general agreement on this.

It is to be hoped that improvement in heart function will itself diminish the incidence of serious arrhythmias, but there is no certainty of this. It is possible that ACE inhibitors have an antiarrhythmic action [6].

The most effective and radical treatment for dilated cardiomyopathy at the present time is cardiac transplantation. Any patient who does not respond rapidly to suitable medical treatment should be assessed for transplantation, bearing in mind that some patients may improve spontaneously for reasons that are not clear. It is possible that such patients have a healing myocarditis. Any patient who responds initially to treatment for heart failure and then relapses, despite adequate continued treatment, should also be assessed for transplantation.

Other methods of treatment are currently under investigation. These are: immunosuppressive agents for patients with suspected acute or sub-acute infective myocarditis leading to dilated cardiomyopathy, the use of beta-adrenergic blocking agents for the treatment of heart failure and the use of anti-viral agents in patients with clear evidence of myocarditis.

Restrictive Cardiomyopathy

In restrictive cardiomyopathy, ventricular expansion and volume in diastole are restricted by abnormal tissue in the myocardium and/or the endocardium.

The most common cause of restrictive cardiomyopathy is endomyocardial fibrosis. It occurs both in the tropics and in temperate climates. The pathology and functional disorders are similar in both types. An immunological disorder of the eosinophil is involved, and there may be hypereosinophilia with involvement of other organs [7].

Pathology of Endomyocardial Fibrosis

In the initial acute inflammatory phase, the endomyocardium is intensely infiltrated with round cells, mainly eosinophils. There is little, if any, fibrosis. In the chronic fibrotic stage, there is dense fibrosis in the ventricular cavities involving mainly the inflow tracts and progressing to obliterate the ventricular cavities. The process is essentially patchy and may involve both ventricles or either one. The dense fibrosis which extends into the myocardium is overlaid by thrombus which readily becomes organised, but often gives rise to embolism. There is endarteritis obliterans in the intramyocardial arterioles in the fibrotic area. The atria are usually greatly dilated and account for much of the gross cardiomegaly that not infrequently occurs [7-9].

Haemodynamics

The haemodynamics of endomyocardial fibrosis are similar to those of constrictive pericarditis, but with certain important differences. The initial filling of the ventricles is rapid and the diastolic pressure low but, as ventricular expansion is halted by the pathological process in endocardium, myocardium or pericardium, filling slows, and diastolic pressure rises. The high diastolic pressure together with the impairment of myocardial function gives rise to congestive heart failure. The differences between restrictive cardiomyopathy (endomyocardial fibrosis) and constrictive pericarditis are threefold. First, since constrictive pericarditis is a generalised process, the diastolic pressures in both ventricles are identical, whereas, since endomyocardial fibrosis is a patchy progress, the diastolic pressures are different. Second, the early diastolic dip of the ventricular pressure pulse is at zero or below in constrictive pericarditis, but above zero in endomyocardial fibrosis because of the myocardial involvement. Third, pulmonary hypertension, which is partly due to severe mitral regurgitation in many cases, is common in endomyocardial fibrosis but rare in constrictive pericarditis. Finally, in constrictive pericarditis the myocardium is usually largely intact so systolic function is retained throughout the disease or until the very late stages.

Relation of Structural and Functional Disorders to Heart Failure

In the acute phase of endomyocardial fibrosis in the tropics, there is often fever; atrial fibrillation is common. The inflammatory (*infective?*) endomyocarditis depresses systolic function and may lead to congestive heart failure, especially if atrial fibrillation is paroxsysmal or established. In the chronic thrombofibrotic phase, congestive heart failure is due partly to severe atrioventricular regurgitation, partly to reduction in left ventricular volume and restriction of inflow, and partly to myocardial fibrosis. Pericardial effusion is common in right-sided tropical endomyocardial fibrosis and aggravates the signs of heart failure.

Influence of Structural and Functional Disorders on Management

In the acute inflammatory phase of endomyocardial fibrosis, in which hypereosinophilia is common and there may be involvement of other organs, treatment with antimetabolic agents may be tried. In the later stages, conventional treatment for heart failure, especially with diuretics, is necessary, and anticoagulants are required to prevent embolism. Surgical treatment, employing endocardectomy and atrioventricular valve replacement, has had some success. In severe intractable cases, cardiac transplantation should be considered.

Amyloid Heart Disease

The amyloid deposits stiffen the myocardium, impeding ventricular relaxation and filling. Amyloid heart disease has diastolic features in common with hypertrophic cardiomyopathy (impaired relaxation) and with constrictive cardiomyopathy (restriction of filling). The amyloid deposits also impair systolic function and, by their relation to intramural arterioles, may cause ischaemia. Treatment other than transplantation is wholly unsatisfactory.

Hypertrophic cardiomyopathy, amyloid heart disease, endomyocardial fibrosis and constrictive pericarditis are examples of diastolic heart disease in which the initial or major abnormalities of function are diastolic.

References

1. Goodwin JF (1982) The frontiers of cardiomyopathy. Br Heart J 48:1–18
2. Goodwin JF (1987) Ergebnisse der Inneren Medizin und Kinderheilkunde, vol 55. Springer, Berlin Heidelberg New York
3. Maron BJ, Epstein SE, Roberts WC (1979) Hypertrophic cardiomyopathy and transmural myocardial infarction without significant atherosclerosis of the external coronary arteries. Am J Cardiol 43:1036
4. Goodwin JF (1988) Pharmacologic treatment of hypertrophic cardiomyopathy; beta blockade or calcium blockade or what? Cardiovasc Drugs Therapy 1:665
5. The CONSENSUS trial study Group (1987) Effects of enalapril on mortality in severe congestive heart failure: results of the co-operative North Scandanavian enalapril revival study (CONSENSUS). N Engl J Med 316:1429
6. Cleland JGS, Dargie HJ (1988) Arrhythmias, catecholamines and electrolytes. Am J Cardiol 62:55a
7. Olsen EGJ, Spry CJF (1979) The pathogenesis of Loffler's endomyocardial disease and its relationship to endomyocardial fibrosis. In: Yu PN, Goodwin JF (eds) Progress in cardiology, vol 8. Lea and Febiger, Philadelphia, p 281
8. Spry CJF, Davies J, Tai TC, Olsen EGJ, Oakley CM, Goodwin JF (1983) Clinical features of fifteen patients with hypereosinophilic syndrome. Q J Med 52:1
9. Davies J, Spry CJF, Sapsford R, Olsen EGJ, Du Perez G, Oakley CM, Goodwin JF (1983) Cardiovascular features of eleven patients with eosinophilic endomyocardial disease. Q J Med 52:23

Pharmacotherapy of Heart Failure

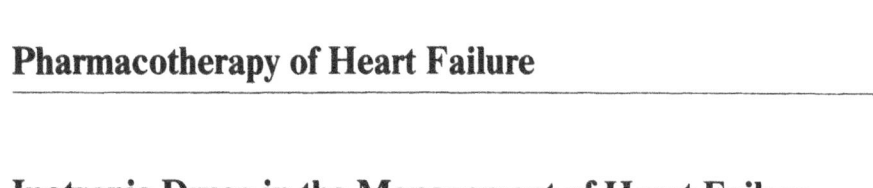

Inotropic Drugs in the Management of Heart Failure

Effects of Different Positive Inotropic Drugs in Congestive Heart Failure

H.-H. ERLEMEIER and W. BLEIFELD

Introduction

The treatment of congestive heart failure is a challenge for modern medicine. Despite the fact that digitalis was introduced into therapy 200 years ago and vasodilators have been used for the last 15 years, the outcome of overt heart failure is still bad [1]. Therefore, many efforts have been undertaken in order to develop new inotropes, but only in recent years have a number of promising compounds emerged. The present article reviews the different action of new inotropic compounds on the myocardium, and the results of first clinical trials are presented.

Pathophysiology

The depression of the myocardial pump function following acute myocardial infarction or during acute failure in the course of congestive cardiomyopathy results in a drop in the arterial blood pressure and a decrease of stroke volume. Several counter-regulation mechanisms are activated to restore the parameters of circulation:

- The Frank-Starling mechanism is initiated by the dilatation of the left ventricle in order to increase the stroke volume [2].
- The release of endogenous catecholamines is followed by an increase of cardiac output via the inotropic and chronotropic effects. In addition, they raise the systemic vascular resistance in order to maintain the arterial blood pressure [3].
- The reduced renal perfusion and the high level of circulating catecholamines activate the release of renin. Renin mediates the transformation from angiotensin I to angiotensin II, which is a potent vasoconstrictor. The action of angiotensin II supports the increase of arterial blood pressure and glomerular filtration [3,4].
- Finally, aldosterone leads to an increase of sodium and fluid retention, which contributes to the increase of preload by enhanced venous return [5].
- The role of other humoral factors such as arginine vasopressin, and atrial natriuretic peptide (ANP) is still under investigation [6,7].

B.S. Lewis, A. Kimchi (Eds.)
Heart Failure Mechanisms and Management
© Springer-Verlag Berlin Heidelberg 1991

All these feed-back systems are effective in maintaining cardiac output and arterial blood pressure in patients with congestive heart failure. However, they cause further myocardial damage:

- Myocardial wall tension becomes increased by the raise of preload and afterload. This may hasten the myocardial impairment [8].
- Pulmonary congestion following the increased left ventricular filling pressure impairs the oxygen exchange.
- Venous congestion may lead to an impairment of liver and renal function and may also impede the digestive system.

Diuretics relieve the symptoms of congestion. However, they usually reduce cardiac output by counteracting the humoral and myocardial feed-back systems [9] and by a shift of the performance state on the function curve to the left. Nevertheless, diuretics are standard in the treatment of congestive heart failure.

Vasodilators decrease afterload and improve cardiac output after acute administration. During long-term therapy, however, the effects of some vasodilators are counteracted by the activation of humoral feed-back systems and tolerance develops [10].

In contrast, the *ACE inhibitors* exert beneficial effects on quality of life and exercise capacity, but they may cause hypotension and renal failure because of the reduction of the angiotensin II level [4,11]. Therefore, the restoration of the impaired myocardial pump function remains the main aim in the therapy of overt heart failure. Thus, the attention is focused on new inotropic compounds.

Biochemistry of Myocardial Contraction

Calcium ions play a major role in the excitation-contraction coupling. Triggered by the depolarization of the myocardial cell, they are released from intracellular stores and bind then to troponin, the receptor protein of the contractile apparatus. Then, the bridging mechanisms between the actin and myosin proteins results in the beginning of myocardial contraction. Most inotropes work on the basis of an increase of the intracellular Ca^{2+} pool [12]: digitalis inhibits the Na^+/K^+ pump, which leads to an increasing intracellular sodium level. These surplus amounts of sodium ions leave the cell via the Na^+/Ca^{2+} pump in exchange for calcium ions [12,13]. The influx of calcium ions into the cell is also mediated by the slow calcium channels. Their activity is controlled by the intracellular cAMP level. The phosphodiesterase inhibitors (PDE inhibitors) block the metabolism of cAMP by inhibition of its degrading enzyme [13].

The beta-adrenoceptor agonists activate the beta-adrenoceptors on the cell surface. As a result, the stimulated receptors are coupled to adenylate cyclase, which leads to an increase of the cAMP level [13,14]. The compounds sulmazole and pimobendane increase the sensitivity of troponin to calcium ions resulting in an inotropic effect despite an unchanged activator-Ca^{2+} pool [13,15]. This seems to be a particularly energy-saving action because steps requiring ATP such as the synthesis of cAMP and the uptake of increased amounts of calcium ions into the intracellular stores are bypassed [15,16].

Clinical Features of Inotropes

The aims of each therapy with inotropes are the improvement of quality of life and exercise capacity, and the prolongation of survival. Therefore, it has to be proved whether or not new inotropic drugs can sustain their acute effects in long-term treatment [17,18].

Dobutamine is a beta-adrenoceptor agonist which has a strong effect on the failing heart, resulting in a marked increase of cardiac output and a decrease of the left ventricular filling pressure [19]. After continuous infusions for over more than 3 days, tolerance developed because of the down-regulation of the beta-receptors [20]. The concept of intermittent weekly infusions with dobutamine in outpatients with advanced cardiac failure has been abandoned because of an increased mortality in the treatment group [21].

Prenalterol and *pirbuterol* are orally active beta-agonists [22,23]. These compounds also led to tolerance development during long-term therapy, despite promising short-term effects [23,24]. In contrast, *xamoterol*, a partial beta-agonist, exerted a sustained increase of exercise capacity and quality of life during a 3-month treatment period [25]. The rate of side effects was lower than with digitalis.

Amrinone was the first PDE inhibitor available. After short-term adminis-tration, it increased cardiac output and decreased afterload [26]. Its inotropic effect on the impaired myocardium is questionable: in contrast to previous observations, Wilmshurst [27] found no effect on the myocardium after in-tracoronary application, whereas after intravenous application a vasodilator-like mode of action was achieved. A high rate of serious side effects and a lack of hemodynamic improvement were observed during long-term oral therapy [28]. Amrinone is therefore not yet available in the oral formulation.

Milrinone and *enoxinome* are PDE inhibitors with similar hemodynamic effects after short-term administration [29,30]. In contrast to amrinone, they were better tolerated during long-term oral treatment. First small studies suggested that both compounds caused a sustained hemodynamic improvement, but larger randomized trials are necessary for a final statement [31,32].

The Ca^{2+} sensitizers *pimobendane* and *sulmazole* exert a weak inhibition of the phosphodiesterase. They also have an inotropic effect which results from direct activation of the Ca^{2+}-binding sites on the contractile proteins. In contrast to pure PDE inhibitors or catecholamines, the positive inotropic effect is not necessarily combined with an increase in intracellular calcium release and sequestration. Thus the latter effect increased the contractile force more econ-omically [33]. When given to patients with severe heart failure on a short-term basis, they improved cardiac output and decreased pulmonary capillary wedge pressure by the same amount as dobutamine [34]. First results from long-term studies suggested a sustained hemodynamic improvement during a 1-month treatment period and at least equal effects compaired to captopril [35,36]. However, these compounds also have to be proven in their efficacy in larger randomized trials.

Digitalis is the oldest inotrope and the first drug applied in congestive heart failure. Despite that, only rare controlled studies have been published. Digitalis exerts only weak hemodynamic effects [37]. The indication for digitalis even in patients with sinus rhythm and coronary artery disease has been controversial [38]. Further work is necessary for a better estimation of benefits and hazards of digitalis treatment.

Disadvantages of Inotropic Therapy

A common side effect of all inotropes which increase the intracellular Ca^{2+} level is serious arrhythmias [13,18]. Inotropes should be given with caution to patients with severe impaired left ventricular function, who are at a particular risk of sudden death. Therefore, the rate of sudden deaths in the running trials should be carefully observed.

Inotropic stimulation may increase the left ventricular wall tension by the rise in the contractile force. This may hasten left ventricular impairment and may shorten survival [17,18,39]. On the other hand, a reduced preload and a decreased diameter of the left ventricle may contribute to a decrease of the wall tension. Therefore, the PDE inhibitors and the Ca^{2+} sensitizers claim to have an advantage over beta-agonists and digitalis because of their vasodilating properties [39].

Several compounds exert an active acceleration of the myocardial relaxation besides their effects during systole. This so-called lusitropic action contributes to the decrease of preload [40]. Although only rare studies on this topic have so far been published, the lusitropic effects have emerged as playing an important role and should be mentioned in making a final statement on each inotrope.

Summary

In the therapy of cardiac failure, digitalis, diuretics and vasodilators are used as standard therapy. Each of these substances, however, has specific disadvantages. In the group of the PDE inhibitors, enoximone and milrinone are promising compounds, whereas oral therapy with amrinone has failed because of severe side effects and the lack of long-term improvement. The beta-adrenoceptor agonists dobutamine, pirbuterol, and prenalterol exhibited tolerance development during long-term therapy. The partial adrenoceptor agonist xamoterol exerted a sustained improvement of exercise capacity and quality of life. Pimobendane and sulmazole work directly on the contractile proteins. Their action has been suggested as favorable from the energetic point of view. Larger randomized studies concerning the new inotropes are now under investigation.

References

1. Rowlands DJ (1988) Cardiac failure: overview. Curr Opinion Cardiol 3:319–320
2. Bleifeld W, Hamm CW (1987) Herz und Kreislauf. Klinische Pathophysiologie. Springer, Berlin Heidelberg New York
3. Cohn JN, Levine B, Francis GS, Goldsmith S (1981) Neurohumoral control mechanisms in congestive heart failure. Am Heart J 102:509–514
4. Badr KF, Ichikawa I (1988) Prerenal failure: a deleterious shift from renal compensation to decompensation. N Engl J Med 319:623–629
5. Davies JO (1984) Mechanisms of salt and water retention in cardiac failure. In: Braunwald E (ed) The myocardium: failure and infarction. HP Publ, New York, pp 80–100
6. Pruszczynski W, Vahanian A, Ardaillon R, Acar J (1984) Role of antidiuretic hormone in impaired water excretion of patients with congestive heart failure. J Clin Endocrinol Metab 58:599–605
7. Drexler H, Hirth C, Stasch JP, Lang RE, Finckh M, Maio G, Just H (1988) Circulatory role of atrial natriuretic peptide in experimental heart failure. Z Kardiol 77 [Suppl 2]:47–50
8. Pfeffer MA, Lamas GA, Vaughan DE, Parisi AF, Braunwald E (1988) Effect of captopril on progressive ventricular dilatation after anterior myocardial infarction. N Engl J Med 319:80–85
9. Brown JJ, Davies DL, Johnson VW, Lever AF, Robertson JIS (1970) Renin relationships in congestive cardiac failure, treated and untreated. Am Heart J 80:329–342
10. Riegger GAJ, Haeske W, Kraus C, Kromer EP, Kochsiek K (1987) Contribution of the renin-angiotensin-aldosterone system to development of tolerance and fluid retention in chronic congestive heart failure during prazosin treatment. Am J Cardiol 59:906–910
11. Packer M, Medina N, Yurshak M (1984) Relation between serum sodium concentration and the hemodynamic and clinical responses to converting enzyme inhibition with captopril in severe heart failure. J Am Coll Cardiol 3:1035–1043
12. Colucci WS, Wright RF, Braunwald E (1986) New positive inotropic agents in the treatment of congestive heart failure. N Engl J Med 314:290–299
13. Scholz H (1984) Inotropic drugs and their mechanisms of action. J Am Coll Cardiol 4:389–397
14. Lefkowitz RJ, Caron MG, Stiles GL (1984) Mechanisms of membrane-receptor regulation. N Engl J Med 310:1570–1579
15. Diederen W, Dämmgen J, Kadatz R (1982) Cardiovascular profile of UDCG 115, a new orally and long lasting cardiotonic compound, not related to beta-mimetics or cardiac glycosides. Naunyn Schmiedebergs Arch Pharmacol 321:R36
16. Diederen W (1984) Improvement of ventricular function in dogs by the cardiotonic drug pimobendan in comparison to the vasodilators captopril and dihydralazin. Cell Calcium 5:312
17. Maskin CS, Le Jemtel TH, Sonnenblick EH (1984) Inotropic drugs for treatment of the failing heart. Cardiovasc Clin 14:1–17
18. Katz AM (1978) A new inotropic drug: its promise and a caution. N Engl J Med 299:1409–1410
19. Kupper W, Waller D, Hanrath P, Bleifeld W (1982) Hemodynamic and cardiac metabolic effects of inotropic stimulation with dobutamine in patients with coronary artery disease. Eur Heart J 3:29–34
20. Unverferth DV, Blanford M, Kates RE, Leier CV (1980) Tolerance to dobutamine after a 72 hour continuous infusion. Am J Med 69:262–266
21. Krell MJ, Kline EM, Bates ER, Hodgson J, Dilworth, Laufer N, Vogel RA, Pitt B (1986) Intermittent ambulatory dobutamine infusions in patients with severe congestive heart failure. Am Heart J 112:787–791

22. Kupper W, Schütt M, Hamm CW, Kuck KH, Hanrath P, Bleifeld W (1983) Haemodynamic and cardiac metabolic effects of the new β_1-agonist prenalterol in patients with cardiac failure. Eur Heart J 4:573-583

23. Colucci WS, Alexander RW, Williams GH, Rude RE, Holman BL, Konstam MA, Wyme J, Mudge GH, Braunwald E (1982) Decreased lymphozyte beta-adrenergic-receptor density in patients with heart failure and tolerance to the beta-adrenergic agonist pirbuterol. N Engl J Med 305:185-190

24. Lambertz H, Meyer J, Erbel R (1984) Long-term hemodynamic effects of prenalterol in patients with severe congestive heart failure. Circulation 69:298-305

25. The German and Austrian xamoterol study group (1988) Double-blind placebo-controlled comparison of digoxin and xamoterol in chronic heart failure. Lancet I:489-493

26. Konstam MA, Cohen SR, Weiland DS, Martin TT, Dhirendra D, Isner JM, Salem DN (1986) Relative contribution of inotropic and vasodilator effects to amrinone − induced hemodynamic improvement in congestive heart failure. Am J Cardiol 57:242-248

27. Wilmshurst PT, Thompson DS, June SM, Dittrich HC, Dawson JR, Walker JM, Jenkins BS, Coltart DS, Webb-Peploe MM (1985) Effects of intracoronary and intravenous amrinone infusions in patients with cardiac failure and patients with near normal cardiac function. Br Heart J 53:493-506

28. Packer M, Medina N, Yurshak M (1984) Hemodynamic and clinical limitations of long-term inotropic therapy with amrinone in patients with severe chronic heart failure. Circulation 70:1038-1047

29. McKay RG, Miller M, Fergason JJ, Momomuwa SI, Sahagian P, Grossman W, Pasternak RC (1986) Assessment of left ventricular end-systolic pressure volume relations with an impedance catheter and transient inferior vena cava occlusion: Use of this system in the evaluation of the cardiotonic effects of dobutamine, milrinone, posicor and epinephrine. J Am Coll Cardiol 8:1152-1160

30. Uretsky BF, Valdes AM, Reddy PS (1986) Positive inotropic therapy for short-term support and long-term management of patients with congestive heart failure: hemodynamic effects and clinical efficacy of MDL 17, 043. Circulation 73 [Suppl III]:III 219-229

31. Weber KT, Janicki JS, Mukesh CJ (1986) Enoximone (MDL 17, 043) for stable, chronic heart failure secondary to ischemic or idiopathic cardiomyopathy. Am J Cardiol 58:589-595

32. Le Jemtel TH, Gumbardo D, Chadwick B, Rutman HJ, Sonnenblick E (1986) Milrinone for long-term therapy of severe heart failure: clinical experience with special reference to maximal exercise tolerance. Circulation 73 [Suppl III]:III 213-218

33. Holubarsch C, Hasenfuss G, Blanchard E, Mulieri LA, Alpert NR, Just H (1985) Myokardiale Mechanik und Energetik unter Isoproterenol und UDCG 115, einer neuen positiv inotropen Substanz. Z Kardiol 74 [Suppl 3]:103

34. Permanetter B, Baumann K, Busch U, Wirtzfeld A (1986) Hämodynamische Effekte von UDCG 115 − BS bei Patienten mit fortgeschrittener myokardialer Insuffizienz. In: Just H, Bussmann W (eds) Vasoaktive Substanzen bei Herzinsuffizienz. Springer, Berlin Heidelberg New York, pp 324-329

35. Renard M, Walter M, Liebens J, Dresse A, Bernard R (1988) Pimobendane (UDCG 115 BS) in chronic congestive heart failure. Chest 93:1159-1164

36. Hauf GF, Grom E, Jähnchen E, Roskamm H (1987) Hemodynamic efficacy of UDCG 115 and captopril in patients with congestive heart failure − a double blind randomized study. Eur Heart J 8 [Suppl 2]:36

37. Gheorghiade M, St Clair J, St Clair C, Beller GA (1987) Hemodynamic effects of intravenous digoxin in patients with severe heart failure initially treated with diuretics and vasodilators. J Am Coll Cardiol 9:849-857

38. Yusuf S, Wittes J, Bailey K, Furberg C (1986) Digitalis − a new controversy regarding an old drug. Circulation 73:14-18

39. Le Jemtel TH, Sonnenblick EH (1983) Should the failing heart be stimulated? N Engl J Med 310:1384-1385

40. Smith VE, Katz AM (1987) Inotropic and lusitropic abnormalities as the basis for heart failure. Heart Failure 1:55-65

Pharmacological Properties and Mechanism of Action of Denopamine in Experimental Animals

T. Nagao, Y. Sasaki, H. Yabana, M. Hoshiyama, and S. Harigaya

Denopamine is a novel phenylethanolamine derivative (Fig. 1). It is a highly selective β_1-agonist and was derived from a study on structure-activity relationships of a β_2-agonist, trimetoquinol, and was designed as an orally active positive inotropic agent with minor side effects. We report here denopamine's pharmacological properties and mechanism of action. Denopamine has been used clinically as a remedy for chronic heart failure in Japan since 1988.

Positive Inotropic Action

In the anesthetized dog, i.v. denopamine caused a positive inotropic effect: its potency was 1/100 that of isoproterenol. The positive inotropic effect of denopamine was stereoselective and the $(-)$-isomer, denopamine, is an active form. The positive inotropic effect of denopamine was inhibited by 1 mg/kg, i.v. practolol. Denopamine caused no significant effects on arterial blood pressure and a small increase in heart rate [1]. As shown in Fig. 2, xamoterol and amrinone caused slightly more potent positive inotropic action than positive chronotropic action, but denopamine showed more selectively positive inotropic effect than xamoterol and amrinone. In the separate experiment, denopamine showed positive lusitropic effect as estimated by Weiss's time constant T together with a positive inotropic effect in anesthetized dogs [2].

In reserpinized dogs, the relative positive inotropic effect of denopamine compared to isoproterenol was almost similar to that in normal anesthetized dogs [1].

When denopamine was administered orally to conscious dogs at doses of 0.1–0.4 mg/kg, LV dp/dt_{max} was increased dose dependently (Fig. 3). Denopamine at a dose of 0.4 mg/kg caused an increase in LV dp/dt_{max} by 65%, and the effect lasted for 5–7 h. Heart rate was not affected at lower doses, and mean blood pressure was not significantly affected either. Changes in plasma levels were paralleled with changes in LV dp/dt_{max} [3].

B.S. Lewis, A. Kimchi (Eds.)
Heart Failure Mechanisms and Management
© Springer-Verlag Berlin Heidelberg 1991

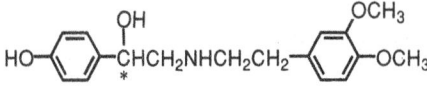

Fig. 1. Chemical structure of denopamine. *Asterisk*, asymmetric center

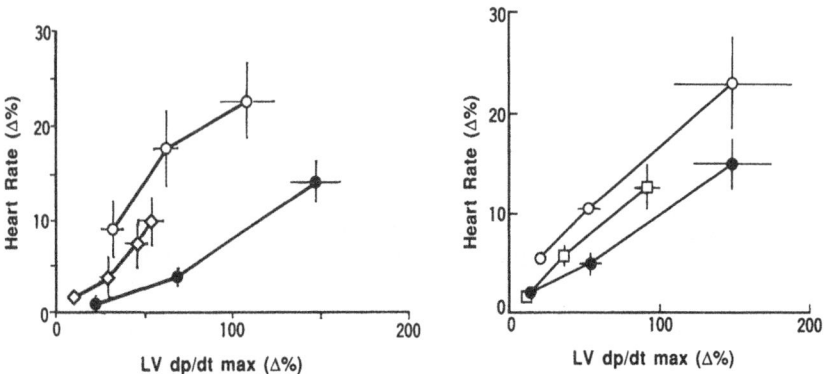

Fig. 2. Relationships between positive inotropic action and positive chronotropic action of denopamine, isoproterenol, xamoterol, and amrinone in pentobarbital-anesthetized dogs. *Solid circles*, denopamine (1–10 μg/kg, i.v.); *open circles*, isoproterenol (0.003–0.03 μg/kg, i.v.); *diamonds*, xamoterol (0.3–10 μg/kg, i.v.); *squares*, amrinone (100–1000 μg/kg, i.v., n = 5)

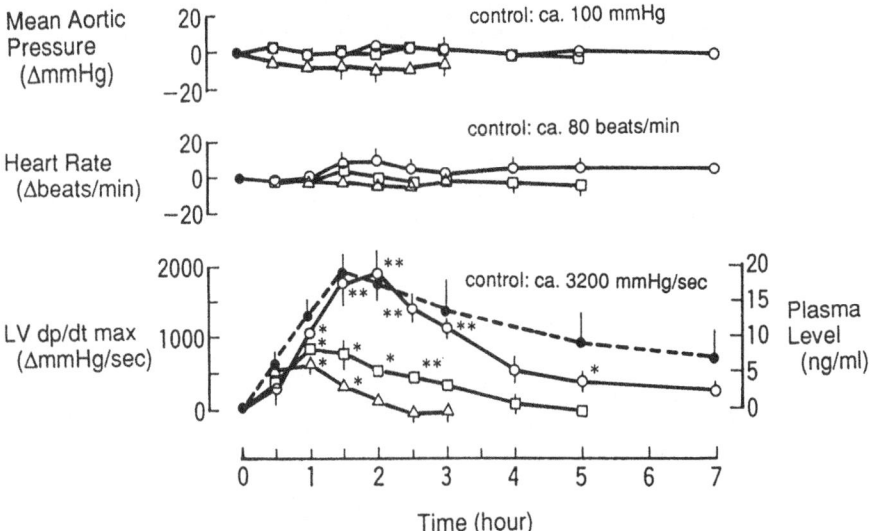

Fig. 3. Time course of actions of oral denopamine on mean aortic pressure, heart rate, LV dp/dt$_{max}$, and plasma levels in conscious instrumented dogs [3]. *Triangles*, 0.1 mg/kg, p.o., n = 5; *open circles*, 0.4 mg/kg, p.o., n = 5; *squares*, 0.2 mg/kg, p.o., n = 5; *solid circles*, plasma level, n = 4

Isolated Cardiac Muscle

Positive inotropic and positive chronotropic actions of denopamine were studied in isolated papillary muscle and right atria of guinea pigs, respectively. As shown in Fig. 4, dose-response curves for the positive inotropic and positive chronotropic actions of denopamine were less steep than those for isoproterenol. pD_2 values of denopamine and isoproterenol for positive inotropy were 7.08 and 8.59, respectively [4]. Maximal response was lower for denopamine (0.83) than isoproterenol (1.00). Xamoterol showed positive inotropy for ten out of 16 (maximal response: 0.27), and negative inotropy for six out of 16. Maximal responses for positive chronotropic effect were 1.00 for isoproterenol, 0.69 for denopamine, and 0.45 for xamoterol, although xamoterol also caused an increase or a decrease in heart rate. Incidentally, maximal response of denopamine in isolated papillary muscle of the cat was the same as that of isoproterenol [5]. Denopamine decreased maximal response of isoproterenol for positive chronotropic action to a level of the maximal response for denopamine itself [6], and the pA_2 value was 6.9 [4].

In the isolated trabeculae muscle of the dog, the shortening effect of denopamine on the time to peak tension was weaker than that of isoproterenol [7]. In the guinea pig papillary muscle, denopamine caused increases in both the rate of the rise in contraction and the rate of the fall in relaxation to a similar extent. Isoproterenol preferably increased the latter, and ouabain rather increased the former [8].

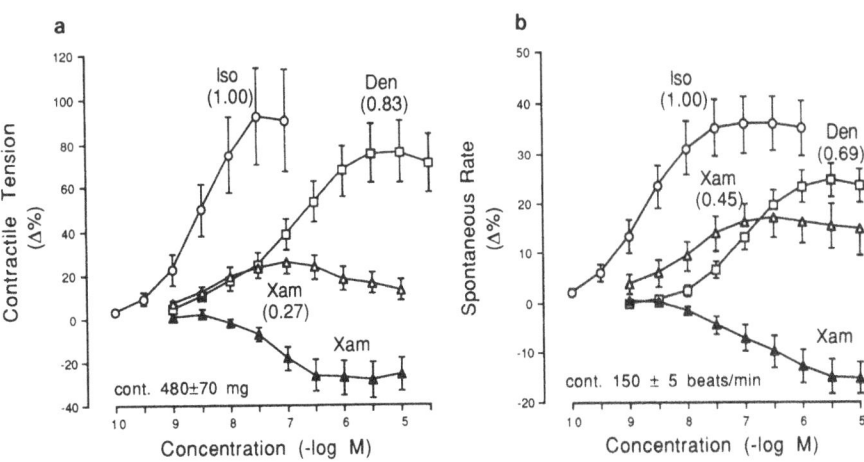

Fig. 4a,b. Positive inotropic and positive chronotropic actions of denopamine (*Den*), isoproterenol (*Iso*), and xamoterol (*Xam*) in the isolated ventricular papillary muscle (**a**) and right atria (**b**) of guinea pig [4]. *Figures in parentheses,* relative value to maximal response of isoproterenol (1.00). $n = 6$–$13 \pm$ SEM

Myocardial Oxygen Consumption

In the halothane-anesthetized dog, denopamine caused a smaller increase in myocardial oxygen consumption (MVO_2) than isoproterenol at given positive inotropy. Especially at lower doses, denopamine increased LV dp/dt_{max} without a significant increase in MVO_2. At the same time, reduction by denopamine of left ventricular diameter both in systole and diastole was more prominent than isoproterenol. Thus, this weak MVO_2-increasing effect of denopamine may be derived from its weak chronotropic effects and a significant reduction of cardiac size [9].

Hemodynamic Effect

Denopamine by i.v. injection to anesthetized dogs increased LV dp/dt_{max}, cardiac output, stroke volume, and decreased total vascular resistance and central venous pressure. An increase in coronary blood flow by denopamine was weaker than that by isoproterenol [9]. Denopamine caused a very weak (1/10 000 that of isoproterenol) vasodilating effect on the femoral artery by intraarterial injection, and the effect was slightly inhibited by propranolol [1].

Arrythmogenic Activity

Denopamine has been reported to have a weaker arrhythmogenic action in both in vitro and in vivo studies than ouabain [5,6]. The arrythmogenic activity of denopamine was also compared with that of catecholamines in conscious dogs 3–4 days after coronary ligation. Denopamine tended to increase non-sinus rhythm from 0.3 to 1 mg/kg, i.v., while ED_{50} for positive inotropic action was 2 $\mu g/kg$, i.v. Noradrenaline, isoproterenol, dobutamine, and dopamine showed dose-dependent arrhythmogenic actions in this preparation. Similarly, the arrythmogenic activity of denopamine was weaker than that of dobutamine and dopamine in halothane-anesthetized dogs [2].

In the isolated guinea pig and cat papillary muscles, denopamine, unlike catecholamines, did not induce dose-related irregular beats [5,8]. Therefore, we further studied the arrythmogenecity of denopamine using isolated cat papillary muscle in comparison with milrinone. Figure 5 shows the effects of denopamine and milrinone on post-contraction evoked by triggered activity. Milrinone showed a smaller increase in contractile force, but the incidence of post-contraction was higher than with denopamine. Thus denopamine showed a different effect on contraction and post-contraction indicating a different property from milrinone.

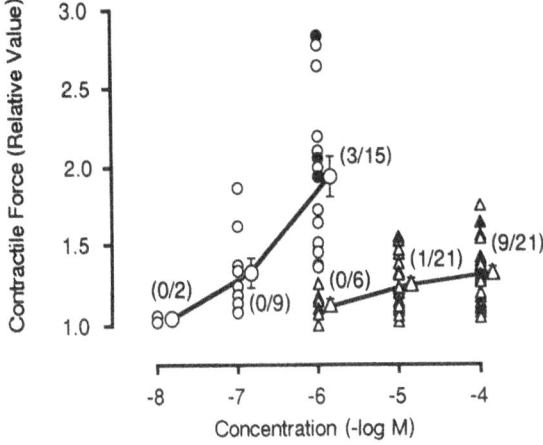

Fig. 5. Effects of denopamine and milrinone on contractile force (1 Hz) and postcontraction evoked by triggered activity (5 Hz, 120 beats) in the isolated cat right papillary muscle. *Open circles,* denopamine; *open triangles,* milrinone; *numbers in parentheses,* incidence of postcontraction; *solid symbols,* postcontraction *larger symbols,* mean of contractile force ± SEM

Tolerance

Since consecutive administration of catecholamines has been shown to cause tolerance, we studied whether denopamine causes desensitization and down-regulation in rats [10]. After consecutive administration, rats were anesthetized, and ED_{50} was obtained by i.v. denopamine or isoproterenol. In the separate experiment with the same dose study B_{max} of the β-adrenoceptor in the heart was obtained by ^{3}H-dihydroalprenolol (DHA) ligand study. Denopamine at a dose of 40 mg kg^{-1} day^{-1} in the diet for 14 days caused no effects on ED_{50} and B_{max}. Incidentally, ED_{50} and ED_{100} for denopamine in rats were 0.77 and 3 mg/kg, p.o., respectively. On the other hand, isoproterenol at doses of 5 and 50 μg/kg, s.c., t.i.d. (ED_{100} = 5 μg/kg, s.c.) caused an increase in ED_{50} and a significant reduction in B_{max}. These results indicate that denopamine, unlike isoproterenol, caused no tolerance and down-regulation at effective doses.

Mechanism of Action

Slow Response

Denopamine 2.8×10^{-7} M induced slow response in the partially depolarized guinea pig papillary muscle with 25 mM K$^+$ [7]. In another study, denopamine and isoproterenol increased the maximal rate of depolarization (V_{max}) of slow response. Moreover, isoproterenol increased the contractile force in normal solution and V_{max} of slow response to a similar extent, while denopamine increased the contractile force more prominently than V_{max}, suggesting that denopamine has a different relationship between Ca influx and contraction from isoproterenol [8].

Affinity and Selectivity for β-Adrenoceptor

We assessed the β_1 selectivity and agonistic property using ^{3}H-DHA in turkey erythrocyte membranes as a β_1 pure preparation and in rat reticulocyte membranes as a β_2 pure preparation [11]. As illustrated in Fig. 6, denopamine is the most selective β_1-agonist, but its intrinsic activity, assessed by Ki shift in the presence and absence of GTP, was lower than full agonists such as isoproterenol and noradrenaline. This means that denopamine is a partial agonist in the radioligand-binding study.

Effects on Adenylate Cyclase, cAMP Levels, and Protein Phosphorylation of Cardiac Muscle

The effects of denopamine and isoproterenol on adenylate cyclase activity in canine sarcolemmal vesicles were studied. Drugs were added to sarcolemmal vesicles in vitro. Denopamine caused a small increase (0.25) in adenylate cyclase activity, as compared with isoproterenol (1.00) [12].

Effects of denopamine, isoproterenol, and milrinone on cAMP levels in different subcellular fractions were studied in the perfused guinea pig heart. The

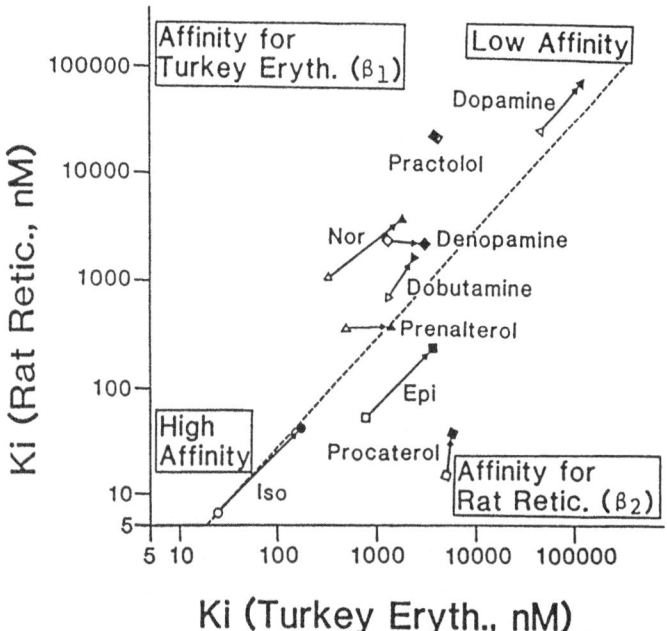

Fig. 6. β_1, β_2 selectivity and agonist property of denopamine and β-adrenergic agents were assessed by means of ^{3}H-DHA binding to turkey erythrocyte (*Eryth.*) and rat reticulocyte (*Retic.*) membranes. Ki shift by GTP (0.1 mM) represents agonist property of the agent [11] *Nor*, norepinephrine; *Epi*, epinephrine; *open symbols*, without GTP; *solid symbols*, with GTP

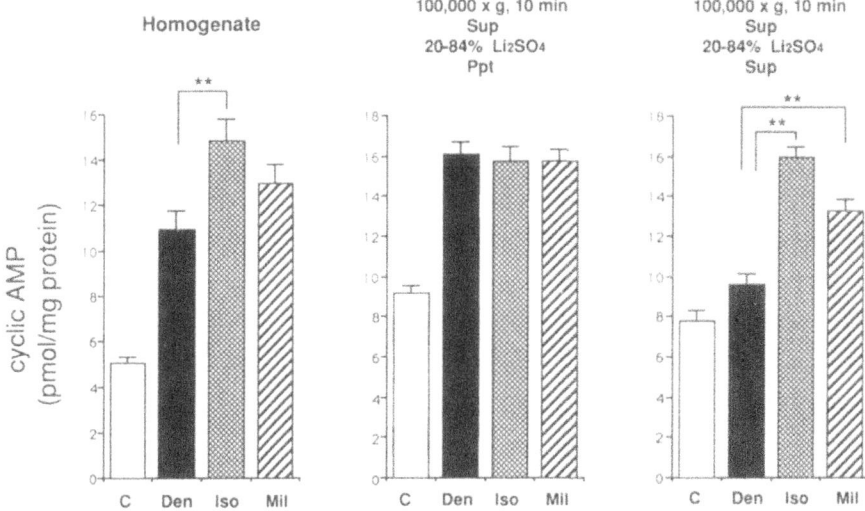

Fig. 7. Effects of denopamine (*Den*), isoproterenol (*Iso*), and milrinone (*Mil*) on cAMP levels in various subcellular fractions of perfused guinea pig hearts at concentrations of equipotent inotropy. $n = 6\text{-}10 \pm$ SEM. *Asterisks*, $P < 0.01$ vs. control (*C*); *Sup*, supernatant; *Ppt*, precipitate

concentration of the drugs was selected to increse dF/dt_{max} to a similar extent. As shown in Fig. 7, in the homogenate fraction, the increasing effect of cAMP levels was isoproterenol > milrinone > denopamine in decreasing order. In the precipitated fraction obtained by adding Li_2SO_4 starting from 20% to 84% to the 100 000 × g supernatant of the homogenate, the elevations of cAMP levels by these drugs were identical. However, in the supernatant fraction remaining after precipitation by Li_2SO_4, denopamine showed a minimal increase in cAMP, and isoproterenol and milrinone caused marked increases. It was speculated that the precipitated fraction worked for cardiac contraction, and other fractions contributed to other effects like an arrhythmogenic effect of these drugs.

Effects of denopamine on the phosphorylation of cardiac muscle proteins were studied in comparison with isoproterenol using perfused guinea pig hearts [13]. Denopamine, like isoproterenol, stimulated phosphorylation of five cardiac proteins including troponin-I and phospholamban. This result is consistent with the earlier finding that the rate of relaxation was increased by both isoproterenol and denopamine.

Summary

Denopamine has an orally active positive inotropic action and causes smaller increases in heart rate and myocardial oxygen consumption. It also increases the rate of relaxation. Denopamine is a highly selective β_1-agonist and is a partial agonist with high intrinsic activity. However, denopamine has a weak stimulating effect on adenylate cyclase and causes a minimal increase in cAMP levels in the heart. These pharmacological properties may contribute to weak arrhythmogenic action and absence of tolerance. Moreover, the pharmacological actions of denopamine described here are consistent with clinical observations.

References

1. Nagao T, Ikeo T, Murata S, Sato M, Nakajima H (1984) Cardiovascular effects of a new positive inotropic agent, $(-)$-(R)-1-(p-hydroxyphenyl)-2-((3,4-dimethoxyphenethyl)amino)ethanol (TA-064) in the anesthetized dog and isolated guinea pig heart. Jpn J Pharmacol 35:415–423
2. Narita H, Yabana H, Kikkawa K, Miyazaki K, Ikeo T, Nagao T (1986) Weak arrhythmogenic property of the new cardiotonic agent denopamine in dogs. Comparison with catecholamines. Jpn J Pharmacol 41:334–344
3. Ikeo T, Nagao T, Suzuki T, Yabana H, Nakajima H (1985) Cardiovascular effects and plasma levels of denopamine (TA-064), a new positive inotropic agent, in chronically instrumented dogs. Jpn J Pharmacol 39:191–199
4. Yabana H, Watanabe H, Nagao T (1989) β-Adrenoceptor selectivity and its partial agonistic action of denopamine. − Comparison with T-0509 and xamoterol −. Jpn J Pharmacol 49 [Suppl]:60P
5. Hosiyama M, Ikeo T, Miyazaki K, Nagao T (1985) Effects of denopamine on contractile force and heart rate, and its arrhythmogenic activity in the isolated cat heart muscle. Jpn Pharmacol Ther 13:6323–6330
6. Narita H, Nagao T, Yabana H, Miyazaki K, Nosaka K, Watanabe H, Hoshiyama M (1988) Weak arrhythmogenecity and partial agonistic property of denopamine. Jpn Pharmacol Ther 16:3089–3100
7. Hoshiyama M, Miyazaki K (1985) Effects of denopamine on electrical and mechanical properties of the isolated canine and guinea pig heart muscles. Jpn Pharmacol Ther 13:6333–6342
8. Sato T, Imanishi S, Arita M (1985) Positive inotropic effect of denopamine (TA-064), a new cardiotonic agent, in guinea pig papillary muscle. − In comparison with isoproterenol and ouabain −. Jpn Pharmacol Ther 13:5727–5736
9. Ikeo T, Nagao T (1985) Effects of denopamine (TA-064), a new positive inotropic agent, on myocardial oxygen consumption and left ventricular dimension in anesthetized dogs. Jpn J Pharmacol 39:179–189
10. Yabana H, Naito K, Nagao T (1986) Effect of chronic administration of denopamine (TA-064), a new positive inotropic agent, on cardiac response of rats to denopamine. Jpn J Pharmacol 42:87–97
11. Naito K, Nagao T, Ono Y, Otsuka H, Harigaya S, Nakajima H (1985) Effect of GTP on the affinity of denopamine, a new cardiotonic agent, for β-adrenergic receptors of turkey erythrocytes and rat reticulocyte membranes. Jpn J Pharmacol 39:541–549
12. Bing RJ, Sasaki Y, Burger W, Chemnitius JM (1984) Cardiac inotropic response of a new β-1-agonist (T-064) with low sarcolemmal adenylate cyclase activation. Curr Therap Res 36:1127–1144
13. Sasaki Y, Yabana H, Nagao T, Takeyama S (1988) Effect of denopamine on the phosphorylation of cardiac muscle proteins in the perfused guinea-pig heart. Biochem Pharmacol 37:679–686

Long-Term Double-Blind Comparative Study of Ibopamine Versus Placebo in the Treatment of Chronic Congestive Heart Failure

J.-G. KAYANAKIS and the French-Benelux Ibopamine Study Group[1]

Introduction

Conventionally, congestive heart failure (CHF) has been treated with digitalis glycosides and diuretics to improve cardiac performance and reduce symptoms of congestion [1–3]. Recently, treatment of CHF has been advanced through the use of vasodilators and in particular angiotensin-converting enzyme inhibitors (ACEs) [4–6]. In addition to improving exercise tolerance and symptoms, a controlled clinical trial in severely disabled (NYHA class IV) CHF patients found a reduction in mortality when enalapril was added to various treatment regimens [7]. Mortality was also shown to be reduced in patients treated with the vasodilator hydralazine in combination with nitrates but not the alpha-blocker prazosin [4]. As the role of vasodilation in CHF has become more clear, the role of inotropy has become increasingly controversial.

This clinical trial was designed to evaluate the benefit of adding ibopamine, a new drug with both vasodilating and inotropic properties, in stable patients with moderate CHF.

Material and Methods

Study Design

The study was a double-blind, randomized, placebo-controlled multicenter trial in adult patients with chronic CHF (NYHA classes II and III). It was conducted in 15 centers in accordance with the declarations of Helsinki and Tokyo. Informed consent was obtained from each patient prior to participation. The study was divided into three parts: an 8-week double-blind trial, a 4-month double-blind extension of the original trial, and lastly a 6-month open treatment period.

During screening, two symptom-limited maximal exercise tolerance tests were performed, and the mean result was used as the baseline determination. The test was performed on an electronically braked upright bicycle with 10-watt increments every minute or on a treadmill using the Naughton exercise protocol.

[1] A complete list of investigators is listed in the Acknowledgements.

B.S. Lewis, A. Kimchi (Eds.)
Heart Failure Mechanisms and Management
© Springer-Verlag Berlin Heidelberg 1991

At randomization, patients received either ibopamine 200 mg t.i.d. or matching placebo and were seen every 2 weeks for the first 8 weeks and then every 2 months thereafter. At each visit the following parameters were recorded: cardiovascular physical examination, clinical status questionnaire, and ECG. At weeks 4, 8, and 24, an exercise tolerance test and NYHA evaluation were done. Safety was evaluated by monitoring all adverse events which occurred regardless of investigator-perceived relationship to study medications, and through serial blood and urine testing.

Concomitant treatment with digoxin, diuretics, antiarrhythmics, and nitrates permitted, but they could not be started or increased during the study.

Patients wee excluded if they had unstable angina, recent myocardial infarction, uncontrolled arrhythmias, primary obstructive valvular disease, insulin-dependent diabetes, and severe renal or hepatic dysfunction.

Parameters of Assessment

Exercise duration, NYHA class, body weight, edema score, and the patient clinical status questionnaire were monitored to assess patient response. The exercise tolerance test was required to be limited by symptoms of exhaustion, shortness of breath, muscular pain, or fatigue, dizziness, or chest pain.

Statistical Methods

Data were pooled after examining for center, study medication, and center by study medication interactions. Data were excluded from centers that had fewer than five patients entered or less than one evaluable patient per drug regimen.

Exercise tolerance results were analyzed for change from baseline using a model with linear effect due to study medication. Two-sided 95% confidence intervals for the average change from baseline were calculated. A 95% confidence interval which does not include zero infers a difference is present at a $p < .05$ confidence level.

Results for NYHA and total symptom score were analyzed based on a change from baseline using three methods. The first was a linear function evaluation which included improvement, no change, and worsening.

A Wilcoxon test was done for analysis of NYHA change at week 24 and at end-point.

The third statistical test examined the 95% confidence intervals of the difference between the two groups of the percentage of patients who improved or worsened.

An "intent to treat" analysis was also done, in which all patients were included, regardless of compliance or number of patients per center.

Results

Demography

One hundred eleven patients were randomized to treatment during the 8 weeks of Phase I (49 to ibopamine and 62 to placebo) (Table 1). Mean age was 59.9 with a range of 25–80 years; 83% of the patients were male. At baseline 54.1% were classified as NYHA class II and 45.9% NYHA class III.

Six centers enrolling a total of 20 patients (seven ibopamine, 13 placebo) did not participate in phases 2 or 3 of the study. This decision was made prior to initiation of the trial. Thus, 60 patients continued into the phase 2 4-month double-blind extension trial (29 ibopamine, 31 placebo). The mean age of this group was 57.7 with a range of 25–74 years; 86% were male; 70% were in NYHA class II and 30% were in NYHA class III. Fifty-one patients completed a total of 24 weeks of coded medication. Fifty patients then entered phase 3 and received 6 months of open labeled ibopamine. Thirty-nine completed 12 months of study.

Table 1. Demographic characteristics of patients entering 8-week phase compared to subset entering 4-month double-blind extension

		Eight weeks ($n = 111$)		Four-month extension ($n = 60$)	
		Placebo ($n = 62$)	Ibopamine ($n = 49$)	Placebo ($n = 31$)	Ibopamine ($n = 29$)
Male	(n)	51	42	26	26
	(%)	82	86	84	90
Female	(n)	11	7	5	3
	(%)	18	14	16	10
Age (years)		60.5	59.3	59.9	55.3
Range (years)		31–80	25–78	31–74	25–73
NYHA class II	(n)	33	27	23	19
	(%)	53	55	74	66
NYHA class III	(n)	29	22	8	10
	(%)	47	45	26	34
Baseline exercise test (min)		9.2	8.8	10.4	11.2
Concomitant medications					
Glycosides	(n)	45	32	22	20
	(%)	73	65	71	72
Diuretic high ceiling	(n)	35	32	17	20
	(%)	56	65	55	69
Diuretic (K^+ sparing)	(n)	34	21	20	14
	(%)	55	43	65	48
Coronary vasodilators	(n)	22	15	14	4
	(%)	36	31	45	14
Antiarrhythmics	(n)	26	28	11	19
	(%)	41	57	36	66

There were no major differences between the two treatment groups regarding etiology of heart disease or concomitant medication during any of the three phases.

Efficacy Evaluation

Phase I

Of the 111 patients entered into the initial 8-week phase, data from 89 were statistically evaluable (placebo 48, ibopamine 41). Data from the remainder (placebo 14, ibopamine eight) were excluded from statistical analysis because of one or more study conduct irregularities: protocol violations (placebo three, ibopamine one), no evaluable on-therapy data (placebo four, ibopamine two), change in baseline diuretic or digoxin during screening (placebo eight, ibopamine seven), use of excluded medication (ibopamine one), inconsistent exercise protocol (ibopamine one), or insufficient number of patients per center on each drug regimen (placebo seven).

Phase II

Of the 60 patients who continued into the second phase of the study, data from 47 patients were statistically evaluable (placebo 26, ibopamine 21). Reasons for exclusion from the statistical data set for 13 patients (placebo five, ibopamine eight) included protocol violations (seven), nonevaluable data (four), and lack of efficacy testing at week 24 (two).

Phase III

Of the 50 patients who continued into the open extension phase, data from 46 patients were evaluable. Reasons for exclusion included no data at month 6 to establish baseline, no data post month 6 (one), and one center had too few patients entered (one).

Exercise Tolerance (Fig. 1)

Phase I

The data from 72 patients who exercised on the bicycle protocol were statistically evaluated. An additional 17 patients who exercised on a treadmill were evaluated separately. At week 8 the placebo group had minimally increased their exercise tolerance by 0.13 min while the ibopamine group had increased by 0.4 min. This result was not statistically different. These results were comparable for the treadmill patients.

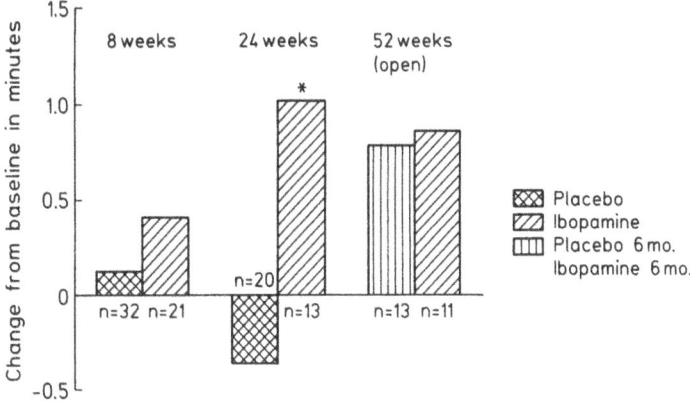

Fig. 1. Exercise tolerance at 8, 24, and 52 weeks on bicycle ergometer. A statistical improvement is present at 24 weeks between ibopamine- and placebo-treated groups. *Asterisk*, $p < 0.05$

Phase II

The data after 24 weeks of therapy from 33 patients who exercised on the bicycle protocol were statistically evaluated. An additional nine patients who exercised on a treadmill were evaluated separately. At week 8 there was minimal improvement of 0.11 min in the placebo group and 0.31 min in the ibopamine group. This was not statistically significant and was similar to the results seen in the larger group during phase I. At week 24 there was a small drop in exercise tolerance in the placebo group of -0.35 min, while in the ibopamine group there was a gain of 1.02 min. The difference between the groups at 24 weeks was statistically significant ($p < .05$). The percentage of placebo patients who increased their exercise tolerance by at least 2 min was 10% at 24 weeks, while the percentage on ibopamine was 31%. No difference was observed in rate pressure product either compared to baseline or between treatment groups.

Phase III

The data after 52 weeks of therapy from 42 patients were evaluated. Exercise tolerance in the previously treated ibopamine patients who continued on ibopamine was maintained with a slight additional improvement of 0.17 min seen at 1 year compared to 24 weeks. The placebo group showed an improvement of 0.56 min after 6 months of open labeled ibopamine compared to the results after 24 weeks on placebo. There was no difference in exercise tolerance between the two groups at the end of this open study. Total improvement at 1 year compared to screening was 0.79 min for the placebo group followed by the ibopamine group, and 0.87 min for the group treated for all 12 months on ibopamine.

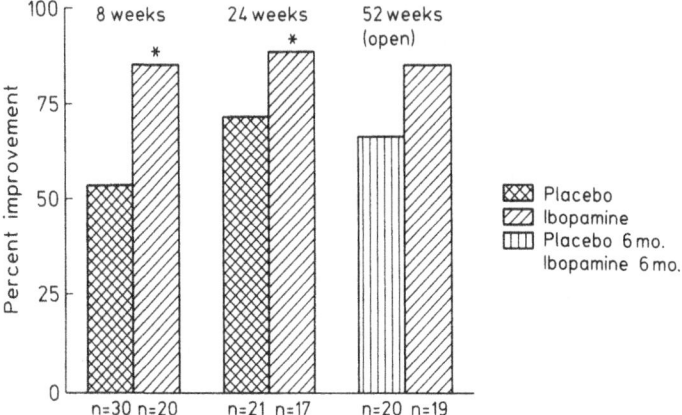

Fig. 2. Symptom score percentage improvement at 8, 24, and 52 weeks. A statistical improvement at 8 and 24 weeks is present between the ibopamine- and placebo-treated groups. *Asterisks*, $p < 0.05$

Total Symptom Score (Fig. 2)

Phase I

Average symptom scores were similar for both treatment groups. At week 8 53% of the placebo group demonstrated a reduction in symptoms, while 85% of the ibopamine group showed a reduction. The difference between the two groups was statistically different ($p < .05$).

Phase II

Average scores were similar for the two groups at baseline. At week 8, 50% of placebo patients had a reduction in symptom score, and 71% had a reduction at week 24. On ibopamine 85% had a reduction at week 8 and 88% at week 24. The difference between groups was statistically significant at both week 8 and week 24 ($p < .05$).

Phase III

At the end of 1 year the percentage of patients treated with ibopamine for 1 year who showed a reduction in symptoms was 84% compared to 70% for the group treated with ibopamine for the last 6 months only.

NYHA Class (Fig. 3)

Phase I

The number of patients who showed an improvement in NYHA class at week 8 was 37% for placebo and 58% for ibopamine. While the difference between the groups was not statistically significant, there was a statistical improvement ($p <$ .05) for the ibopamine group compared to baseline. Patients who were NYHA class III at baseline showed the most improvement. The percentage improvement of class III patients randomized to ibopamine was 56% compared to 28% on placebo. No difference between the groups was seen in the NYHA class II patients.

Phase II

At week 8, 42% of placebo patients showed an improvement in NYHA class, and 40% improved at week 24. This compared to 71% at week 8 and 70% at week 24 for the ibopamine group. The difference between the two treatment arms was statistically significant at end-point analysis (last on treatment assessment). As in the 8-week portion of the study, patients who were in NYHA class III at baseline showed the most improvement; 43% on placebo improved compared to 100% on ibopamine.

Phase III

At the end of 1 year, the patients treated on ibopamine throughout showed maintenance of the improvement present at 6 months; 68% improved at 6 months compared to 64% at 1 year. In patients initially on placebo, 42% were improved

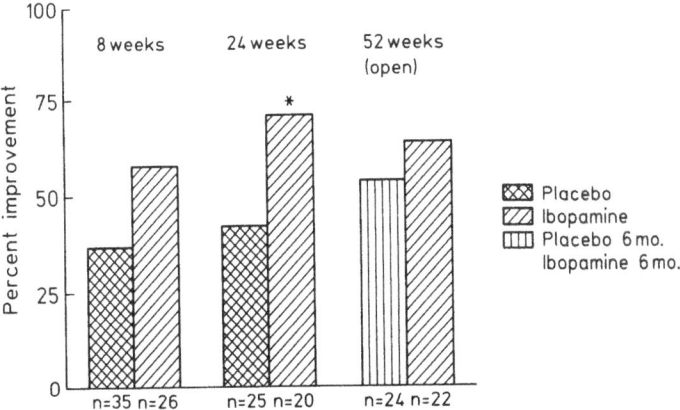

Fig. 3. NYHA class percentage improvement at 8, 24, and 52 weeks. A statistical improvement is present at 8 and 24 weeks between the ibopamine- and placebo-treated groups. *Asterisk, $p < 0.05$*

at 6 months. After switching to ibopamine, 54% improved their NYHA class. Both groups shared similar improvement in NYHA at 1 year (placebo-ibopamine 54%, ibopamine-ibopamine 64%).

Safety Results

During the 8- and 24-week placebo-controlled phases of this study, frequent adverse clinical events occurred in both treatment groups (87% placebo, 83% ibopamine). These events were most often associated with the cardiovascular, respiratory, and general body systems (Table 2).

Table 2. Reason for concluding study

| | Eight weeks | | | | Twenty-four weeks | | | |
| | Placebo | | Ibopamine | | Placebo | | Ibopamine | |
	(n)	(%)	(n)	(%)	(n)	(%)	(n)	(%)
Completed	44	71	36	73	25	80.6	25	93.5
Clinical event	6	9.7	9	18.3	3	9.6	3	10.3
Insufficient effect	6	9.7	3	6.1	3	9.6	0	
Noncompliance	3	4.8	0		0		1	3.4
Death (within 48 h)	3	4.8	1	1.8	0[a]		0	

[a] One patient on placebo suffered myocardial infarction and died 11 days later.

During the 8-week period, 21 patients on placebo experienced a severe cardiovascular or respiratory event compared to 17 on ibopamine. During the 4-month extension, six patients on placebo compared to three on ibopamine had a severe cardiovascular or respiratory event. Ibopamine was associated with more frequent withdrawal from the study because of complaints of abdominal pain, nausea, and vomiting than placebo (one placebo, four ibopamine). Increased arrhythmias were seen in both treatment groups and were the reason for early withdrawn in one patient on placebo and two patients on ibopamine. One patient on placebo was withdrawn following an acute myocardial infarction. This patient subsequently died 11 days later.

Increased levels of liver transaminases that reached at least twice the normal levels occurred in both treatment groups (five placebo, six ibopamine). In most instances, these were minimally elevated or returned to previous levels on subsequent testing. Two patients treated with ibopamine were discontinued during the 4-month extension period for elevated LFTS. In one patient, the ALAT rose to 408 IU (NL 0-33), and the ASAT rose to 154 IU (NL 0-21). By 3 weeks after discontinuing ibopamine the LFTS were normal. A relationship to ibopamine was considered possible after hepatitis A and B were ruled out. The second patient, concomitantly treated with amiodarone, continued to have abnormal LFTs until amiodarone was also discontinued. The cause of the

Table 3. Severe cardiovascular and respiratory events

	Placebo (n)	Ibopamine (n)
Eight-week phase		
Worsening CHF	5	1
Arrhythmias	3	3
CVA	1	1
Angina	0	1
Hypertension	0	1
Dyspnea	4	1
Pulmonary edema	1	1
Pneumonia	1	1
Cough	1	2
Syncope	3	0
Four-month extension	0	1
Worsening CHF	2	1
Syncope	0	1
Cough	1	0
Arrhythmia	1	0
Myocardial infarction	1	0
Dyspnea		

elevated LFTs in this patient was considered possibly related to amiodarone or the combination of amiodarone and ibopamine.

A total of four patients died during the double-blind treatment or within 48 h after stopping treatment. There were three deaths in the placebo group due to pulmonary edema, cerebrovascular accident (CVA), and sudden death; and one in the ibopamine group due to sudden death. An additional four patients (two placebo, two ibopamine) died within 30 days of stopping therapy. The causes included acute myocardial infarction and sudden death 11 and 17 days post therapy in placebo patients, and CVA and acute CHF 13 and 11 days after stopping ibopamine. One additional patient committed suicide during the open ibopamine extension period. He had a history of depression.

There were no overall trends in hematology and renal or liver function parameters that could be attributed to treatment with ibopamine. The incidence of abnormal on-therapy values and transitions from normal pretherapy to abnormal on-therapy values for serum electrolytes, protein electrophoresis, and other blood chemistries including fasting blood glucose were similar for the two treatment groups.

Discussion

Ibopamine is a prodrug which, when hydrolyzed by serum esterases, is converted to N-methyldopamine (epinine). It has been marketed in Italy since

1984 for the treatment of CHF and is under development in other parts of the world.

Animal pharmacology indicates that this compound produces a selective activation of peripheral (vascular) dopamine receptors as well as beta- and alpha-adrenergic stimulation [8]. In conscious dogs, ibopamine has been shown to induce a significant reduction in systemic vascular resistance as well as a decrease in renal vascular resistance via dopaminergic and beta-adrenergic activation [9]. In addition, a direct positive inotropic activity has been demonstrated and attributed to its beta-agonism. The combination of afterload reduction and positive inotropy leads in humans to enhancement of hemodynamic performance [10].

A consistent decrease in systemic vascular resistance and an increase in cardiac index has been observed, usually without alteration in heart rate or blood pressure. The peak response is seen at 1–2 h and lasts approximately 4 h [11–13]. Ibopamine has also been shown to reduce serum norepinephrine levels [14,15].

Few studies have examined the long-term effect of ibopamine in a controlled, double-blinded fashion. This study examined the response of clinical symptoms, NYHA class, and exercise tolerance after 8 weeks and 24 weeks of therapy. The final open phase evaluated whether improvement would continue to be maintained up to 52 weeks.

During this study, a benefit in this population of stable chronic CHF patients was observed with ibopamine as compared to placebo. The benefit was present in both clinical symptoms as well as in exercise tolerance. Interestingly, the benefit in exercise tolerance appeared only after 8 weeks of treatment; this may be due to small hemadynamic changes occurring over time leading to a cumulative effect in exercise tolerance or to slow changes that take place in the peripheral vasculature resulting in improved oxygen delivery to the exercising skeletal muscles.

The magnitude of increase in exercise time at 24 weeks in ibopamine patients was similar to what has been reported during chronic digoxin therapy [16] but less than that reported for patients on ACE therapy [16].

In a previous study [17] ibopamine was shown to be safely substituted for digoxin in a group of stable CHF patients on chronic digoxin therapy. Those patients showed no deterioration in clinical symptoms or exercise tolerance after 4 weeks of ibopamine compared to patients continued on digoxin. This present study evaluated the additive benefit of ibopamine to digoxin and diuretics and found an improvement in exercise tolerance afte 24 weeks.

Other groups have also studied ibopamine in patients with moderate CHF and have found similar results [18,19]. These previous studies have been limited by shorter periods of observation and fewer patients.

In the open phase of this study, maintenance of clinical benefit appeared up to 1 year of therapy. Small additional increments of improvement were also seen in the group who were switched at 24 weeks from placebo to ibopamine.

The safety of chronic ibopamine administration was evaluated through careful monitoring of adverse events and serial laboratory testing. During both the 8- and 24-week blinded phases of this study, there was no evidence of increased incidence of clinically significant arrhythmias or other cardiovascular or respiratory complaints from patients on ibopamine compared to placebo. This study was small and not designed to assess mortality. However, deaths were infrequent and observed no more often on ibopamine than placebo. The combination of the inotropic and vasodilative activities of ibopamine were well tolerated in this population for up to 12 months, and no increased toxicity was noted. Two large open labeled and safety studies (311 and 1007 patients) similarly found good tolerability and lack of trends of serious toxicity [20,21].

Summary

In this double-blind, randomized, placebo-controlled study, treatment with ibopamine resulted in increased exercise tolerance, improvement in NYHA class, and reduction in symptoms of CHF. These changes showed improvement in NYHA class and clinical symptoms at week 8 and improvement in both clinical findings and exercise tolerance at week 24.

In general, patients tolerated ibopamine well for periods up to 1 year. There was no evidence of increased arrhythmias or sudden deaths. Gastrointestinal complaints tended to occur more frequently with ibopamine, while patients on placebo tended to drop from the study more frequently for insufficient therapeutic response.

Conclusions

Our study suggests that ibopamine provides added benefit when given in combination with digoxin and diuretics to patients with moderate CHF. The results of this study need to be confirmed by additional double-blind, long-term trials in order to verify our results, in particular to the maintenance of improvement up to 52 weeks. The place of this compound in the treatment of CHF will be determined by its very good safety profile and tolerability in patients on conventional therapy.

Acknowledgements. The ibopamine trial study group consisted of the following investigators. The city in which their institution is located is shown in parentheses. The trial was supported by a clinical grant from Smith Kline & French Laboratories. *France*: P. Bernasconi, A. Pleskof (Amiens); R. Germain, P.H. Germain (Strasbourg); Y. Grosgogeat, M. Komajda (Paris); J.G. Kayanakis, L. Larouchi (Bayonne); M. Marquet (Gap); J. Medvedowsky, C. Barnay (Aix en Provence); P.H. Morand, J.P. Camous, P. Gibelin (Nice); G. Motte, B. Raffestin, P. Escourou (Clamart); R. Rocher (Bourges); A. Serradimigni, M. Benichou, F. Philip (Marseille); J.P. Normand, B. Lancelin, D. Bet (Versailles); M. Schleman, P.H. Tournadre, E. Apoil, E. Riva (Smith Kline & French Laboratories). *Belgium*: E. Balthazar, J.P. Lanckman, R. Van Der Schueren, Ledune, Hamoude (Jumet); G. Dereume, B. Tremblay, A. Shita (Tournai). *Switzerland*: B. Ruedi, J.F. Enrico, C. Jornod (Neufchatel); U. Sigwart, M. Grbic, M. Blanc (Lausanne).

References

1. Parmley WW (1979) Circulatory function and control. In: Beeson PB, McDermott W, Wyngarden SB (eds) Cecil textbook of medicine. Saunders, Philadelphia, pp 1063–1072
2. Braunwald E (1980) Pathophysiology of heart failure. In: Braunwald E (ed) Heart disease. Saunders, Philadelphia, pp 453–471
3. Zelis R, Flaim SF, Liedtke AJ, Nellis SH (1981) Cardiocirculatory dynamics in the normal and failing heart. Ann Rev Physiol 43:455–476
4. Cohn JN, Archibald DG, Ziesche S et al. (1986) Effect of vasodilator therapy and mortality in chronic congestive heart failure: results of a Veterans Administration cooperative study. N Engl J Med 314:1547–1552
5. Captopril Multicenter Research Group (1983) A placebo-controlled trial of captopril in refractory chronic congestive heart failure. J Am Coll Cardiol 2:755–763
6. Captopril Multicenter Research Group (1985) A cooperative multicenter study of captopril in congestive heart failure: hemodynamic effects and long-term effects. Am Heart J 110:439–447
7. Consensus Trial Study Group (1989) Effects of enalapril on mortality in severe congestive heart failure. Results of the cooperative North Scandinavian Enalapril Survival Study. N Engl J Med 316:1429–1435
8. Casagrande C, Ghiradi P, Marchetti G (1985) Ibopamine (Review). New Drugs Annual Cardiovasc Drugs 3:173–193
9. Itoh H, Kohli J, Rajfer S, Goldberg LI (1985) Comparison of the cardiovascular actions of dopamine and epinine in the dog. J Pharmacol Exp Ther 233:1, 87–93
10. Ren JH, Leithe ME, Huss P, Unverferth DV, Leier CV (1983) The effects of ibopamine on cardiovascular and renal function in normal human subjects. Curr Ther Res 34:667–675
11. Ren JH, Unverferth DV, Leier CV (1984) The ibopamine congener, ibopamine, in congestive heart failure. J Cardiovasc Pharmacol 6:748–755
12. Leier CV, Ren JH, Huss P, Unverferth DV (1986) Hemodynamic effects of ibopamine, a dopamine congener, in patients with congestive heart failure. Pharmacotherapy 6:35–40
13. Dei Cas L, Manca C, Bernardini B, Vasini G, Visiolo O (1982) Non-invasive evaluation of the effects oral ibopamine (SB7505) on cardiac and renal function in patients with congestive heart failure. J Cardiovasc Pharmacol 4:436–440
14. Nakano T, Morimoto Y, Kakuta Y, Konishi T, Kodera T, Kanamaru M, Takezawa H (1986) Acute effects of ibopamine hydrochloride on hemodynamics, plasma catecholamine levels, renin activity, aldosterone, metabolism and blood gas in patients with severe congestive heart failure. Arzneimittelforschung 36(11,12):1829–1894
15. Rajfer S, Rossen J, Douglas FL, Goldberg LI, Karrison T (1986) Effects of long-term therapy with oral ibopamine on resting hemodynamics and exercise capacity in patients with heart failure: relationship to the generation of N-methyldopamine and plasma norepinephrine levels. Circulation 73(4):740–748
16. The Captopril-Digoxin Multicenter Research Group (1988) Comparative effects of therapy with captopril and digoxin in patients with mild to moderate heart failure. JAMA 259(4):539–544
17. Cavalli A, Riva E, Schleman M, Abbondati G, Fucella LM, Smith Kline and French Laboratories Ibopamine Group Ibopamine as a substitute for digitalis in patients with congestive heart failure on chronic digoxin therapy. Int J Cardiol (in press)
18. Cantalli I, Lolli C, Bomba E, Brunelli D, Bracchetti D (1986) Sustained oral treatment with ibopamine in patients with chronic congestive heart failure. Curr Ther Res 36:900–911
19. Gavazzi A, Mussiai A, Bramucci E (1986) Hemodynamic evaluation during exercise test after acute and chronic ibopamine treatment in patients with congestive heart failure. Arzneimittelforschung 36(I) 2a:366–370
20. Ferrari V, Sher D, Marchetti G (1986) A survey of 311 patients receiving ibopamine mainly during hospital treatment for severe congestive heart failure. Arzneimittelforschung [Suppl 36(I)]:398–405
21. Sher D, Ferrari V (1986) Ibopamine post-marketing surveillance. Arzneimittelforschung 37(II):873–900

Angiotensin Converting Enzyme Inhibitors

Neuroendocrine-Renal Relationships in Heart Failure: Effect of Captopril

J. McMurray, J. McLay, and A.D. Struthers

Introduction

The haemodynamic effects of angiotensin converting enzyme (ACE) inhibitors have been extensively examined in patients with chronic heart failure. The renal effects of these drugs have, however, been less well studied [1]. The relatively few studies that have evaluated the renal actions of ACE inhibitors in chronic heart failure have shown an acute fall in urinary sodium excretion [2-4]. The present study was designed to investigate the mechanism, or mechanisms, of this early sodium-retaining effect of ACE inhibitors.

Patients and Methods

With ethical committee approval, 15 patients aged 51-86 (mean 71) years were studied after having given written informed consent. The primary cause of heart failure was coronary artery disease in 12, hypertension in two and valvular disease in one. All patients were receiving diuretics: 14 frusemide (range, 40-120 mg/day; mean, 77 mg) and one bendrofluazide. Many were on additional cardiac medications: two digoxin, six oral nitrates, one prazosin and three calcium channel blockers. The dose of all medications was, as far as possible, kept constant during the study.

Protocol. Patients took their usual diuretic (and other medications) in the morning of day 0 of the study. They were admitted to the ward in the afternoon of day 0. At 2200 hours on day 0 the patients were given a 300 mg oral dose of lithium carbonate; this was to enable evaluation of segmental nephron function as described below. On study day 1 a light breakfast was permitted, but caffeine-containing beverages were avoided. Patients were then asked to empty their bladders at 0900 hours and to rest supine on a bed. An intravenous cannula was sited in an antecubital vein. A placebo tablet was then administered in a single blind fashion. Every 15 min for the next 2.5 h blood pressure and heart rate were recorded by a semi-automatic sphygmomanometer (Critikon, Tampa, Florida, USA). At the end of this 2.5-h (i.e. at 1130 hours) venous blood was collected for measurement of electrolytes, creatinine and neurohormonal activity (see below). Patients were then asked to empty their bladders, and the urine voided was

B.S. Lewis, A. Kimchi (Eds.)
Heart Failure Mechanisms and Management
© Springer-Verlag Berlin Heidelberg 1991

collected for later analysis. At this point the patient's usual diuretic was given. At 1400 and 2200 hours 6.25 mg or 25 mg captopril was given; a second dose of 300 mg lithium carbonate was also given at 2200 hours. Day 2 of the study was conducted as day 1 except that 12.5 mg or 25 mg captopril was given in a single-blind manner at 0900 hours instead of placebo. Patients were discharged in the evening of day 2. This protocol therefore permitted comparison of renal sodium handling after placebo (day 1) with renal sodium handling after captopril (day 2); the protocol also allowed correlation of renal function with systemic haemodynamics and neuroendocrine activity after each treatment.

Laboratory Measurements. Serum and urinary sodium and lithium were measured by flame emission photometry using an internal caesium standard (Instrumentation Laboratories, Model 943, Milan, Italy). Serum and urinary creatinine were measured by a modified Jaffe reaction on an autoanalyser (Cobas Bio, Roche Diagnostica, Basel, Switzerland). Plasma renin activity (PRA; CIS UK Ltd, High Wycombe, Buckinghamshire, UK), aldosterone (Serono Diagnostics, Woking, Surrey, UK) and atrial natriuretic factor (ANF; Amersham International, Aylesbury, Buckinghamshire, UK) were measured using commercially available radioimmunoassay kits. Plasma noradrenaline was assayed by the double isotope radioenzymatic method of Brown and Jenner (1981) [5].

Measures of Segmental Nephron Function. Clearance was calculated as urinary concentration × urinary flow rate/plasma concentration. Creatinine clearance was used as a measure of glomerular filtration rate (GFR). Fractional clearance (excretion) was calculated as clearance/creatinine clearance. The following parameters were derived using the lithium method [6]. Fractional excretion of lithium = proximal tubular outflow; sodium clearance/lithium clearance = distal nephron outflow.

Statistical Analysis. Values following placebo were compared to values following captopril by paired t test; $p < 0.05$ was taken as statistically significant. All results are given as mean ± one standard error of mean.

Results

Minimum blood pressure after placebo was 119 ± 6/72 ± 3 and after captopril was 95 ± 6/59 ± 3 mmHg ($p < 0.01$). The renal function results are shown in Table 1. Creatinine clearance was similar on the two treatment days (57 ± 4 after placebo and 57 ± 7 ml/min after captopril; NS). Fractional sodium excretion was lower after captopril than after placebo ($p < 0.01$), i.e. overall tubular sodium reabsorption increased. Both proximal and distal nephron outflows were lower after captopril than after placebo ($p < 0.001$ and $p < 0.01$, respectively), i.e. both proximal and distal nephron sodium reabsorption increased. Table 2 shows the neurohormonal measurements. Noradrenaline levels were not different on the 2 treatment days. As expected, PRA increased ($p < 0.001$) and aldosterone decreased ($p < 0.01$) with captopril. ANF levels were lower after captopril than after placebo ($p < 0.02$).

Table 1. Renal function after placebo and after captopril

	Placebo	Captopril
Ccr (ml/min)	57 ± 4	57 ± 7
FENa (%)	0.86 ± 0.18	0.34 ± 0.06[a]
FELi (%)	23.6 ± 2.2	15.7 ± 2.6[b]
CNa/CLi (%)	3.98 ± 0.81	2.59 ± 0.41[a]

Ccr, Creatinine clearance; *FENa*, sodium fractional excretion; *FELi*, lithium fractional excretion; *CNa*, sodium clearance; *CLL*, lithium clearance.
[a] $p < 0.01$.
[b] $p < 0.001$.

Table 2. Neurohormonal measurements after placebo and after captopril

	Placebo	Captopril
PRA (ng ml^{-1} h^{-1})	4.2 ± 4.7	68.3 ± 153.5[c]
Aldosterone (pg ml^{-1})	264 ± 71	114 ± 24[b]
Noradrenaline (pg ml^{-1})	793 ± 62	731 ± 73
ANF (pmol l^{-1})	80 ± 14	61 ± 11[a]

[a] $p < 0.02$.
[b] $p < 0.01$.
[c] $p < 0.001$.

Discussion

The current results confirm previous observations that acute administration of captopril and other ACE inhibitors can result in sodium retention in chronic heart failure [2–4]. We have now shown that this response is, at least in part, due to increased proximal and distal nephron sodium reabsorption. At first sight these changes may seem paradoxical. Aldosterone and angiotensin II are usually considered to be antinatriuretic. Aldosterone acts on the distal nephron and studies in experimental animals show that angiotensin II has a direct proximal tubular effect [7]. We have recently confirmed this effect of angiotensin II in man [8]. Pharmacological interruption of the RAAS (Renin-Angiotensin-Aldosterone system) in these patients, however, resulted in sodium retention.

What is the explanation for this apparent contradiction? Four possibilities are worthy of consideration. Firstly, the haemodynamic response to ACE inhibition could account for the acute antinatriuresis. ACE inhibition dissociates renal blood flow (RBF) from GFR so that, usually, RBF increases while GFR remains unchanged, i.e. filtration fraction falls [1,9]. If, however, renal perfusion pressure falls (due to a decrease in systemic blood pressure) below a certain limit, the "autoregulatory breakpoint", GFR falls progressively, i.e. GFR becomes flow dependent. The values for creatinine clearance found in the present study were typical of previous GFR measurements and did not change with captopril, a finding also consistent with previous observations [2,9,10]. Furthermore, the autoregulatory breakpoint in man is between 55 and 60 mmHg, and minimum mean arterial pressure, even after captopril, remained above this level in our study. Therefore, if a haemodynamic mechanism (i.e. one dependent on a fall in renal perfusion pressure) did account for the fall in sodium excretion it must have resulted from a change in some other variable than GFR. Such filtration-independent mechanisms have been proposed; theoretically a reduction in renal interstitial pressure, for example, could account for our finding [11–13].

A second possible explanation is that captopril may have reduced the natriuretic response to the patient's diuretic therapy, and that this led to the fall in sodium excretion from day 1 to day 2. There is evidence from animal experiments, studies in hypertensive patients and in patients with chronic heart failure that both captopril and enalapril have this effect [14–16]. Several points argue against this possibility in the current study. Our patients were studied on both days 1 and 2, over 20 h after their last dose of diuretic, i.e. when little if any continuing diuretic effect should have been present. Furthermore, between the clearance study on day 1 and that on day 2 the patients had received only two doses of captopril, the first of which was given 2.5 h after the diuretic and therefore at a time by which much of the natriuretic effect would have been achieved. Our results also show that proximal tubular sodium excretion increased after captopril, a response out of keeping with inhibition of the known segmental nephron sites of action of loop diuretics.

A third explanation is based on long-standing observations of the effect of very high concentrations of angiotensin II on sodium transport by isolated proximal tubules in vitro. In contrast to the widely appreciated effect of lower doses of angiotensin II (see above), high levels of this hormone may actually inhibit sodium reabsorption in this part of the nephron [17,18]. Conceivably patients with heart failure could have very high intrarenal levels of angiotensin II, and reduction of these levels by ACE inhibition could paradoxically increase sodium reabsorption. This explanation is favoured by another group who found very similar findings to our own in patients with chronic renal failure treated with enalapril [19].

A final explanation, which we believe has not previously been proposed, is that the antinatriuresis could have been caused by an acute fall in ANF levels after captopril. The fall in ANF presumably reflects the well-described falls in cardiac filling pressures that are seen after administration of captopril. ANF has pronounced inhibitory effects on proximal and distal nephron sodium reabsorption in man [20–22]. Clearly, therefore, the enhanced tubular sodium reabsorption seen after captopril could be explained by a reduced effect of ANF. It is also possible that a combination of these explanations could explain our findings. For example, the effect of ANF is dependent on renal perfusion pressure [23]. The falls in both mean arterial pressure (the haemodynamic mechanism) and ANF following captopril could therefore interact synergistically to reduce urinary sodium excretion.

In summary, we have shown that introduction of captopril may be associated with increased proximal and distal nephron sodium reabsorption in patients with chronic heart failure. This tubular antinatriuresis occurred without a change in GFR and without sympathetic activation and despite interruption of the RAAS. The fall in sodium excretion seen acutely with captopril could be explained by a renal haemodynamic mechanism, antagonism of the effect of loop diuretics, inhibition of a (paradoxical) pro-natriuretic effect of very high intrarenal concentrations of angiotensin II, a fall in plasma ANF levels or by some combination of these mechanisms.

References

1. Gans ROB, Hoorntje SJ, Donker AJM (1988) Renal effects of angiotensin-I converting enzyme inhibitors. Neth J Med 32:247–264
2. Pierpont GL, Francis GS, Cohn JN (1981) Effect of captopril on renal function in patients with congestive heart failure. Br Heart J 46:522–527
3. Mujais SK, Fouad FM, Textor SC, Tarazi RC, Bravo EL, Hart N, Gifford RW (1984) Transient renal dysfunction during initial inhibition of converting enzyme in congestive heart failure. Br Heart J 52:63–71
4. Crozier IG, Ikram H, Nicholls MG, Jans S (1987) Acute haemodynamic, hormonal and electrolyte effects of ramipril in severe congestive heart failure. Am J Cardiol 59:155D–163D
5. Brown MJ, Jenner DA (1981) Novel double isotope technique for enzymatic assay of catecholamines permitting high precision, sensitivity and plasma sample capacity. Clin Sci 61:591–598
6. Solomon LR, Atherton JC, Bobinski H, Hillier V, Green R (1988) The effect of low dose infusion of atrial natriuretic peptide on renal function in man. Clin Sci 75:403–410
7. Hall JE (1986) Control of sodium excretion by angiotensin II: intrarenal mechanisms and blood pressure regulation. Am J Physiol 250:R960–R972
8. Seidelin PH, McMurray J, Struthers AD (1989) Mechanism of the antinatriuretic action of physiological doses of angiotensin in man. Clin Sci 76:419–425
9. Cleland JGF, Dargie HJ, Gillen G, Robertson I, East BW, Ball SG, Morton JJ, Robertson JIS (1986), Captopril in heart failure: a double blind study of the effects on renal function. J Cardiovasc Pharmacol 8:700–706
10. Ribstein J, Mimran A (1986) Acute renal effects of captopril in patients with congestive heart failure. J Clin Hypertens 3:238–244
11. Roman RJ (1988) Pressure-diuresis in volume expanded rats: tubular reabsorption in superficial and deep nephrons. Hypertension 12:177–183
12. Roman RJ, Cowley AW, Garcia-Estan J, Lombard JH (1988) Pressure diuresis in volume expanded rats: cortical and medullary hemodynamics. Hypertension 12:168–176
13. Romero JC, Knox FG (1988) Mechanisms underlying pressure related natriuresis: the role of the renin-angiotensin and prostaglandin systems. Hypertension 11:724–738
14. DiNicolantonio R, Morgan TO (1987) Captopril attenuates diuretic and natriuretic actions of furosemide but not atrial natriuretic peptide. Clin Exp Hypertens [A] A9:19–32
15. Cleland JGF, Gillen G, Dargie HJ (1988) The effects of frusemide and angiotensin-converting enzyme inhibitors and their combination on cardiac and renal haemodynamics in heart failure. Eur Heart J 9:132–141
16. Flapan AD, Davies E, Williams BC, Edwards CRW, Shaw TRD (1989) Captopril does not potentiate the action of loop diuretics in patients with cardiac failure. Br Heart J 61:87
17. Harris PJ, Young JA (1977) Dose dependent stimulation and inhibition of proximal tubular sodium reabsorption of proximal tubular sodium reabsorption by angiotensin II in the rat kidney. Pfluegers Arch 367:295–297
18. Schuster VL, Kokko JP, Jacobson HR (1984) Angiotensin II directly stimulates transport in rabbit proximal convoluted tubules. J Clin Invest 73:507–515

19. Kamper A, Leyssac PP, Holstein-Rathlou NH (1989) Renal tubular function during ACE inhibition in patients with chronic renal failure. International symposium on ACE inhibition, London, 1989, Abstract F051
20. Biollaz J, Bidiville J, Diezi J, Waeber B, Nussberger J, Brunner-Ferber F, Gomez HJ, Brunner H (1987) Site of action of a synthetic atrial natriuretic peptide evaluated in humans. Kidney Int 32:537–546
21. Thomson K (1984) Lithium clearance: a new method for determining proximal and distal tubular reabsorption of sodium and water. Nephron 37:217–223
22. McMurray J, Seidelin PH, Struthers AD (1989) Evidence for a proximal and distal nephron action of atrial natriuretic factor in man. Nephron 51:39–43
23. Davis CL, Briggs JP (1987) Effect of reduction in renal artery pressure on atrial natriuretic peptide-induced natriuresis. Am J Physiol 252:F146–F153

Nitrate Therapy

The In Vitro Metabolism
of Nitrovasodilators and Their Conversion
into Vasoactive Species*

M. Feelisch and E. Noack

Introduction

Despite the extensive therapeutic use of nitrovasodilators and a good knowledge of the hemodynamic alterations that lead to improved myocardial performance, until recently surprisingly few data were available concerning their mode of action at the molecular level. It is now well documented that the pharma codynamic action of these compounds is mediated by the activation of the soluble isoenzyme of guanylate cyclase (sGC; E.C. 4.6.1.2). Relaxation studies with isolated vessel preparations revealed the involvement of at least two independent mechanisms of sGC stimulation: one is an indirect endothelium-related process and the second leads to sGC stimulation on bypassing the endothelium-dependent process. Acetylcholine, ATP, and bradykinin, for example, have a vasodilatory effect only in the presence of an intact endothelial layer while nitrovasodilators such as nitrite (NO_2^-), glyceryl trinitrate (GTN), or sodium nitroprusside (SNP) are relaxant agents in any case. That is why the existence of a humoral endothelium-derived relaxing factor (EDRF) which mediates sGC activation by the endothelium-dependent vasodilators had been postulated. The subsequent rise in cytosolic cGMP concentration induces a complex cascade of protein phosphorylations, finally resulting in smooth muscle relaxation [12,34].

   Although the chemical nature of the potential active metabolite is still the subject of controversy, it now seems well established that nitrovasodilators must be metabolized prior to reveal vasodilator activity [3,29]. Brien et al. [4] recently demonstrated that GTN biotransformation and tissue cGMP elevation precede the onset of GTN-induced relaxation. Whether the conversion of nitrovasodilators into vasoactive compounds is achieved by enzymatic and/or nonenzymatic steps is yet unknown. Besides the proposed interaction with a specific organic nitrate receptor [35], three major hypothesis concerning the mode of action of organic nitrates have been put forward (Fig. 1): (1) In an early concept, NO_2^- formed intracellularly upon enzymatic degradation was regarded as the ultimate active metabolite [17]. This concept was, however, contradicted by the fact that NO_2^- only displays vasodilator effectiveness at concentrations much higher than those needed for organic nitrates itself. It is, therefore, highly unlikely that the

*This work was in part supported by the Deutsche Forschungsgemeinschaft (SFB 242, coronary heart disease, Düsseldorf) and by a scholarship from SKD, Göttingen, FRG.

B.S. Lewis, A. Kimchi (Eds.)
Heart Failure Mechanisms and Management
© Springer-Verlag Berlin Heidelberg 1991

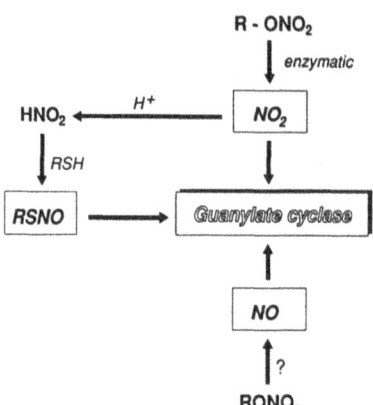

Fig. 1. Proposed modes of action of organic nitrates

comparably low amounts of NO_2^- arising upon intracellular cleavage of organic nitrates would have any effect on sGC activity, the more so as basal NO_2^- concentrations in the smooth muscle are assumed to be in the micromolar range. (2) Ignarro and coworkers [23] developed an elegant hypothesis according to which released NO_2^- should react with thiol groups to form S-nitrosothiols (RSNO). Because they produced hemodynamic effects similar to organic nitrates, nitrosothiols were for a long time regarded as the common active principle of sGC stimulation by nitrovasodilators. (3) Murad and colleagues [24] proposed that the nitric oxide free radical (NO) was the terminal activator of sGC. By which molecular process(es) NO should be liberated from nitrovasodilators remained obscure.

The aim of the current study was to cast some light on the mechanism of nitrovasodilator-induced sGC activation by testing the reliability of these three hypothesis from a biochemical point of view and to clarify whether or not one common metabolite is responsible for the sGC-activating properties of all nitrovasodilators. In broken cell preparations, organic nitrates were found to require the presence of the SH-containing amino acid cysteine to induce enzyme stimulation, whilst other nitrovasodilators such as SNP, NO_2^- or SIN-1, the active metabolite of molsidomine, thiol-independently increase sGC activity. Previous studies in our laboratory had shown that incubation with thiols other than cysteine always resulted in the decomposition of GTN whilst a concomitant activation was only seen with a few compounds [9]. This indicated that thiol-induced degradation of organic nitrates does not necessarily give rise to sGC activation. With these results in mind it seemed promising to search for a metabolite which is only produced in the presence of one of these "active" thiols. We suggested that under certain conditions enzyme activation is preceded by a nonenzymatic step which is needed to generate the active metabolite. By directly monitoring the formation of NO_2^-, NO_3^-, RSNO, and NO we investigated whether the pattern of metabolites arising upon incubation of GTN with several thiol compounds differs fundamentally from that of GTN with cysteine. By using identical experimental conditions these data could be directly compared with enzyme activation.

Materials and Methods

A crude extract of sGC from rat liver was prepared according to Steurer and Schütz [39] and Ignarro et al. [22]. The activity of sGC was determined according to the method of Kimura et al. [27] and cGMP formed was estimated by radioimmunoassay. The generation of NO_2^- and NO_3^- resulting from the decomposition of nitrovasodilators was simultaneously monitored by means of HPLC and expressed as initial rate [8,30].

NO release was measured by a difference-spectrophotometric technique based on the rapid NO-induced conversion of oxyhemoglobin (HbO_2) to methemoglobin (MetHb) [8,16]. Because of the 1:1 stoichiometry of the underlying reaction ($HbO_2 + NO \rightarrow MetHb + NO_3^-$) [6], the continuous time-dependent recording of the methemoglobin concentration mirrors the rate of NO formation. This method is highly sensitive, specific for NO, and does not suffer from interference by dissolved oxygen or released NO_2^-. The selectivity and accuracy of this indirect method was verified by chemiluminescence [7].

Formation of RSNO compounds was monitored by HPLC with small modifications of the method described by Fung et al. [13]. Peak identity was verified by comparison with crystalline S-nitrosothiols. Calibration was performed every day with a 50 μM solution of the respective RSNO compound. Stability of S-nitrosothiols was determined in phosphate buffer pH 7.40 at 37°C. Decomposition rates were calculated from the slope of the photometrically recorded absorbance changes at 335 nm after correction of background absorbance for thiols and NO_2^-. Aqueous NO solutions were prepared as follows: Double distilled water was deaerated by sonification and bubbling with argon. This water was then filled into an all-glass system that had been previously purged with oxygen-free argon. After flushing with argon for 60 min, gas flow was switched to NO by means of a three-way stopcock. Nitric oxide ($> 99.9\%$) was passed over solid KOH and bubbled through a concentrated aqueous solution of potassium hydroxide to remove trace amounts of higher nitrogen oxides. The concentration of NO-saturated water at 25°C was 1.8 mM determined by HPLC as NO_2^-.

Erythrityl tetranitrate was purchased from Chemische Fabrik Tempelhof Preuss & Temmler, Berlin, FRG, and stored in absolute ethanol. Glycerol mononitrates were provided by Mack, Illertissen, FRG, teopranitols, were from Schwabe, Karlsruhe, FRG. All other organic nitrates were from Schwarz Pharma, Monheim, FRG. Amyl nitrite was obtained from Fluka, Switzerland, and SNP from Merck, Darmstadt, FRG. Sydnonimines and furoxans were a generous gift of Cassella, Frankfurt, FRG. Aqueous solutions of nitrovasodilators were prepared just before use. Thiol compounds were of the highest grade available and had been further purified to HPLC purity when necessary. 3-Mercaptopicolinic acid was a kind gift of Dr. DiTullio, SK&F Research Laboratories, Philadelphia, USA. N-acetyl-D,L-penicillamine thionitrite was prepared according to Field et al. [11]. Synthesis and separation of crystalline S-nitrosothiols of L-cysteine, N-acetyl-L-cysteine, L-glutathione, L-homocysteine and L-cysteamine was achieved by modification of published procedures [5,15,31]. Identity of prepared nitrosothiols was verified by elementary analysis (within 30 min after preparation). UV/VIS, mass spectroscopy (m^+ -30), and HPLC.

Data are presented as means ± SEM. Differences were assessed by using Student's two-tailed t test for paired variables and were regarded as statistically significant when $p > 0.05$. Calculation of EC_{50} values was assessed by using the logit transformation according to Hafner et al. [14].

Results

Formation of NO_2^-

With all organic nitrates considerable formation of NO_2^- was seen in the presence of cysteine. The rate of NO_2^- generation was linearly dependent on the concentration of both thiol and organic nitrate (0.01–100 mM cysteine, $r = 0.996$, $n = 14$; 0.05–2 mM GTN, $r = 0.993$, $n = 13$). By determining the rates of NO_2^- formation at varying pH, we provided evidence that NO_2^- formation is due to a nucleophilic attack of the thiolate anion (RS⁻) on the nitrate ester (data not shown). The rate of NO_3^- formation is considerably lower and thiol-independently brought about by alkaline hydrolysis of the nitrate ester bond.

A close correlation exists between the rates of cysteine-induced NO_2^- formation from different organic nitrates and the half-maximal stimulation by the respective compounds of the isolated sGC ($r = 0.997$, $p < 0.001$, $n = 11$; Fig. 2). At first glance one may be tempted to consider this as clue for a causal linkage between both processes. Furthermore, the rate of GTN decomposition in the presence of several thiol compounds closely corresponded to the rate of NO_2^- formation (data not shown). On investigating more than 60 thiol compounds as potential substitutes for cysteine, we found some of these compounds to induce remarkably higher rates of NO_2^- formation with GTN when compared to cysteine, while being ineffective as costimulators at the sGC (inset in Fig. 2).

Formation of S-Nitrosothiols

To examine the RSNO theory we tested the action of several S-nitrosothiols on sGC. On a molar comparison, the enzyme stimulation observed was higher in precisely those compounds which were less stable under the given conditions. This led us to conclude that not the intact RSNO compound but, rather, a metabolite produced by its decomposition must be responsible for enzyme stimulation. A direct comparison with authentic NO confirmed that this metabolite is most probably NO itself, as this radical is the strongest activator of sGC so far tested (Fig. 3).

In contrast to the lack of enzyme activation, GTN surprisingly revealed a small amount of RSNO formation with all thiol compounds tested (GTN 2 mM,

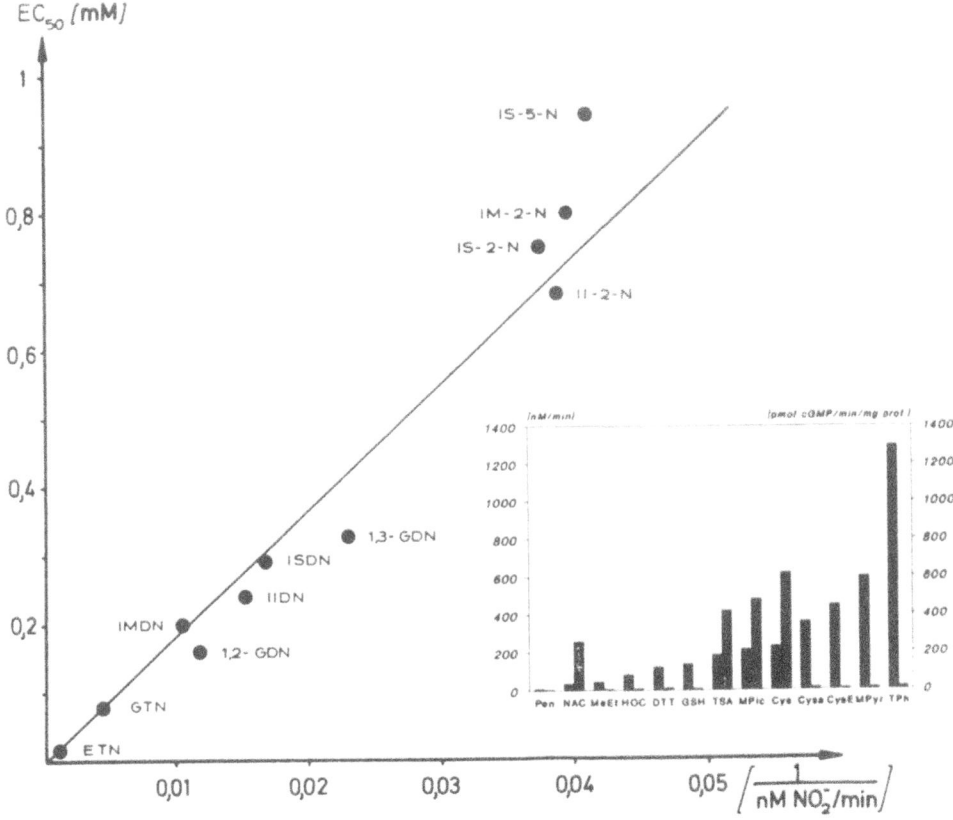

Fig. 2. Comparison between the rate of cysteine-induced NO_2^- formation and the sGC activating potency of different organic nitrates (NO_2^-: organic nitrates 0.2 mM, cysteine 1 mM; sGC: cysteine 5 mM). Abbreviations: *ETN*, erythrityl tetranitrate; *GDN*, glyceryl dinitrate; *GTN*, glyceryl trinitrate; *IIDN*, isoidide dinitrate; *IMDN*, isomannide dinitrate; *ISDN*, isosorbide dinitrate; *II-2-N*, isoidide 2-mononitrate; *IM-2-N*, isomannide 2-mononitrate; *IS-2-N*, isosorbide 2-mononitrate; *IS-5-N*, isosorbide 5-mononitrate. *Inset:* Comparison of NO_2^- formation rate with sGC activation by GTN in the presence of different thiols (NO_2^-: GTN 0.2 mM, thiols 1 mM; sGC: GTN 0.5 mM, thiols 5 mM). Abbreviations: *Cys*, L-cysteine; *CysE*, L-cysteine methylester; *Cysa*, L-cysteamine; *DTT*, 1,4-dithiothreitol; *GSH*, L-glutathione; *HOC*, L-homocysteine; *MeEt*, mercaptoethanol; MPic, 3-mercaptopicolinic acid, *MPyr*, mercaptopyruvic acid; *NAC*, N-acetyl-L-cysteine; *Pen*, L-penicillamine; *TPh*, thiophenol; *TSA*, thiosalicylic acid

thiols 20 mM, p $<$ 0.01, n = 5). At pH 7.40, RSNO formation from GTN and cysteine was so weak that it could account for neither NO formation nor enzyme activation. A quantitative comparison showed that RSNO formation is likely to be due to an equilibrium reaction between NO_2^- and the thiol compound. Thus, both intermediary formed S-nitrosothiols and nitrite ions are unlikely to account for the sGC-stimulating action of organic nitrates.

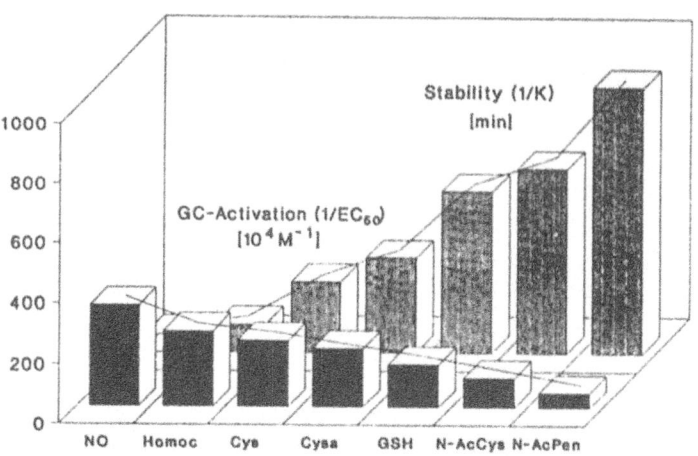

Fig. 3. Relationship between stability and sGC-stimulating potency of S-nitrosothiols. Abbreviations: *Cys*, L-cysteine-SNO; *Cysa*, L-cysteamine-SNO; *GSH*, L-glutathione-SNO; *Homoc*, L-homocysteine-SNO; *N-AcCys*, N-Acetyl-L-cysteine-SNO; *N-AcPen*, N-acetyl-DL-penicillamine-SNO; *NO*, nitric oxide

Formation of NO

In addition to the generation of NO_2^- we measured a pronounced formation of NO from organic nitrates and cysteine. As with NO_2^-, the rate of NO formation correlated well with the stimulatory potency of the respective nitrates at the isolated sGC ($r = 0.994$, $p < 0.001$, $n = 14$; Fig. 4). Enzyme stimulation was higher (corresponding EC_{50} values were, accordingly, lower) the more NO was liberated per unit of time. The greatest NO liberation was observed with GTN, followed by the group of dinitrates and mononitrates. In contrast to the formation of NO_2^- and RSNO, generation of NO was only measurable with those thiol compounds which also mediate enzyme activation. The relationship between the rate of formation of NO and the concentration of cysteine had the same sigmoid characteristic as found at the sGC [8], whereas the rate of NO_2^- formation was linearly dependent on the concentration of cysteine. When organic nitrates were incubated at concentrations which induced just half-maximal enzyme stimulation (EC_{50}), a nearly identical rate of NO liberation was recorded for each compound (inset in Fig. 4).

Additional experiments confirmed the significance of NO for enzyme stimulation: NO formation increased with higher temperature and at alkaline pH, and this was paralleled by a concomitant leftward shift of the concentration/response curves at the sGC. Addition of methylene blue or related dyes reduced both NO formation and enzyme activation in a concentration-dependent manner with no significant influence on the initial formation of NO_2^- ($n = 3$). In accordance with its scavenging effect on generated NO, the presence of 10–100 μM oxyhemoglobin (but not methemoglobin) completely abolished enzyme stimulation by all organic nitrates.

EC_{50} (mM)

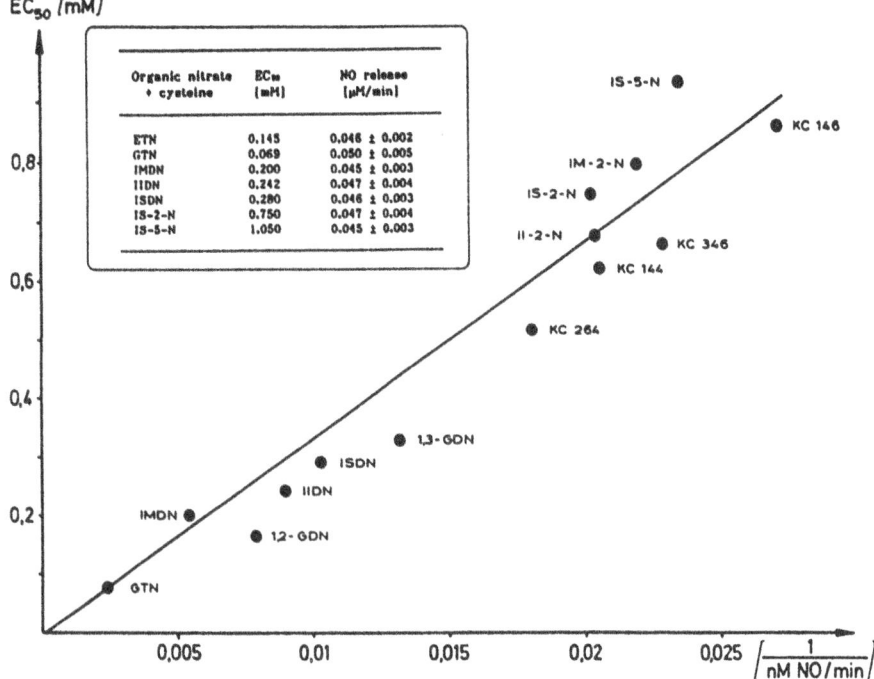

Fig. 4. Correlation between the rate of cysteine-mediated NO release from different organic nitrates and the extent of sGC stimulation (NO: organic nitrates 1 mM, L-cysteine 5 mM, 37°C, pH 7.70, $n = 7$; sGC: L-cysteine 5 mM, 37°C, pH 7.40, $n = 3$). Abbreviations: KC-xxx, isomeric teopranitols; all other abbreviations as in Fig. 2). *Inset*: Uniform NO release from different organic nitrates at their EC_{50} concentration

Mechanism of Interaction Between Organic Nitrates and Thiols

It was obvious that for cleavage of organic nitrates to NO_2^-, SH-containing compounds of either structure seemed to be sufficient, while for the additional formation of NO (and concomitant activation of sGC) a supplementary factor was apparently required, because only very few of more than 60 thiols tested were active in both respects, namely cysteine and its N-acetyl analogue, thiosalicylic acid, and 3-mercaptopicolinic acid. Structural differences are thought to account for these few thiols not only decomposing organic nitrates to NO_2^- but, simultaneously, to NO as well. As an essential feature for this metabolism, indeed a common chemical structure could be determined: a mercapto group separated by two carbon atoms from a carbonyl function, oriented in plane. Besides these steric requirements, additional electronical parameters may be limiting, as an isomeric compound of the "active" 3-mercaptopicolinic acid (2-mercaptonicotinic acid) was found to be ineffective, although meeting the structural demands described above.

Another close relationship exists between the formation rates of NO_2^- and NO from various organic nitrates (Fig. 5). With cysteine as the thiol compound, the

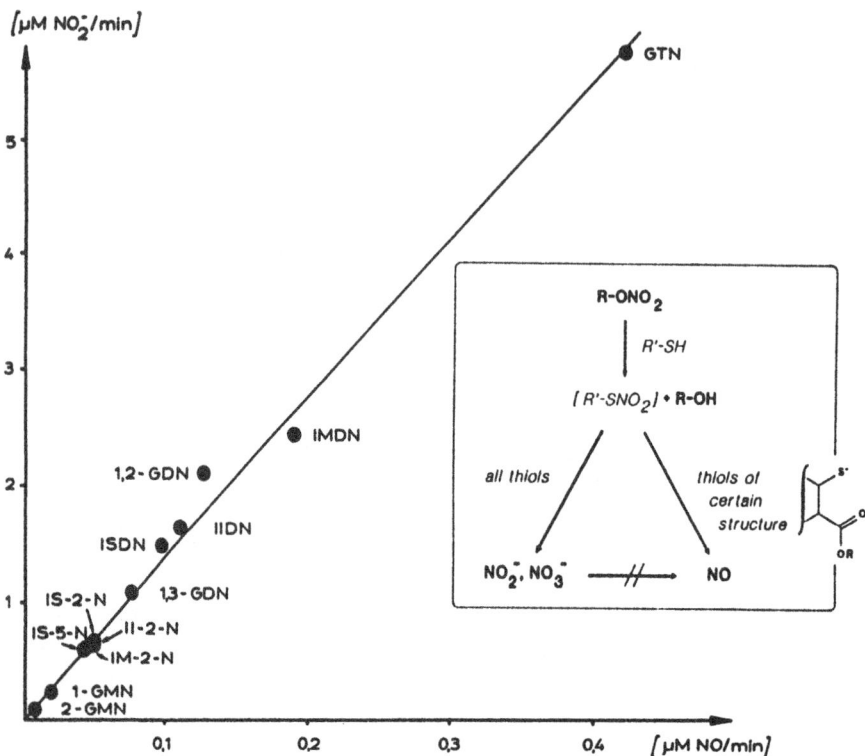

Fig. 5. Relationship between the formation rates of NO and NO_2^- from GTN and cysteine. Conditions in both assays: organic nitrates 1 mM, cysteine 5 mM, 37°C, n = 3 (NO_2^-), n = 7 (NO). Abbreviations: *GMN*, glyceryl mononitrate; all other abbreviations as in Fig. 2. *Inset:* Proposed mechanism of the reaction between thiols and organic nitrates. Abbreviations: *R-OH*, alcohol; *R-ONO₂*, organic nitrate; *R-SH*, thiol; *R-SNO₂*, thionitrate

conversion rates were at a constant ratio of 14:1 regardless of the structure of the organic nitrate. Reduction of the NO_2^- generated to NO was experimentally excluded, as neither definite amounts of NO_2^- (1, 10, 100 μM) were reduced by cysteine (1 mM, pH 7.4, 37°C, 1 h) nor was any formation of NO measurable under these conditions (n = 3). We, therefore, assume that in the course of the reaction between organic nitrate and SH-containing compound a common thiol-specific intermediate arises which decomposes with the release of NO_2^- and – under special circumstances – of NO, too. A thionitrate ($RSNO_2$), i.e., a thioester which may arise upon transesterification from the organic nitrate to the respective thiol, appears to be the most likely candidate for such an intermediate. A carbonyl function in a distinct spatial orientation towards the mercapto group (as in cysteine or thiosalicylic acid) may favor an intramolecular rearrangement of this intermediate, which stabilizes by splitting off NO.

NO Release from Other Nitrovasodilators

Comparative measurements with other nitrovasodilators uniformly confirmed the dependence of enzyme stimulation on the rate of NO release. The pathway of NO formation, however, is different for each class of compound.

Amyl nitrite, a representative of organic nitrites, releases NO only in the presence of thiols, although it was apparently less discriminating in respect to the chemical structure of the SH compound, as NO liberation was detected with all thiols tested. Interestingly, at the same time a strong nonlinear formation of S-nitrosothiols was observed. The net rate of NO liberation depended on the RSNO concentration at the time and its rate of decomposition under the prevailing conditions.

SNP spontaneously releases NO in a nonlinear manner, seemingly independent of pH over a wide range, plateauing at higher concentrations [8], probably because a certain limit for the dissociation of NO from the pentacyano complex has been attained.

Sydnonimines such as SIN-1 are highly unstable in aqueous solution and pH-dependently hydrolyze to the ring-opened "A"-forms; these in turn spontaneously decompose with the release of NO. NO formation appeared to be initiated by molecular oxygen (data not shown). Those sydnonimines with the highest release of NO were the most effective stimulators of sGC. The presence of cysteine (5 mM) enhanced neither NO formation nor enzyme activation. Besides NO, NO_2^- and NO_3^- are also generated, the rate not correlating with sGC stimulation.

As representatives of a new vasodilator group, furoxans were also tested as potential NO liberators. None of these compounds liberated NO spontaneously, but all did after addition of thiols. The rate of NO formation closely correlated with enzyme activation. Again, those compounds with the highest rate of NO release caused the strongest enzyme activation [10]. Upon incubation with thiol compounds, furoxans formed S-nitrosothiols, the initial rates of which ran in parallel with the measured rates for NO formation.

Discussion

In this study we present the first evidence that neither NO_2^- nor nitrosothiols directly activate sGC but that they do so by decomposition to NO. Collectively, our data strongly support the concept that NO is the ultimate enzyme-stimulating metabolite of all nitrovasodilators.

Organic nitrates were decomposed to a considerable extent to NO_2^- by all tested thiols, whereas sGC activation was only observed in the presence of a few compounds. The seemingly close correlation between NO_2^- generation from and sGC stimulation by organic nitrates in the presence of cysteine clearly demonstrated that a good correlation between two parameters does not necessarily indicate a cause-effect relationship. Our data are consistent with a study by

Romanin and Kukovetz [37], demonstrating that comparable amounts of NO_2^- were formed from GTN with either cysteine or its methyl ester, whereas sGC activation was only observed with cysteine. The specific need of organic nitrates for cysteine to activate sGC clearly demonstrates that, in addition to the formation of NO_2^-, this compound must have yet another function for enzyme activation. Thus, the denitration rate is an unsuitable parameter for determining the actions of organic nitrates, because NO_2^- formation is not coupled to activation of the target enzyme, sGC.

The close correlation between the rate of NO liberation and the extent of sGC stimulation, the uniform rate of NO release at enzymatically equipotent concentrations, and the inhibitory effects of methylene blue and oxyhemoglobin confirmed that NO plays a crucial role in activation of sGC by nitrovasodilators. Given the observed pH-dependence, nitrosothiols are unlikely to be the precursors of NO formation and sGC stimulation by organic nitrates. S-nitrosothiols are, however, intermediates in the thiol-induced formation of NO from organic nitrites and furoxans. The inverse correlation between stability and sGC stimulating potency of several nitrosothiols clearly demonstrates that these compounds do not directly activate sGC. It is much more likely that NO formed during decomposition of these unstable compounds is responsible for enzyme activation, and this is supported by the fact that authentic NO was the strongest activator of sGC. In contrast to a published procedure for the synthesis of nitrosothiols [21], we found that NO does not react with thiols directly.

As a resume of the experimental data dealing with the mechanism of NO liberation from different nitrovasodilator classes, we propose the following scheme (Fig. 6):

All nitrovasodilators have to penetrate the membrane of the smooth muscle cell first in order to be metabolized intracellularly. NO already released in the plasma compartment presumably does not account for the vasodilatory effect of these drugs because of its extremely short half-life in the presence of oxygen (5.6 s in air-saturated aqueous buffer [26]). It is rather unlikely that NO generated intraluminally from nitrovasodilators can cross the endothelial layer to reach the underlying smooth muscle in concentrations able to induce marked relaxation. Organic nitrates will be degraded to the alcohols and NO_2^-/NO_3^- in both enzymatic and nonenzymatic steps. The enzymatic pathway is mainly catalyzed by glutathione S-transferase [18] and a so-called "nitrate-forming enzyme" [40], the nonenzymatic one by free thiols present in the cytosol [9]. In both cases a thionitrate may be the common intermediate. NO_2^- and NO_3^- interchange with extracellular compartments [36] without affecting enzyme activity. Of all thiols present within the smooth muscle cell, only cysteine or its N-acetyl analogue (either free or at the active site of any enzyme) are also able to induce NO liberation. Organic nitrites and furoxans react intracellularly with all available thiols (presumably predominantly with glutathione) to form S-nitrosothiols which — as thermodynamically unstable compounds — decompose to NO by radical cleavage. S-nitrosothiols, which may be formed from organic nitrates in plasma [13], decompose by the same route to NO after entering the cell. SNP releases NO spontaneously and sydnonimines by an oxygen-dependent radical

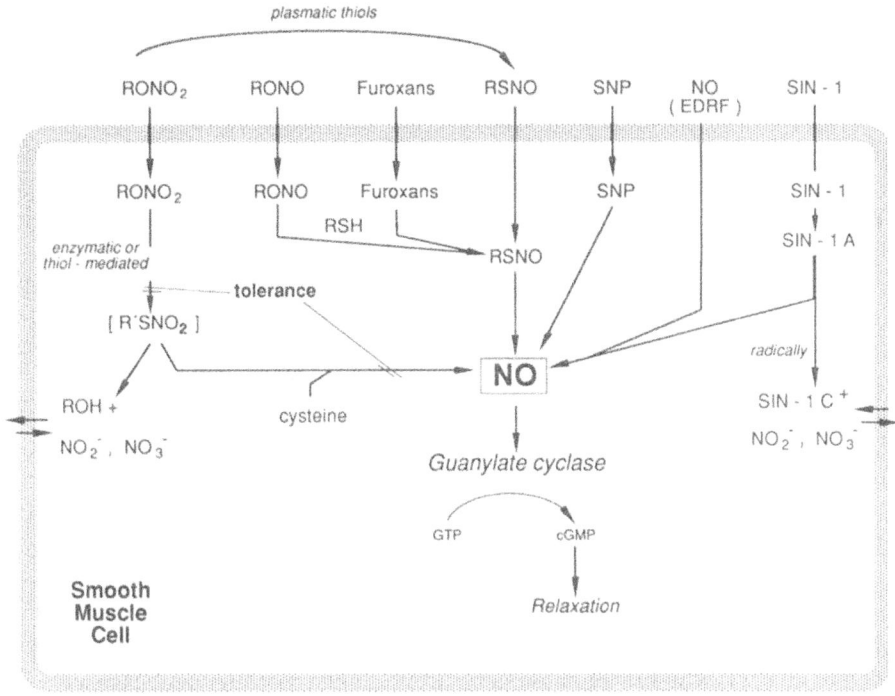

Fig. 6. Proposed scheme of sGC activation with respect to the different pathways of NO formation from nitrovasodilators. Abbreviations: *EDRF*. endothelium-derived relaxing factor: *Furoxans*. 3,4-disubstituted furazan-2-oxides: *NO*, nitric oxide: *RONO*. organic nitrite: *RONO₂*, organic nitrate: *RSH* thiol: *RSNO*, nitrosothiol: *SIN-1*, active metabolite of molsidomine: *SNP*, sodium nitroprusside

process following base-catalyzed hydrolysis to the ring-opened A forms. Simultaneously arising NO_2^- and NO_3^- do not account for sGC stimulation.

The apparent similarities between the denitration profile in vitro and the biotransformation in vivo led us to conclude that the nonenzymatic metabolism of organic nitrates and other nitrovasodilators may also play an essential role in their pharmacodynamic action in vivo. Two mutually independent pathways exist for their decomposition, one leading to NO formation and thus to enzyme activation and the other leading to NO_2^- formation. Although the latter pathway predominates, it only represents an inactivation step. One may assume that, within the smooth muscle cell, a combination of enzymatic and nonenzymatic processes operate the output of which depends on both the concentration of free thiols and prevailing enzymatic activity. It is conceivable that the reactions observed in vitro are a projection of the enzymatic metabolism in vivo. If so, these processes may be of similar importance for other biological processes which are controlled by thiol- and haem-containing enzymes.

A better understanding of the structural determinants that govern the reaction between organic nitrates and thiols is an important prerequisite for rational drug design. We here present new data concerning the chemical mechanism of NO and NO_2^- formation from organic nitrates which strongly suggest that thionitrates ($RSNO_2$) are formed transiently. Such chemical species had previously been postulated to represent the intermediates in the enzymatic decomposition of organic nitrates by glutathione S-transferase [25] and in a chemical reaction of organic nitrates with thiols, which gives rise to NO_2^- [41,43]. We here propose that thionitrates represent the common intermediates of both NO_2^-/NO_3^- and NO formation from organic nitrates, which easily explains the close relationship between the formation rates of NO_2^- and NO. Certain structural features seem to induce a shift of the decomposition profile of this intermediate from NO_2^- to NO formation.

The lack of cross-tolerance between classical organic nitrates and thiol-independent nitrovasodilators such as SNP or SIN-1 [28,33], together with the recent demonstration that the NO-induced relaxation of rabbit aortic rings remains unaffected by nitrate tolerance [38], indicates that a decrease in biotransformation of organic nitrates rather than desensitization of sGC triggers the development of nitrate tolerance. Thus, apart from possible alterations of the target enzyme sGC itself [2,42], tolerance is likely to be related to an intracellular event such as depletion of cysteine stores and/or diminished activity of an as yet unidentified enzyme which converts organic nitrates to NO. In recent studies by Ahlner et al. [1] with bovine mesenteric arteries and by Hütter et al. [19] with a working rat heart preparation, a biphasic concentration/response curve for GTN was described. Two sites of biotransformation seem to exist: a high-affinity component of an enzymatic nature and a low-affinity component [2] which may be represented by the nonenzymatic, cysteine-dependent NO formation. The enzymatic route of bioactivation in intact cells is presumably much more effective than the nonenzymatic one but suffers from rapid desensitization on exposure to high concentrations of organic nitrates. Upon high-dose exposure to GTN, the enzymatic capacity is likely to be down-regulated so that only the nonenzymatic pathway of NO formation remains operating, resulting in decreased effectiveness of organic nitrates but no alteration in the response to those nitrovasodilators which spontaneously liberate NO. Whether or not nitrate tolerance is the result of impaired biotransformation to NO by vascular tissue needs further investigation.

Much effort was spent in the past to identify the chemical nature of the "endothelium-derived relaxing factor" (EDRF). Some groups recently provided evidence that EDRF is identical with NO [20,32]. That means that the endothelium-dependent vasodilators are acting in the same way as the nitrovasodilators, namely, by formation of NO. In the light of this discovery it becomes clear that synthetic nitrovasodilators imitate a physiological process of blood vessel regulation. From this point of view they thus represent different pro-drugs of EDRF and so should no longer be regarded as empirical therapeutics but as physiologically and rationally established drugs. The use of nitrovasodilators may be regarded as causal therapy, inasmuch as these compounds are suitable substitutes for an endogenous factor under pathophysiological conditions which are accompanied by endothelial dysfunction and decreased production and/or effectiveness of EDRF.

Summary

Recent evidence suggests that the heterogeneous group of "nitrovasodilators" act through a common mechanism, i.e. the generation of nitric oxide (NO). These compounds thus represent pro-drugs which mimic a physiological mechanism of endothelial controlled vasodilatation. Elucidation of the chemical pathways by which NO is generated from these compounds is crucial for understanding the mechanisms of soluble guanylate cyclase (sGC) activation and the subsequent vasodilatation. We therefore investigated the in vitro metabolism of organic nitrates and nitrites, S-nitrosothiols, furoxans, sydnonimins, and nitroprusside using difference-spectrophotometry, chemiluminescence, and HPLC techniques in direct comparison to enzyme activation. As cysteine is known to act as an essential cofactor for sGC stimulation by organic nitrates, measurements were performed in the presence and absence of related thiol compounds. Completely different ways of "bioactivation" were demonstrated depending on the chemical nature of both nitrovasodilator and thiol component. Organic nitrates, nitrites, and furoxans required a preceding interaction with a mercapto group to liberate NO, while sydnonimins, S-nitrosothiols, and nitroprusside spontaneously released NO. Enzyme activation always closely correlated with the rate of NO generation. The reaction of organic nitrates with cysteine seemed to be highly specific, because SH compounds with slightly different steric and electronical characteristics decomposed organic nitrates to nitrite ions (NO_2^-) only without generating NO or affecting sGC activity. We suggest that these new data will help in designing new drugs which better meet the therapeutic requirements while not inducing tolerance.

Acknowledgement. We would like to thank Mrs I. Beier for skilful technical assistance.

References

1. Ahlner J, Axelsson KL, Ekstam Ljusegren M, Grundström N, Andersson RGG (1987) Demonstration of a high-affinity component of glyceryl trinitrate-induced vasodilation in the bovine mesenteric artery. J Cycl Nucl Prot Res 11:445–456
2. Bennett BM, Schröder H, Hayward LD, Waldman SA, Murad F (1988) Effect of in vitro organic nitrate tolerance on relaxation, cyclic GMP accumulation and guanylate cyclase activation by glyceryl trinitrate and the enantiomers of isoidide dinitrate. Circ Res 63:693–701
3. Brien JF, McLaughlin BE, Breedon TH, Bennett BM, Nakatsu K, Marks GS (1986) Biotransformation of glyceryl trinitrate occurs concurrently with relaxation of rabbit aorta. J Pharmacol Exp Ther 237(2):608–614
4. Brien JF, McLaughlin BE, Kobus SM, Kawamoto JH, Nakatsu K, Marks GS (1988) Mechanism of gyceryl trinitrate-induced vasodilation. I. Relationship between drug biotransformation, tissue cyclic GMP elevation and relaxation of rabbit aorta. J Pharmacol Exp Ther 244(1):322–327
5. Cantoni C, Bianchi MA, Beretta G (1975) Stabilita di nitrosoderivati (nitrosotioli, nitrosofenoli e nitrosoemoglobina) a pH alkalino (Ital). Ind Aliment 14(7–8):79–81
6. Doyle MP, Hoekstra JW (1981) Oxidation of nitrogen oxides by bound dioxygen in hemoproteins. J Inorg Biochem 14:351–358
7. Feelisch M, Noack E (1987) Nitric oxide formation from nitrovasodilators occurs independently of hemoglobin or non-heme iron. Eur J Pharmacol 142:465–469

8. Feelisch M, Noack E (1987) Correlation between nitric oxide formation during degradation of organic nitrates and activation of guanylate cyclase. Eur J Pharmacol 139:19-30

9. Feelisch M, Noack E, Schröder H (1988) Explanation of the discrepancy between the degree of organic nitrate decomposition, nitrite formation and guanylate cyclase stimulation. Eur Heart J 9(Suppl A):57-62

10. Feelisch M, Noack E (1989) Thiol-induced generation of nitric oxide (NO) accounts for the vasodilatory action of furoxans (abstr). Naunyn Schmiedebergs Arch Pharmacol 339(Suppl):R67

11. Field L, Dilts RV, Ravichandran R, Lenhert PG, Carnahan GE (1978) An unusually stable thionitrite from N-acetyl-D,L-penicillamine. X-ray crystal structure of 2-(acetylamino)-2-carboxy-1,1-dimethylethyl thionitrite. J Chem Soc Chem Comm 1157:249-252

12. Fiscus RR, Rapoport RM, Murad F (1984) Endothelium-dependent and nitrovasodilator-induced activation of cyclic GMP-dependent protein kinase in rat aorta. J Cycl Nucl Prot Phosph Res 9(6):415-425

13. Fung HL, Chong S, Kowaluk E, Hough K, Kakemi M (1988) Mechanisms for the pharmacological interaction of organic nitrates with thiols. Existence of an extracellular pathway for the reversal of nitrate vascular tolerance by N-acetylcysteine. J Pharmacol Exp Ther 245(2):524-530

14. Hafner D, Heinen E, Noack E (1977) Mathematical analysis of concentration-response relationship. Method for the evaluation of the EC_{50} and the number of binding sites per receptor molecule using the logit transformation. Arzneimittelforschung 27:1871-1873

15. Hart TW (1985) Some observations concerning the S-nitroso and S-phenylsulfonyl derivates of L-cysteine and glutathione. Tetrahedr Lett 26(16):2013-2016

16. Haussmann HJ, Werringloer J (1987) Mechanism and control of the denitrosation of N-nitrosodimethylamine. In: Bartsch H, O'Neill IK, Schulte-Herman R (eds) Relevance of N-nitroso compounds to human cancer: exposure and mechanisms. IARC, Lyon, pp 109-112

17. Hay M (1883) The chemical nature and physiological action of nitroglycerin. Practitioner 30:422-433

18. Heppel LA, Hilmoe RJ (1950) Metabolism of inorganic nitrite and nitrate esters. II. The enzymatic reduction of nitroglycerin and erythritol tetranitrate by glutathione. J Biol Chem 183:129-138

19. Hütter J, Schmidt M, Rittler J (1988) Effects of sulfhydryl-containing compounds on nitroglycerin-induced coronary dilation in isolated working rat hearts. Eur J Pharmacol 156:215-222

20. Ignarro LJ (1989) Endothelium-derived nitric oxide:actions and properties. FASEB J 3:31-36

21. Ignarro LJ, Gruetter CA (1980) Requirement of thiols for activation of coronary arterial guanylate cyclase by glyceryl trinitrate and sodium nitrite. Possible involvement of S-nitrosothiols. Biochim Biophys Acta 631:221-231

22. Ignarro LJ, Kadowitz PJ, Baricos WH (1981) Evidence that regulation of hepatic guanylate cyclase activity involves interactions between catalytic site SH-groups and both substrate and activator. Arch Biochem Biophys 208(1):75-86

23. Ignarro LJ, Lippton H, Edwards JC, Baricos WH, Hyman AL, Kadowitz PJ, Gruetter CA (1981) Mechanism of vascular smooth muscle relaxation by organic nitrates, nitrites, nitroprusside and nitric oxide: evidence for the involvement of S-nitrosothiols as active intermediates. J Pharmacol Exp Ther 218:739-749

24. Katsuki S, Arnold W, Mittal C, Murad F (1977) Stimulation of guanylate cyclase by sodium nitroprusside, nitroglycerin and nitric oxide in various tissue preparations and comparison to the effects of sodium azide and hydroxylamine. J Cycl Nucl Res 3:23-35

25. Keen JH, Habig WH, Jakoby WB (1976) Mechanism of the several activities of glutathione-S-transferases. J Biol Chem 251:6183-6188

26. Kelm M, Feelisch M, Spahr R, Piper HM, Noack E, Schrader J (1988) Quantitative and kinetic characterization of nitric oxide and EDRF from cultured endothelial cells. Biochem Biophys Res Commun 154(1):236-244

27. Kimura H, Mittal CK, Murad F (1975) Activation of guanylate cyclase from rat liver and other tissues by sodium azide. J Biol Chem 250(20):8016-8022

28. Kukovetz WR, Holzmann S (1986) Mode of action of nitrates with regard to vasodilation and tolerance. Z Kardiol 75(Suppl 3):8-11

29. Kuropteva ZV, Pastushenko ON (1985) Change in paramagnetic blood and liver complexes in animals under the influence of nitroglycerin (Russ). Dokl Akad Nauk SSSR 281(1):189–192

30. Leuenberger U, Gauch R, Rieder K, Baumgartner E (1980) Determination of nitrate and bromide in foodstuffs by high-performance liquid chromatography. J Chromatogr 202:461–468

31. Mirna A, Hofmann K (1969) Über den Verbleib von Nitrit in Fleischwaren. I. Umsetzung von Nitrit mit Sulfhydrylverbindungen. Fleischwirtschaft 10:1361–1366

32. Moncada S, Palmer RMJ, Higgs EA (1988) The discovery of nitric oxide as the endogenous nitrovasodilator. Hypertension 12:365–372

33. Mülsch A, Busse R, Bassenge E (1988) Desensitization of guanylate cyclase in nitrate tolerance does not impair endothelium-dependent responses. Eur J Pharmacol 158:191–198

34. Murad F (1987) Cyclic guanosine monophosphate as a mediator of vasodilation. J Clin Invest 78:1–5

35. Needleman P, Johnson EM (1975) The pharmacological and biochemical interaction of organic nitrates with sulfhydryls: possible correlations with the mechanism of tolerance development, vasodilation and mitochondrial and enzyme reactions. In: Needleman P (ed) Handbook of experimental pharmacology, vol 40. Springer, Berlin Heidelberg New York, pp 97–114

36. Parks NJ, Krohn KA, Mathis CA, Chasko JH, Geiger KR, Gregor ME, Peek NF (1981) Nitrogen-13-labeled nitrite and nitrate: distribution and metabolism after intratracheal administration. Science 212(3):58–61

37. Romanin C, Kukovetz WR (1988) Guanylate cyclase activation by organic nitrates is not mediated via nitrite. J Mol Cell Cardiol 20:389–396

38. Slack CJ, McLaughlin BE, Nakatsu K, Marks GS, Brien JF (1988) Nitric oxide-induced vasodilation of organic nitrate-tolerant rabbit aorta. Can J Physiol Pharmacol 66:1344–1346

39. Steurer G, Schütz W (1984) Guanylate cyclase stimulation by nitro-compounds is dependent on free Ca. Experientia 40:970–971

40. Tsuruta H, Hasegawa H (1970) Studies on nitroglycol poisoning – On some properties of an enzyme which decomposes nitroglycol into inorganic nitrate. Ind Health 8:99–118

41. Tsuruta H, Hasegawa H (1970) Studies on nitroglycol poisoning – Decomposition mechanism of nitroglycol by nitrite forming enzyme. Ind Health 8:119–140

42. Waldman SA, Rapoport RM, Ginsburg R, Murad F (1986) Desensitization to nitroglycerin in vascular smooth muscle from rat and human. Biochem Pharmacol 35(20):3525–3531

43. Yeates RA, Laufen, H Leitold M (1985) The reaction between organic nitrates and sulfhydryl compounds – A possible model system for the activation of organic nitrates. Mol Pharmacol 28:555–559

The Role of Nitrates in Congestive Heart Failure

J. ABRAMS

Introduction

The use of intravenous nitroglycerin (NTG) and long-acting nitrates in acute and chronic congestive heart failure (CHF) has been popular since the introduction of vasodilator therapy for CHF in the early 1970s. Although the angiotensin-converting enzyme (ACE) inhibitors have become extremely popular as "unloading" agents in CHF, current evidence suggests that nitrates may be comparably effective to these agents. It is of interest that both classes of drugs exert their effects on the venous and arterial sides of the circulation in heart faiure, with a subsequent reduction in preload and afterload of the heart. This discussion relates only to the patient with CHF *and* depressed left ventricular contractile or systolic function (e.g., ejection fraction less than 35%–40%).

The nitrates are beneficial in improving the disordered hemodynamics in the heart failure state. They consistently reduce pulmonary capillary wedge, pulmonary artery, and right atrial pressures. Although salutory nitrate effects on stroke volume and cardiac output are modest, cardiac pump performance is usually increased [1,2]. In addition, the nitrates appear to enhance long-term exercise performance [3,4]; of the vasodilator drugs, only the ACE inhibitors have been shown to have a similar positive effect on exercise tolerance in CHF [5]. Finally, oral nitrates have been shown to improve survival in patients with class II or III congestive heart failure when used in conjunction with hydralazine (V-Heft trial) [6].

Mechanisms of Action

Nitroglycerin and the long-acting nitrates are relaxants of vascular smooth muscle and induce vasodilatation of the veins and arteries and, in high doses, the arterioles or resistance vessels (Fig. 1). Nitrate effects on the arterial circulation (afterload reduction) are critical to improvement of cardiac function in CHF. A pure venodilator would lead to a reduction in cardiac output, but the decrease in arterial impedance and systemic vascular resistance that occurs with nitrates results in an augmentation of stroke volume and cardiac output. After nitrate administration, the circulating blood volume is redistributed away from the lungs and heart towards the abdominal and splanchnic circulations as well as to the

B.S. Lewis, A. Kimchi (Eds.)
Heart Failure Mechanisms and Management
© Springer-Verlag Berlin Heidelberg 1991

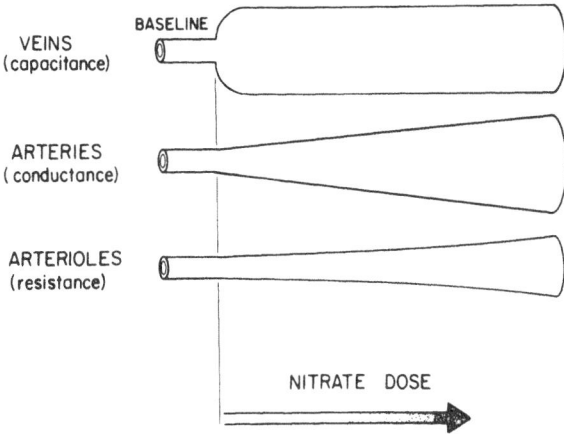

Fig. 1. Hemodynamic effects of nitrates on the major vascular beds. At very low doses the venous capacitance vessels are nearly maximally dilated. The systemic arteries begin to dilate at low doses; this is further accentuated with higher doses of nitrates. Systolic blood pressure begins to fall even in the absence of an effect on resistance vessels. Arteriolar vasodilatation occurs only with very high nitrate concentrations, which are probably not achieved with usual clinical doses of these drugs. (From [27] with permission)

extremities. There is a decrease in return of blood to the right heart, resulting in a fall in preload of both right and left ventricles. Pulmonary artery systolic pressure falls, in part due to direct pulmonary artery vasodilatation. The decrease in right heart pressures appears to be a unique feature of this group of vasodilators. Nitroglycerin compounds favorably effect the pressure-volume relationships of the left ventricle, perhaps in part because of altered pericardial restraining forces and/or a smaller right ventricular volume [7].

Acutely, nitrates do not improve exercise tolerance in heart failure subjects; this is similar to the ACE inhibitors. However, *long-term* administration of both classes of drug results in enhanced aerobic performance in patients with CHF [3,4]. It may be that a sustained reduction in left ventricular filling pressure allows for a "training effect," such that patients are able to exercise better over time following chronic nitrate administration.

Clinical Studies

Many clinical investigations carried out in the 1970s and early 1980s have documented the benefits of nitrates in patients with heart failure. In particular, oral isosorbide dinitrate (ISDN) and 2% NTG ointment have been shown to be effective as long-acting nitrate therapy [1]. Oral ISDN therapy results in long-term benefits on exercise tolerance (over a period of 12 weeks) in controlled trials [3,4]. Sustained hemodynamic improvement at rest is manifest by a decrease in left ventricular filling pressure, a lower pulmonary artery pressure and resistance, with variable effects on arterial pressure, systemic vascular resistance, and cardiac output. Improvement in exercise hemodynamics during chronic nitrate therapy presumably reflects a dominant decrease in left ventricular preload.

In the acute setting, intravenous NTG is extremely effective in improving the disordered hemodynamics in heart failure, producing a reduction in pulmonary wedge pressure and an improvement in cardiac output. Data with transdermal NTG patches in CHF is sparse [8-12]. Limited information documents the rapid appearance of vascular attenuation or tolerance, often within 24 h of patch application [9-12]. There is also a blunted hemodynamic response with long-term NTG patch therapy [8]. It appears that intermittent application of NTG patches allows for sustained vascular responsiveness [12]. Large doses of the patches may be necessary for a beneficial clinical effect [9-11] (see below).

Benefits of Nitroglycerin Therapy

Nitrates should be considered for use in addition to digitalis and diuretics in patients who continue to have signs and/or symptoms of CHF. As mentioned, several long-term studies document that administration of oral ISDN results in continued improvement in both hemodynamics and exercise performance [3,4].

The United States Veterans Administration Cooperative Trial (V-Heft) demonstrated a substantial reduction in mortality in CHF when oral 40 mg ISDN q.i.d. was administered in conjunction with 75 mg hydralazine q.i.d., compared to a placebo control group as well as another cohort of patients treated with prazosin 5 mg q.i.d. [5] (Fig. 2). There were mortality benefits of greater than 20% for up to 3 years in this study; the difference from placebo was a 38% reduction in deaths at 12 months. This was the first major trial with any drug documenting improvement in mortality in patients with CHF. Similar data in class IV CHF patients has been subsequently shown for enalapril [13].

Problems with Nitrate Therapy

The usual nitrate side effects of headache and hypotension appear to be less of a problem in heart failure. In general, patients with CHF tolerate nitrates quite well. Reflex tachycardia and hypotension are infrequent.

Nitrate resistance has been documented in several studies. This appears to be a primary failure of peripheral vasodilatation, such that hemodynamic parameters are unperturbed by nitrate administration [14-16]. Patients who are resistant to nitrates tend to be quite ill, often with severe biventricular CHF. Even very large doses may be ineffective.

Nitrate tolerance remains a major problem in the treatment of CHF as well as angina pectoris. At the present, all experts recommend an interval approach to nitrate therapy. This involves pulsed dosing employing a nitrate-free interval

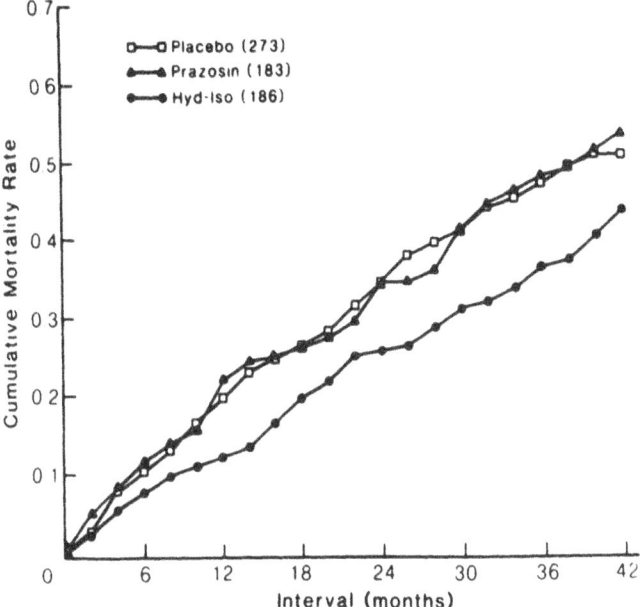

Fig. 2. Survival curves for patients with congestive heart failure (Class II-III) who were given a regimen of either placebo, prazosin 5 mg q.i.d., or the combination of hydralazine 75 mg q.i.d. and Isosorbide Dinitrate 40 mg q.i.d. Note that the placebo and Prazosin mortality curves are identical. There is a significant reduction from mortality of 20-30% for the nitrate-hydralazine group at 12, 24, and 36 months. (From [6] with permission)

(one or more) throughout a 24-h period. Thus, oral ISDN [17] t.i.d. or NTG ointment application, or NTG patch therapy with an 8- to 12-h off period [12], is recommended. Tolerance has been well documented in patients given large doses of transdermal NTG but may be avoidable with an intermittent or interval approach [12]. Acute administration of N-acetylcysteine has been shown to reverse hemodynamic tolerance to prolonged intravenous NTG infusion in CHF, but this therapy is experimental and impractical [18]. Carefully designed dosing strategies must be employed to avoid the vexing problem of nitrate tolerance. An interval or on-off performance approach is strongly recommended to provide protracted nitrate efficacy in CHF subjects.

Nitrate Dosage

In general, rather large amounts of nitrates are necessary for patients with CHF. Thus, 2.5-5 cm NTG ointment, 40-80 mg oral ISDN, and 20-40 mg per 24 h transdermal NTG patches are recommended. Therapy should be started with smaller doses to make sure that nitrates are well tolerated, and that a fall in blood pressure does not occur.

Acute Myocardial Infarction

Intravenous NTG and other long-acting nitrates are effective drugs for controlling left ventricular failure associated with acute myocardial infarction; in addition, there are considerable animal and human data indicating that the *early* administration of intravenous NTG has important beneficial effects. This drug has previously been shown to reduce infarct size and decrease complications of acute myocardial infarction [19–23]. Pooled data from a number of small trials using intravenous NTG within the first 24–48 h of infarction has demonstrated a striking reduction in early mortality compared to placebo [24]. Important new data suggest that early administration of intravenous NTG also results in protection against the adverse remodeling that occurs (infarct expansion, wall thinning) in many patients following an acute myocardial infarction [25]. In addition to a meta-analysis showing that in-hospital mortality is reduced in acute myocardial infarction when intravenous NTG is started within the first few hours after the event [24], a recent large trial demonstrates that long-term mortality (1-year) has been found to be lower in anterior wall infarction initially treated for 48 h with an intravenous NTG drip [25].

Additional therapy with buccal NTG after an initial 48-h NTG infusion for 6 weeks has been shown to result in further improvement in left ventricular size and function, as well as enhanced exercise performance [26].

Summary

Nitrates are extremely effective agents for adjunctive therapy of CHF. These drugs are safe, easy to use, and well tolerated. Nitrates have been shown to be truly cardioprotective, in addition to having beneficial effects on improving the disordered hemodynamics and reduced exercise tolerance in CHF. Exciting recent data also suggest that early administration of intravenous NTG following an acute myocardial infarction may have important short- and long-term benefits.

References

1. Abrams J (1979) Pharmacology of nitroglycerin and long-acting nitrates and their usefulness in the treatment of chronic congestive heart failure. In: Gould L, Reddy CVR (eds) Vasodilator therapy for cardiac disorders. Futura, Mount Kisco, NY, pp 129–168
2. Herman B, Charlap S, Frishman WH (1989) Nitrates in congestive heart failure. Med Clin North Am 73:361–371
3. Leier CV, Huss P, Magorien RD, Unverferth DV (1983) Improved exercise capacity and differing arterial and venous tolerance during chronic isosorbide dinitrate therapy for congestive heart failure. Circulation 67:87–822
4. Franciosa JA, Cohn JN (1980) Sustained hemodynamic effects without tolerance during long-term isosorbide dinitrate treatment in chronic left ventricular failure. Am J Cardiol 45:650–654
5. Abrams J (1988) A reappraisal of nitrate therapy. JAMA 259:396–401

6. Cohn JN et al. (1986) Effect of vasodilator therapy on mortality in chronic congestive heart failure. Results of a Veterans Administration cooperative study. N Engl J Med 374:1547–1552

7. Smith ER, Smiseth OA, Kingma I, Manyari D, Belenkie I, Tyberg JV (1984) Mechanisms of action of nitrates. Role of changes in venous capacitance and in the left ventricular diastolic pressure-volume relation. Am J Med 76(6A):14

8. Sharpe DN, Coxon R (1984) Nitroglycerin in a transdermal therapeutic system in chronic heart failure. J Cardiovasc Pharmacol 6:76–82

9. Olivari MT, Carlyle PF, Levine B, Cohn JN (1983) Hemodynamic and hormonal response to transdermal nitroglycerin in normal subjects and in patients with congestive heart failure. J Am Coll Cardiol 2:872–878

10. Jordan RA, Seth L, Henry DA, Wilen MM, Franciosa JA (1985) Dose requirements and hemodynamic effects of transdermal nitroglycerin compared to placebo in patients with congestive heart failure. Circulation 71:980–985

11. Elkayam U, Roth A, Henriquez B, Weber L, Tonnemacher D, Rahimtoola SH (1985) The hemodynamic and hormonal effects of high-dose transdermal nitroglycerin in patients with chronic congestive heart failure. Am J Cardiol 56:555–559

12. Sharpe N, Coxon R, Webster M, Luke R (1987) Hemodynamic effects of intermittent transdermal nitroglycerin in chronic congestive heart failure. Am J Cardiol 59:895–899

13. Effects of enalapril on mortality in severe congestive heart failure. Results of the Cooperative North Scandinavian Enalapril Survival Study (Consensus). N Engl J Med 316:1429–1435

14. Armstrong PW, Moffat JA, Marks GS (1982) Arterial-venous nitroglycerin gradient during intravenous infusion in man. Circulation 66:1273

15. Magrini F, Niarchos AP (1980) Ineffectiveness of sublingual nitroglycerin in acute left ventricular failure in the presence of massive peripheral edema. Am J Cardiol 45:841

16. Kulick D, Roth A, McIntosh N, Rahimtoola SH, Elkayam U (1988) Resistance to isorsorbide dinitrate in patients with severe chronic heart failure: incidence and attempt at hemodynamic prediction. J Am Coll Cardiol 12:1023–1028

17. Elkayam U, Jamison M, Roth A, Kulick D, Vasquez J, Rahimtoola SH (1989) Oral isosorbide dinitrate in chronic heart failure: tolerance development to four times daily versus three times daily regimen. J Am Coll Cardiol 13:1784

18. Packer M, Lee WH, Kessler P, Medina Yushak M (1986) Induction of nitrate tolerance in human heart failure by continuous intravenous infusion of nitroglycerin and reversal of tolerance by N-acetylcysteine, a sulfhydryl donor. J Am Coll Cardiol 7:27A

19. Flaherty JT, Becker LC, Bulkley BH (1983) A randomized prospective trial of intravenous nitroglycerin in patients with acute myocardial infarction. Circulation 68:576–584

20. Flaherty JT (1983) Comparison of intravenous nitroglycerin and sodium nitroprusside in acute myocardial infarction. Am J Med [Suppl] 74:53–60

21. Bussman WD, Passek D, Seidel W, Kaltenback M (1981) Reduction of CK and CK-MB indexes of infarct size by intravenous nitroglycerin. Circulation 63:615–622

22. Jugdutt BI, Becker LC, Hutchins C (1980) Effects of intravenous nitroglycerin on collateral blood flow and infarct size in the conscious dog. Circulation 63:17–28

23. Jugdutt BI, Sussex BA, Warnica JW, Rossan RLS (1983) Persistent reduction in left ventricular asynergy in patients with acute myocardial infarction by intravenous infusion of nitroglycerin. Circulation 68:1264–1273

24. Yusuf S, Collins R, MacMahon S, Peto R (1988) Effect of intravenous nitrates on mortality in acute myocardial infarction: an overview of the randomized trials. Lancet II:1088–1092

25. Jugdutt BI, Warnica JW (1988) Intravenous nitroglycerin therapy to limit myocardial infarct size, expansion, and complications: effect of timing, dosage, and infarct location. Circulation 78:906–919

26. Jugdutt BI, Warnica JW (1988) Tolerance with intravenous nitroglycerin in acute myocardial infarction. J Am Coll Cardiol 11:43A

27. Abrams J (1985) Hemodynamic effects of nitroglycerin and long-acting nitrates. Am Heart J 110:216

Isosorbide Dinitrate and Nitroglycerin Oral Spray in Heart Failure

A. Schneeweiss, A. Marmor, L. Reisin, and J.S. Alpert

Introduction

Nitrates are widely used for the treatment and prevention of heart failure and angina pectoris. Even the traditionally most rapid method of administration, the sublingual tablet, takes at least 2 min until the onset of effect. Usually this takes longer because 2 min is the time required from the moment of dissolution by nitrates, administered in the form of sublingual tablets, to reach peak plasma levels [1]. An additional period is, however, required for dissolution of the tablet, which must take place at least partially before absorption begins. This period shows interpatient variability, which may involve further delay of the onset of action.

Several forms of oral spray are available in which the active compound (isosorbide dinitrate, ISDN; or nitroglycerin, NTG) is kept as a solution in a spray container. These were planned to avoid the delay required for dissolution of sublingual tablets. ISDN spray was found effective in a variety of cardiovascular diseases: it relieves pain in patients with chronic stable or unstable angina pectoris and produces hemodynamic and symptomatic improvement in patients with acute exacerbation of congestive heart failure and pulmonary edema.

Nitrate Oral Spray in Congestive Heart Failure

The superiority of nitrate oral spray is in the immediate treatment of acute episodes of the diseases for which nitrates are used. In congestive heart failure, an acute episode usually presents as acute pulmonary edema. Nitrates have substantially improved the management of acute pulmonary edema. The nitrate-induced hemodynamic improvement in this condition results mainly from venodilation and is accompanied by clinical improvement [1–6]. As the rapidity of drug administration plays a major role in the management of acute pulmonary edema, the usual routes of administration of nitrates are the intravenous and sublingual ones. Sublingual administration of a tablet of nitrate is often not practical in very dyspneic patients. Moreover, dissolution of the tablets takes about 2 min, before significant absorption begins [7].

ISND spray appears to be the optimal method for very rapid treatment. We studied two patients with acute pulmonary edema in whom hemodynamic

B.S. Lewis, A. Kimchi (Eds.)
Heart Failure Mechanisms and Management
© Springer-Verlag Berlin Heidelberg 1991

improvement occurred within 1 min after administration of ISDN spray. The patients, both with chronic congestive heart failure, were studied by Swan-Ganz catheter for hemodynamic evaluation. Both developed acute pulmonary edema while the catheter was in place and during chronic treatment with diuretics only. In both, ISDN spray produced immediate hemodynamic improvement, evident by decreases in wedge pressure and increases in cardiac output, within 60 s. Further hemodynamic improvement, associated with symptomatic improvement, was observed at 5 min.

In a larger and more recent study, the hemodynamic effects of ISDN spray were evaluated in eight patients with acute deterioration of chronic congestive heart failure [8]. All cardiovascular drugs were discontinued at least 3 days prior to the study, and a Swan-Ganz catheter was introduced. During hospitalization, the patients developed symptoms and hemodynamic signs of acute deterioration of the chronic condition. They were tachypneic, dyspneic, or orthopneic. One squirt of ISDN spray (equal to 1.25 mg ISDN) produced hemodynamic improvement which became evident in all patients within 1 min and reached a peak within 5.2 min from administration. The drug decreased the pulmonary arterial pressure from $57 \pm 13/29 \pm 10$ mmHg to $40 \pm 7/22 \pm 5$ mmHg and pulmonary capillary wedge pressure from 25 ± 10 mmHg to 17 ± 6 mmHg and increased cardiac index from 2.1 to 3.0 l min^{-1} m^{-2}. Systemic and pulmonary vascular resistances were reduced. All the changes were statistically significant. They were associated with symptomatic relief. The fact that hemodynamic effect was achieved within a period shorter than that required to start an intravenous line indicates that ISDN spray may be beneficial for emergency treatment of acute deterioration in chronic congestive heart failure.

In a recent trial, we compared the magnitude and time course of the hemodynamic effect of a new formulation of an aqueous solution of ISDN spray to those of sublingual NTG tablets in 12 patients with chronic congestive heart failure. The patients received, in a random order, ISDN spray 2.5 mg or sublingual NTG 0.8 mg. Hemodynamic measurements were performed before and at 1, 3, 5, 10, 20, 30, and 60 min after each drug. The second drug was given only after return of the hemodynamic parameters to baseline, plus a washout period of 2 h. The hemodynamic variables measured were comparable at baseline. Both drugs produced hemodynamic improvement, including a decrease in pulmonary capillary wedge pressure (PCWP), right atrial pressure (RAP), and systemic and pulmonary vascular resistances. Only ISDN spray significantly increased cardiac output. The onset of action of ISDN spray was significantly more rapid than that of NTG. This was evident primarily in the decrease in PCWP. With ISDN spray, the decrease started at 1 min after administration, and at 3 min a decrease of 8.6 mmHg was already found. The corresponding value for sublingual NTG was 1.6 mmHG. The difference between ISDN and NTG was highly significant ($p < 0.02$). The peak effect of ISDN spray on PCWP and RAP was greater than that of NTG.

Nitrates can also produce arterial dilation, but this requires moderate to high doses [8–11]. Therefore, it is obvious that nitrates would be especially effective in patients with heart failure whose main hemodynamic impairment is pulmonary congestion, that is, elevated left ventricular filling pressure in the presence of only a minimal decrease in cardiac output. Nevertheless, most studies of nitrates in heart failure have involved mainly patients with both elevated left ventricular filling pressure and reduced cardiac output. In a previous study, we have demonstrated the superiority of ISDN oral spray over sublingual tablets in patients with this combined hemodynamic impairment [10]. However, no report on the comparative effect of these two formulations in patients with predominant pulmonary congestion (where venodilation is the main expected beneficial effect) has been reported.

We compared the time course of the hemodynamic effect of 5 mg ISDN in the forms of sublingual tablet and oral spray in 15 patients with isolated chronic pulmonary congestion (pulmonary arterial end-diastolic pressure of 15 mmHg or more in the presence of normal or only slightly reduced cardiac index). Both formulations produced significant reductions in the pulmonary arterial end-diastolic pressure. The effect of ISDN tablets (sublingually) became evident at 10 min after administration and was maximal at 30 min. The effect of ISDN oral spray became evident at 3 min and reached a peak at 10 min. The magnitude of the hemodynamic responses was similar. These findings indicate that ISDN oral spray is superior to ISDN sublingual tablets for rapid relief of pulmonary congestion.

Nitrate Oral Spray in Angina Pectoris

The same principles that apply to the use of nitrate oral spray in heart failure are also valid for angina pectoris. The antianginal effect of ISDN spray was assessed in patients with exercise-induced angina pectoris in order to determine and quantify its time course. Ten patients (mean age 58.9 ± 6.2 years) were included in the study. All had chronic stable angina pectoris. The length of time to onset of angina and to appearance of a 1.0-mm ST segment depression was determined; the time to disappearance of pain and of ST segment depression after discontinuation of exercise was also measured. ISDN spray delayed the onset of angina and electrocardiographic ischemic changes in all patients. Exercise time to pain was 5.1 ± 1.4 min with placebo and 7.2 ± 1.3 min with ISDN ($p < 0.001$). Time to appearance of ST segment depression was 7.1 ± 1.5 min with placebo and 10.2 ± 1.2 min with ISDN. Time to disappearance of pain after discontinuation of exercise was shortened from 3.2 ± 0.8 min on placebo to 2.1 ± 0.8 min with ISDN ($p < 0.001$). Time to disappearance of ST segment depression was shortened from 4.2 ± 0.6 to 2.5 ± 0.8 min, ($p < 0.005$). Two patients experienced transient headache, and one patient had transient dizziness with slight decrease in blood pressure after ISDN. All patients completed the study without experiencing major adverse effects.

In a recent trial, Bachmann and Gansser (unpublished data) found that the new formulation of the hydrophilic spray of ISDN has been shown to act more rapidly on the coronary arteries than the older lipophilic spray, as evaluated by quantitative coronary angiography.

Conclusion

Nitrate oral spray, and particularly the new formulation of hydrophilic ISDN spray, are the most rapid methods for achieving the therapeutic effect of nitrates in heart failure.

References

1. Armstrong PW, Armstrong JA, Marks GS (1979) Blood level after sublingual nitroglycerin. Circulation 59:585–589
2. Morrison RA, Wiegand UW, Jähnchen DE et al. (1983) Isosorbide dinitrate kinetics and dynamics after intravenous, sublingual, and percutaneous dosing in angina. Clin Pharmacol Ther 33:747–756
3. Doyle E, Chasseaud LF, Taylor T (1980) Measurement of plasma concentrations of isosorbide dinitrate. Biopharm Drug Dispos 1:141–147
4. Robinson BF (1968) Mode of action of nitroglycerin in angina pectoris. Correlation between hemodynamic effects during exercise and prevention of pain. Br Heart J 30:295–302
5. Sandler G, Ilani MA, Lawson CW (1963) Glyceryl trinitrate in angina pectoris. Lancet 1:1130–1136
6. Kattus AA, Alvaro AB, Coulson A (1975) Effectiveness of isosorbide dinitrate and nitroglycerin in relieving angina pectoris during uninterrupted exercise. Chest 67:640–646
7. Detry JR, Bruce RA (1971) Effect of nitroglycerin on "maximal" oxygen intake and exercise electrocardiogram in coronary heart disease. Circulation 43:155–163
8. Schneeweiss A, Marmor A, Plich M, Alpert JS (1987) ISDN spray in congestive heart failure. Am J Cardiol 59(8):848–852
9. Chiche P, Bligadoo S (1979) Nitrates, "pharmacological phlebotomy" and pulmonary edema. Am Heart J 97(3):408
10. Strauer BE, Scherpe A (1978) Ventricular function and coronary hemodynamics after intravenous nitroglycerin in coronary artery disease. Am Heart J 95:210
11. Franciosa JA, Cohn JN (1974) Hemodynamic effects of orally administered isosorbide dinitrate in patients with congestive heart failure. Circulation 50:1020

Improved Left Ventricular Geometry and Function by Prolonged Nitroglycerin Therapy After Acute Myocardial Infarction*

B.I. Jugdutt, B.L. Michorowski, and W.J. Tymchak

Introduction

Early therapy with intravenous nitroglycerin (NG) during acute myocardial infarction reduces infarct expansion experimentally and clinically [1,2]. However, the healing process after myocardial infarction takes place over 6 weeks in the dog model, with early expansion and late thinning [3,4], and even longer in humans [4]. The aim of this study was therefore to test the hypothesis that prolonged reduction of preload and afterload during the healing phase after a first anterior transmural acute myocardial infarction (ATAMI) might further improve left ventricular (LV) geometry and function [5,6].

Methods

The protocol is shown in Fig. 1. A total of 43 consecutive patients admitted to the coronary care unit with a "first" ATAMI were evaluated. Informed consent was obtained if inclusion and exclusion criteria were met. The patients were given low-dose intravenous NG infusion therapy for up to 48 h after onset of typical chest pain of infarction. At 48 h patients were randomized to either buccal NG (group 1) or placebo (group 2) for 6 weeks. During the first 48 h clinical data, electrocardiograms, ST segment maps, hemodynamics, two-dimensional echocardiograms, and data on serial creatine kinase (CK) and CK-MB were obtained. After 48 h clinical data, electrocardiograms and echocardiograms were collected at 2, 4, 6, 8, and 10 days and at 6, 12, and 24 weeks. Further inclusion criteria were age under 75 years, heart rate over 60 beats/min, systolic blood pressure between 110 mmHg and 200 mmHg, sinus rhythm, and no past history or electrocardiographic evidence of infarction. Exclusion criteria included heart block, cardiogenic shock, rheumatic or valvular or congenital heart disease, other contraindications to NG therapy, concomitant use of calcium channel blockers or β-blockers or drugs that might alter parameters being measured after NG.

The dose of intravenous NG infusion was titrated to decrease mean blood pressure by 10% but not below 80 mmHg. The dose of buccal NG (Nitrogard-SR, Syntex) was 1–3 mg three times a day in three divided doses given at 800, 1300,

*Supported in part by a grant from the Canadian Heart Foundation, Ottawa, Ontario, Canada.

B.S. Lewis, A. Kimchi (Eds.)
Heart Failure Mechanisms and Management
© Springer-Verlag Berlin Heidelberg 1991

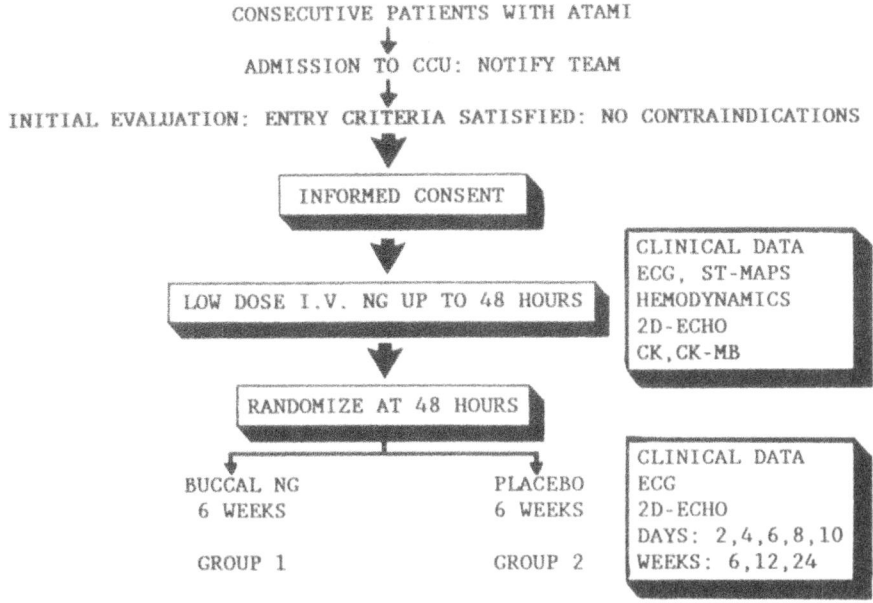

Fig. 1. The protocol. *CK*, Creatine kinase; *CCU*, coronary care unit; *ECG*, electrocardiogram; *2D-ECHO*, two-dimensional echocardiogram

and 1800 hours with an 8-h washout period to avoid vascular tolerance. The initial dose was titrated so that mean blood pressure did not fall by more than 10%. The placebo group received 2 mg nonactive buccal tablets (Syntex).

As described previously [2] and shown in Fig. 2, serial echocardiograms were used to measure: (a) the endocardial surface area of LV asynergy, defined as akinesis plus dyskinesis; (b) LV ejection fraction; and (c) LV geometry (expansion index, thickness ratio, peak regional shape distortion). Expansion index was defined as the ratio of asynergy containing endocardial segment length to normal segment length. The midpoint of the papillary muscles provided landmarks for segment lengths. Thickness ratio was measured as the ratio of thicknesses of middle asynergic and normal zones.

All data were coded, and final analysis was carried out in blinded fashion at the end of the study. Serial data were analyzed using analysis of variance (ANOVA) and multiple-measures ANOVA. Values are expressed as mean ± standard deviation. Statistical significance was assumed at a level of $p < 0.05$.

Results

Baseline Data. All 43 patients entered in the study with a first ATAMI received intravenous NG over the first 48 h. Thereafter, they were randomly allocated to

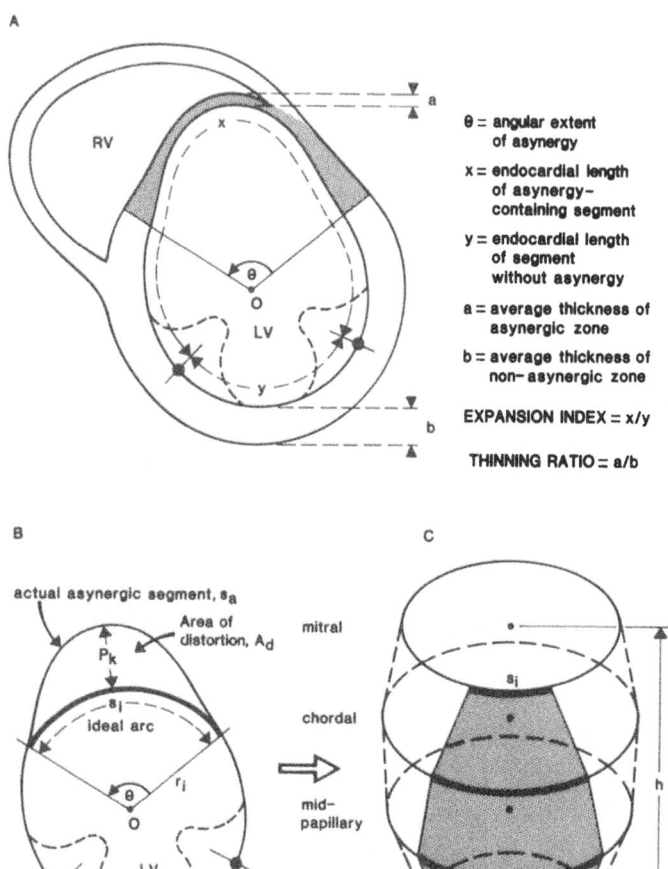

Fig. 2. A Method of calculating expansion index and thinning or thickness ratio. A middle left ventricular (*LV*) section at end-diastole from a patient with anterior infarction; asynergy and regional shape distortion are shown. LV segment lengths were measured from the midpoints of papillary muscle landmarks. *RV*, right ventricle. **B** Method of quantifying regional shape distortion on the endocardial outline of a middle papillary left ventricular section at end-diastole. The center (*O*) of the ideal circle and radius were computed using points from the nonasynergic segment. The angular extent of asynergy (*θ*) was measured and the ideal arc of asynergy (*S_i*) computed using the nonasynertic segment and center (*O*), thus replacing the actual distorted asynergic segment (*S_a*). The areas of the regional shape distortion (*A_d*) and the ideal section (*A_i*) were measured. Peak distortion (*P_k*) was computed from the angular distribution of the average distances, within 5° windows, between pairs of corresponding points at intersections of radials with actual and ideal segments, respectively. **C** Total left ventricular asynergy (*stippled area*) was computed as percentage surface area of the endocardial shell constructed from the four short-axis sections and height (*h*) derived from the average long-axis length of the apical four- and two-chamber views

buccal NG ($n = 23$, group 1) or buccal placebo ($n = 20$; group 2). The baseline data for the two groups were similar in terms of sex (78% versus 85% men), age (61 versus 57 years), body surface area (1.9 versus 1.9 m²), interval from chest pain to admission (13 versus 13 h), interval from chest pain to NG infusion (15 versus 15 h); average NG dose (71 versus 77 µg/min), interval from admission to the first echocardiogram (24 versus 23 h), and admission Killip class score (1.3 versus 1.4). At 2 days, there was no difference between the two groups in blood pressure (systolic 111 versus 115 mmHg; diastolic 74 versus 74 mmHg; mean 87 versus 88 mmHg), heart rate (84 versus 87 beats/min), heart rate × mean blood pressure (7.6 versus 8.0 mmHg × beats/min × 10^3), or Killip class score (1.3 versus 1.4). Also, there was no difference between the two groups in peak CK (2583 versus 2174 IU/l) or CK infarct size (52 versus 46 gEq).

Clinical Follow-up. At 24 weeks, the functional class score (New York Heart Association) was less in the NG than placebo group (1.3 ± 0.4 versus 1.8 ± 0.6; $p < 0.005$). There were also fewer deaths at 24 weeks in the NG group, but the difference was not statistically significant (0/23 versus 3/20). There was no statistically significant difference in resting hemodynamics for the two groups at 2 days, 10 days, 6 weeks, 12 weeks, or 24 weeks.

Effect on LV Function. Asynergy decreased similarly between admission and 48 h with intravenous NG in the two groups. Thus, total regional LV asynergy in the two groups was similar initially and after randomization at 2 days. However, total LV asynergy was persistently lower in the buccal NG group compared to placebo at 6 weeks (14% versus 21%; $p < 0.05$) and after buccal NG was discontinued, at 12 and 24 weeks. LV ejection fraction, computed by the modified Simpson's rule, in the two groups was similar initially and at 2 days but was higher in the buccal NG group compared to placebo at 6, 12, and 24 weeks; at 24 weeks the mean values were 51% versus 40% ($p \leq 0.05$, by multiple-measures ANOVA).

Effect on LV Geometry. Figure 3 shows the increase in the expansion index after randomization in the placebo group, but this did not change in the buccal NG group. This divergence was significant at 6 weeks and persisted at 12 and 24 weeks ($p \leq 0.05$). Similarly, the thickness ratio was persistently unchanged in the buccal NG group but decreased in the placebo group, the divergence being significant at 6, 12, and 24 weeks ($p \leq 0.05$). Figure 4 shows the effect on LV volume normalized to body surface area. There was no significant change after randomization in the buccal NG group but a persistent increase in the placebo group. This divergence was statistically significant ($p \leq 0.05$) at 6, 12, and 24 weeks. A similar effect of NG was seen on normalized LV diameters at the different short-axis levels and on the peak regional shape distortion.

Summary

The results of this study indicate that prolonged NG therapy after a first ATAMI decreased LV volume, decreased infarct expansion, decreased infarct thinning,

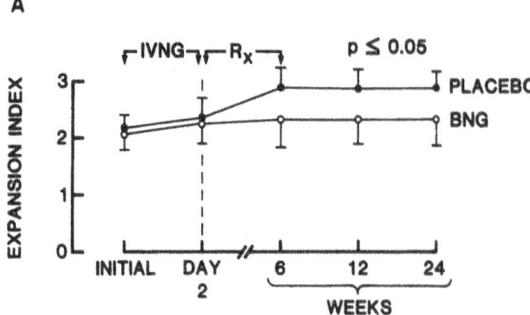

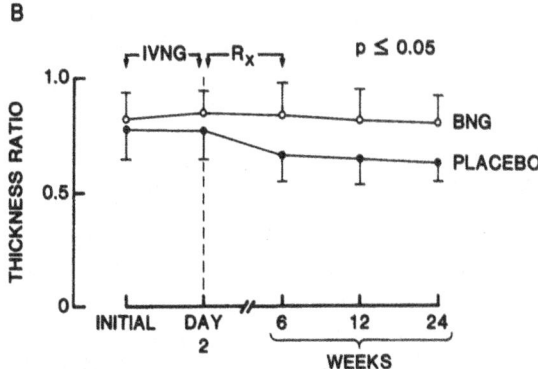

Fig. 3. Effect of treatment on infarct expansion (**A**) and thinning (**B**) IV NG, Intravenous nitroglycerin; BNG, buccal nitroglycerin

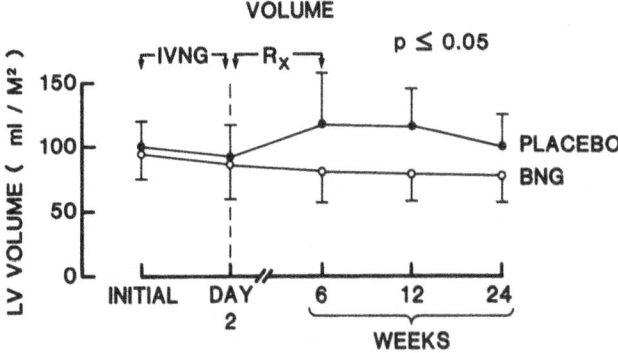

Fig. 4. Effect of treatment on LV volume. Abbreviations as in Fig. 3

decreased LV asynergy, and increased LV ejection fraction. Prolonged NG therapy during early and late phases of healing after ATAMI preserves LV topography and function. These beneficial effects on early and late remodeling with prolonged NG therapy might prevent LV aneurysm formation. The most likely mechanisms include prolonged reduction of preload, afterload, LV volume, and LV wall stress.

References

1. Jugdutt BI (1985) Delayed effects of early infarct-limiting therapies on healing after myocardial infarction. Circulation 72:907–914
2. Jugdutt BI, Warnica JW (1988) Intravenous nitroglycerin therapy to limit myocardial infarct size, expansion and complications: effect of timing, dosage and infarct location. Circulation 78:906–910
3. Jugdutt BI, Amy RW (1986) Healing after myocardial infarction in the dog: changes in infarct hydroxyproline and topography. J Am Coll Cardiol 7:91–102
4. Jugdutt BI (1987) Left ventricular rupture threshold during healing after myocardial infarction in the dog. Can J Physiol Pharmacol 65:307–316
5. Michorowski BL, Tymchak WT, Jugdutt BI (1987) Improved left ventricular function and topography by prolonged nitroglycerin therapy after acute myocardial infarction (abstract). Circulation 76 [Suppl]:IV–128
6. Jugdutt BI, Michorowski BL, Tymchak WJ (1989) Improved left ventricular function and topography by prolonged nitroglycerin therapy after acute myocardial infarction. Z Kardiol [Suppl 3]78:(in press)

Hemodynamic Effects of a Subchronic Therapy with 120 mg Isosorbide Dinitrate Slow-Release in Coronary Artery Disease and Left Heart Failure

R. Wolf, A. Nötges, U. Traber, and R. Sinn

The hemodynamic effects of nitrates in patients with left ventricular dysfunction and both acute and chronic heart failure are well documented [1,12]. However, the development of hemodynamic tolerance during long-term treatment with oral nitrates remains a subject of debate [6,7]. This has two clinically important implications [2–4]:

1. Cardiac unloading by long-acting nitrates would increase exercise tolerance.
2. The progression of the degree of heart failure would be prevented or delayed.

Thus, we investigated the hemodynamic effect of a subchronic (3-week) treatment with 120 mg isosorbide dinitrate (ISDN) in slow-release (SR) form in patients with mild or moderate chronic left heart failure after myocardial infarction. In a subgroup of patients hemodynamic measurements were performed after a 1-year treatment with 120 mg ISDN SR.

Patients and Methods

Eighteen patients (13 male; age: range 48–73, mean 62.2 years) with proven myocardial infarction in the chronic stage were investigated. All patients were in a stable clinical condition with symptoms of chronic left heart failure in NYHA functional class II-III. No patient showed signs of persistent post-infarction ischemia, and there was no indication for bypass grafting or percutaneous transluminal coronary angioplasty by angiographic and nuclear studies in any case.

After Swan-Ganz catheterization, the hemodynamics were measured at rest and during symptom-limited exercise by supine bicycle ergometry before, 2 and 10 h after intake of lx 120 mg ISDN SR orally. In 16 patients hemodynamic measurements were performed after a 3-week therapy with 120 mg ISDN per day using an identical exercise protocol.

No patient received long-term nitrates or vasodilators within 10 days before both hemodynamic investigations; basic drug therapy was unchanged.

Diuretics were given at the end of each investigation when indicated. In six of 16 patients hemodynamic measurements could be performed after a 1-year treatment with 120 mg ISDN SR.

B.S. Lewis, A. Kimchi (Eds.)
Heart Failure Mechanisms and Management
© Springer-Verlag Berlin Heidelberg 1991

Results

Left Ventricular Filling Pressure at Rest

Before the subchronic treatment was initiated, ISDN significantly reduced left ventricular filling pressure (LVFP = mean capillary wedge pressure) from 18.9 ± 8.1 to 12.1 ± 5.9 and 12.2 ± 4.6 mmHg 2 and 10 h after intake, respectively ($p < 0.0005$). After a 3-week therapy a decrease of LVFP from 20.6 ± 8.9 before ISDN to 11.7 ± 5.8 and 13.0 ± 3.8 mmHg after application was observed ($p < 0.025$) (Fig. 1).

LVFP During Exercise

Mean exercise capacity was 52 ± 25 watt. LVFP increased to 31.2 ± 10.5 mmHg and was significantly reduced to 19.0 ± 10.1 and 23.5 ± 11.0 mmHg 2 and 10 h after 120 mg ISDN SR, respectively ($p < 0.25$). LVFP 2 h after intake was significantly decreased compared to LVFP 10 h after ISDN ($p < 0.05$). After 3 weeks LVFP significantly decreased from 33.1 ± 14.4 mmHg to 20.5 ± 10.4 and

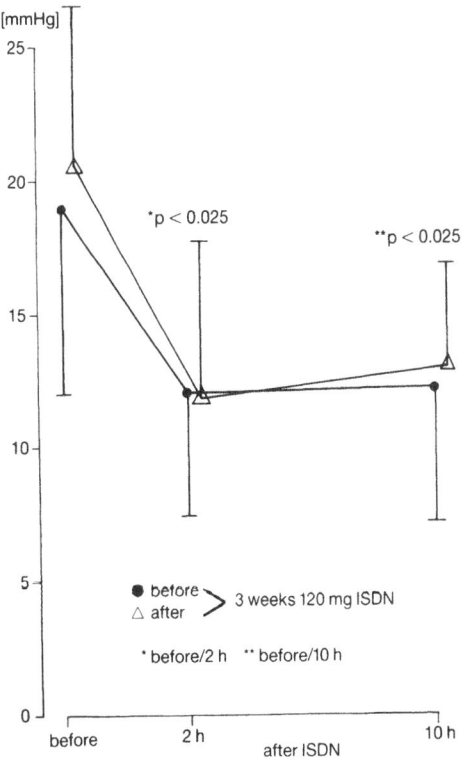

Fig. 1. LVFP at rest before (*circles*) and after (*triangles*) a subchronic (3-week) therapy with 120 mg ISDN SR

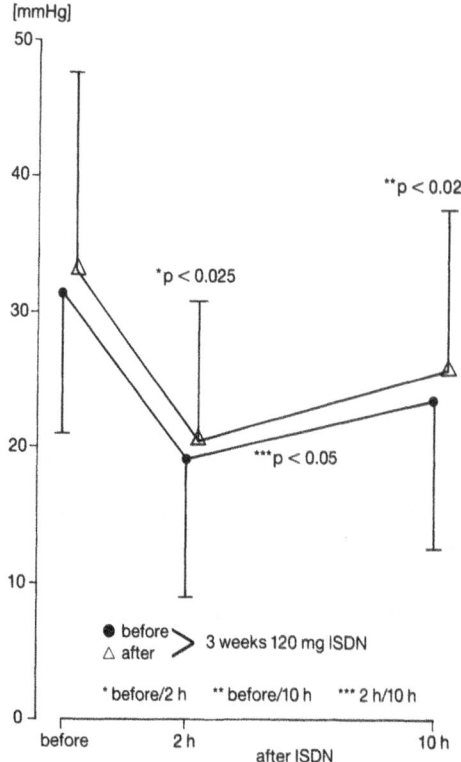

Fig. 2. LVFP during exercise before (*circles*) and after (*triangles*) a subchronic (3-week) therapy with 120 mg ISDN SR

25.8 ± 11.7 mmHg 2 and 10 h after ISDN, respectively ($p < 0.0025$). LVFP 10 h after ISDN was significantly increased compared to 2 h after intake ($p < 0.05$) (Fig. 2).

Mean Pulmonary Artery Pressure at Rest

Before subchronic therapy was initiated, ISDN significantly decreased mean pulmonary artery pressure (MPAP) from 29.4 ± 11.1 to 20.6 ± 6.5 and 21.2 ± 5.5 mmHg 2 and 10 h after application, respectively ($p < 0.0005$). After 3 weeks a significant reduction of MPAP from 31.4 ± 11.4 mmHg before ISDN to 21.7 ± 6.5 and 23.3 ± 4.8 mmHg after intake was registered ($p < 0.0025$) (Fig. 3).

MPAP During Exercise

MPAP increased to 46.8 ± 12.9 mmHg and was significantly reduced to 32.7 ± 12.7 and 39.4 ± 11.6 mmHg 2 and 10 h after 120 mg ISDN SR, respectively ($p < 0.0005$). MPAP 10 h after intake was significantly increased compared to 2 h after ISDN ($p < 0.05$). After a 3-week treatment MPAP was significantly reduced by ISDN from 53.3 ± 19.9 mmHg to 39.2 ± 15.5 and 46.0 ± 18.6 mmHg

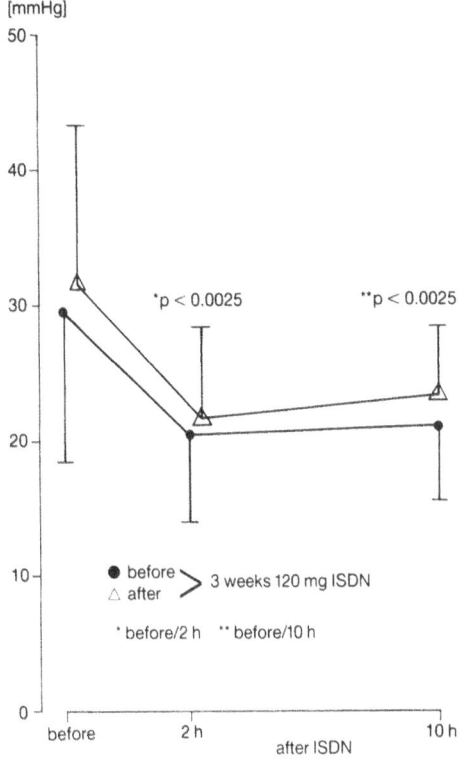

[mmHg]

Fig. 3. MPAP at rest before (*circles*) and after (*triangles*) a subchronic (3-week) therapy with 120 mg ISDN SR

2 and 10 h after intake, respectively ($p < 0.0005$). Ten hours after ISDN application MPAP significantly increased compared to 2 h after intake ($p < 0.05$) (Fig. 4).

Cardiac Output and Heart Rate at Rest and During Exercise

Figure 5 demonstrates that the reduction of LVFP by ISDN was not associated with significant changes of cardiac index both at rest and during exercise. However, the relationship between LVFP and cardiac index can be expressed by two log functional curves. This indicates "optimal" LV filling pressures at rest and during exercise. No significant changes of heart rate at rest and during exercise were observed both before and after a 3-week treatment (Table 1).

LVFP During Exercise after 1-Year Treatment with 120 mg ISDN SR

In six patients ISDN markedly reduced LVFP from 38.7 ± 14.6 mmHg to 27.0 ± 7.0 and 32.1 ± 7.0 mmHg after 2 and 10 h, respectively, after 1 year. This decrease was comparable to LVFP reduction before long-term treatment was initiated (Table 2).

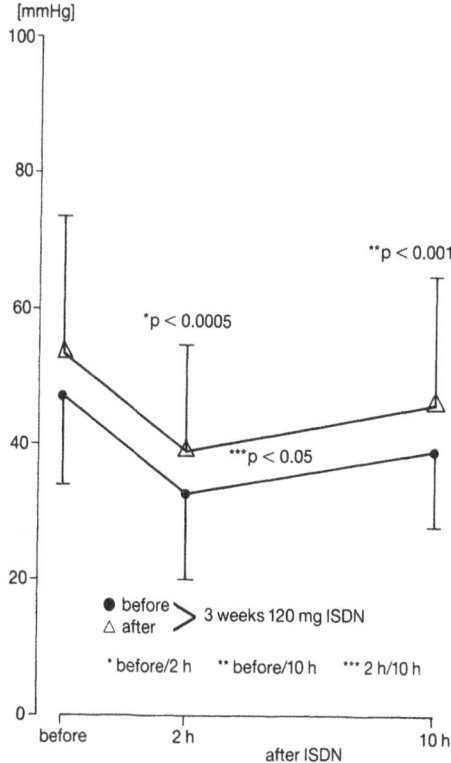

Fig. 4. MPAP during exercise before (*circles*) and after (*triangles*) a subchronic (3-week) therapy with ISDN SR

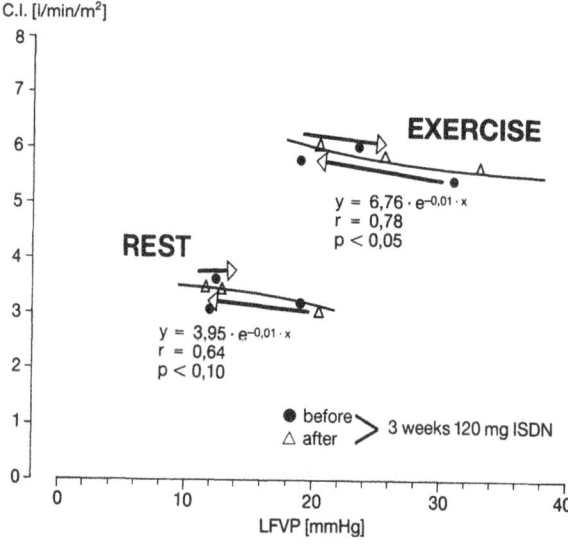

Fig. 5. Cardiac index and LVFP at rest and during exercise before (*circles*) and after (*triangles*) a subchronic (3-week) therapy with ISDN SR. *Arrows* indicate changes of the control values before ISDN intake 2 and 10 hours after ISDN. For all variables log functional curves can be calculated

Table 1. Heart rate before and after a subchronic (3-week) therapy with 120 mg ISDN SR

		Before	After 3 weeks
Rest	Before	70.7 ± 14.7	68.0 ± 12.8
	2 h after ISDN	73.1 ± 12.5	71.4 ± 12.8
	10 h after ISDN	73.3 ± 12.3	73.1 ± 11.8
Exercise	Before	115.6 ± 16.0	112.1 ± 14.3
	2 h after ISDN	111.1 ± 15.1	110.1 ± 12.5
	10 h after ISDN	115.4 ± 17.0	115.9 ± 15.5

Table 2. LVFP during exercise before and after 1-year treatment with 120 mg ISDN SR ($n = 6$)

	Before	After 1 year
Before ISDN	39.3 ± 11.0	38.7 ± 14.6
2 h after ISDN	29.7 ± 13.5	27.0 ± 7.0
10 h after ISDN	33.0 ± 11.8	32.1 ± 7.0

Discussion

Progression of LV dilatation and of the clinical syndrome of congestive heart failure provides important prognostic relevance [10,11]. Both the combination of vasodilators and ISDN and the treatment with angiotensin-converting enzyme inhibitors in patients with congestive heart failure could improve LV function, exercise tolerance, and prognosis [2-5,11). The results presented indicate that a chronic preload reduction at rest and during exercise by ISDN may represent the hemodynamic mechanism for improving LV dysfunction. Cardiac unloading by 120 mg ISDN in SR form could be documented over 10 h after intake and was reproducible after a 1-year treatment in a smaller subgroup. The vasodilating effect of nitrates with increasing arterial compliance and venous capacitance in mild heart failure might be preferable to a long-term treatment with diuretics [1,4,8,9]. In conclusion, our results indicate that there is no significant evidence for the development of nitrates tolerance or reflex sympathetic activity using this treatment regimen in chronic left heart failure.

References

1. Abrams J (1985) Hemodynamic effects of nitroglycerin and long-acting nitrates. Am Heart J 110:216–224
2. Cohn JN, Archibald DG, Ziesche S et al. (1986) Effect of vasodilator therapy on mortality in chronic congestive heart failure. N Engl J Med 314:1547–1552
3. Cohn JN, Archibald DG, Francis GS et al. (1987) Veterans administration cooperative study on vasodilator therapy of heart failure: influence of prerandomization variables on the reduction of mortality by treatment with hydralazine and isosorbide dinitrate. Circulation 75 IV:49–54
4. Cohn JN (1987) Role of nitrates in congestive heart failure. Am J Cardiol 60:39–43
5. The Consensus Trial Study Group (1987) Effects of enalapril on mortality in severe congestive heart failure. N Engl J Med 316:1429–1435
6. Franciosa JA, Cohn JN (1980) Sustained hemodynamic effects without tolerance during long-term isosorbide dinitrate treatment of chronic left ventricular failure. Am J Cardiol 45:648–654
7. Kulick D, Roth A, McIntosh N, Rahimtoola SH, Elkayam U (1988) Resistance to isosorbide dinitrate in patients with severe chronic heart failure: incidence and attempt at hemodynamic prediction. J Am Coll Cardiol 12:1023–1028
8. Nelson GI, Silke B, Ahuja RC, Hussain M, Taylor SH (1983) Hemodynamic advantages of isosorbide dinitrate over frusemide in acute heart-failure following myocardial infarction. Lancet 1:730–733
9. Nelson GI, Silke B, Forsyth DR, Verma SP, Hussain M, Taylor SH (1983) Hemodynamic comparison of primary venous or arteriolar dilatation and the subsequent effect of furosemide in left ventricular failure after acute myocardial infarction. Am J Cardiol 52:1036–1040
10. Pfeffer MA, Lamas GA, Vaughan DE, Parisi AF, Braunwald E (1988) Effect of captopril on progressive ventricular dilatation after anterior myocardial infarction. N Engl J Med 319:80–86
11. Pfeffer MA, Pfeffer JM (1987) Ventricular enlargement and reduced survival after myocardial infarction. Circulation 75 (Suppl IV):93–97
12. Williams DO, Bommer WF, Miller RR, Amsterdam EA, Mason DT (1977) Hemodynamic assessment of oral peripheral vasodilator therapy in chronic congestive heart failure: prolonged effectiveness of isosorbide dinitrate. Am J Cardiol 39:84–90

Calcium Antagonists

Calcium Antagonists in the Management of Heart Failure

A. KIMCHI and B.S. LEWIS

Introduction

Calcium channel blocking drugs produce several direct cardiovascular effects: (a) peripheral vasodilatation, due to smooth muscle relaxation; (b) coronary dilatation, which increases coronary blood flow and in patients with myocardial ischemia may improve ventricular function following the relief of reversible regional myocardial asynergy; (c) decreased myocardial contractility and reduced left ventricular (LV) function; and (d) depression of the specialized conduction tissue, causing sinus bradycardia and atrioventricular conduction delay. Since calcium channel blockers reduce vascular tone, they offer promise as vasodilators in the management of heart failure [1–7]. However, their negative inotropic effect, although usually counterbalanced by sympathetic stimulation in patients with normal or moderate LV function, presents a real problem in their use, since in certain patients with severe congestive heart failure such compensation may be impaired due to attenuation of the baroreceptor response, an already abnormally high level of circulating catecholamines, and a limited cardiac reserve.

Clinical Experience with First-Generation Calcium Antagonists in Heart Failure

A number of clinical studies have evaluated the hemodynamic effects of the first-generation calcium antagonists verapamil, diltiazem, and nifedipine in patients with congestive heart failure.

Verapamil

Of the calcium antagonists in common use, verapamil exerts the strongest negative inotropic effect clinically, and should be avoided if possible in patients with ventricular dysfunction [8], although it has been shown that intravenous verapamil may lower systemic vascular resistance in certain patients with heart failure and improve indexes of LV performance [9]. The severity of the underlying state of ventricular dysfunction may influence these effects [10]. In 22 patients who

B.S. Lewis, A. Kimchi (Eds.)
Heart Failure Mechanisms and Management
© Springer-Verlag Berlin Heidelberg 1991

had a wedge pressure of less than 18 mmHg, intravenous verapamil (0.145 mg kg^{-1} bolus followed by 0.005 mg kg^{-1}, min^{-1} reduced mean arterial pressure and systemic vascular resistance, while cardiac and stroke index increased. In contrast, in patients with a mean capillary wedge pressure above 18 mmHg, administration of verapamil was associated with hemodynamic deterioration manifested by a decrease of both stroke work index and cardiac index, an abrupt increase in wedge pressure, and clinical evidence of heart failure and dyspnea.

Comparison of verapamil with nifedipine in hypertensive patients with heart failure [11] showed that nifedipine persistently reduced systemic vascular resistance, mean arterial pressure, mean pulmonary wedge pressure, and LV diastolic diameter. Verapamil reduced systemic vascular resistance and mean arterial pressure but was not effective with regard to the wedge pressure or LV diastolic diameter.

Because of its effects on the specialized conducting pathways, verapamil is an effective anti-arrhythmic drug and may have potential benefit in patients in whom heart failure is associated with supraventricular tachyarrhythmia. This, however, was not the case in three infants with supraventricular tachycardia and congestive heart failure given verapamil intravenously [12]. Thus, when verapamil is needed for the rapid control of supraventricular arrhythmia in patients with compromised LV function, it is best given with calcium pretreatment [13].

The unloading vasodilating effect of verapamil may be insufficient to offset its intrinsic depression of LV contractility. In addition, the depressive effect of verapamil on sinus node automaticity and atrioventricular nodal conduction may blunt the baroreceptor-induced sympathetic reflex mechanism which would help maintain cardiac output during vasodilatation in patients with depressed LV function.

Diltiazem

Walsh et al. [14] studied the hemodynamic effects of intravenous diltiazem in eight patients with advanced congestive heart failure. Diltiazem (100 to 200 µg kg^{-1} min^{-1} over 40 min) increased stroke index by 50% and cardiac index by 20%. Heart rate decreased by 23%, mean arterial pressure by 18%, and wedge pressure by 34%. Oral diltiazem (90–120 mg, every 8 h for 24 h) produced similar hemodynamic effects in seven patients.

Marked slowing of the heart rate (from 68 ± 12 to 55 ± 9 beats/min) was confirmed [15] in eight patients with coronary disease and impaired LV function who received diltiazem (0.5 mg kg^{-1}) intravenously. Mean aortic pressure and systemic vascular resistance decreased, whereas pulmonary vascular resistance showed no change. End-systolic volume diminished, in keeping with the increase in stroke volume and ejection fraction.

In a comparative study [16] both diltiazem (90 mg) and nifedipine (20 mg) were found to produce small increases in stroke index with little change in LV filling pressure, but stroke work index decreased only with nifedipine. On the other hand, heart rate decreased with diltiazem but not with nifedipine. Despite a possible lesser negative inotropic effect, diltiazem has been associated with clinical deterioration in patients with heart failure [17,18], usually in association with a pronounced fall in heart rate or the appearance of transient junctional arrhythmias [17].

Nifedipine

The most extensively studied calcium channel blocking drug in patients with congestive heart failure has been nifedipine [19–42]. Because of its potent peripheral vasodilator effect, it was initially accepted with enthusiasm in the treatment of patients with LV dysfunction. In contrast to verapamil, the vasodilator effect of nifedipine induces reflex sympathetic mechanisms which maintain or increase the cardiac output, and there is little direct effect on heart rate to limit this response. Sublingual nifedipine was effective in acute pulmonary edema [19] with a fall in systemic vascular resistance, systemic arterial pressure, an increase in stroke volume and cardiac output, and a fall in pulmonary capillary wedge pressure. A larger dose of nifedipine (20 mg sublingually) produced a significant increase in cardiac index [20], associated with a fall in mean arterial pressure, systemic vascular resistance, and LV end-diastolic pressure. A similar dose of nifedipine improved cardiac performance in eight patients with mild to moderate heart failure [22]. Pulmonary arterial pressure and pulmonary vascular resistance were not altered in this study.

A detailed analysis of both systolic and diastolic measurements of LV function [27] examined the effects of nifedipine in relation to baseline measurements of LV function in 32 patients. Although nifedipine decreased systemic vascular resistance in all patients, the most striking decreases occurred in patients who had dilated ventricles (end-diastolic volume greater than 90 ml m^{-2}) and impaired baseline LV function. In these patients, the decrease in systemic and pulmonary vascular resistance was associated with an increase in cardiac index of 25%, compared to a negligible change in patients with a normal LV end-diastolic dimension. In patients with increased initial end-diastolic volumes there was a downward shift of the diastolic pressure-volume curve, but this may have been the consequence of a decrease in external ventricular constraint since indexes of LV relaxation and compliance did not change significantly.

Following the initial enthusiasm regarding the role of nifedipine in patients with heart failure, several reports appeared describing patients in whom nifedipine produced severe hemodynamic and clinical deterioration [21,23,26]. Elkayam et al. [38] found that in 6 of 31 patients with severe chronic congestive heart failure, administration of the drug resulted in significant hemodynamic deterioration. Nifedipine caused a smaller increase in cardiac index than nitroprusside [31], although the decrease in mean blood pressure was greater with nifedipine. Hydralazine too [32] appeared better than nifedipine as an afterload-reducing drug in patients with severe heart failure.

Second-Generation Calcium Antagonist Drugs

The second-generation calcium antagonists were developed to provide drugs which have a more potent vasodilator effect (both coronary and peripheral), with a lesser effect on myocardial contractility.

Nisoldipine

Nisoldipine is a second-generation calcium channel blocking agent of the 1-4-dihydropyridine family [43] and is four to ten times more potent than nifedipine as a calcium antagonist in vascular smooth muscle. However, in isolated heart preparations, nisoldipine is only equipotent to, or even less potent than nifedipine in its negative inotropic effect. Nisoldipine has relative specificity for dilatation of the coronary vascular bed and little effect on heart rate [43-52]. These characteristics suggest that the drug may prove superior to other calcium channel blockers in the treatment of patients with LV dysfunction.

To determine the effects of nisoldipine in patients with severe LV dysfunction, Kimchi et al. studied the hemodynamic changes after oral nisoldipine in 14 patients (mean age 72 years) with severe congestive heart failure [53]; in terms of the New York Heart Association classification, 3 patients were of class 3 and 11 of class 4. Baseline hemodynamics included a mean LV ejection fraction of 26% $\pm$ 14%, cardiac index of 1.98 $\pm$ 0.34 l min^{-1} m^{-2}, and wedge pressure of 26 $\pm$ 8 mmHg. Control hemodynamic measurements and radionuclide ventriculography were obtained after heart rate, blood pressure, wedge pressure, and cardiac output had been stable for at least 1 h. An oral dose of nisoldipine (5, 10, or 20 mg in double-blind fashion) was administered according to random assignment, and hemodynamic measurements were repeated at 30 min and at 1, 2, 3, 4, 5, 6, 7, and 8 h thereafter. Radionuclide imaging was repeated 2 and 3 h following nisoldipine administration. Figure 1 illustrates the temporal hemodynamic changes, over the entire study period, for four selected patients who showed a salutary hemodynamic response after administration of nisoldipine. The increase in cardiac index in these patients was associated with a drop in arterial pressure and decrease in pulmonary capillary wedge pressure. The peak systemic hemodynamic effect of nisoldipine (maximal fall in systemic vascular resistance) varied in its time of onset in each individual patient, occurring on the average 2.8 $\pm$ 1.6 h after the administration of the drug. Because of this wide individual variation, the hemodynamic changes produced by the drug were analyzed in each patient at the time of the peak effect on systemic vascular resistance (Table 1). At this time, there was a significant decrease in mean arterial pressure, wedge pressure, and mean pulmonary arterial pressure. As a result of the increase in stroke index, cardiac index increased from 2.0 $\pm$ 0.3 to 2.6 $\pm$ 0.6 l min^{-1} m^{-2}. LV ejection fraction increased from 26% $\pm$ 14% to 29% $\pm$ 15%.

Acute administration of nisoldipine may therefore be efficacious in certain patients with chronic congestive heart failure. Improved LV function with nisoldipine may be associated with a reduction in mean pulmonary capillary

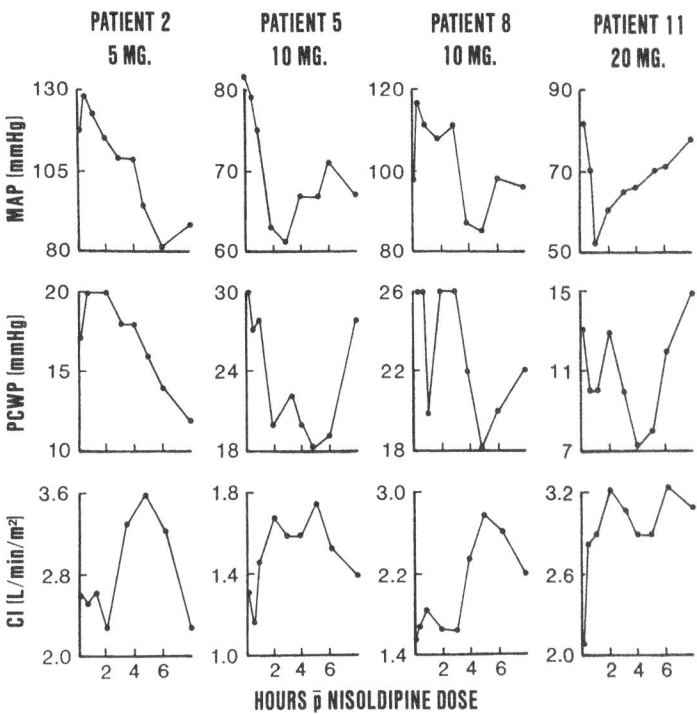

Fig. 1. Effect of nisoldipine on mean arterial pressure (*MAP*), mean pulmonary capillary wedge pressure (*PCWP*), and cardiac index (*CI*), for four selected individual patients who showed a salutary hemodynamic response after nisoldipine administration. (From [53])

Table 1. Peak hemodynamic effects of nisoldipine. (Adapted from [53])

	HR	MAP	RAP	PAP	PCW	SVR	LVEF	CI	SI
Control	82	89	10	35	26	1921	26	2.0	25
	±13	±14	± 5	±10	± 8	± 425	±14	±0.3	± 6
Nisoldipine	79	74[b]	9	31[a]	21[b]	1243[b]	29[b]	2.6[b]	34[b]
	±11	±12	± 4	± 7	± 6	± 320	±15	±0.6	± 8

HR, heart rate (bpm); *MAP*, mean arterial pressure (mmHg); *RAP*, mean right atrial pressure (mmHg); *PAP*, mean pulmonary arterial pressure (mmHg); *PCW*, mean pulmonary capillary wedge pressure (mmHg); *SVR*, systemic vascular resistance (dyne s^1 cm^{-5}); *LVEF*, left ventricular ejection fraction (%), *CI*, cardiac index (l min^{-1} m^{-2}); *SI*, stroke index (ml m^{-2}). Values are mean ±1 SD.
[a] $p < 0.05$.
[b] $p < 0.01$.

wedge pressure and measurements related to afterload. Similar results were obtained by other investigators. Klepzig and Strauer[54] showed that intravenous nisoldipine (6 µg kg^{-1}) in 15 patients with class III heart failure resulted in pronounced afterload reduction with improvement of the cardiac and stroke index. Kiowski et al. [55] studied the effects of nisoldipine in 14 patients with chronic congestive heart failure at rest and during submaximal exercise before and after 3 μg kg^{-1} intravenous nisoldipine and after 4 weeks of oral nisoldipine (20 mg bid). Systemic vascular resistance decreased both at rest and during exercise, while stroke volume and ejection fraction increased. Schmidt et al. [56] studied the hemodynamic effects of nisoldipine in ten patients with acute cardiac failure after myocardial infarction. In all ten patients there was a significant fall in aortic pressure and total peripheral resistance 1 h after injection, while cardiac and stroke index increased. No side-effects were observed.

Nienaber et al. [57] compared the acute hemodynamic effects of nisoldipine and nifedipine in six patients with congestive heart failure and found that at doses titrated to produce a similar 20% decrease in systemic vascular resistance (0.2 μg kg^{-1} min^{-1} for nisoldipine and 0.6 μg kg^{-1} min^{-1} for nifedipine), nisoldipine produced a significantly greater increase in cardiac index than nifedipine (24% ± 14% versus 10% ± 6%). Nisoldipine was also associated with a greater decrease in wedge pressure (23% ± 18% versus 10% ± 21%) and in pulmonary vascular resistance (21% ± 9% versus 6% ± 20%). Importantly, LV ejection fraction increased with nisoldipine (+ 16 ± 8%) but was unchanged with nifedipine (+ 1 ± 9%). This suggested that the myocardial depressant effect of nisoldipine was less than that of nifedipine in patients with congestive heart failure. However, hemodynamic deterioration may occur with nisoldipine in patients who have an initial severe hemodynamic and neuroendocrine abnormality [58], and renin release is potentiated.

The effect of nisoldipine on LV function and contractility [59] was studied by Lewis et al. in nine patients with moderate to severe ischemic heart failure and a baseline resting LV ejection fraction of less than 40%. Patients with angina pectoris or with evidence of reversible ischemia on exercise treadmill testing were excluded from the study, since a beneficial effect of nisoldipine on reversible ischemia would alter and improve regional and global ventricular function and would make the mechanism of action of the calcium channel blocking drug on hemodynamics and myocardial contractility difficult to interpret. Ventricular loading conditions were altered by sublingual nitroglycerin to facilitate construction of LV pressure-volume and LV stress-shortening curves for assessment of LV contractility. Nisoldipine (0.12 μg kg^{-1} min^{-1} intravenously) decreased mean arterial pressure and systemic vascular resistance by 18%, while heart rate was essentially unchanged. Cardiac and stroke index increased in seven of the nine patients. Ejection fraction was 21% ± 8% in the control state and increased to 24% ± 9% during administration of nisoldipine.

Examination of the LV end-systolic pressure-volume relation (Fig. 2) showed that in the control state the curve was located far to the right of normal with large LV end-systolic volumes at rather low end-systolic pressures, indicating depressed LV contractility. During administration of nisoldipine, there was a small downward shift of the curve, implying some decrease in LV contractility. On the other hand, the stress-shortening relation (Fig. 3) showed that during treatment with nisoldipine, the curve passed through the control points, suggesting that contractility was essentially unaltered by the drug.

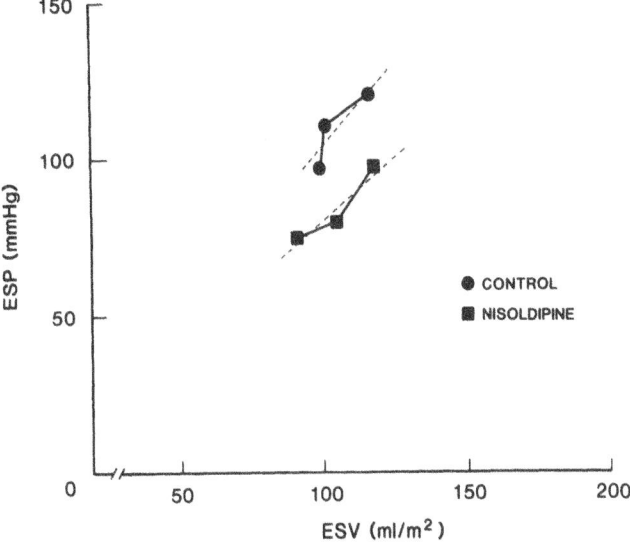

Fig. 2. Left ventricular end-systolic pressure (*ESP*) – volume (*ESV*) relationship before (control) and during infusion of nisoldipine in seven patients. Both curves are displaced far to the right, indicating decreased ventricular function. With nisoldipine the curve is displaced slightly downwards. (From [59])

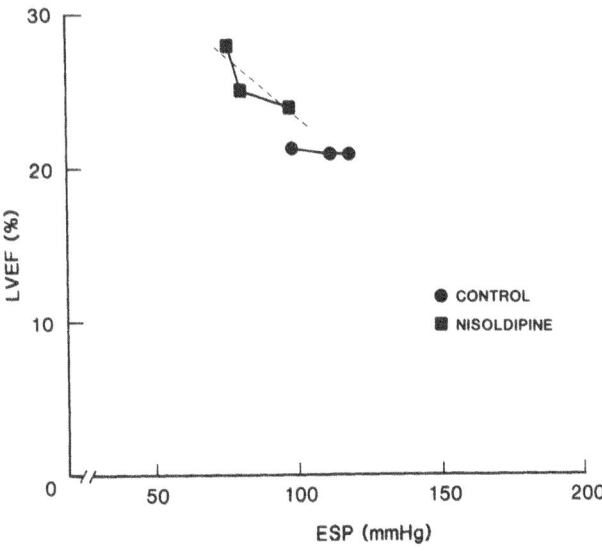

Fig. 3. Left ventricular end-systolic pressure (*ESP*) – shortening (*LVEF*) relationship in seven patients in the control state and during infusion of nisoldipine. The curve with nisoldipine passes through the control data points, indicating no change in ventricular inotropic state. (From [59])

Other Newer Calcium Antagonists

Several newer calcium antagonists, many apparently having a very high selectivity ratio for vascular as opposed to myocardial effects, have now been evaluated in patients with congestive heart failure. Studies with nitrendipine [60], nicardipine [61,62], felodipine [63–67], and PN 200-110 [68] have all demonstrated an acute beneficial hemodynamic effect in patients with heart failure.

Clinical Implications and Future Directions

At present the first-line therapy of congestive heart failure appears to consist of treatment with diuretics and vasodilators such as nitrates hydralazine or angiotensin-converting enzyme inhibitors, which may prolong life in patients with severe ventricular dysfunction [69,70]. However, in patients in whom LV dysfunction may be associated with myocardial ischemia or hypertension, the newer calcium antagonists and their potent coronary vasodilator effect may be useful. Calcium antagonists may also have a role in patients with diastolic LV dysfunction, such as hypertrophic cardiomyopathy, and in selected patients with pulmonary hypertension. Patients with cardiac failure and supraventricular tachyarrhythmia may benefit from calcium channel blockers (such as verapamil or diltiazem) which control the ventricular rate and improve cardiac output. Since the early administration of calcium antagonists may alter the progression of some forms of heart failure [71], calcium antagonists may have a role in the management of certain patients with lesser degrees of ventricular dysfunction (New York Heart Association classes 1 and 2).

In summary, despite the potential beneficial effects of calcium antagonists, there is a continued plea for caution regarding the use of these agents in patients. Although some patients with congestive heart failure may benefit from both the short- and long-term administration of these medications, in other studies hemodynamic deterioration may occur, particularly in those patients with an initially severe hemodynamic and neuroendocrine abnormality and in those who receive relatively large doses of the calcium antagonist.

Summary

The vasodilator effect of calcium channel blocking drugs has led to considerable interest concerning their possible role in the management of patients with heart failure. Their negative inotropic effect, however, is a potential drawback and perhaps the crucial question regarding their use. Although the negative inotropic effect is usually counterbalanced by sympathetic stimulation in patients with normal or moderate LV function, experience with the first-generation calcium antagonists verapamil, diltiazem, and nifedipine demonstrated that in patients with severe congestive heart failure such compensation may be impaired and inadequate in preventing hemodynamic deterioration following administration of the drug. Second-generation calcium channel blocking drugs such as the dihydrophyridine derivative nisoldipine are significantly more potent vasodilators, so that in the doses used they decrease arteriolar resistance and increase the forward cardiac and stroke output with a smaller myocardial depressant effect. These compounds may have a role in the management of patients in whom heart failure is related to myocardial ischemia or hypertension, and particularly in patients with lesser degrees of ventricular dysfunction. Long-term studies are required to assess the clinical benefit of chronic use and their effect on exercise tolerance and longevity.

Acknowledgements. We are indebted to Becky Kimchi and Noga Lewis for their assistance throughout the preparation of this manuscript.

References

1. Low RI, Takeda P, Mason DT, DeMaria AN (1982) The effects of calcium channel blocking agents on cardiovascular function. Am J Cardiol 49:547–553
2. Ellrodt AG, Singh BN (1983) Clinical applications of slow channel blocking compounds. Pharmacol Ther 23:1–43
3. Schwartz A, Matlib MA, Balwierczak J, Lathrop DA (1985) Pharmacology of calcium antagonists. Am J Cardiol 55:3C–7C
4. Josephson MA, Singh BN (1985) Use of calcium antagonists in ventricular dysfunction. Am J Cardiol 55:81B–88B
5. Baughman K (1986) Calcium channel blocking agents in congestive heart failure. Am J Med 80(Suppl 2B):46–50
6. Colucci WS (1987) Usefulness of calcium antagonists for congestive heart failure. Am J Cardiol 59:52B–58B
7. O'Rourke RA, Walsh RA (1987) Experience with calcium antagonist drugs in congestive heart failure. Am J Cardiol 59:64B–69B
8. Lewis BS, Mitha AS, Gotsman MS (1975) Immediate hemodynamic effects of verapamil in man. Cardiology 60:366–376
9. Ferlinz J, Citron PD (1983) Hemodynamic and myocardial performance characteristics after verapamil use in congestive heart failure. Am J Cardiol 51:1339–1345
10. Chew CYC, Hecht HS, Collett JT, McAllister RG, Singh BN (1981) Influence of severity of ventricular dysfunction on hemodynamic responses to intravenously administered verapamil in ischemic heart disease. Am J Cardiol 47:917–922
11. Guazzi MD, Cipolla C, Bella PD, Fabbiocchi F, Montorsi P, Sganzerla P (1984) Disparate unloading efficacy of the calcium channel blockers, verapamil and nifedipine, on the failing hypertensive left ventricle. Am Heart J 108:116–123
12. Epstein ML, Kiel EA, Victorica BE (1985) Cardiac decompensation following verapamil therapy in infants with supraventricular tachycardia. Pediatrics 75:737–740
13. Weiss AT, Lewis BS, Halon DA, Hasin Y, Gotsman MS (1983) The use of calcium with verapamil in the management of supraventricular tachyarrhythmias. Int J Cardiol 4:275–280
14. Walsh RW, Porter CB, Starling MR, O'Rourke RA (1984) Beneficial hemodynamic effects of intravenous and oral diltiazem in severe congestive heart failure. J Am Coll Cardiol 3:1044–1050

15. Materne P, Legrand V, Vandormael M, Collignon P, Kulbertus HE (1984) Hemodynamic effects of intravenous diltiazem with impaired left ventricular function. Am J Cardiol 54:733-737
16. Packer M, Lee WH, Medina N, Yushak M (1985) Comparative negative inotropic effects of nifedipine and diltiazem in patients with severe left ventricular dysfunction (abstract). Circulation 72 (Suppl III):III-275
17. Packer M, Kessler PD, Lee WH (1987) Calcium-channel blockade in the management of severe chronic congestive heart failure: a bridge too far. Circulation 75 (Suppl V):V56-64
18. Strauss WE, Egan T, McIntyre KM, Parisi AF (1985) Combination therapy with diltiazem and propranolol: precipitation of congestive heart failure. Clin Cardiol 8:363-366
19. Polese A, Fiorentini C, Olivari MT, Guazzi MD (1979) Clinical use of a calcium antagonist agent (nifedipine) in acute pulmonary edema. Am J Med 66:825-830
20. Klugmann S, Fioretti A, Salvi A, Camerini F (1980) Afterload reducing agents in congestive cardiomyopathy: a study with a calcium antagonist drug: nifedipine. Eur Heart J 1:49-52
21. Gillmer DJ, Kark P (1980) Pulmonary oedema precipitated by nifedipine. Br Med J 280:1420-1421
22. Matsumoto S, Ito T, Sada T, Takahashi M, Su KM, Ueda A, Okabe F, Cato M, Sekine I, Ito Y (1980) Hemodynamic effects of nifedipine in congestive heart failure. Am J Cardiol 46:476-480
23. Brooks N, Cattell M, Pidgeon J, Balcon R (1980) Unpredictable response to nifedipine in severe cardiac failure. Br Med J 281:1324
24. Cantelli I, Pavesi PC, Naccarella F, Bracchetti D (1981) Comparison of acute hemodynamic effects of nifedipine and isosorbide dinitrate in patients with heart failure following acute myocardial infarction. Int J Cardiol 1:151-163
25. Ludbrook PA, Tiefenbrunn AJ, Sobel BE, Reed FR (1981) Influence of nifedipine on left ventricular systolic and diastolic function. Relationships to manifestations of ischemia and congestive failure. Am J Med 71:683-692
26. Robson RH, Vishwanath MC (1982) Nifedipine and beta-blockade as a cause of cardiac failure. Br Med J 284:104
27. Ludbrook PA, Tiefenbrunn AJ, Reed FR, Sobel BE (1982) Acute hemodynamic responses to sublingual nifedipine: dependence on left ventricular function. Circulation 65:489-498
28. Cantelli I, Pavesi PC, Parchi C, Naccarella F, Bracchetti D (1983) Acute hemodynamic effects of combined therapy with digoxin and nifedipine in patients with chronic heart failure. Am Heart J 106:308-315
29. Elkayam U, Weber L, Torkan B, Berman D, Rahimtoola SH (1983) Acute hemodynamic effect of oral nifedipine in severe chronic congestive heart failure. Am J Cardiol 52:1041-1045
30. Leier CV, Patrick TJ, Hermiller J, Pacht KD, Huss P, Magorien RD, Unverferth DV (1984) Nifedipine in congestive heart failure: effects on resting and exercise hemodynamics and regional blood flow. Am Heart J 108:1461-1468
31. Elkayam U, Weber L, Torkan B, McKay CR, Rahimtoola SH (1984) Comparison of hemodynamic responses to nifedipine and nitroprusside in severe chronic congestive heart failure. Am J Cardiol 53:1321-1325
32. Elkayam U, Weber R, McKay CR, Rahimtoola SH (1984) Differences in hemodynamic response to vasodilation due to calcium channel antagonism with nifedipine and direct-acting agonism with hydralazine in chronic refractory congestive heart failure. Am J Cardiol 54:126-131
33. Magorien RD, Leier CV, Kolibash AJ, Barbush TJ, Unverferth DV (1984) Beneficial effects of nifedipine on rest and exercise myocardial energetics in patients with congestive heart failure. Circulation 70:884-890
34. Elkayam U, Weber L, Campese VM, Massry SG, Rahimtoola SH (1984) Renal hemodynamic effects of vasodilation with nifedipine and hydralazine in patients with heart failure. J Am Coll Cardiol 4:1261-1267
35. Fifer MA, Colucci WS, Lorell BH, Jaski BE, Barry WH (1985) Inotropic, vascular and neurodocrine effects of nifedipine in heart failure: Comparison with nitroprusside. J Am Coll Cardiol 5:731-737
36. Miller AB, Conetta DA, Bass TA (1985) Sublingual nifedipine: acute effects in severe chronic congestive heart failure secondary to idiopathic dilated cardiomyopathy. Am J Cardiol 55:1359-1362

37. Gertz MA, Falk RH, Skinner M, Cohen AS, Kyle RA (1985) Worsening of congestive heart failure in amyloid heart disease treated by calcium channel-blocking agents. Am J Cardiol 55:1645–

38. Elkayam U, Weber L, McKay C, Rahimtoola S (1985) Spectrum of acute hemodynamic effects of nifedipine in severe congestive heart failure. Am J Cardiol 56:560–566

39. Kubo SH, Fox SC, Prida XE, Cody RJ (1985) Combined hemodynamic effects of nifedipine and nitroglycerin in congestive heart failure. Am Heart J 110:1032–1034

40. Agostoni PG, DeCesare N, Doria E, Polese A, Tamborini G, Guazzi MD (1986) Afterload reduction: a comparison of captopril and nifedipine in dilated cardiomyopathy. Br Heart J 55:391–399

41. Elkayam U, Roth A, Hsueh W, Weber L, Freidenberger L, Rahimtoola SH (1986) Neurohumoral consequences of vasodilator therapy with hydralazine and nifedipine in severe congestive heart failure. Am Heart J 111:1130–1138

42. Lefkowitz CA, Moe GW, Armstrong PW (1987) A comparative evaluation of hemodynamic and neurohumoral effects of nitroglycerin and nifedipine in congestive heart failure. Am J Cardiol 59:59B–63B

43. Kazda S, Garthoff B, Meyer H, Schlossmann K, Stoepel K, Towart R, Vater W, Wehinger E (1980) Pharmacology of a new calcium antagonistic compound, isobutyl methyl 1,4-dihydro-2,6-dimethyl-4-(2-nitrophenyl)-3,5-pyridine dicarboxylate (Nisoldipine, Bay K 5552). Arzneimittelforschung 30(II):2144–2162

44. Vogt A, Neuhaus KL, Kreuzer H (1980) Hemodynamic effects of the new vasodilator drug Bay K 5552 in man. Arzneimittelforschung 32(II):2162–2164

45. Warltier DC, Meils CM, Gross GJ, Brooks HL (1981) Blood flow in normal and acutely ischemic myocardium after verapamil, diltiazem and nisoldipine (Bay K 5552), a new dihydropyridine calcium antagonist. J Pharmacol Exp Ther 218:296–302

46. Maxwell GM, Crompton S, Rencis V (1982) Effect of nisoldipine upon the general and coronary hemodynamics of the anesthetized dog. J Cardiovasc Pharmacol 4:393–397

47. Vogt A, Kreuzer H (1983) Hemodynamic effects of nisoldipine in chronic congestive heart failure. Arzneimittelforschung 33(I):877–879

48. Serruys W, Suryapranata H, Planellas J, Wijns W, Vanhaleweyk GLJ, Soward A, Jaski BE, Hugenholtz PG (1985) Acute effects of intravenous nisoldipine on left ventricular function and coronary hemodynamics. Am J Cardiol 56:140–146

49. Soward AL, DeFeyter PJ, Hugenholtz PG, Serruys PW (1986) Coronary and systemic hemodynamic effects of intravenous nisoldipine. Am J Cardiol 58:1199–1203

50. Soward AL, DeFeyter PJ, Hugenholtz PG, Serruys PW (1986) Maintenance of increased coronary blood flow in excess of demand by nisoldipine administered as an intravenous infusion. Am J Cardiol 58:1204–1208

51. Kimchi A, Ellrodt AG, Shah PK, Riedinger MS, Berman DS, Swan HJC, Murata GH (1985) Salutary hemodynamic effects of nisoldipine (Bay K 5552), a new calcium channel blocker, in patients with severe chronic congestive heart failure (abstract). J Am Coll Cardiol 5:420

52. Kimchi A, Ellrodt AG, Charuzi Y, Shell W, Murata GM (1985) Salutary hemodynamic and sustained clinical beneficial effects of nisoldipine, a new calcium channel blocker, in patients with recurrent ischemia and severe heart failure. Am Heart J 110:496–498

53. Kimchi A, Ellrodt AG, Shah PK, Riedinger MS, Charuzi Y, Berman DS, Swan HJC (1987) Hemodynamic effects of nisoldipine in patients with severe heart failure. In: Hugenholtz PG, Meyer J (eds) Nisoldipine 1987. Springer, Berlin Heidelberg New York, pp 307–314

54. Klepzig M, Strauer BB (1985) Nisoldipine for treatment of heart failure? (abstract). Eur J Clin Invest 1985; 15:A11

55. Kiowski W, Erne P, Pfisterer M, Muller J, Burkart F (1985) Hemodynamic effects of nisoldipine in patients with severe left ventricular failure (abstract). Circulation 72(Suppl):III-407

56. Schmidt WG, Essen RV, Flachskampf FA, Schmitz E (1986) Hemodynamic effects of nisoldipine in acute cardiac failure after myocardial infarction (abstract). J Am Coll Cardiol 72:180A

57. Nienaber CA, Spielmann RP, Clausen A (1985) Acute hemodynamic response to intravenous nisoldipine in ischemic cardiomyopathy – comparison with nifedipine (abstract). Circulation 72[Suppl]:III-407

58. Barjon J-N, Rouleau J-L, Bichet D, Juneau C, De Champlain J (1987) Chronic renal and neurohumoral effects of the calcium entry blocker nisoldipine in patients with congestive heart failure. JACC 9:622–630
59. Lewis BS, Shefer A, Merdler A, Flugelman MY, Hardoff R, Halon DA (1987) Acute effects of intravenous nisoldipine on hemodynamics and left ventricular function in cardiac failure. In: Hugenholtz PG, Meyer J (eds) Nisoldipine 1987. Springer, Berlin Heidelberg New York, pp 315–323
60. Olivari MT, Levine TB, Cohn JN (1984) Acute hemodynamic effects of nitrendipine in chronic congestive heart failure. J Cardiovasc Pharmacol 6(Suppl):S1002–S1005
61. Lahiri A, Robinson CW, Tovey J, Caruana MP, Kohli RS, Harlow BJ, Raftery EB (1984) Intravenous nicardipine in patients with chronic heart failure: a nuclear stethoscope study. Postgrad Med J 60 (Suppl 4):35–38
62. Lahiri A, Robinson CW, Kohli RS, Caruana MP, Raftery EB (1986) Acute and chronic effects of nicardipine on systolic and diastolic left ventricular performance in patients with heart failure: a pilot study. Clin Cardiol 9:257–261
63. Timmis AD, Campbell S, Monaghan MJ, Walker L, Jewitt DE (1984) Acute haemodynamic and metabolic effects of felodipine in congestive heart failure. Br Heart J 51:445–451
64. Timmis AD, Smyth P, Kenny JF, Campbell S, Jewitt DE (1984) Effects of vasodilator treatment with felodipine on haemodynamic responses to treadmill exercise in congestive heart failure. Br Heart J 52:314–320
65. Emanuelsson H, Hjalmarson A, Holmberg S, Waagstein F (1985) Acute haemodynamic effects of felodipine in congestive heart failure. Eur J Clin Pharmacol 28:489–493
66. Timmis AD, Jewitt DE (1985) Studies with felodipine in congestive heart failure. Drugs 29 (Suppl 2):66–75
67. Tweddel AC, Hutton I (1986) Felodipine in ventricular dysfunction. Eur Heart J 7:54–60
68. Greenberg B, Siemienczuk D, Broudy D (1987) Hemodynamic effects of PN 200-110 in congestive heart failure. Am J Cardiol 59:70B–74B
69. Cohn JN, Archibald DG, Ziesche S, Franciosa JA, Harston WE, Tristani FE, Dunkman WB, Jacobs W, Francis GS, Flohr KH, Goldman S, Cobb FR, Shah PM, Saunders R, Fletcher RD, Loeb HS, Hughes VC, Baker B (1986) Effect of vasodilator therapy on mortality in chronic congestive heart failure. Results of a veterans administration cooperative study. N Engl J Med 314:1547–1552
70. Consensus Trial Study Group (1987) Effects of enalapril on mortality in severe congestive heart failure: results of the co-operative North Scandinavian enalapril survival study. N Engl J Med 316:1429–1435
71. Lossinitzer K, Janke J, Hein B, Stauch M, Fleckenstein A (1975) Disturbed myocardial calcium metabolism: a possible pathogenetic factor in the hereditary cardiomyopathy of the Syrian hamster. In: Fleckenstein A, Dona G (eds) Pathophysiology and morphology of myocardial cell alteration. Univ Park, Baltimore, pp 207–217 (Recent advances in studies on cardiac structure and metabolism, vol 6)

A Critical Appraisal of the Role of Calcium Antagonists in the Management of Patients with Ischemic Heart Disease*

W.G. NAYLER

Introduction

Chirac was probably the first investigator to describe the consequences of coronary artery ligation when, almost 300 years ago, he reported that hearts stop beating soon after coronary artery occlusion [1]. Chirac was describing the consequences of experimentally induced coronary insufficiency in dogs, but naturally occurring occlusions occur in man with equally undesirable consequences. The occlusions can occur for a variety of reason, such as coronary artery spasm, thrombosis, and atheroma. Inadequate perfusion can be triggered by other events, including a sustained increase in heart rate without an accompanying increase in coronary blood flow. Such a condition is encountered when the coronary vasculature is either stenosed, maximally dilated, or atheromatous. Severe systemic hypotension – such as that which occurs during shock or excessive vasodilator therapy – can also promote underperfusion.

This paper is not concerned with elaborating the causes of inadequate coronary perfusion, but rather with considering the conditions under which the calcium antagonists can be used effectively to protect the ischemic heart. These are the conditions under which the ischemic insult would otherwise result in cell death, tissue necrosis, and "pump" failure. Before considering the role of the calcium antagonists in the management of such patients with ischemic heart disease, however, there is a need to consider the cascade of events which is triggered by inadequate coronary perfusion, particularly with respect to the time course of these events.

Ischemia-Induced Changes in Myocardial Structure, Chemistry, and Function

Structure. The myocardium survives relatively short episodes of ischemia without exhibiting gross ultrastructural damage [2]. However, even after only 2–3 min subtle changes can be detected – for example, glycogen granules disappear from the cytosol after only a few minutes of ischemia. Within 20 min (Table 1)

*This research was supported by a grant from the National Health and Medical Research Council of Australia.

B.S. Lewis, A. Kimchi (Eds.)
Heart Failure Mechanisms and Management
© Springer-Verlag Berlin Heidelberg 1991

Table 1. Time course of some of the ischemia-induced changes in the myocardium

Minutes of ischemia	Change	
3	Glycogen↓	
	H⁺↑	
5	ATP↓	
	CP↓ ↓	
	H⁺↑ ↑	
20	Ultrastructural changes	Reversible
	Mitochondrial swelling	
	Margination of nuclear chromatin	
	Cell swelling	
	Biochemical changes	
	CP↓ ↓ ↓ ↓	
	ATP↓ ↓	
	H⁺↑ ↑ ↑ ↑	
	Glycogen↓ ↓ ↓ ↓ ↓	
	Noradrenaline↓	
60	Ultrastructural and biochemical changes	Irreversible
	Mitochondrial disruption	
	Myofibrillar lysis	
	Membrane disruption	
	SR disruption	
	ATP + CP↓ ↓ ↓ ↓ ↓	
	Noradrenaline↓ ↓	
	H⁺↑ ↑ ↑ ↑	

Note: The up/down arrows indicate direction of change: H^+ increases ($\uparrow$); ATP, CP, glycogen, noradrenaline decrease ($\downarrow$).

evidence of cell swelling begins to appear, the mitochondria begin to swell, and there is evidence of margination of the nuclear chromatin [3]. The sarcolemma remains intact, however, and if large radioactively tagged molecules are introduced into the extracellular medium, they remain excluded from the cytosol [4]. Increasing the duration of the ischemic event by only another 10 min to 30 min, results in readily demonstrable morphological changes. The mitochondrial matrix clears, the sarcoplasmic reticulum shows signs of disruption and vacuolization, and the sarcolemma, although intact, begins to bulge away from the underlying cytoplasm and myofibrils. Extending the ischemic episode beyond 30 min (Table 1) precipitates obvious evidence of damage. The myofibrils, which until now have remained well aligned, begin to show evidence of lysis and disruption. The sarcolemma may tear away from the underlying Z bands, and the mitochondria become overtly swollen. Nevertheless, identifiable sarcolemmal discontinuities are rare.

Reperfusion. Without reperfusion potentially viable cells die and necrose [3]. Reperfusion, on the other hand, can either hasten the expression of ischemia-induced lethal injury or prevent tissue which is not yet lethally injured from becoming irreversibly damaged. The reperfusion-induced events which can be responsible for accelerating and exaggerating the ischemia-induced damage revolve around an uncontrolled gain in water, with consequent tissue edema [5], disruption of the already fragile cell membrane [5], an apparently uncontrolled gain in Na^+ [6], a burst of free radical production [7], an uncontrolled increase in tissue calcium [6,8,9], and a loss of nucleotide precursors [10].

Metabolic Consequences of Ischemia and Reperfusion

Ischemia. Inadequate coronary perfusion causes a progressive loss of adenosine triphosphate (ATP) and creatine phosphate (CP). ATP depletion occurs at a relatively rapid rate, not only because its rate of production is severely impaired, but also because the heart continuous to use ATP as a substrate for the various ATPase enzymes which are responsible for maintaining ionic homeostasis. Within 15 min of the commencement of an ischemic episode the ATP content of the heart is halved (Table 2), and within 30 min practically all the ATP has been utilized. The CP reserves are depleted at an even faster rate (Table 2).

The heart uses ATP as its primary energy source, and its production is primarily by oxidative metabolism – a process which yields 38 molecules of ATP for every molecule of glucose which is metabolized. The heart has some capacity for anaerobic metabolism, but it is an inefficient process, yielding only three molecules of ATP for each molecule of glucose derived from glycogen, and only two molecules of ATP for each molecule of glucose derived from the extracellular space. There is another serious hazard associated with a switch to anaerobic glycolysis in that it generates protons which, in the absence of perfusion, accumulate and render the heart severely acidotic [11].

The involvement of ATP in the deleterious consequences of inadequate perfusion is quite widespread. The hydrolysis of ATP produces adenosine diphosphate (ADP) and inorganic phosphate (P_i) as well as energy. In the absence of oxidative phosphorylation this ADP is converted by adenylate kinase

Table 2. Rate of depletion of cardiac adenosine triphosphate (ATP) and creatine phosphate (CP) reserves during normothermic ischemia (μmol/g dry wt)

Minutes of ischemia	ATP	CP
0	23.8 ± 2.6	35.3 ± 1.6
5	14.2 ± 1.3 (40%)	6.1 ± 0.7 (80%)
15	9.4 ± 0.9 (61%)	4.2 ± 0.5 (88%)
30	5.2 ± 1.0 (78%)	3.8 ± 0.4 (89%)
60	4.8 ± 0.6 (80%)	3.2 ± 0.2 (91%)

Data obtained from isolated, retrogradely perfused rat hearts, maintained at 37°C irrespective of flow. Results are mean ± SEM of six experiments. Numbers in parenthesis refers to percentage reduction, relative to the pre-ischemic controls.

to ATP and adenosine monophosphate (AMP). While the production of ATP from this source delays the exhaustion of the ATP reserves, it provides a source of AMP which can be dephosphorylated to adenosine. The cell membrane is permeable to adenosine, which moves out of the cell along its concentration gradient.

The loss of adenosine has at least two important consequences: (a) it depletes the cellular pool of purines, thereby limiting the potential for ATP resynthesis upon reperfusion; and (b) once adenosine appears in the extracellular space it can be further degraded to hypoxanthine and xanthine, both of which provide a substrate for free radial production. The enzymes required for this process are contained in the vascular endothelium [12].

The protons, ammonium ions, and phosphates produced by the degradation of adenine nucleotides and CP, as well as the glycolytic intermediates produced by the anaerobic metabolism of glycogen and glucose, accumulate intracellularly, resulting in a substantially raised tissue osmolarity [5]. At the same time, and because of inadequate ATP as substrate for the associated ATPase enzymes, cytosolic Ca^{2+} begins to rise — at a stage when there is as yet no detectable rise in total tissue Ca^{2+} [13]. This early rise in cytosolic Ca^{2+} is significant because of its potential role as an activator of endogenous proteases and phospholipases. Activation of these enzymes must result in a loss of membrane integrity, and in so doing establish a situation in which uncontrolled Ca^{2+} influx is difficult to avoid upon reperfusion.

Reperfusion. This promotes an entirely new set of conditions. Prior to reperfusion the myocytes are osmolotically swollen and ATP-depleted, and their limiting membranes (the sarcolemma) although fragile are probably intact. Reperfusion adds another complication in that it supplies the ischemia-damaged tissue with an unlimited supply of Ca^{2+} which crosses the sarcolemma either in exchange for Na^+, through the slow Ca^{2+} channels, or by passive diffusion. Much of this Ca^{2+} remains in the cytosol, since its accumulation by the sarcoplasmic reticulum is an energy-dependent process. In addition, some of the Ca^{2+} accumulates in the mitochondria, where it impairs oxidative phosphorylation [14,15].

As soon as cytosolic Ca^{2+} rises above the level needed to activate the endogenous phospholipases (particularly phospholipase A_2) and the endogenous proteases, and as soon as significant quantities of free radicals are generated, the continuity of the sarcolemma — already rendered fragile because of the ischemia-induced cell swelling — is destroyed, resulting in an uncontrolled influx of Ca^{2+} [14,15].

Consequences of Uncontrolled Ca^{2+} Gain

An uncontrolled entry of Ca^{2+}, particularly when it is preceded by ATP depletion, osmotic swelling, and membrane fragility, signals cell death and tissue necrosis [3]. Free radical generation is augmented, phospholipase and protease activation ensures loss of membrane ultrastructure and continuity, and the mitochondria become overloaded with Ca^{2+} and accordingly cannot regenerate sufficient ATP [15] to ensure the recovery of homeostasis with respect to Ca^{2+} or Na^+. The sarcoplasmic reticulum becomes severely damaged and loses its capacity to store Ca^{2+}. The cytoskeleton of the cells is also damaged [8].

Against this background it is logical to question whether drugs which either limit Ca^{2+} entry or have an energy-sparing effect on the heart can be used either to prevent or to attenuate the damage caused by such an uncontrolled gain in Ca^{2+}. In view of the potent pharmacological properties of the Ca^{2+} antagonists, we and others [16] have explored their use as cardioprotective agents under these conditions.

Experimental Studies with Calcium Antagonists

Before considering the significance of the data obtained from the various clinical studies in which calcium antagonists have been used to treat patients with ischemic heart disease, it is useful to consider the results obtained from experimental studies with animals. Some of these results are summarized in Table 3 [17–37].

Studies with verapamil, nifedipine, and diltiazem have all shown that these drugs can limit ischemia – reperfusion injury [16]. This ability to protect applies irrespective of whether the model is that of regional, global, or low-flow ischemia and largely irrespective of which species (rat, rabbit, dog, cat, pig) has been used, *provided* that the drug has been used as a prophylactic agent or administered early during reperfusion, and that a well developed collateral circulation is present.

The various indices of protection which have been used include restoration of tension generating capacity upon reperfusion [16], restoration of mitochondrial ATP-generating activity [15], preservation of ultrastructure [3,38], attenuation of the ischemia-induced acidosis [39], reduction in calcium overload [16], attenuation of the ischemia-induced mobilization of endogenous noradrenaline [40], and reduction in infarct size [23]. In addition to providing clear evidence of protection, the experimental studies have highlighted the desirability of prophylactic therapy and pointed towards a strong correlation between protection, reduction in Ca^{2+} overload, and preservation of the energy-rich phosphate reserves [9].

The basis of the protective effect of the calcium antagonists is multifactorial, with some beneficial effects appearing soon after their administration while other benefits are apparent only after long-term treatment. This division between immediate and long-term beneficial effects is summarized in Table 4. Probably the energy sparing effects predominate early during calcium antagonist therapy whereas the effect on the vasculature and atheroma require longer treatment periods. The experimental studies have also revealed the multifactorial nature of the mechanisms which contribute to the ability of these drugs to reduce infarct size. Some of these mechanisms are included in Fig. 1.

Table 3. Experimental studies of the effect of calcium antagonists on infarct size

Model	Duration of ischemia	Index of damage	Starting time for therapy	Response	Reference
Verapamil					
Anesthetized dog	2 h	ST segment	15 min postocclusion	+	[17]
Anesthetized dog	20 min	ST segment	At occlusion	+	[18]
Anesthetized dog	40 min	Histology	Preocclusion	+	[19]
Anesthetized dog	up to 2 h	ST segment	15 min postocclusion	+	[20]
Anesthetized dog	15–90 min	ST segment	30 min preocclusion	+	[21]
Anesthetized dog	8 h	Tetrazolium	60 min postocclusion	+	[22]
Anesthetized dog	24 h	Tetrazolium	15 min postocclusion	+	[23]
Anesthetized dog	72 h	Histology	15 min postocclusion	0	[24]
Anesthetized dog	72 h	Tetrazolium	During ischemia	+	[25]
Conscious dog	24 h	Tissue + plasma CK	5 h postischemia	0	[26]
Nifedipine					
Conscious dog	24 h	Tissue CK	30 min postocclusion	+	[27]
Anesthetized rabbit	1 h	Infarct size	5 min postocclusion	0	[28]
Anesthetized dog	24 h	Infarct size	10 min postocclusion	+	[29]
Anesthetized baboon	2 h	Infarct size	1 h postocclusion	0	[30]
Diltiazem					
Anesthetized dog	0.5–24 h	ECG/histology	15 min postocclusion	+	[31]
Anesthetized rat	48 h	Tissue CK	30 min preocclusion	+	[32]
Anesthetized pig	75 min	Infarct size	30 min preocclusion	+	[33]
Nicardipine					
Anesthetized dog	3 months	Infarct size	1 min preocclusion	+	[34]
Nisoldipine					
Anesthetized dog	6 h	Infarct size	15 min postocclusion	+	[35]
Conscious dog	24 h	Infarct size	48 h preocclusion	+	[36]
Tiapamil					
Anesthetized baboon	12 h	Tissue CK	20 min postocclusion	+	[37]

+, 0 denote the presence and absence of protection, respectively. *CK*, tissue creatine kinase.

Table 4. Basis of the protective effect of calcium antagonists

Immediate consequences	Delayed consequences
Energy-sparing effect	Slowed atheroma
Reduction in systemic vascular resistance	Slowed hypertrophy in hypertensives
Slowed heart rate	
Negative inotropy	
Biochemical effects	
Slowed loss of adenosine precursors	
Improved mitochondrial function	
Reduced Ca^{2+} overload	
Attenuated proton accumulation	
Slowed release of catecholamines	
Direct effect on coronary vasculature	
Dilation, without "steal"	
Reduced transcapillary leakage	
Electrical activity	
Attenuated reperfusion-induced arrhythmias	
Reduced ventricular ectopics	
Blood	
Slowed platelet aggregation	
Others	
Attenuation of the coronary vasoconstriction effect of endothelin	

Clinical Trial Data

The cardiovascular properties of the calcium antagonists – energy preservation, vasodilation (in peripheral and coronary vasculature), slowed platelet aggregation [41], attenuated catecholamine mobilization [40], slowed Ca^{2+} overload, purine preservation, slowed atheroma formation, reduced incidence of arrhythmias and etopic beats [42] – together with their well-documented ability to protect hearts against the deleterious effects of ischemia and reperfusion during experimental studies (Table 3) and their ability to prevent transcoronary macromolecular leakage [43], provide a sound rationale for using these agents in the clinical setting. The experimental data also provided guidelines for the successful use of these drugs – as prophylactic therapy at the appropriate dose level.

    Three major postinfarction clinical trials with calcium antagonists have now been reported.

Verapamil. In the Danish verapamil trial 1436 patients [44] were treated with verapamil very early after the onset of acute myocardial ischemia, with intravenous therapy being started immediately after coronary care admission.

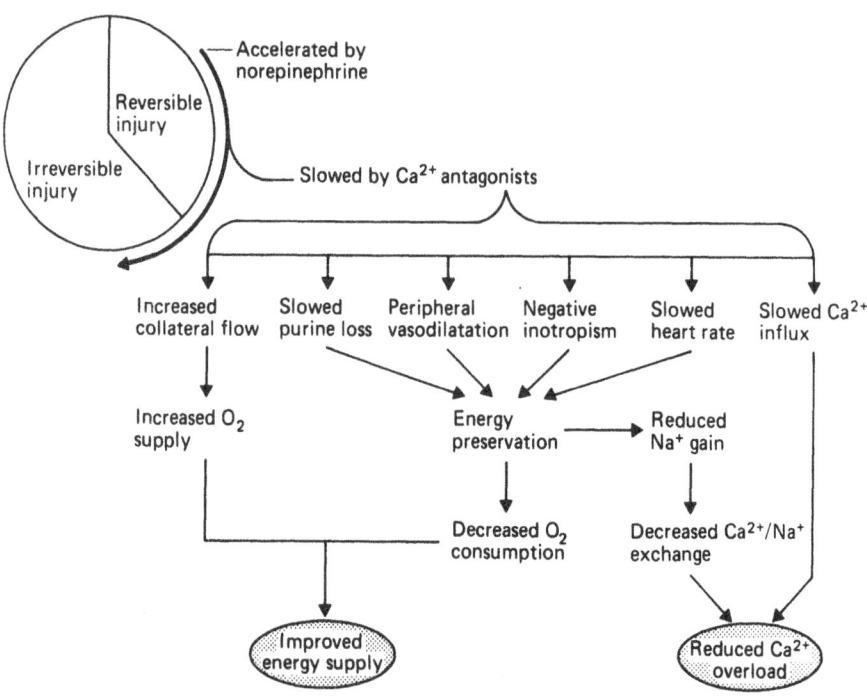

Fig. 1. Schematic representation of the mechanisms involved in the Ca²⁺-antagonist-induced protection of the ischemic myocardium [16]

During the first 6 months of therapy several important points emerged. These were: (a) there was no significant reduction in mortality or rate of reinfarction; and (b) verapamil contributed to excess death during the first few weeks of therapy, due to cardiogenic shock and pulmonary edema. These early findings indicate that verapamil should not be administered early during acute myocardial infarction, particularly if the ischemic episode has resulted in severe left ventricular dysfunction. It is interesting to note, however, that patients who have remained on verapamil therapy [45] have shown a reduced rate of reinfarction (3.9% in the verapamil group and 6.1% in the placebo group) during the subsequent months (Table 5). An increase in early deaths in verapamil-treated patients is not peculiar to the Danish study. A similar effect was described by Crea et al. [46] in a relatively small group of patients with transmural infarctions (Table 6). Here, as with the Danish study, early complications included heart failure and atrioventricular block. Another verapamil study is that of Bussman et al. [47]. This was a small study, and verapamil therapy was started about 8 h after infarction. Based on creatine kinase data, this trial revealed evidence of protection, and it is worth noting that the patients admitted to the trial were those *without left ventricular failure* — that is, the patients had suffered a "mild infarction."

Nifedipine. Several nifedipine trials have been undertaken. The first of these trials, the Norwegian multicenter trial [48], lasted for 6 weeks and failed to provide

Table 5. Mortality and reinfarction in the Danish multicenter verapamil study. (From [45])

Treatment period	Mortality		Reinfarction (%)	
	Verapamil	Placebo	Verapamil	Placebo
1 week	6.4	5.6	3.2	2.1
2 weeks	1.8	2.1	1.0	0.9
3 weeks	1.5	0.6	0	0.8
22–180 days	3.7	6.4[a]	3.9	6.1[b]

[a] $p < 0.05$.
[b] $p < 0.03$.

Table 6. Clinical trials with calcium antagonists in myocardial infarction patients

Calcium antagonist	Patient number, treatment arm	Time to treatment	Index of response	Follow-up time	Reference
Verapamil	717 Verapamil 719 Placebo	4 h	Mortality	6 months	[44, 45]
	25 Verapamil 25 Placebo	8 h	CK release	2 weeks	[47]
	29 Verapamil 25 Placebo	7 ± 5 h	CK release	2 days	[46]
Nifedipine	115 Nifedipine 112 Placebo	$5.5. \pm 2.9$ h	CK release	6 weeks	[48]
	89 Nifedipine 82 Placebo	4.6 ± 0.1 h	CK release; mortality	6 months	[48]
	64 Nifedipine 68 Placebo	8.0 ± 2.5 h	Mortality; reinfarction	8 weeks	[54]
	595 Nifedipine 562 Placebo	Admission to CUU	Mortality	1 month	[49]
Diltiazem	289 Diltiazem 282 Placebo	24–72 h	Reinfarction	14 days	[51]
	1234 Diltiazem 1232 Placebo	24–72 h	Reinfarction	12–15 months	[52]

Time to treatment refers to time interval between onset of severe chest pain and introduction of calcium antagonist therapy. CK release refers to plasma creatine kinase.

evidence of protection. In this study therapy was initiated 5.5 h (on average) after the onset of symptoms and hence at a time when tissue injury would be well established. Of the other nifedipine trials (Table 5) one [49] is of particular interest because it, like the Danish verapamil trial, revealed an increase in early deaths associated with therapy. In the case of nifedipine two factors could have been responsible: (a) enhanced left ventricular malfunction and (b) underperfusion due to the vasodilatory properties of the drug. One of the other nifedipine trials also warrants attention. This is the prospective double-blind randomized trial of Gerstenblith et al. [50], which was based on the assumption that persistent angina often progresses to infarction in patients who are placed on traditional medical treatment (beta-blockade and long-acting nitrates). Based on a 4-month follow-up period this study showed that adding nifedipine to conventional therapy was beneficial in that it reduced the incidence of death, myocardial infarction, or the need for by-pass surgery.

Diltiazem. The recently completed, randomized double-blind trial with diltiazem differs in two important aspects from the earlier trials with either verapamil or nifedipine. Firstly, only patients with non-Q wave infarction were admitted to the trial. Secondly, treatment was delayed for up to 72 h. The trial, although limited in its duration (14 days) failed to show any change in mortality, but the rate of reinfarction was reduced [51,52]. Continuation of the trial for almost 2 years has shown the maintenance of this reduction in the rate of reinfarction in patients who did not exhibit severe left ventricular dysfunction at the time of infarction.

Relevance of Experimental Studies to the Clinical Situation

Although experimental studies have shown that calcium antagonists can ameliorate the damage caused by ischemia and reperfusion provided that the drugs are used in appropriate doses and at the appropriate times, the results of the clinical trials are less certain. There may be several reasons for this apparent discrepancy, but the most important would seem to be the presence or absence of severe left ventricular dysfunction, the acute nature of the ischemic episode, the pathology of the artery wall, and the failure to use the drugs prophylactically, before the initial infarction. On a long-term basis the outcome looks more promising, but additional investigations are needed to detemine whether the reduced rate of reinfarction associated with the long-term usage of these drugs can be attributed directly to the calcium-antagonist-reduced limitation of Ca^{2+} entry into the jeopardized cells, or whether it is due to their ability to slow the development of atherosclerosis [53] and to protect the endothelium [54]. Hence, future investigations should be aimed at establishing whether it is the immediate or long-term effects of these drugs which are of crucial importance to their use in the management of patients with ischemic heart disease. Possibly other interventions, such as thombolytic therapy [55,56], should be made during the acute stages of infarction, with calcium antagonists being used to prevent reinfarction during the successive months.

Summary

From a purely theoretical point of view calcium antagonists should be useful in the management of patients with ischemic heart disease. They improve the supply of oxygen and substrate to the risk area, accelerate removal of H^+ and other by-products of anaerobic glycolysis, and slow the loss of adenosine precursors. They also have an energy-sparing effect, slow lysosomal enzyme release, inhibit platelet aggregation, and protect the vascular endothelial cells. They also attentuate reperfusion-induced arrhythmias, slow the ischemia-reperfusion induced displacement of endogenous noradrenaline, and diminish Ca^{2+} accumulation during postischemic reperfusion. Laboratory studies, using a variety of species, models of infarction, and reperfusion protocols have confirmed the anticipated usefulness of these drugs in limiting infarct size, provided that the drugs have been either used prophylactically or administered early upon reperfusion. In the clinical setting the situation is less clear, possibly because in the earlier trials the calcium antagonists were not used prophylactically, the danger of underperfusion was not recognized, and sufficient care was not taken to avoid complications due to the negative inotropic effect of the calcium antagonists in patients in whom left ventricular function was already depressed. Existing trial data provides evidence, however, of the ability of calcium antagonists to have a beneficial effect in patients with ischemic heart disease, provided that these drugs are used prophylactically. On a long-term basis other beneficial effects of these drugs must be considered, including their ability to retard atherosclerosis and to slow platelet aggregation.

References

1. Chirac P (1668) de moto cordis. Adverseria Analytica, pp 121-134
2. Brauwald E, Kloner RA (1982) The stunned myocardium: prolonged, postischemic ventricular dysfunction. Circulation 66:1146-1149
3. Nayler WG, Elz JS (1986) Reperfusion injury: laboratory artifact or clinical dilemma. Circulation 74:215-221
4. Bourdillon PDV, Poole-Wilson PA (1981) Effects of ischaemia and reperfusion on calcium exchange and mechanical function in isolated rabbit myocardium. Cardiovasc Res 15:121-130
5. Steenbergen C, Hill ML, Jennings RB (1985) Volume regulation and plasma membrane injury in aerobic, anaerobic and ischemic injury in vitro. Effects of osmotic cell swelling on plasma membrane integrity. Circ Res 57:864-875
6. Shen AC, Jennings RB (1972) Myocardial calcium and magnesium in acute ischemic injury. Am J Pathol 67:417-433
7. Weisfeldt ML (1987) Reperfusion and reperfusion injury. Clin Res 11:13-20
8. Murphy JG, Marsh JD, Smith TW (1987) The role of calcium in ischemic myocardial injury. Circulation 75 (Suppl V):V15-V24
9. Nayler WG (1983) Calcium and cell death. Eur Heart J 4 (Suppl C):33-41
10. de Jong JW, Harmeson E, de Tombe PP, Keijzer E (1982) Nifedipine reduced adenine nucleotide breakdown in ischaemic rat heart. Eur J Pharm 81:89-96
11. Poole-Wilson PA (1978) Measurement of myocardial intracellular pH in pathological states. J Mol Cell Cardiol 10:511-526
12. Jarasch ED, Grund C, Bruder G (1981) Localization of xanthine oxidase in mammary gland epithelium and capillary endothelium. Cell 25:67-82
13. Steenbergen C, Murphy E, Levy L, London RE (1987) Elevation of cytosolic free calcium concentration early in myocardial ischemia in perfused rat heart. Circ Res 60:700-707
14. Nayler WG (1982) Protection of the myocardium against post-ischaemic reperfusion damage. J Thorac Cardiovasc Surg 84:897-905
15. Nayler WG, Ferrari R, Williams A (1980) Protective effect of pretreatment with verapamil, nifedipine and propranolol on mitochondrial function in the ischemic and reperfused myocardium. Am J Cardiol 46:242-248

16. Nayler WG (1987) Calcium antagonists and the ischemic myocardium. Int J Cardiol 15:267-285
17. Smith HJ, Singh BN, Nisbet HD, Norris RM (1979) Effects of verapamil on infarct size following experimental coronary occlusion. Cardiovasc Res 9:569-578
18. Wende W, Bleifeld W, Meyer J, Stuhlen HW (1975) Reduction of the size of acute experimental myocardial infarction by verapamil. Bas Res Cardiol 70:198-200
19. Reimer KA, Lowe J, Jennings RB (1977) Effects of the calcium antagonist verapamil on necrosis following temporary coronary artery occlusion in dogs. Circulation 55:581-587
20. Smith HJ, Singh BN, Norris RM, Nispet HD, John MB, Hurley PJ (1977) The effect of verapamil on experimental myocardial ischemia with a particular reference to regional blood flow and metabolism. Aust NZ J Med 7:114-121
21. da Luz PL, de Barros LFM, Leite JJ, Pileggi F, de Court LV (1980) Effect of verapamil on regional coronary and myocardial perfusion during acute coronary occlusion. Am J Cardiol 45:269-275
22. de Boer LWV, Strauss W, Kloner RA, Rude RE, Davis RF, Maroko PR, Braunwald E (1980) Autoradiographic method for measuring the ischemic myocardium at risk: effects of verapamil on infarct size after experimental coronary artery occlusion. Proc Natl Acad Sci USA 77:6119-6123
23. Yellon DM, Hearse DJ, Maxwell MP, Chambers DE, Downey JM (1983) Sustained limitation of myocardial necrosis 24 hours after coronary artery occlusion: verapamil infusion in dogs with small myocardial infarcts. Am J Cardiol 51:1409-1413
24. Reimer KA, Jennings RB (1984) Verapamil in two reperfusion models of myocardial infarction. Temporary protection of severely ischemic myocardium without limitation of ultimate infarct size. Lab Invest 51:655-666
25. Lo H-M, Kloner RA, Braunwald E (1985) Effect of intracoronary verapamil on infarct size in the ischemic reperfusion canine heart: critical importance of the timing of treatment. Am J Cardiol 56:672-677
26. Karlsberg RP, Henry PD, Ahmed SA, Sobel BE, Roberts R (1977) Lack of protection of ischemic myocardium by verapamil in conscious dogs. Eur J Pharm 42:339-346
27. Henry PO, Shuchleib R, Borda LJ, Roberts R, Williamson JR, Sobel BE (1978) Effects of nifedipine on myocardial perfusion and ischemic injury in dogs. Circ Res 43:372-380
28. Foster E, de Jong D, Connelly C, Apstein CS (1984) Failure of nifedipine and reperfusion to reduce infarct size relative to region at risk as measured by NADH fluorophotography. Circulation 70:506-512
29. Lamping KA, Christensen CW, Pek LR, Warltier DG, Gross GJ (1984) Effects of nicoandil and nifedipine on protection of ischemic myocardium. J Cardiovasc Pharm 6:536-542
30. Geary GC, Smith GT, Suehiro GT, McNamara JJ (1982) Failure of nifedipine therapy to reduce myocardial infarct size in the baboon. Am J Cardiol 49:331-338
31. Nakamura M, Kikuchi Y, Senda Y, Yamada A, Koiwaya Y (1980) Myocardial blood flow following experimental coronary occlusion. Effects of diltiazem. Chest 78(Suppl):205-209
32. Flaim SF, Zelis R (1981) Diltiazem pretreatment reduces experimental myocardial infarct size in rat. Pharmacology 23:281·286
33. Klein HH, Schubotbe M, Nebendahl K, Kruezer H (1984) The effect of two different diltiazem treatments on infarct size in ischemic, reperfused porcine hearts. Circulation 69:1000-1005
34. Alps BJ, Calder C, Wilson A, Scott-Park FM (1983) The beneficial effect of nicardipine on the healing of myocardial infarcts in dogs. Arzneimittelforschung 33:1638-1646
35. Crottogini AJ, Depaoli JP, Barra JG, Fischer EC, Chatruc MR, Pichel RH, de la Fuente L (1985) The effect of the new calcium antagonist nisoldipine (Bay K5552) on myocardial infarct size limitation in conscious dogs. Am Heart J 110:753-760
36. Tumas J, Deth R, Kloner RA (1985) Effect of nisoldipine, a new calcium antagonist, on myocardial infarct size and cardiac dynamics following acute myocardial infarction. J Cardiovasc Pharmacol 7:361-367
37. Rogers GG, Rosendorff C, Shimell CJ, Coull A (1982) Effects of tiapamil on hemodynamics and myocardial salvage during myocardial infarction in the baboon. Cardiology 69(Suppl 1):58-67
38. Nayler WG (1981) The role of calcium in the ischemic myocardium. Am J Pathol 102:262-268
39. Kirkels J Hans, Ruigrok TJC, van Echteld CJ, Meijler FL (1987) Protective effect of pretreatment with calcium antagonist anipamil on the ischemic-reperfused rat myocardium: a phosphorus-31 nuclear magnetic resonance study. J Am Coll Cardiol 11:1087-1093

40. Nayler WG, Sturrock WJ (1985) The inhibitory effect of calcium antagonists on the depletion of cardiac norepinephrine during postischemic reperfusion. J Cardiovasc Pharm 7:581–587

41. Ware JA, Johnson PC, Smith M, Salzman EW (1986) Inhibition of human platelet aggregation and cytoplasmic calcium response by calcium antagonists: studies with Aequorin and Quin 2. Circ Res 59:39–42

42. Kaumann AJ, Aramendia P (1968) Prevention of ventricular fibrillation induced by coronary ligation. J Pharmac Exp Ther 164:326–332

43. MacDonagh PF, Roberts DJ (1986) Prevention of transcoronary macromolecular leakage after ischemia-reperfusion by the calcium entry blocker nisoldipine. Direct observations in isolated rat hearts. Circ Res 58:127–136

44. The Danish Study Group (1984) Verapamil in acute myocardial infarction. Eur Heart J 5:516–528

45. The Danish Study Group (1986) The Danish studies on verapamil in acute myocardial infarction. Br J Clin Pharmac 21:197S–204S

46. Crea F, Deanfield J, Crean P, Sharom M, David G, Maseri A (1985) Effects of verapamil in preventing post-infarction angina and reinfarction. Am J Cardiol 55:900–904

47. Bussmann WD, Seher W, Gruengras M (1984) Reduction of creatine kinase and creatine kinase MB indexes of infarct size by intravenous verapamil. Am J Cardiol 54:1224–1230

48. Sirnes PA, Overskeid K, Pedersen TR et al. (1984) Evolution of infarct size during the early use of nifedipine in patients with acute myocardial infarction. The Norwegian nifedipine multicenter trial. Circulation 4:638–644

49. Wilcox RG, Hampton JR, Banks DC et al. (1986) Trials of early nifedipine in patients with suspected myocardial infarction (the Trent study). Proc Br Cardiol Soc 506

50. Gerstenblith G, Ouyang P, Achuff SC et al. (1982) Nifedipine in unstable angina. A double-blind randomized trial. N Engl J Med 306:885–890

51. Gibson RS, Boden WE, Theroux P et al. (1986) Diltiazem and reinfarction in patients with non-Q wave myocardial infarction: results of a double-blind randomized, multicenter trial. N Engl J Med 315:423–429

52. Moss AJ, Abrams J, Albuquerque NM, Bigger JT et al. (1988) The effect of diltiazem on mortality and reinfarction after myocardial infarction. N Engl J Med 319:385–392

53. Parmely WW, Blumlein S, Sievers R (1985) Modification of experimental atherosclerosis by calcium channel blockers. Am J Cardiol 55:165B–171B

54. Muller JE, Morrison HJ, Stone PH et al. (1984) Nifedipine therapy for patients with threatened and acute double-blind, placebo-controlled comparison. Circulation 69:740–747

55. Braunwald E (1987) The path to myocardial salvage by thrombolytic therapy. Circulation 76(Suppl II):II-2–II-7

56. Ritchie JL, Cerqueira M, Maynard C, Davis K, Kennedy W (1988) Ventricular function and infarct size: the western Washington intravenous steptokinase in myocardial infarction trial. J Am Coll Cardiol 11:689–697

Central and Renal Hemodynamic Effects of Diltiazem in Chronic Heart Failure

D.L. KULICK and U. ELKAYAM

Introduction

There has been recent interest in attempting to use the arterial vasodilating activity of calcium channel blocking drugs to decrease left ventricular (LV) afterload in patients with severe heart failure (CHF). However, unlike other vasodilators used in the treatment of CHF, calcium channel blocking drugs possess intrinsic negative inotropic activity as well; clinical studies have shown that both verapamil [1] and nifedipine [2,3] may lead to marked clinical deterioration in patients with severe CHF. Diltiazem, the third presently available calcium channel blocking agent, has less intrinsic negative inotropic effect than verapamil and nifedipine [4,5] and has been shown in one study to be acutely beneficial in patients with severe CHF [6].

Patients and Methods

In order to further assess the efficacy and safety of diltiazem in patients with severe CHF, we studied ten patients with chronic CHF due to severe LV systolic dysfunction (mean LV ejection fraction 0.22 ± 0.08); nine of the ten patients had dilated cardiomyopathy, and one had LV dysfunction due to coronary artery disease. All patients were in New York Heart Association functional class III or IV. A balloon flotation thermodilution catheter was inserted into the pulmonary artery the day prior to study; patients were allowed to continue their usual oral dose of digitalis throughout the study, but all other cardioactive and vasodilating agents were withheld for at least 24 h.

On the day of the study, four consecutive baseline measurements of central hemodynamics were obtained 1 h apart to assess baseline stability; determination of renal blood flow and glomerular filtration rate by measurement of inulin and sodium para-amino hippurate clearances was performed with each baseline. Patients were then given a single oral dose of 60 mg diltiazem, and repeat central and renal hemodynamic parameters were measured over the next 8 h. Mixed venous blood was sampled for determination of plasma catecholamine levels and renin concentration at baseline, as well as at 1, 2, and 4 h following drug administration; plasma diltiazem levels were measured 2 h following drug administration. The following day, the entire protocol was repeated, using a single 90-mg dose of diltiazem.

B.S. Lewis, A. Kimchi (Eds.)
Heart Failure Mechanisms and Management
© Springer-Verlag Berlin Heidelberg 1991

Results

No significant differences were noted in the four consecutive baseline measurements on either day for any central or renal hemodynamic variables measured; therefore all postdrug measurements were compared to the mean of the four baselines. For each central hemodynamic parameter, a 95% confidence interval was computed for each patient from the four baseline values. Figure 1 depicts the group values for central and renal hemodynamics before and after administration of 60 and 90 mg diltiazem. As can be seen, the heart rate was significantly ($p < 0.05$) slowed at 4 h (79 ± 14 versus 86 ± 10 beats/min), 6 h (78 ± 12 beats/min), and 8 h (77 ± 9 beats/min) following 60 mg diltiazem; no significant effect on heart rate was noted following 90 mg diltiazem. Similarly, the pulmonary vascular resistance was significantly reduced 4 h following the 60-mg dose (165 ± 74 versus 231 ± 108 dyne s^{-1} cm^{-5}), but this effect was not observed following 90 mg. No changes for the group were noted for any other central hemodynamic parameters following either dose. Both renal blood flow and glomerular filtration rate were depressed at baseline, and no significant changes in renal hemodynamics were noted following either diltiazem dose (Fig. 2.).

Figures 3 and 4 demonstrate the individual responses of pulmonary artery wedge pressure (PAW) and stroke volume index (SVI) to 90 mg diltiazem. Changes were considered to be due to drug effect if they exceeded the 95% confidence interval calculated for each patient from the four baseline measurements, for at least two consecutive measurements. As shown, following 90 mg diltiazem, SVI increased in three patients (numbers 3, 5, and 6) and fell in one (number 7); one patient demonstrated a persistent rise in PAW (number 8). None of these hemodynamic changes were associated with any change in the patients' clinical status.

At baseline, patients had markedly elevated plasma hormone levels. The mean plasma epinephrine ranged from 215 ± 309 to 287 ± 406 pg/ml (normal 42 ± 35), norepinephrine from 837 ± 481 to 1132 ± 987 pg/ml (normal 148 ± 45), and plasma renin concentration from 13 ± 23 to 27 ± 51 ng/ml per hour (normal 2.5 ± 0.6); none of these three plasma hormone levels were affected by administration of either dose of diltiazem. Plasma diltiazem levels following 60 mg ranged from 13 to 173 ng/ml (mean 76 ± 57) and following 90 mg from 40 to 246 ng/ml (mean 88 ± 70).

Discussion

Owing to their arterial vasodilating effects, there has been considerable recent interest in exploring the value of calcium channel blocking agents in the management of severe LV systolic dysfunction, with the notion that this vasorelaxing action might outweigh the intrinsic negative inotropy of these agents. In clinical usage, verapamil has been demonstrated to be deleterious in patients with severe LV dysfunction [1]. Similarly, nifedipine has been shown to be potentially harmful in a substantial number of patients with severe LV dysfunction, resulting

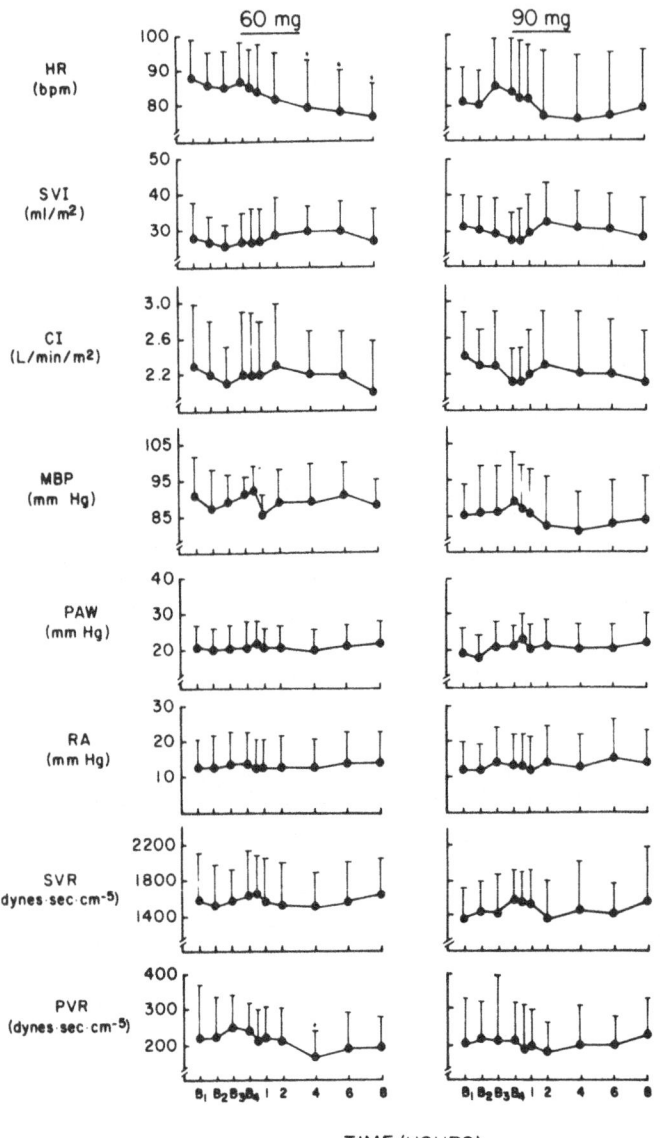

Fig. 1. Sequential effects of 60 mg and 90 mg diltiazem on heart rate (*HR*), stroke volume index (*SVI*), cardiac index (*CI*), mean blood pressure (*MBP*), mean pulmonary artery wedge pressure (*PAW*), mean right atrial pressure (*RA*), systemic vascular resistance (*SVR*), and pulmonary vascular resistance (*PVR*). B_1–B_4 are four consecutive baselines taken 1 h apart

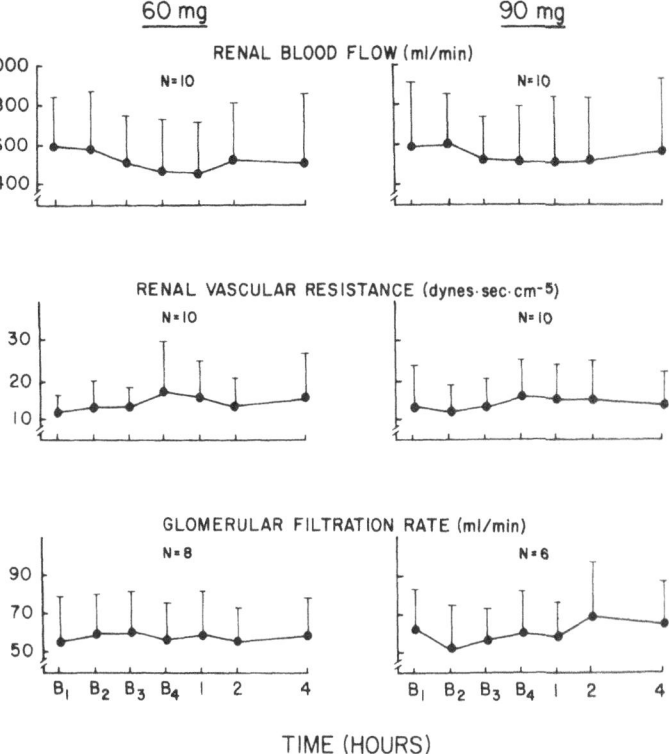

Fig. 2. Sequential effects of 60 mg and 90 mg diltiazem on renal blood flow, renal vascular resistance, and glomerular filtration rate

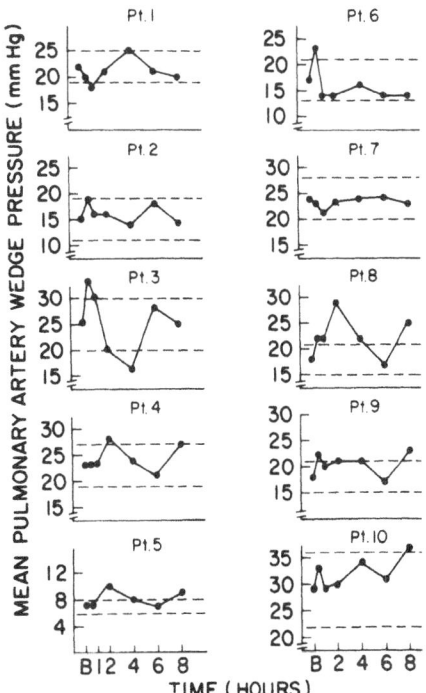

Fig. 3. Individual responses of mean pulmonary artery wedge pressure to 90 mg diltiazem. Baseline (*B*) is reported as the mean value of four consecutive measurements obtained 1 h apart. *Broken lines,* 95% confidence intervals computed for each patient from all four baseline values

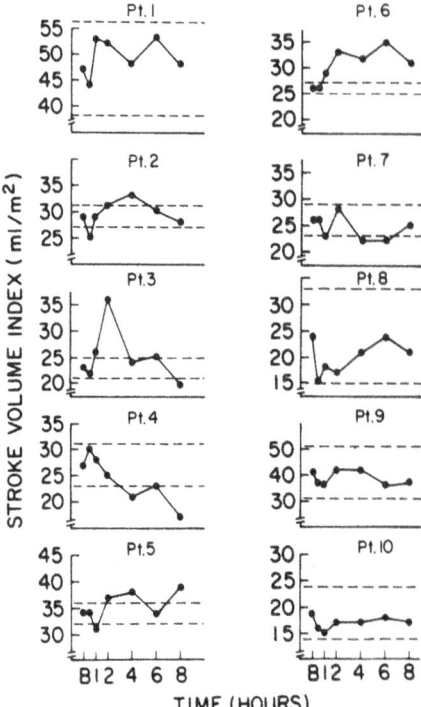

Fig. 4. Individual responses of stroke volume index to 90 mg diltiazem. Abbreviations and symbols as in Fig. 3

in occasional profound hypotension and hemodynamic deterioration [2,3,7]; furthermore, in patients who tolerate the drug, nifedipine has been demonstrated to be less effective than conventional vasodilators in direct comparisons [8,9]. Diltiazem, the third presently available calcium antagonist, possesses the least negative inotropy of the three [4,5] and has been recently evaluated in patients with CHF. In the present study, we found weak and mostly insignificant hemodynamic effects following administration of typical clinical doses of 60 and 90 mg diltiazem. In ten patients with severe LV dysfunction, there was no change overall in either LV filling pressure or stroke volume, nor was any significant change in systemic vascular resistance observed. Examining the data for individual patients however, one finds distinct heterogeneity; following a 90-mg dose of diltiazem, three of ten patients exhibited hemodynamic improvement, as reflected by a sustained rise in SVI. Two of ten patients hemodynamically worsened, as reflected by a sustained rise in PAW or fall in SVI; neither of these two patients exhibited any worsening in clinical status despite these changes.

Walsh et al. [6] administered diltiazem to a small group of patients with comparably severe depression of LV function and, in contrast to our study, found significant hemodynamic improvement with this agent. There are several possible explanations for the observed discrepancies between the two studies. In addition to some methodological differences, the dose of diltiazem employed in the study of Walsh et al. was higher than that in the present study (the majority of their patients received 120 mg); while the possibility of the higher dose being responsible for the observed benefit cannot be excluded, we observed no correlation between plasma diltiazem levels and change in LV SVI in our patients. Finally, in half of the patients in the study of Walsh et al. coronary artery disease was the cause of CHF, and diltiazem-induced relief of ischemia may have contributed to the benefits they noted. While both our study and that of Walsh et al. demonstrate relative safety of diltiazem in patients with severe LV dysfunction, these are both small series of patients, and an occasional patient may still experience clinical deterioration following diltiazem administration; in addition, these are both acute studies, and the safety of chronic diltiazem administration in patients with severe LV dysfunction remains to be evaluated.

Impaired renal blood flow is often observed in patients with CHF and is partly responsible for the sodium retention seen in this state [10]. While certain commonly employed vasodilators may augment renal blood flow [11–13], we were unable to demonstrate a selective beneficial effect on renal hemodynamics following diltiazem administration. In addition, patients with severe CHF commonly have elevated plasma catecholamine and renin levels, which may be of prognostic importance [14,15]; our patients had markedly elevated levels of these hormones, which were not affected by diltiazem administration.

Conclusion

The administration of 60–90 mg diltiazem to ten patients with severe LV dysfunction resulted in weak and essentially insignificant effects on central and renal hemodynamics, although individual patients did show marked variability in response. Based on these findings, diltiazem cannot be recommended as primary vasodilator therapy for CHF; however, if a calcium channel antagonist is indicated for another clinical situation (e.g., arrhythmia control, relief of ischemia) in a patient with concomitant LV dysfunction, diltiazem appears to be the safest of the available agents within this class. However, the occasional hemodynamic worsening which we observed suggests that diltiazem therapy may not be free of risk in this subset of patients.

References

1. Chew CY, Hecht HS, Collett JT, McAllister RG, Singh BN (1981) Influence of severity of ventricular dysfunction on hemodynamic responses to intravenously administered verapamil in ischemic heart disease. Am J Cardiol 47:917–922
2. Elkayam U, Weber L, McKay CR, Rahimtoola SH (1985) Spectrum of acute hemodynamic effects of nifedipine in severe congestive heart failure. Am J Cardiol 56:560–566
3. Brooks N, Cattell M, Pidgeon J, Balcon R (1980) Unpredictable response to nifedipine in severe cardiac failure. Br Med J 281:1324
4. Henry PD (1980) Comparative pharmacology of calcium antagonists: nifedipine, verapamil, and diltiazem. Am J Cardiol 46:1047–1058

5. Stone PH, Antman EM, Muller JE, Braunwald E (1980) Calcium channel blocking agents in the treatment of cardiovascular disorders. II. Hemodynamic effects and clinical applications. Ann Intern Med 93:886–904
6. Walsh RA, Porter CB, Starling MR, O'Rourke RA (1984) Beneficial hemodynamic effects of intravenous and oral diltiazem in severe congestive heart failure. J Am Coll Cardiol 3:1044–1050
7. Packer M, Lee WH, Medina N, Yushak M (1985) Comparative negative inotropic effects of nifedipine and diltiazem in patients with severe left ventricular dysfunction (abstract). Circulation 72:III-275
8. Elkayam U, Weber L, Torkan B, McKay CR, Rahimtoola SH (1984) Comparison of hemodynamic responses to nifedipine and nitroprusside in severe chronic congestive heart failure. Am J Cardiol 53:1321–1325
9. Elkayam U, Weber L, McKay CR, Rahimtoola SH (1984) Differences in hemodynamic response to vasodilation due to calcium channel antagonism with nifedipine and direct-acting agonism with hydralazine in chronic refractory congestive heart failure. Am J Cardiol 54:126–131
10. Leithe ME, Margorien RD, Hermiller JB, Unverferth DV, Leier CV (1984) Relationship between central hemodynamics and regional blood flow in normal subjects and in patients with congestive heart failure. Circulation 69:57–64
11. Cogan JJ, Humphreys MH, Carlson CJ, Rapaport E (1980) Renal effects of nitroprusside and hydralazine in patients with congestive heart failure. Circulation 61:316–323
12. Creager MA, Halperin JL, Bernard DB, Faxon DP, Melidossian CD, Gavras H, Ryan TJ (1981) Acute regional circulatory and renal hemodynamic effects of converting-enzyme inhibition in patients with congestive heart failure. Circulation 64:483–489
13. Elkayam U, Weber L, Campese VM, Massry SG, Rahimtoola SH (1984) Renal hemodynamic effects of vasodilation with nifedipine and hydralazine in patients with heart failure. J Am Coll Cardiol 4:1261–1267
14. Cohn JN, Levine TB, Francis GS, Goldsmith S (1981) Neurohumoral control mechanisms in congestive heart failure. Am Heart J 102:509–514
15. Cohn JN, Levine TB, Olivari MT, Garberg V, Lura D, Francis GS, Simon AB, Rector T (1984) Plasma norepinephrine as a guide to prognosis in patients with chronic congestive heart failure. N Engl J Med 311:819–823

Nisoldipine: Vasodilatory Effects of a Second-Generation Dihydropyridine

S. Jost, W. Rafflenbeul, D. Gulba, H. Hecker, P. Jost, and P.R. Lichtlen

Introduction

The vascular specificity of the second-generation dihydropyridine calcium antagonist nisoldipine is well known; systemic and coronary vascular resistance is
substantially attenuated by nisoldipine whereas myocardial contractility remains
virtually unaffected [1–7]. Therefore, nisoldipine has proven to be effective in the
treatment not only of coronary artery disease [8] but also of heart failure [9–12].
Vasodilation of epicardial coronary stenoses is regarded as another important
antianginal mechanism, since in the presence of a high-grade stenosis in
epicardial coronary arteries the perfusion of the compromised myocardium is
dependent mainly on the resistance of the stenosis [13,14]. Dilation of coronary
stenoses was also documented in several studies with the first-generation dihydropyridine nifedipine [15,16].

The present study investigated the influence of intravenous administration of
two different doses of nisoldipine on angiographically normal and stenotic
epicardial coronary arteries as well as on coronary and systemic resistance vessels.

Patients and Methods

A total of 26 patients with coronary artery disease were consecutively assigned to
two treatment groups for 0.5 mg (group A; 1 woman, 12 men; ages 34–59, mean
54 ± 12 years) or 1.0 mg nisoldipine (group B; 1 woman, 12 men; ages 43–66,
mean 54 ± 8 years). In group A four patients had more than one major coronary
artery diseased with high-grade stenoses (> 50% diameter reduction) versus nine
patients in group B. Three patients in group A had previously undergone PTCA
and/or coronary bypass grafting versus ten patients in group B.

All vasoactive drugs (except nitroglycerin preparations) had been withheld
for at least 16 h prior to the study, which was undertaken at the beginning of a
diagnostic coronary angiography. With the help of an injection pump nisoldipine
was continuously infused over 4 min into the inferior caval vein. Before and 2, 4,
7, 10, and 15 min after onset of the infusion angiograms of the left coronary artery
were taken in identical angiographic projections; on the 35-mm cinefilms
the mean diameters of all 111 angiographically normal coronary segments and the
minimal diameters of 24 stenotic segments were measured with a computer-as-

B.S. Lewis, A. Kimchi (Eds.)
Heart Failure Mechanisms and Management
© Springer-Verlag Berlin Heidelberg 1991

sisted contour analysis system (CAAS). In one patient in group B with all segments diffusely sclerotic, coronary vasomotility was not assessed. In eight patients of group A and nine in group B blood samples were taken from the right femoral vein. Nisoldipine plasma levels were determined by gas chromatography with use of the electron-capture detection technique [17]. Coronary sinus oxygen saturation was assessed in six patients in group A and seven in group B. Systolic and diastolic aortic pressure as well as heart rate were measured in all patients.

In the angiograms end-diastolic frames presenting the coronary arteries in identical positions were selected for quantitative assessment. Coronary segments assigned for analysis had to be free of overlap with other coronary arteries and structures such as bones or diaphragm; furthermore, only segments running nearly parallel to the image plane without considerable shortening effects were selected. Division of the left coronary artery into segments was based on the recommendations of the American Heart Association [18].

In a specially constructed cinevideo converter the frames were magnified 2.8-fold, converted into video format and digitized in a matrix size of 512×512 pixels [19,20]. These data were transferred to a PDP 11/24 minicomputer and to a video monitor for control of the segment contour analysis procedure by the analyzer; the latter could interfere with the procedure with the help of a terminal and a writing tablet (for details see [19,20]). Calibration of the cineframes was performed with the aid of the tip of the coronary catheter of known size. Correction for pin-cushion distortion was available [19]. The vessel-contour detection algorithm is described in detail elsewhere [19,20]. Perpendicular to a center line established in the coronary segment, densitometric measurements were made; the vessel contours were defined on the basis of the weighted sum of the first and second derivative functions of the resulting brightness profile. From the distances between the right and left contour points a diameter function was computed along the center line. The mean diameter of a segment was interpolated from measurements in distances of about 0.1 mm along the center line. The minimal diameter of a stenosis was read from the diameter function.

The one-sample t test was used to test the null hypothesis that the change in mean value of a parameter over a given time interval was zero. Linear regression and Pearson correlation coefficients were used to analyze the relationship between two continuous variables.

Results

The individual courses of the changes in mean diameter of angiographically normal epicardial coronary segments in the two groups are depicted in Fig. 1. The differences in mean segment diameters compared to control values were expressed as percentage changes. Individual values were obtained by averaging the diameter changes of all segments analyzed in the patient. In group A the individual maximal dilation ranged from 3% to 20%, in group B from 7% to 36%. In most patients these maxima were not attained before the end of the study

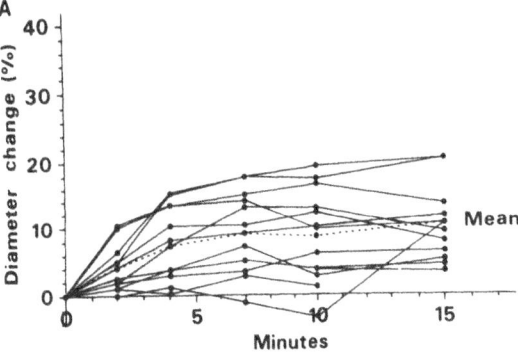

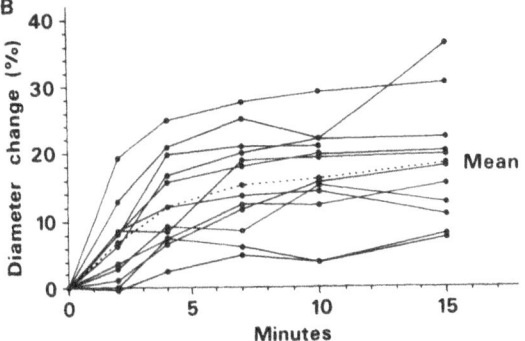

Fig.1A,B. Individual diameter changes in angiographically normal coronary segments averaged for all segments analyzed per patient. **A** Group A. *n* = 13. **B** Group B. *n* = 12

period. Therefore, with both doses the curves of the mean values showed a plateau after the end of the drug infusion, with the tendency to further increase; the average maxima of 11% ± 6% in group A and 18% ± 9% in group B were measured in the 15th min (see Table 1).

The average values of the nisoldipine plasma levels after both doses are presented in Fig. 2. Maximal values were obtained at the end of the infusion, i.e., in the 4th min; these averaged 8 ± 4 ng/ml in group A and 17 ± 7 ng/ml in group B (Table 1). Since in both groups coronary dilation revealed a hysteresis compared to the nisoldipine plasma levels, a correlation between these parameters was not possible at all measurement times of the protocol. However, in group A a significant correlation was found between the individual maximum values of plasma levels and coronary dilation ($r = 0.89$, $p < 0.01$); in contrast, with the higher dose no such correlation existed ($r = -0.19$, NS; Fig. 3).

The minimal diameters of 15 (eight patients) and 9 coronary stenoses (six patients) were assessed in group A and B respectively. The initial minimal diameters of the analyzed lesions and the respective diameters of maximal change with nisoldipine are presented in Fig. 4. The diagonal here represents the level of no diameter change. Eleven stenoses in group A and eight in group B showed a diameter increase after the drug; maximal dilation of these narrowings ranged from 5% to 80% in group A and from 15% to 70% in group B. In four stenoses in group A and in one in group B a slight diameter reduction was observed.

Table 1. Mean values of nisoldipine plasma levels, dilation of angiographically normal coronary segments, coronary sinus oxygen saturation, systolic and diastolic aortic pressures, heart rate, and rate-pressure product with 0.5 mg (group A) and 1.0 mg (group B) intravenous nisoldipine

	Group		Time (min)							
			0	1	2	3	4	7	10	15
Plasma level (ng/ml)	A	(n = 8)	0.0±0.0	0.8±0.7	4.0±2.1	5.8±3.0	7.9±3.6	6.1±3.0	5.2±1.7	4.3±0.9
	B	(n = 9)	0.0±0.0	2.1±3.7	10.9±6.0	13.3±6.0	16.9±7.1	12.0±2.5	10.7±2.1	9.1±2.6
Coronary dilation (%)	A	(n = 13)	—	—	4.3±3.3[b]	—	7.7±5.5[c]	9.3±6.3[c]	8.7±7.1[c]	10.6±5.6[c]
	B	(n = 12)	—	—	7.0±5.9[b]	—	12.7±6.9[c]	15.6±7.2[c]	16.3±7.4[c]	18.1±9.0[c]
Coronary sinus oxygen saturation (%)	A	(n = 6)	31.9±6.6	28.8±4.0	31.6±5.7	36.2±4.3	35.0±5.8	37.9±6.2[a]	38.1±7.0[a]	40.2±6.6[b]
	B	(n = 7)	33.2±5.8	31.6±7.0	40.0±8.9	45.8±7.0[b]	43.7±10.7[a]	42.3±9.3[a]	41.8±8.2[a]	42.3±6.8[b]
Systolic aortic pressure (mmHg)	A	(n = 13)	137±21	133±20	124±21[c]	113±18[c]	109±18[c]	108±17[c]	111±17[c]	115±17[c]
	B	(n = 13)	143±19	131±18[c]	114±16[c]	102±12[c]	96±12[c]	99±13[c]	102±14[c]	108±13[c]
Diastolic aortic pressure (mmHg)	A	(n = 13)	75±9	73±10	68±10[c]	64±9[c]	61±9[c]	59±7[c]	63±8[c]	67±9[b]
	B	(n = 13)	74±11	69±12[b]	62±9[c]	55±9[c]	51±9[c]	52±9[c]	54±10[c]	58±9[b]
Heart rate (min^{-1})	A	(n = 13)	72±12	75±8	78±8[a]	80±8[a]	84±9[b]	81±7[b]	81±6[a]	81±7[a]
	B	(n = 13)	70±10	72±8[a]	85±10[c]	89±11[c]	91±15[c]	90±12[c]	87±12[c]	85±10[c]
Rate-pressure product (10^3 mmHg min^{-1})	A	(n = 13)	10.0±2.6	10.0±2.1	9.8±2.1	9.1±1.8[a]	9.2±1.9	8.8±1.8[a]	9.0±1.8	9.5±2.2
	B	(n = 13)	10.2±2.0	9.7±1.9[a]	9.8±1.7	9.2±1.6[a]	8.9±2.0[b]	9.0±1.8[a]	9.0±2.0[a]	9.3±1.7

Statistical significance measured against t_0.

[a] $p < 0.05$.

[b] $p < 0.01$.

[c] $p < 0.001$.

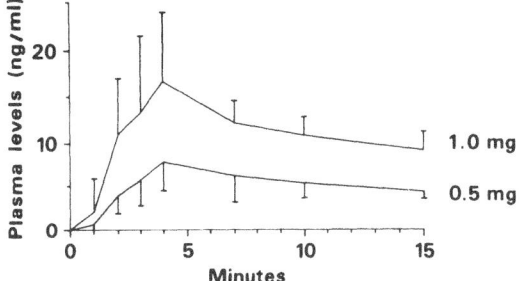

Fig. 2. Average course of the nisoldipine plasma levels during the study period in eight patients of group A and nine patients of Group B

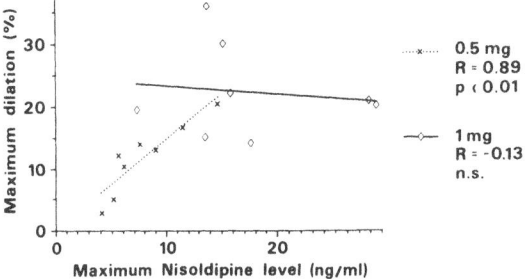

Fig. 3. Correlation in both groups between the individual maximal nisoldipine plasma levels and the respective maximal coronary dilation

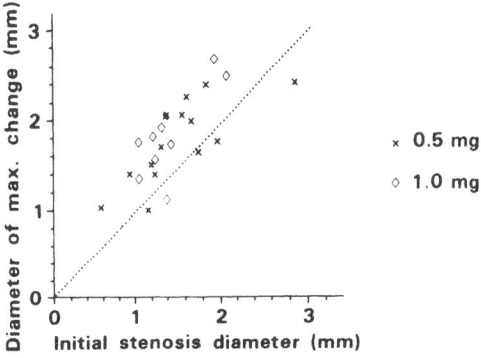

Fig. 4. Maximal changes in minimal diameters of 24 coronary stenoses (group A, $n = 15$; group B, $n = 9$) during the observation period

With both doses of nisoldipine significant changes in coronary venous oxygen saturation were measured (Fig. 5). In group A, the average oxygen saturation increased from $32\% \pm 7\%$ saturation to a maximum of $40\% \pm 7\%$ in the 15th min ($p < 0.01$; Table 1); in group B saturation rose from $33\% \pm 6\%$ to $46\% \pm 7\%$ in the 3rd min ($p < 0.01$) and persisted at a significantly elevated level at least for the rest of the investigation (15th min: $42\% \pm 7\%$; $p < 0.01$). With both doses, significant correlations were found between the individual courses of the changes in coronary sinus oxygen saturation and of the respective average dilation of angiographically normal coronary segments. In group A the individual regression coefficients of these correlations ranged from 0.64 to 0.93 (mean 0.81 ± 0.10), in group B from 0.22 to 0.89 (mean 0.66 ± 0.25; $p < 0.05$).

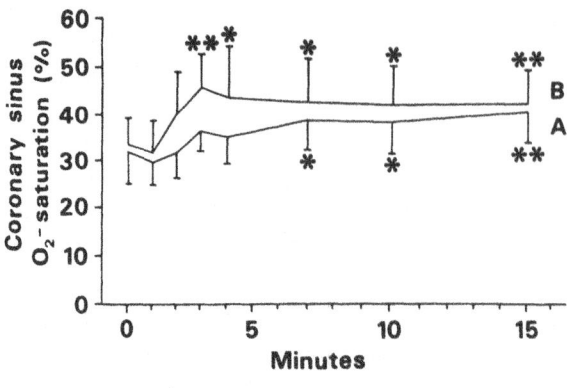

Fig. 5. Mean values of coronary sinus oxygen saturation with 0.5 mg ($n = 6$) and 1.0 mg ($n = 7$) nisoldipine

*p ‹ 0.05, **p ‹ 0.01 compared to control

The changes in systolic and diastolic aortic pressure and in heart rate are presented in detail in Table 1. With both doses of nisoldipine systolic and diastolic pressure decreased significantly ($p < 0.001$); this effect was most pronounced in the 4th or 7th min. At 15 min the diastolic pressure ($p < 0.01$) and particularly the systolic pressure ($p < 0.001$) were still markedly lowered in both groups (Table 1). As a result of the adrenergic counterregulation, heart rate increased significantly in both groups ($p < 0.01$). The rate-pressure product was significantly lowered by both doses of nisoldipine ($p < 0.05$; Table 1).

Discussion

The dilation of those epicardial coronary stenoses which are still capable of vasomotility, i.e., reduction of proximal coronary resistance, plays an important role among the mechanisms of action of antianginal drugs [13,14,15,21,22]. In addition to nitrocompounds [15,21–23], calcium antagonists, particularly nifedipine, have proven to be potent dilators of epicardial coronary arteries and particularly of stenoses [15,16,24]; these compounds also represent powerful drugs in the treatment of vasospasm of largely normal and stenotic epicardial coronary arteries [25]. The vasodilatory efficacy of the new dihydropyridine calcium antagonist nisoldipine on angiographically normal as well as stenotic epicardial coronary arteries is demonstrated in the present study; this effect was most profound after the dose of 1 mg. Since some coronary stenoses are concentric in nature, i.e., they consist of a circumferential atherosclerotic plaque, not all obstructions analyzed showed vasodilation with nisoldipine. Furthermore, it must be noted that the standard deviation of the automatic analysis system CAAS in repeated obstruction diameter measurements in different end-diastolic cineframes in identical angiographic projections (as performed in this study) amounts to about 0.2 mm [20]. Therefore, only changes in obstruction diameters of about 20% or more can be considered reliable.

The maximal drug plasma levels observed with both doses of nisoldipine were considerably lower than comparably effective plasma levels of nifedipine [24,26]. Nisoldipine plasma levels determined at the time of the maximal coronary dilation corresponded to the values usually measured after oral administration of this drug [27]. After the end of the infusion of both doses of nisoldipine the dilation of epicardial coronary arteries tended to increase further to the end of the study period despite declining plasma levels. Since no active metabolites of nisoldipine are known, this hysteresis seems to be a consequence of the high receptor affinity of the compound, which was confirmed in recent receptor binding studies [28,29]. Due to the different courses of nisoldipine plasma levels and coronary dilation a correlation between these parameters at the individual measurement times was not possible. Only with the lower dose did a correlation exist on the basis of the time-independent maximal values, which may also be due to the strong receptor affinity of nisoldipine. As can be concluded from Fig. 3, the correlation between maximal nisoldipine plasma levels and maximal coronary dilation ceased at concentrations above 15 ng/ml. A possible explanation is that even at these low nisoldipine plasma levels a prolonged saturation of most of the available receptors occurred, so that the corresponding maximal coronary dilation could not be further increased by higher drug concentrations.

In recent studies with intravenous nifedipine [24,26] a significant correlation between plasma levels and coronary dilation was found at all measurement times of the protocol, which was quite similar to that in the present study [24]. The hysteresis of the coronary dilation in relation to nisoldipine plasma levels in the present study is in contrast to these results obtained with nifedipine. The persistence of the coronary dilation after nisoldipine is also in contrast to the courses of the hemodynamic changes, which run nearly parallel to the plasma levels, as was demonstrated in this study as well as by other investigators [27]. In the presence of calcium antagonists the reactive catecholamine release following the systemic pressure drop obviously counteracts this drop in systemic resistance but is not able to antagonize considerably the vasodilation of coronary arteries [30].

Dilation of the epicardial coronary arteries paralleled dilation of the coronary arterioles, as indicated by a rise in coronary sinus oxygen saturation. A drop in coronary resistance can be beneficial in coronary artery disease due to the associated rise in myocardial perfusion. Whereas vasodilating drugs such as dipyridamole or chromonar tend to induce a coronary "steal" phenomenon [31,32], calcium antagonists such as nifedipine increase blood supply not only to uncompromised myocardium but also to poststenotic ischemic regions [33,34]. In dogs, nisoldipine enhanced coronary collateral flow to poststenotic regions with a comparable distribution to epicardial and endocardial layers [35]. While in previous clinical studies with intravenous nifedipine coronary blood flow was increased for only a few minutes [36,37], in the present study both dosages of nisoldipine caused a prolonged rise in the coronary venous oxygen saturation, probably due to the slower dissociation of nisoldipine from the binding site [28,29].

Systolic and diastolic blood pressure were substantially reduced with both doses of nisoldipine; at the end of the observation period the pressure values were still markedly lowered. Afterload reduction is an important oxygen-sparing mechanism because it is associated with a considerable drop in myocardial wall tension. In addition, the rate-pressure product declined – particularly after the higher dose – which is also associated with a decrease in myocardial oxygen consumption. Since myocardial contractility is fairly unaffected by nisoldipine, the afterload reduction can result in an increase of ejection fraction and cardiac output, which can be advantageous in heart failure [2,9–12].

Summary

The vasodilatory effect of the second-generation dihydropyridine calcium antagonist nisoldipine on epicardial coronary arteries as well as on coronary and systemic resistance vessels was tested. Two, 4, 7, 10, and 15 min after onset of an intravenous infusion (4 min) of 0.5 mg (13 patients, group A) or 1.0 mg nisoldipine (13 patients, group B) diameter changes of angiographically normal and stenotic epicardial coronary arteries were analyzed with a computer-assisted contour detection system (CAAS). After both doses the maximal increase in mean diameters of normal coronary segments was achieved not before the 15th min, averaging $11\% \pm 6\%$ in group A ($p < 0.001$) and $18\% \pm 9\%$ in group B ($p < 0.001$). Eleven of 15 coronary stenoses in group A and 8 of 9 in group B dilated to 5%–80% and 15%–70% respectively.

Simultaneously the nisoldipine plasma levels were determined in eight patients in group A and nine patients in group B. These were maximal at the end of the infusion (4th min) with an average of 8 ± 4 ng/ml in group A and 17 ± 7 ng/ml in group B. A significant correlation between nisoldipine plasma levels and dilation of normal coronary segments was obtained only with the individual maxima of these parameters and only in group A ($p < 0.01$). The hysteresis of the coronary dilation in relation to the drug plasma levels may be due to the high receptor affinity of nisoldipine.

As a result of the vasodilatory effects of nisoldipine on systemic resistance vessels, systolic and diastolic pressures were profoundly reduced in the patients of either group ($p < 0.001$). Furthermore, both doses of nisoldipine induced a rise in heart rate ($p < 0.01$) and a slight drop in the rate-pressure product ($p < 0.05$).

Acknowledgement. The drug plasma levels were kindly determined by Dr. Gertrud Ahr, Bayer, Wuppertal, FRG. The secretarial assistance of Mrs. Katharina Marx is gratefully acknowledged.

References

1. Kazda S, Garthoff N, Meyer H et al. (1980) Pharmacology of a new calcium antagonistic compound, isobutyl methyl 1,4-dihydro-2, 6-dimethyl-4-(2-nitrophenyl)-3, 5-pyridine-dicarboxylate (nisoldipine, Bay K 5552). Drug Res 30 (II):2144–2162
2. Serruys PW, Suryapranata H, Planellas J et al. (1985) Acute effects of intravenous nisoldipine on left ventricular function and coronary hemodynamics. Am J Cardiol 56:140–146

3. Soward AL, De Feyter PJ, Hugenholtz PG et al. (1986) Coronary and systemic hemodynamic effects of intravenous nisoldipine. Am J Cardiol 58:1199-1203

4. Godfraind T, Egleme C, Finet M et al. (1987) The actions of nifedipine and nisoldipine on the contractile activity of human coronary arteries and human cardiac tissue in vitro. Pharmacol Toxicol 61:79-84

5. Kiowski W, Pfisterer M, Burkart F (1988) Vasodilating and myocardial effects of nisoldipine. In: Lichtlen PR, Hugenholtz PG (eds) Nisoldipine 1988. Schattauer, Stuttagart, pp 58-66

6. Schipke JD, Burkhoff D, Alexander J Jr, Schaefer J, Sagawa K (1988) Effect of nisoldipine on coronary resistance, contractility and oxygen consumption of the isolated blood-perfused canine left ventricle. J Pharmacol Exp Ther 244:1000-1004

7. Godfraind T, Morel N, Wibo M (1988) Mechanisms of the vascular selectivity of nisoldipine. In: Lichtlen PR, Hugenholtz PG (eds) Nisoldipine 1988. Schattauer, Stuttgart, pp 25-37

8. Lam J, Chaitman BR, Crean P et al. (1985) A dose-ranging placebo-controlled, double-blind trial of nisoldipine in effort angina: duration and extent of antianginal effects. J Am Coll Cardiol 6:447-452

9. Kiowski W, Erne P, Pfisterer M et al. (1987) Arterial vasodilator, systemic and coronary hemodynamic effects of nisoldipine in congestive heart failure secondary to ischemic or dilated cardiomyopathy. Am J Cardiol 59:1118-1125

10. Nienaber CA, Spielmann RP, Aschenberg W et al. (1987) Comparison of the acute hemodynamic response to intravenous nisoldipine (Bay K 5552) and intravenous nifedipine for left ventricular dysfunction secondary to myocardial infarction. Am J Cardiol 60:836-841

11. Aschenberg W, Hobuß M, Schofer J, Bleifeld W (1988) Acute and chronic hemodynamic effects of oral nisoldipine versus captopril in ischemic congestive heart failure. In: Lichtlen PR, Hugenholtz PG (eds) Nisoldipine 1988. Schattauer, Stuttgart, pp 77-81

12. Gurne O, Rousseau MF, van Eyll C, Hanet C, Pouleur H (1990) Spontaneous progression of left ventricular dysfunction in ischemic heart disease: a preventive role for nisoldipine?

13. Logan SE (1975) On the fluid mechanics of human coronary artery stenoses. IEEE Trans Biomed Eng 22:327-334

14. Mates RE, Gupta RI, Bell AC et al. (1978) Fluid dynamics of coronary artery stenosis. Circ Res 42:152-162

15. Rafflenbeul W, Lichtlen P (1983) Quantitative coronary angiography – evidence of a sustained increase in vascular smooth muscle tone in coronary artery stenosis. Z Kardiol [Suppl III] 72:87-91

16. Lichtlen P, Rafflenbeul W (1985) Effects of calcium antagonists on fixed and dynamic obstructions in patients with severe coronary artery disease. In: Fleckenstein A, Van Breemen CR, Hoffmeister F (eds) Cardiovascular effects of dihydropyridine-type calcium antagonists and agonists. Springer, Berlin Heidelberg New York, pp 381-407

17. Ahr G, Wingender W, Kuhlmann J (1987) Pharmacokinetics of nisoldipine. In: Hugenholtz PG, Meyer J (eds) Nisoldipine 1987. Springer, Berlin Heidelberg New York, pp 59-66

18. Austen WG, Edwards JE, Frye RL et al. (1975) A reporting system on patients evaluated for coronary artery disease: report of the Ad Hoc Committee for Grading of Coronary Artery Disease, Council on Cardiovascular Surgery, American Heart Association. Circulation [Suppl] 51:5-40

19. Reiber JHC, Serruys PW, Kooijman CJ et al. (1985) Assessment of short-, medium- and long-term variations in arterial dimensions from computer-assisted quantitation of coronary cineangiograms. Circulation 71:280-288

20. Reiber JHC, van Eldik-Helleman P, Visser-Akkerman N et al. (1988) Variabilities in measurement of coronary arterial dimensions resulting from variations in cineframe selection. Cathet Cardiovasc Diagn 14:221-228

21. Rafflenbeul W, Urthaler F, Russell RO et al. (1980) Dilatation of coronary artery stenoses after isosorbide dinitrate in man. Br Heart J 43:546-549

22. Brown BG, Bolson E, Petersen RB et al. (1981) The mechanisms of nitroglycerin action: stenosis vasodilatation as a major component of the drug response. Circulation 64:189-197

23. Jost S, Rafflenbeul W, Knop I et al. (1989) Drug plasma levels and coronary vasodilation after isosorbide dinitrate chewing capsules. Eur Heart J 10 [Suppl F]:137-141

24. Jost S, Rafflenbeul W, Mogwitz B et al. (1989) Coronary vasodilation with dihydropyridines – a pharmacokinetic study. Eur Heart J 10 [Suppl F]: 147–152
25. Heupler FA Jr, Proudfit WL (1979) Nifedipine therapy for refractory coronary arterial spasm. Am J Cardiol 44:789–803
26. Nellessen U, Rafflenbeul W, Jost S et al. (1987) Diameter changes of large epicardial coronary arteries after sublingual or intravenous administration of nifedipine; correlation to plasma levels. Z Kardiol 76:329–339
27. Graefe KH, Ziegler R, Wingender W et al. (1988) Plasma concentration-response relationships for some cardiovascular effects of dihydropyridines in healthy subjects. Clin Pharmacol Ther 43:16–22
28. Pan M, Janis RA, Triggle DJ (1983) Comparison of the equilibrium and kinetic binding characteristics of tritiated calcium channel inhibitors, nisoldipine, nimodipine, nitrendipine and nifedipine. Pharmacologist 25:202
29. Janis RA, Shrikhande AV, Greguski R et al. (1985) Review of nisoldipine binding studies. In: Hugenholtz PG, Meyer J (eds) Nisoldipine 1987. Springer, Berlin Heidelberg New York, pp 27–35
30. Heusch G, Deussen A (1984) Nifedipine prevents sympathetic vasoconstriction distal to severe coronary stenoses. J Cardiovasc Pharmacol 6:378–383
31. Nakamura M, Nakagaki O, Nose Y, Fukumaya T, Kikuchi Y (1978) Effects of nitroglycerin and dipyridamole on regional myocardial blood flow. Basic Res Cardiol 73:482–496
32. Warltier DC, Gross GJ, Brooks HL et al. (1980) Coronary steal-induced increase in myocardial infarct size after pharmacologic coronary vasodilation. Am J Cardiol 46:83–90
33. Lichtlen P, Engel HJ (1976) Coronary dynamics of various antianginal drugs at rest and during exercise measured by the precordial xenon residue detection technique. In: Lichtlen PR (ed) Coronary angiography and angina pectoris. Thieme, Stuttgart, pp 365–377
34. Heusch G, Guth BD, Seitelberger R et al. (1987) Attenuation of exercise-induced myocardial ischemia in dogs with recruitment of coronary vasodilator reserve by nifedipine. Circulation 75:482–490
35. Warltier DC, Meils CM, Gross GJ et al. (1981) Blood flow in normal and acutely ischemic myocardium after verapamil, diltiazem and nisoldipine (Bay K 5552), a new dihydropyridine calcium antagonist. J Pharmacol Exp Ther 228:296–302
36. Schanzenbächer P, Liebau G, Deeg P et al. (1983) Effect of intravenous and intracoronary nifedipine on coronary blood flow and myocardial oxygen consumption. Am J Cardiol 51:712–717
37. Kaltenbach M, Schulz W, Kober G (1979) Effects of nifedipine after intravenous and intracoronary administration. Am J Cardiol 44:832–836

Acute Hemodynamic Effects
of Nisoldipine in Patients with Coronary Artery Disease
and Reduced Left Ventricular Function

S. Ghio, S. De Servi, E. Bramucci, L. Angoli, P. Cioffi, L. Piatti, and G. Specchia

Nisoldipine is a calcium channel blocking agent with dihydropyridinic structure, chemically derived from the first calcium antagonist dihydropyridine nifedipine. Its pharmacological properties differ from those of the parent drug in that nisoldipine appears to be a more potent and selective vasodilator of vascular smooth muscle, thus showing at equihypotensive doses less depressant effects upon myocardial contractility [1]. The possibility to achieve effective vasodilation in the coronary circulation [2] without the risk of a negative inotropic action would be extremely useful in the treatment of patients with coronary artery disease (CAD) and reduced myocardial contractile function. The present study was undertaken to further elucidate the acute hemodynamic effects of nisoldipine in patients with CAD and impaired left ventricular function.

Materials and Methods

Patient Selection. Thirteen patients (12 men and 1 woman; mean age 54 ± 12 years) were selected among those undergoing diagnostic cardiac catheterization in our laboratory. All patients had a previous Q wave myocardial infarction, diagnosed on the basis of a typical enzyme curve (creatine kinase and lactic dehydrogenase) and evolving electrocardiographic abnormalities, and all showed clinical signs of heart failure (NYHA class II or III). Patients with associated valvular heart disease were excluded from the study. Informed written consent was obtained before the study.

Cardiac Catheterization and Data Acquisition. Cardiac catheterization was performed with patients in fasting state, premedicated with diazepam (10 mg per os), through the femoral percutaneous approach. Vasodilator therapy, including nitrates and calcium antagonists, was discontinued 12 h before the study; no patient was taking digitalis. After selective coronary arteriography an 8-F micromanometer tipped catheter was advanced to the left ventricle (LV) for injection of contrast media and simultaneous LV pressure measurements. The micromanometer system was calibrated electronically after equilibration against the pressure recorded via the fluid-filled catheter. The zero-pressure reference was set at midchest. Left ventriculography was performed under control conditions and after nisoldipine in 30° RAO projection, injecting 40–45 ml contrast

B.S. Lewis, A. Kimchi (Eds.)
Heart Failure Mechanisms and Management
© Springer-Verlag Berlin Heidelberg 1991

media (iopamidol) at 8–12 ml/s. Films were exposed at 50 frames per second using a 35-mm cine camera. The simultaneous pressure curve was recorded at 250 mm/s paper speed together with the ECG, and a timing reference system marked the paper at the time of each cine exposure.

Protocol. Hemodynamic parameters were determined under control conditions (at least 15 min after coronary angiography); then the first left ventriculography was performed. After a pause of 15 min to allow dissipation of the hemodynamic effects of the contrast media, nisoldipine was administered (6 μg/kg over 3 min). Seven to ten minutes after nisoldipine administration, hemodynamic measurements were repeated, and the second left ventriculography was performed.

Data Analysis. The first available, adequately opacified, non-postextrasystolic beat was chosen for analysis. LV contours were traced manually with a light pen upon a digitizer interfaced with a Tagarno projector and a Digital PDP 11/23 computer. LV volumes were calculated according to the Dodge method. End-diastolic (EDVI) and end-systolic (ESVI) volumes were selected as the ones with the maximum and minimum volumes, respectively, and ejection fraction (EF) was calculated as (EDVI − ESVI)/EDVI. Quantitative segmental wall motion was studied according to the Stanford method [3]. Starting from the anterior aortoventricular junction the LV was divided into five areas (in clockwise direction: anterobasal, anterolateral, apical, diaphragmatic, and posterobasal), and an area ejection fraction (AEF) was calculated as: (end-diastolic area − end-systolic area)/end-diastolic area. In all patients the relationship between each LV area and the extent of coronary artery disease was assessed; if an area was supplied by a diseased coronary vessel, it was defined as a CAD area. Pressure and volume data were matched every 20 ms in the interval between minimal diastolic and peak a wave pressure and fitted using a least squares technique to the monoexponential function: $P = beKV$, where P = LV pressure (mmHg), V = LV volume (ml), e = base of the natural log, b = data constant, and K = rate constant of the function, which was used as an index of LV chamber stiffness. The intercept on the pressure axis at zero volume was derived by exponential extrapolation and was used to indicate the relative position of the curve on the P-V plot. Peak LV pressure, end-diastolic pressure, minimal diastolic pressure, peak positive dP/dt and maximum $dP/dt/P$ were obtained on-line, mediated over a four- to six-beat period. LV relaxation was analyzed off-line in terms of peak negative dP/dt and T, time constant of the exponential LV pressure decay during isovolumic relaxation. T was computed in the interval between peak negative dP/dt and the time at which pressure fell 5 mmHg above the following end-diastolic pressure, according to the method of Raff and Glantz [4], as the negative inverse slope of the linear function of dP/dt versus P.

Statistical Analysis. Data are expressed as mean ± standard deviation. Group data obtained before and after nisoldipine were compared using the paired t test. Linear regression analysis was also performed to look for significant relationships between variables.

Results

Systolic Function. Intravenous administration of nisoldipine induced a significant decrease in LV systolic pressure (from 122.2 ± 17.4 to 98.4 ± 13.2 mmHg, $p < .001$; Table 1). Heart rate increased (from 72.6 ± 12.4 to 82.2 ± 12.6 bpm, $p < .005$). Peak positive dP/dt decreased (from 1074 ± 195 to 964 ± 207 mmHg s⁻¹, $p < .001$). Maximum positive $dP/dt/P$ did not change significantly (from 21.7 ± 4.0 to 22.9 ± 4.1 s⁻¹, NS). EF increased markedly (from 33.6 ± 10.1 to 44.8 ± 13.1, $p < .001$). A EF increased by an average of 5% in the 6 normokinetic non-CAD areas, 9% in the 5 normokinetic CAD areas, 35% in the 13 dissinergic non-CAD areas, and 29% in the 36 dissinergic CAD areas ($p < .05$; Fig. 1).

Diastolic Function. EDVI did not change after nisoldipine (from 143.7 ± 37.6 to 144.2 ± 35.5 ml m⁻², NS; Table 2). Both end-diastolic and minimal diastolic pressures were slightly but significantly reduced (from 21.9 ± 7.4 to 19.0 ± 16.1

Table 1. Systolic hemodynamics and LV function before and after nisoldipine

	Control	Nisoldipine	Change (%)	p
LV systolic pressure (mmHg)	122.2 ± 17.4	98.4 ± 13.2	−20	< .001
Heart rate (beats min⁻¹)	72.6 ± 12.4	82.2 ± 12.6	+ 13	< .005
Peak positive dP/dt (mmHg s⁻¹)	1074 ± 195	964 ± 207	−10	< .001
Maximum $dP/dt/P$ (s⁻¹)	21.7 ± 4.0	22.9 ± 4.1	+ 0.1	NS
Ejection fraction	33.6 ± 10.1	44.8 ± 13.1	+ 33	< .001

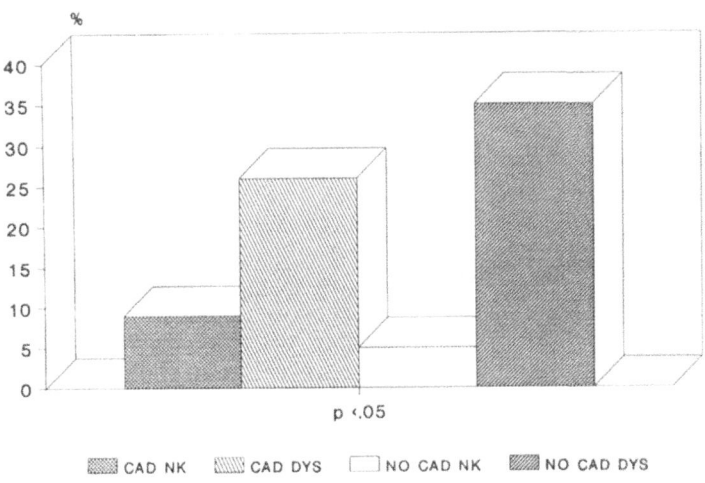

Fig. 1. Percentage change in area ejection fraction after nisoldipine in normokinetic areas supplied by diseased coronary vessels (*CAD NK*), dyssinergic areas supplied by diseased coronary vessels (*CAD, DYS*), normokinetic areas supplied by normal coronary vessels (*NO CAD NK*). and dyssinergic areas supplied by normal coronary vessels (*NO CAD DYS*)

Table 2. Diastolic hemodynamics and LV volumes before and after nisoldipine

	Control	Nisoldipine	Change (%)	p
LV end-diastolic volume (ml m^{-2})	143.7 ± 37.6	144.2 ± 35.5	$+ 0.1$	NS
LV end-diastolic pressure (mmHg)	21.9 ± 7.4	19.0 ± 16.1	-13	$< .05$
LV minimal diastolic pressure (mmHg)	9.7 ± 2.8	8.2 ± 2.5	-15	$< .05$
Peak negative dP/dt (mmHg s^{-1})	945 ± 143	822 ± 171	-13	$< .05$
T constant of isovolumic relaxation (ms)	48.7 ± 10.6	40.2 ± 9.2	-17	$< .02$
Rate constant K of LV passive P-V relation (mmHg s^{-1})	0.013 ± 0.009	0.013 ± 0.008	0.0	NS
Pressure intercept of LV P-V relation (mmHg)	1.7 ± 1.5	1.1 ± 0.9	$- 3.5$	NS

mmHg, $p < .05$, and from 9.7 ± 2.8 to 8.2 ± 2.5 mmHg, $p < .05$, respectively). Peak negative dP/dt decreased (from 945 ± 143 to 822 ± 171 mmHg s^{-1}, $p < .05$). The T constant of isovolumic relaxation also decreased from 48.7 ± 10.6 to 40.2 ± 9.2 ms, $p < .02$). The extent of decrease in T was more evident at higher baseline T levels ($Y = 25.7 - 0.7 X$, $r = 0.66$, $p < .05$), and it was not significantly related to changes in heart rate ($r = -0.34$), systolic pressure ($r = -0.19$), or end-diastolic pressure ($r = -0.41$) (Fig. 2). The mean correlation coefficients of the diastolic fit to the monoexponential function $P = beKV$ were 0.91 for control data and 0.88 for nisoldipine data. The rate constant K of this function did not change (from .013 $\pm$ .009 to .013 $\pm$ .008 mmHg s^{-1}, NS); the intercept b of this curve decreased, although not significantly (from 1.7 ± 1.5 to 1.1 ± 0.9 mmHg, NS).

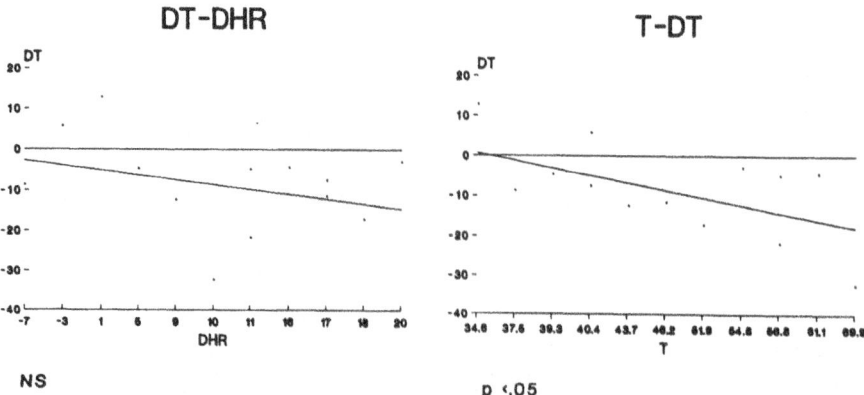

Fig. 2. Correlation between increase in heart rate and decrease in T (DT-DHR) and between baseline relaxation rate and change in relaxation after nisoldipine (T-DT)

Discussion

In our patients the acute administration of nisoldipine reduced peak systolic pressure by an average 25%, and a reflex increase in heart rate was observed. The contractility index maximum $dP/dt/P$ did not change significantly. Since an increase in contractility is expected in relation to an increase in heart rate [5], the lack of increase in maximum $dP/dt/P$ in our patients might be interpreted as a slightly negative inotropic effect of nisoldipine. Negative inotropic effects were not observed in a previous study [2], most likely because the authors reported the effects of the drug in patients with globally preserved LV function (mean EF = 0.51), whereas we investigated a population of patients with a reduced myocardial contractile function (mean EF = 0.33). EF increased in all patients, by an average of 30%. Segmental wall motion analysis showed that regional EF increased in hypokinetic areas, where they supplied by normal or abnormal coronary arteries, suggesting that the improvement in systolic contraction was due to the reduction in load and wall tension rather than to any effect of nisolpidine on the coronary circulation.

A slight but significant decrease in LV filling pressures was observed after nisolpidine. A previous report indicates that nisoldipine reduces cardiac preload in patients with chronic heart failure [6]. We did not measure venous tone, and it is impossible to ascertain from our data whether the LV diastolic pressure decrease was secondary to a direct action of nisoldipine on venous smooth muscle or a consequence of the improvement in relaxation rate. Indeed the T constant of isovolumic relaxation decreased by an average of 16.6%, and this effect was more pronounced in patients with a greater impairment of relaxation under control conditions. It must be said that spontaneous heart rate was higher after nisolpidine than in control conditions, and this would bias a comparison of T values obtained before and after the drug. We do not believe, however, that the decrease in T in our data may be simply explained by the increase in heart rate for two reasons: (a) in the original study of Weisfeldt [7] the relationship between T and heart rate was such that for a 50% increase in heart rate an 8% decrease in T was observed, whereas we noted a 16.6% decrease in T in association with a 14% increase in heart rate; (b) no significant relationship was found in our data between heart rate and T changes.

Furthermore, even if we had studied the patients at matched paced heart rate, it would have been impossible to correct for the increase in circulating cathecolamines and neurally released cathecolamines, which is also part of the general sympathetic activation elicited by a rapid reduction in afterload. Cathecolamines accelerate intracellular inactivation mechanisms [8], and this is the most likely explanation for the decrease in T in our data.

It is interesting to note, however, that the marked improvement in relaxation rate after nisoldipine administration partially contrasts with the lack of increase of the contractility index maximum $dP/dt/P$ which suggests, as discussed above, a slightly negative inotropic effect of nisoldipine. Contraction and relaxation are two strictly interrelated processes: biochemical mechanisms leading to calcium influx during contraction and calcium efflux during relaxation must be coupled to avoid calcium depletion or accumulation into the cell. Even though this coupling is variable and probably different in CAD and non-CAD patients [9], interventions which impair contractility (such as intracoronary calcium antagonists) also impair LV relaxation [10]. Studies aimed at evaluating the direct effects of nisoldipine on myocardial function (i.e., with intracoronary administration of the drug) are clearly required to establish the specific action of nisoldipine upon myocardial relaxation.

Finally, the rate constant of diastolic P-V relation was not changed after nisoldipine, but the intercept of the curve on the pressure axis was slightly reduced, indicating a downward displacement of the whole curve. Such modifications are probably related to the reduction in preload and changes in the external constraints to the LV, namely the right ventricle and the pericardium [11], whereas LV distensile properties were left unmodified by the drug.

In conclusion, our study demonstrates that the acute intravenous administration of nisoldipine in patients with CAD and impaired LV function determines a marked reduction in LV afterload without inducing overt depressant effects upon myocardial contractility and significantly improving LV relaxation.

References

1. Kazda S, Garthoff B, Meyer H, Schossmann K, Stoepel K, Towart R, Vater W, Wehinger E (1980) Pharmacology of a new calcium antagonistic compound, isobutyl methyl 1,4 dihydro-2,6 dimethyl-4-(2 nitrophenyl)-3,5 pyridinedicarboxylate (nisoldipine, Bay K 5552). Arzneimittelforschung 30(II)12:2144
2. Serruys PW, Suryapranata H, Planellas S, Wijns W, Vanhaleweyk GLS, Soward A, Jaski B, Hugenholtz PG (1985) Acute effects of intravenous nisoldipine on left ventricular function and coronary hemodynamics. Am J Cardiol 56:140
3. Ingels NB, Daughters GT, Stinson EB, Alderman EL (1980) Evaluation of methods for quantitating left ventricular segmental wall motion in man using myocardial markers as a standard. Circulation 61:966
4. Raff GL, Glantz SA (1981) Volume loading slows left ventricular isovolumic relaxation rate. Evidence of load-dependent relaxation in the intact dog heart. Circ Res 48:813
5. Covell SW, Ross S, Taylor R, Sonnenblick EH, Braunwald E (1967) Effects of increasing frequency of contraction on force-velocity relation of left ventricle. Cardiovasc Res 1:2
6. Vogt A, Kreutzer H (1983) Hemodynamic effects of nisoldipine in chronic congestive heart failure. Arzneimittelforschung 33:877
7. Weiss SL, Frederiksen JW, Weisfeldt ML (1976) Hemodynamic determinants of the time course of fall in canine left ventricular pressure. J Clin Invest 58:751
8. Nayler WG, Williams A (1978) Relaxation in heart muscle: some morphological and biochemical considerations. Eur J Cardiol [Suppl] 7:35
9. Rousseau MF, Pouleur H, Detry JMR, Brasseur LA (1981) Relationship between changes in left ventricular inotropic state and relaxation in normal subjects and in patients with coronary artery disease. Circulation 64:736
10. Rousseau MF, Veriter F, Detry JMR, Brasseur LA, Pouleur H (1980) Impaired early left ventricular relaxation in coronary artery disease. Effects of intracoronary nifedipine. Circulation 62:764
11. Alderman EL, Glantz SA (1976) Acute hemodynamic interventions shift the diastolic pressure-volume curve in man. Circulation 54:662

Acute and Chronic Effects of Nisoldipine in Patients with Chronic Heart Failure

M. Metra, S. Nodari, T. Guaini, R. Danesi, C. Ceconi, R. Ferrari, and L. Dei Cas

Introduction

In patients with heart failure, excessive rise in systemic vascular resistance leads to further impairment of left ventricular (LV) systolic function. Thus arterial vasodilators have been introduced as agents to improve hemodynamics. Calcium antagonists are among the most powerful arterial vasodilating drugs and have been proposed as myocardial unloading agents in the treatment of patients with depressed LV function [7,9,10,15]. However, their use has yielded controversial results, and in some studies a significant percentage of patients showed hemodynamic deterioration after acute or chronic administration [1,3,4,13], due to the negative inotropic activity and neurohumoral activation consequent to the excessive fall in peripheral resistances. To overcome these limitations new calcium antagonists with a more selective action on smooth muscle have been synthesized. Nisoldipine is a new dihydropyridine derivative characterized by a more potent action on peripheral vascular smooth muscle and by a longer half-life than the parent compound nifedipine [5]. This drug therefore seems particularly useful for the treatment of patients with heart failure as it presents a more selective action on peripheral resistances with less direct negative inotropic effects. Nisoldipine has been shown to exert favorable acute hemodynamic effects [11,17–19]; however, its effect during chronic treatment and on exercise capacity are still partially unsettled.

The aim of our study was to assess the acute and chronic effects of nisoldipine on the central rest and exercise hemodynamics and exercise capacity of patients with chronic heart failure.

Patients and Methods

The study group consists of ten patients (nine men and one woman; mean age 54 ± 11 years) with chronic congestive heart failure; all the patients were clinically stable at least 3 months before entry into the study. Five patients were in New York Heart Association functional class II and five in class III. The cause of heart failure was idiopathic cardiomyopathy in six patients and ischemic heart disease in four. No patients had angina or clinical or electrocardiographic signs of acute myocardial ischemia in the 3 months before the study. All patients had severe LV

B.S. Lewis, A. Kimchi (Eds.)
Heart Failure Mechanisms and Management
© Springer-Verlag Berlin Heidelberg 1991

dysfunction (LV ejection fraction < 0.35) and mild to moderate impairment of exercise capacity (maximal $VO_2 < 25$ ml kg^{-1} min^{-1}).

Each patient underwent right heart catheterization using a triple lumen Swan-Ganz catheter inserted percutaneously through an antecubital vein and positioned in the pulmonary artery. Measured hemodynamic variables included systolic and diastolic pulmonary artery pressure (PAS and PAD), pulmonary capillary wedge pressure (PCWP), and mean right atrial pressure (RAP). Cardiac output (CO) was determined in triplicate by the thermodilution technique. When PAD was identical to PCWP, the former was used as an index of the PCWP itself. Systolic and diastolic arterial blood pressure (SBP and DBP) was automatically obtained by cuff sphygmomanometry using the Dinamap 845 vital signs monitor. Heart rate (HR) was obtained from a continuously monitored electrocardiogram. The derived hemodynamic parameters of cardiac index (CI), stroke volume index (SVI), mean systemic and pulmonary arterial pressures (MAP and PAP), and systemic and pulmonary vascular resistances (SVR and PVR) were calculated according to the standard formulas [20].

During the hemodynamic study each patient underwent a maximal symptom-limited bicycle exercise testing with respiratory gas monitoring. Exercise testing was carried out with the patient in the sitting position starting at a workload of 20 W with workload increments of 20 W every 2 min up to the apperance of limiting dyspnea or fatigue; no patient complained of angina during the test. The electrocardiogram and the respiratory parameters, oxygen consumption (VO_2), CO_2 production, and minute ventilation were monitored continuously during the test. Hemodynamic measurements were obtained at rest, during the last minute of each workload increment, and at maximal exercise.

A supine resting hemodynamic study was performed in every patient to evaluate the acute effects of 10 and 20 mg oral nisoldipine and to assess the individual optimal dose. This dose was defined as the one which determined the greatest hemodynamic improvement without significant side effects. Two patients did not tolerate the dose of 20 mg; one had previous atrial fibrillation and presented excessive tachycardia after nisoldipine 20 mg, and the other complained of intense headache and had a skin rash with the 20-mg dose.

The day after the supine resting hemodynamic study each patient underwent a maximal symptom-limited bicycle exercise test before and 1 h after the administration of the individual optimal dose of nisoldipine.

All patients were reevaluated by right heart catheterization and exercise testing after 2–3 months of chronic therapy with nisoldipine (20 mg bid in eight patients and 10 mg bid in two). Exercise testing was performed 1 h after the last administered dose of nisoldipine and after 24 h of washout from this drug.

Blood samples for the determination of plasma norepinephrine and epinephrine were obtained with the patient in the sitting position at rest and at maximal exercise before and after acute and chronic nisoldipine therapy and nisoldipine washout. Plasma catecholamine concentrations were measured by high-pressure liquid chromatography.

Digitalis, diuretics, and antiarrhythmic drugs were kept constant throughout the chronic phase of the study. Diuretics were always administered at least 12 h

before each hemodynamic evaluation. All vasodilators were withheld at least 72 h
before entry into the study.

Results are expressed as mean ± standard deviation. The paired student's *t*
test was used to evaluate significativity. A *p* value of < 0.05 was considered
indicative of statistical significance.

Results

The supine resting hemodynamic response to nisoldipine is presented in Fig. 1.
This drug induced significant hemodynamic changes which persisted up to 5 h
after its administration. The CI and SVI were significantly increased, with the
peak effect occurring after 1 h (from 3.06 ± 0.46 to 4.42 ± 1.55 l min^{-1} m^{-2} and
from 45 ± 9 to 59 ± 17 ml/beat per square meter). Concomitantly, the MAP
decreased progressively from 97 ± 8 to a nadir of 85 ± 11 mmHg at 3 h, and the
SVR declined from 1328 ± 180 to a nadir of 873 ± 238 dyne sec^{-1} cm^{-5} after 1 h.
The reduction in MAP and SVR persisted throughout the 6-h observation period
with significant values up to 5 h after nisoldipine administration. The HR and
right atrial and pulmonary pressures were not significantly changed.

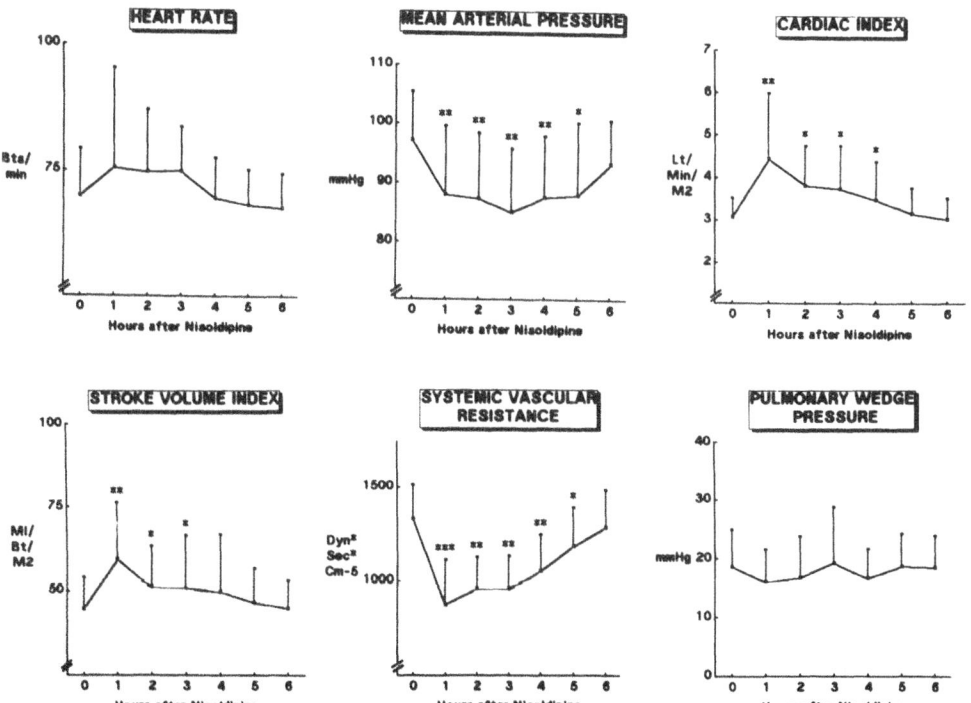

Fig. 1. Time course of the supine resting hemodynamic changes induced by the acute oral administration of 20 mg nisoldipine. *$p < 0.05$; **$p < 0.01$; ***$p < 0.001$ versus control data

The results obtained at rest in the sitting position were similar to those previously observed (Fig. 2). The acute administration of nisoldipine induced a significant increase in CI and SVI (2.41 ± 0.91 to 3.24 ± 1.51 l min^{-1} m^{-2} and 32 ± 12 to 38 ± 17 ml/beat per square meter) with a concomitant reduction in MAP and SVR (96 ± 10 to 81 ± 5 mmHg and 1839 ± 535 to 1192 ± 403 dyne s^{-1} cm^{-5}, respectively). In the sitting position, HR was slightly but significantly increased (from 77 ± 12 to 87 ± 18 beats/min) after the acute administration of nisoldipine. The right atrial and pulmonary pressures did not change significantly, similarly to the results obtained in the supine position.

At restudy after 2–3 months of therapy with oral nisoldipine, resting CI (3.11 ± 1.22 l min^{-1} m^{-2}), SVI (46 ± 14 ml/beat per square meter), MAP (89 ± 9 mmHg), and SVR (1345 ± 467 dyne s^{-1} cm^{-5}) were still changed from baseline but were not significantly different from the values observed after acute administration. HR, on the other hand, significantly decreased (72 ± 9 beats/min) from the values obtained after acute nisoldipine administration and was not significantly different from the baseline.

Withdrawal of nisoldipine caused a fall in resting CI (2.59 ± 0.99 l min^{-1} m^{-2}) and SVI (38 ± 14 ml/beat per square meter) with a concomitant rise in MAP (100 ± 14 mmHg) and SVR (1784 ± 644 dyne s^{-1} cm^{-5}).

At maximal exercise (Fig. 3) the acute administration of nisoldipine caused a significant increase in CI (6.77 ± 2.53 to 7.32 ± 2.65 l min^{-1} m^{-2}) and SVI (45 ±

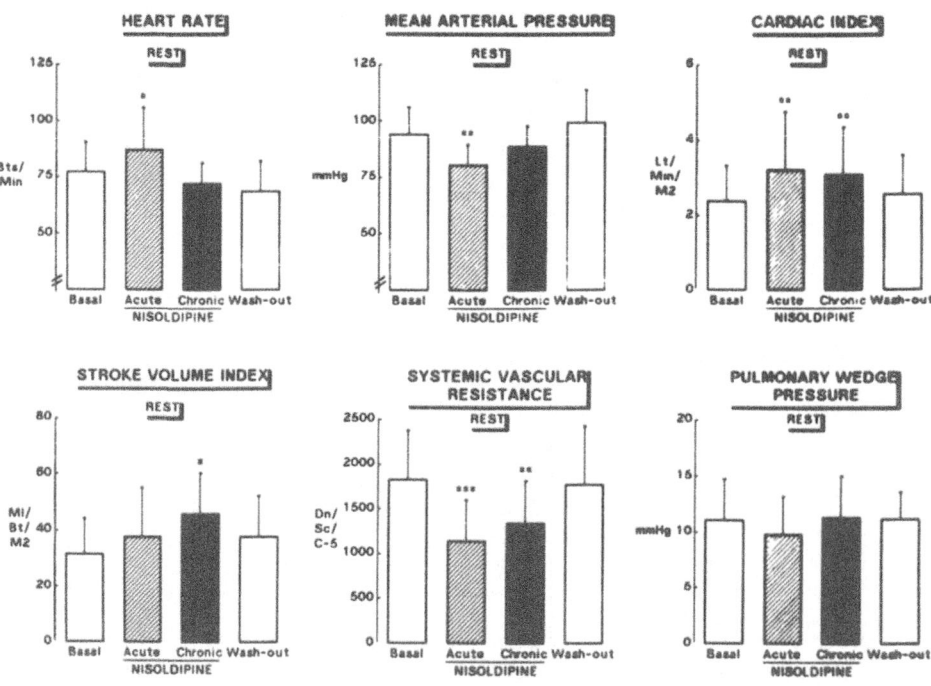

Fig. 2. Sitting resting hemodynamic data at baseline, after acute and chronic nisoldipine administration and 24 h after withdrawal of this drug (wash-out). (Significance as in Fig. 1)

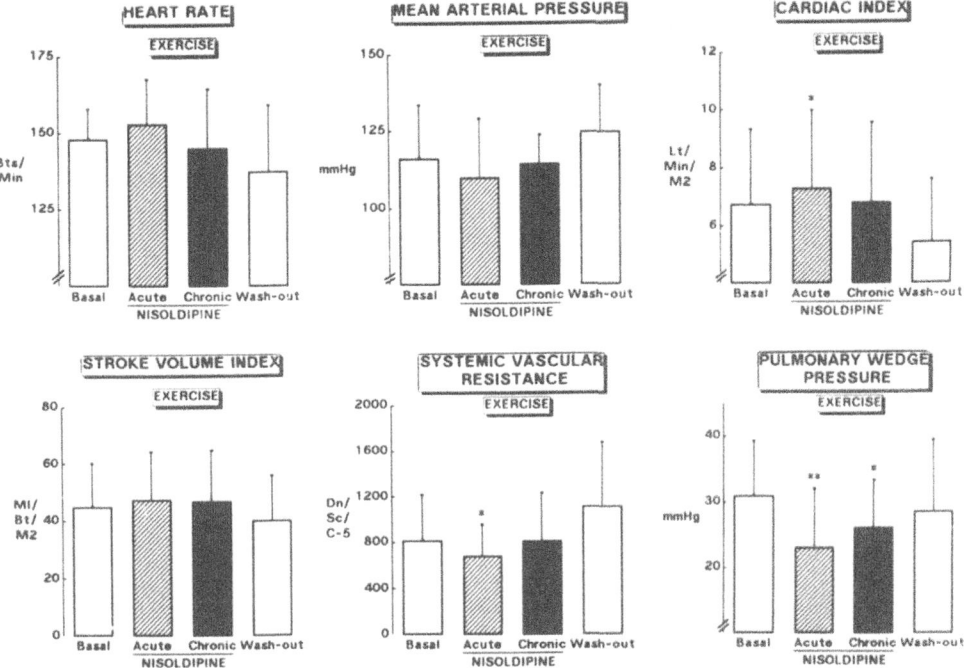

Fig. 3. Sitting maximal exercise hemodynamics at baseline, after acute and chronic nisoldipine administration and 24 h after the withdrawal of this drug (wash-out). (Significance as in Fig. 1)

16 to 48 $\pm$ 17 ml/beat per square meter) with a reduction in SVR (817 $\pm$ 392 to 685 $\pm$ 264 dyne s^{-1} cm^{-5}). Maximal HR, MAP, and RAP were not significantly changed. Differently from the results obtained at rest, PAP and PCWP were significantly reduced from the control values (39 $\pm$ 11 to 30 $\pm$ 9 and 32 $\pm$ 9 to 25 $\pm$ 8 mmHg, respectively).

After chronic therapy the exercise hemodynamic response to nisoldipine was less evident and the CI (6.83 $\pm$ 2.71 l min^{-1} m^{-2}) and SVI (50 $\pm$ 18 ml/beat per square meter) were not significantly different from the control values obtained at maximal exercise. Also the pulmonary pressures, because of the interindividual variability in their response, did not significantly change from the control values. The maximal exercise SVR, on the other hand, was still significantly reduced (813 $\pm$ 416 dyne s^{-1} cm^{-5}).

Nisoldipine withdrawal caused slight rebound changes in exercise hemodynamics. The SVR rose over control values (1114 $\pm$ 559 dyne s^{-1} cm^{-5}) while the exercise CI was slightly decreased (5.45 $\pm$ 2.12 l min^{-1} m^{-2}).

Exercise capacity, evaluated both as maximal exercise duration and maximal VO$_2$, was not significantly changed during either acute or chronic nisoldipine therapy (Fig. 4).

Plasma norepinephrine levels increased, though not significantly, after acute and chronic nisoldipine therapy (from 389 $\pm$ 108 to 580 $\pm$ 195 and 561 $\pm$ 130 pg/ml at rest and from 1856 $\pm$ 1776 to 1882 $\pm$ 1485 and 2441 $\pm$ 1142 pg/ml at

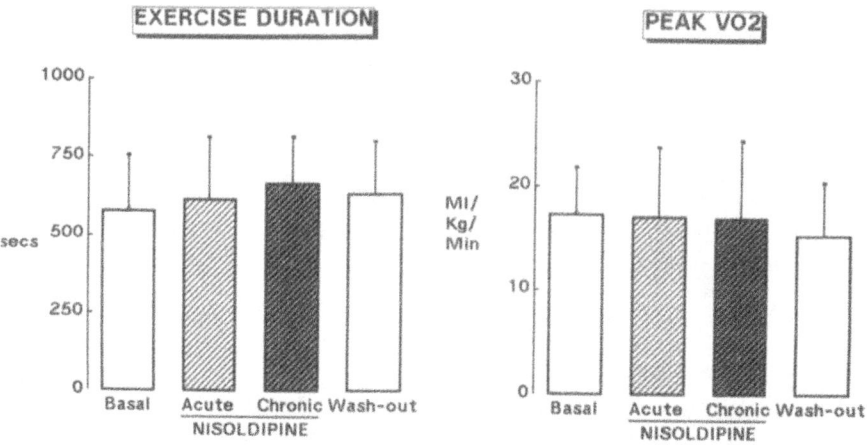

Fig. 4. Maximal exercise performance, evaluated both as total exercise duration and maximal oxygen uptake at baseline, after acute and chronic nisoldipine therapy, and 24 h after the withdrawal of this drug (wash-out)

maximal exercise); on the other hand, no significant change in epinephrine plasma concentrations was noted.

Discussion

Despite their potential usefulness as peripheral unloading agents calcium antagonists have often yielded disappointing results both in the acute and chronic therapy of the patients with heart failure. These findings have been related both to the negative inotropic activity and to the neurohumoral activation consequent to the peripheral vasodilation. The negative inotropic activity can cause an hemodynamic impairment already evident after the acute administration of these compounds while the neurohumoral activation might cause hydrosaline retention and an attenuation of the drug vasodilatatory activity during chronic treatment. To overcome these limits new calcium antagonists with a greater vascular selectivity have recently been synthesized. Nisoldipine is one of the most powerful and selective calcium antagonists on vascular smooth muscle. Because of its high selectivity for peripheral vessels this drug has been shown to be almost completely devoid of any negative inotropic activity when administered at the usual therapeutic doses [16,17]. Thus, nisoldipine should be particularly useful for the treatment of the patients with heart failure.

Our results point out the beneficial effects of the acute administration of nisoldipine on both the rest and, above all, the exercise hemodynamics of patients even with advanced heart failure. These results can be compared with those observed after the acute administration of nifedipine. Although our patients had severely depressed LV function, none presented hemodynamic deterioration after nisoldipine, whereas it has been shown that nifedipine can adversely affect the hemodynamics of a significant percentage of patients with heart failure [3,4,14]. These results are consistent with experimental studies which have shown that nisoldipine, in comparison with nifedipine, is four to ten times more potent in inhibiting the contractions of smooth muscle with a weaker negative inotropic activity on the myocardium [5]. Clinical studies have already shown the beneficial acute hemodynamic effects of nisoldipine in patients with both mild and severe heart failure studied both at rest and submaximal exercise [6,11,19]. Our results show that the beneficial hemodynamic effects of nisoldipine are maintained, or even more evident, also during maximal exercise. While no effect on the LV filling pressures was evident at rest, this parameter was significantly reduced at maximal exercise. Though an improvement in diastolic function has been reported with nisoldipine [17], the lack of effect of this drug on the right atrial and pulmonary pressures at rest suggests that, in patients with heart failure, it acts mainly as an arterial vasodilator. This lack of effect of nisoldipine on the pulmonary pressures at rest has also been noted in other studies [6,16].

Nisoldipine confirmed its beneficial hemodynamic activity also during chronic therapy, however this drug did not significantly modify the exercise capacity, and a slight attenuation of its hemodynamic effects at maximal exercise was observed. Moreover, a tendency for a rebound change in CI and SVR was noted 24 h after nisoldipine withdrawal. The presence of rebound changes after the abrupt withdrawal of a peripheral vasodilator has been interpreted as indirect evidence of the activation of vasoconstrictive neurohumoral mechanisms [12]. It has recently been reported that nisoldipine therapy can cause an excessive increment in plasma norepinephrine and vasopressin during a water load causing a decrease in water excretion and fluid retention [2], and, also in our study, a tendency of plasma norepinephrine to increase after both acute and chronic nisoldipine therapy has been noted. Thus, it may be that nisoldipine activates neurohumoral vasoconstrictor mechanisms which attenuate its efficacy during chronic therapy. However, it has also been shown that the neurohumoral response to peripheral vasodilation is blunted in advanced heart failure [8], and this would favor the use of "pure" vasodilators such as nisoldipine. The lack of effects of nisoldipine on the exercise capacity can be explained by the effects of this drug on the regional distribution of blood flow. While nisoldipine is known to be able to selectively increase coronary blood flow [17,18], it has recently been demonstrated in patients with angina pectoris that it does not increase the blood flow to skeletal muscles [16], and this may account for its lack of effects on exercise capacity.

We used a relatively high dose [2,6] of nisoldipine (20 mg bid) in the attempt to obtain a greater hemodynamic improvement. It is possible that with these doses the weak negative inotropic activity of nisoldipine becomes evident thus preventing the CI to increase enough to counteract the arteriolar vasodilation, with a consequent decrease in tissue blood flow and an activation of neurohumoral vasoconstrictor forces. An excessive increment in the dose of nisoldipine administered intravenously may cause no additional improvement of the CI with, however, further reduction of the MAP and SVR [11]. Thus, it seems that during chronic treatment nisoldipine can be more effective when used in lower doses than those which can acutely induce the maximal hemodynamic changes.

Summary

We studied the acute and chronic effects of nisoldipine in ten patients with chronic heart failure (LV ejection fraction < 0.35; maximal $VO_2 < 25$ ml kg^{-1} min^{-1}). Each patient was evaluated at rest and during maximal bicycle exercise, before and after acute and chronic (2–3 months) oral nisoldipine and 24 h after nisoldipine withdrawal. Blood samples for the measurement with high-pressure liquid chromatography of plasma levels of norepinephrine and epinephrine were obtained at the time of the hemodynamic evaluations. Nisoldipine was administered at the maximal tolerated dosage (20 mg b.i.d. in eight patients and 10 mg in two); all the other vasodilators were withheld. At rest, nisoldipine induced an acute increase of CI and SVI with a reduction of MAP and SVR without a significant change in RAP or PCWP. At maximal exercise acute nisoldipine significantly increased CI and reduced SVR and PCWP. Chronic nisoldipine still improved the resting CI and SVI with a decrease in MAP and SVR; at exercise, hemodynamic changes were attenuated, and SVR and CI were not different from pretreatment values. After nisoldipine withdrawal a slight further reduction in CI and increase in SVR were noted. Exercise tolerance did not change significantly. Plasma norepinephrine levels increased, though not significantly, after acute and chronic nisoldipine; no significant change of epinephrine was noted. The presence of rebound changes after nisoldipine withdrawal and the increment of norepinephrine levels suggest that nisoldipine, despite its acute beneficial effects, when administered at the maximal vasodilator doses, can activate neurohumoral mechanisms which can attenuate its chronic efficacy.

References

1. Agostoni PG, De Cesare U, Doria E, Polese A, Tamborini G, Guazzi MD (1986) Afterload reduction: a comparison of captopril and nifedipine in dilated cardiomyopathy. Br Heart J 55:391–399
2. Barjon JN, Rouleau JC, Bichet D, Joneau C, De Champlain J (1987) Chronic renal and neurohumoral effects of the calcium entry blocker nisoldipine in patients with congestive heart failure. J Am Coll Cardiol 9:622–630
3. Elkayam N, Weber L, Mc Kay C, Rahimtoola S (1985) Spectrum of acute hemodynamic effects of nifedipine in severe congestive heart failure. Am J Cardiol 56:560–566
4. Fifer WA, Colucci WS, Lorell BH, Jaski BE, Barry WH (1985) Inotropic, vascular and neuroendocrine effects of nifedipine in heart failure: comparison with nitroprusside. J Am Coll Cardiol 5:731–737
5. Kazda S, Garthoff B, Meyer H, Schlossmann K, Stoepel K, Towart R, Vater V, Wehinger E (1980) Pharmacology of a new calcium antagonistic compound, isobutyl methyl 1,4 dihydro-2,6-dimethyl-4-(2-nitrophenyl)-3,5 pyridinedicarboxylate (nisoldipine, Bay K 5552). Arzneimittelforschung 30 (II) 12:2144–2162

6. Kiowski W, Erue P, Pfisterer M, Mueller J, Buehler FR, Burkart F (1987) Arterial vasodilator, systemic and coronary hemodynamic effects of nisoldipine in congestive heart failure secondary to ischemic or dilated cardiomyopathy. Am J Cardiol 59:1118–1125

7. Leier CV, Patrick TJ, Hermiller J, Pacht KD, Huss P, Magorien R, Unverferth DV (1984) Nifedipine in congestive heart failure: effects on resting and exercise hemodynamics and regional blood flow. Am Heart J 108:1461–1468

8. Levine TB, Francis GS, Goldsmith SR, Cohn JN (1983) The neurohumoral and hemodynamic response to orthostatic tilt in patients with congestive heart failure. Circulation 67:1070–1075

9. Ludbrook PA, Tiefenbrunn AJ, Reed FR, Sobel BE (1982) Acute hemodynamic responses to sublingual nifedipine: dependence on left ventricular function. Circulation 65:489–498

10. Magorien RD, Leier CV, Kolibash AJ, Barbush TJ, Unverferth DV (1984) Beneficial effects of nifedipine on rest and exercise myocardial energetics in patients with congestive heart failure. Circulation 70:884–890

11. Moe GW, Karlinsky SJ, Frankel D, Armstrong PW (1988) Intravenous nisoldipine in severe congestive heart failure. J Cardiovasc Pharmacol 12:160–166

12. Packer M, Meller J, Medina N, Yushak M, Gorlin R (1981) Determinants of drug response in severe chronic heart failure. 1. Activation of vasocostrictor forces during vasodilator therapy. Circulation 66:506–514

13. Packer M, Kessler PD, Lee WH (1987) Calcium channel blockade in the management of severe chronic congestive heart failure: a bridge too far. Circulation 75 [Suppl V]:V56–V64

14. Packer M, Lee WA, Medina N, Yushak M, Bernstein JL, Kessler PD (1987) Prognostic importance of the immediate hemodynamic response to nifedipine in patients with severe left ventricular dysfunction. J Am Coll Cardiol 10:1303–1311

15. Polese A, Fiorentini C, Olivari MT, Guazzi MD (1979) Clinical use of a calcium antagonistic agent (nifedipine) in acute pulmonary edema. Am J Med 66:825–830

16. Ram J, Freedman SB, Ogasawara S, Thomson A, Kelly DT (1989) Effects of nisoldipine on systemic and leg blood flow, oxygen transport and metabolism, and hemodynamics during exercise in effort angina pectoris. Am J Cardiol 63:802–806

17. Serruys PW, Suryapranata H, Planellas J, Wijns W, Vanhaleweyk GLJ, Soward A, Jaski BE, Hugenoltz PG (1985) Acute effects of intravenous nisoldipine on left ventricular function and coronary hemodynamics. Am J Cardiol 56:140–146

18. Soward AL, De Feyter PJ, Hugenoltz PG, Serruys PW (1986) Coronary and systemic hemodynamic effects of intravenous nisoldipine. Am J Cardiol 58:1199–1203

19. Vogt A, Kreuzer H (1983) Hemodynamic effects of nisoldipine in chronic congestive heart failure. Arzneimittelforschung 33:877–878

20. Yang SS, Bentivoglio LG, Maranhao V, Goldberg H (1978) From cardiac catheterization data to hemodynamic parameters, 2nd edn. Davis, Philadelphia

Cardiac Arrhythmias in Heart Failure

Arrhythmogenic Effects of Inotropic Agents Acting via Cyclic AMP and the Calcium Channel

L.H. OPIE and M.G. WORTHINGTON

Introduction

It is well established that increases of intracellular cyclic AMP and free cytosolic calcium may have inotropic implications. At the same time we have proposed hypotheses that abnormal elevations of cyclic AMP and also of calcium may be arrhythmogenic in certain circumstances. Because inotropic agents are used in the therapy of congestive heart failure, and because arrhythmias are thought to be an important mode of death in patients with heart failure, the following brief review of our hypotheses in relation to the arrhythmogenic qualities of cyclic AMP and of calcium is appropriate and relevant to the topic of this volume.

Role of Cyclic AMP in Arrhythmias

Adenosine $3',5'$-cyclic monophosphate (cyclic AMP) may be the second messenger of one serious pathological effect of β-adrenergic stimulation, namely the provocation of cardiac arrhythmias such as fatal ventricular fibrillation [3,5,8]. The first evidence for the arrhythmogenic role of cyclic AMP was indirect. In 1971, Ueda and Okumura found that inhibition of phosphodiesterase activity by chloroform and other anesthetic agents was associated with experimental ventricular arrhythmias [10]. In 1978, Podzuweit et al. reported studies on a baboon model in which the left anterior descending coronary artery was ligated, and sudden death due to ventricular fibrillation followed about 35 min later [9]. Cyclic AMP values in minidrill biopsies taken repetitively from the ischemic tissue consistently showed a rise starting 5–10 min before fibrillation. A similar association between increased tissue cyclic AMP and ventricular fibrillation was found in a cat model [2]. We have proposed that the increased tissue cyclic AMP may be either the direct cause of ventricular fibrillation or at the least an important precipitating factor. That cyclic AMP is an arrhythmogenic agent is shown by the following (for references see [6]):

1. The rise of cyclic AMP in ischemic tissue associated with the onset of ventricular fibrillation in baboon and pig models

B.S. Lewis, A. Kimchi (Eds.)
Heart Failure Mechanisms and Management
© Springer-Verlag Berlin Heidelberg 1991

2. The effects of isoproterenol in increasing tissue cyclic AMP and precipitating ventricular tachycardia and fibrillation in an otherwise stable pig heart model with a small infarct
3. The dose-response curve linking increases in tissue cyclic AMP with the decrease in the ventricular fibrillation threshold in the isolated rat heart model
4. The shift of the dose-effect curve to the right and the delay in the rise of tissue cyclic AMP during β_1-adrenergic stimulation by the β_1-adrenergic antagonist agent atenolol
5. The opposite effects of theophylline
6. The effect of addition of dibutyryl cyclic AMP (or of cyclic AMP plus theophylline) in decreasing the fibrillation threshold of the isolated rat heart
7. The effect of dibutyryl cyclic AMP in precipitating spontaneous arrhythmias in the coronary ligated rat heart
8. The effect of coronary artery ligation in the rat heart in elevating tissue cyclic AMP and in decreasing the fibrillation threshold
9. The effect of the antiarrhythmic agent amiodarone in elevating the ventricular fibrillation threshold while decreasing tissue cyclic AMP after coronary ligation in the rat heart
10. The effect of infusions of dibutyryl cyclic AMP beyond the edge of the infarct in provoking arrhythmias
11. The electrophysiological properties of dibutyryl cyclic AMP especially in the presence of a high external K^+.

Role of Calcium in Ischemic Arrhythmias

The possible role of calcium in ischemic ventricular fibrillation was first revealed by the findings that verapamil could inhibit this arrhythmia in dogs. Verapamil is, however, a relatively nonspecific agent, also having sodium-blocking qualities especially at high concentrations. Further work on an isolated heart preparation has shown an antiarrhythmic effect of l-verapamil, dl-verapamil, nifedipine, diltiazem, and tiapamil. A possible role for calcium influx in early ischemic arrhythmias is also supported by the data linking intracellular cyclic AMP with ventricular fibrillation. Nonetheless, such arguments are essentially indirect. More convincing proof for the role of calcium now comes from two sources. Firstly, there is increasing evidence that cytosolic calcium concentrations may be enhanced in acute ischemia. Secondly, intracellular injections to calcium cause inward currents, which might predispose to the electrophysiological phenomena of DADs and the transient inward current (I_{ti}). In some circumstances, abnormal oscillations of calcium early in myocardial ischemia could predispose to ventricular arrhythmias. Alternatively, a sustained rise in cytosolic calcium concentration could provoke an inward depolarizing current, thereby increasing ischemic depolarization and the likelihood of currents between nonischemic and ischemic zones. However, because DADs are energy dependent, and because I_{ti}

is abolished by lack of ATP, it seems unlikely that the mechanism relating calcium to early ischemic arrhythmias is directly related to the formation of DADs, unless these were being formed in nonischemic or mildly ischemic or borderline tissue. Other proposed mechanisms for calcium-related arrhythmogenesis are shown in Fig. 1. (For references to the above statements see [7]).

Arrhythmogenic Risks of Inotropic Agents

Virtually all positively inotropic agents have potential arrhythmogenic side effects. These are best established in the case of agents stimulating the formation of cyclic AMP such as the β-adrenergic agonists and, secondly, in the case of digitalis. However, exactly similar arguments to those applying for the β-adrenergic agonists also apply to phosphodiesterase inhibitors. It is true that intracellular compartmentation of cyclic AMP has not only been proposed but is highly likely; nonetheless, thus far no experimental situations have been found in

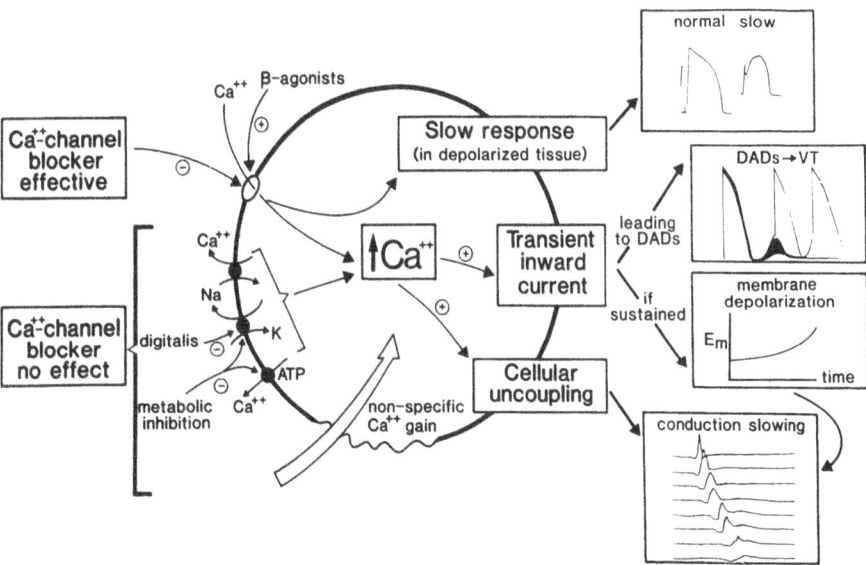

Fig. 1. Cell calcium and arrhythmias. Assuming that intracellular calcium does increase during ischemia, there are a number of potential mechanisms by which the calcium current could be arrhythmogenic: (a) calcium influx might elicit slow responses; (b) an additional increase in cytosolic calcium could activate oscillatory inward current flow and precipitate DADs; (c) if the calcium activation of this inward current were sustained, then accelerated depolarization might increase injury current across the ischemic boundary and precipitate fibrillation; (d) through promoting depolarization and increasing the coupling resistance between cells, a raised cytosolic [Ca^{2+}] might also slow conduction and increase the likelihood of reentry. Ca^{2+} channel blockers should be effective against the effects of a gain of intracellular calcium resulting from enhanced Ca^{2+} entry through the calcium channel. However, these agents should not benefit the consequences of sodium pump or metabolic inhibition or nonspecific Ca^{2+} gain except by their anti-ischemic effect. For further details, see [1]

which an elevation of cyclic AMP has achieved an inotropic effect without arrhythmogenic side effects. A specific example is the effect of forskolin, which was thought to increase cyclic AMP without causing arrhythmias in the isolated rat heart [4]. However, contractility was not measured in these experiments. We have repeated these experiments with, in addition, measurements of left ventricular pressure and have shown that while forskolin can cause cyclic AMP to increase without arrhythmias, it is necessary to give a high enough concentration of forskolin to induce large increments of cyclic AMP which simultaneously have a positive inotropic and arrhythmogenic effect. Our data on forskolin therefore confirm (a) compartmentation of cyclic AMP and (b) that cyclic AMP can be elevated without arrhythmogenic or positive inotropic effects [11]. Higher concentrations $(3 \times 10^{-6} M)$ of forskolin have *both* positively inotropic *and* arrhythmogenic effects, yet the major effect on pressure is an increase in diastolic rather than of systolic pressure. Forskolin is not an appropriate inotropic agent in the rat model.

Summary

There are close links between increments of intracellular cyclic AMP and of calcium. Both are thought to have positive inotropic implications. The hypotheses developed in Cape Town suggest that both cyclic AMP and calcium may be arrhythmogenic and promote arrhythmias at the same time as having their positive inotropic effect. An apparent exception to the rule, showing that cyclic AMP can substantially be increased by forskolin without arrhythmias in the isolated rat heart, is explained by an accumulation of compartmentalized cyclic AMP which has neither arrhythmogenic nor inotropic consequences.

References

1. Coetzee WA, Dennis SC, Opie LH et al. (1987) Calcium channel blockers and early ischemic ventricular arrhythmias: electrophysiological versus anti-ischemic effects. J Mol Cell Cardiol 19 (Suppl II):77–97
2. Corr PB, Witkowski FX, Sobel BE (1978) Mechanisms contributing to malignant dysarrhythmias induced by ischemia in the rat. J Clin Invest 61:109–119
3. Lubbe WF, Podzuweit T, Daries PS, Opie LH (1978) The role of cyclic adenosine monophosphate in adrenergic effects on ventricular vulnerability to fibrillation in the isolated perfused rat heart. J Clin Invest 61:1260–1269
4. Manning AS, Kinoshita K, Buschmans E, Coltart DJ, Hearse DJ (1985) The genesis of arrhythmias during myocardial ischemia. Dissociation between changes in cyclic adenosine monophosphate and electrical instability in the rat. Circ Res 57:668–675
5. Opie LH, Nathan D, Lubbe WF (1979) Biochemical aspects of arrhythmogenesis and ventricular fibrillation. Am J Cardiol 43:131–148
6. Opie LH, Muller C, Nathan D, Daries P, Lubbe WF (1980) Evidence for role of cyclic AMP as second messenger of arrhythmogenic effects of beta-stimulation. In: Hamet P, Sands H (eds) Advances in cyclic nucleotide research, vol 12. Raven, New York, pp 63–69

7. Opie LH, Coetzee WA, Dennis SC, Thandroyen FT (1988) A potential role of calcium ions in early ischemic and reperfusion arrhythmias. Ann NY Acad Sci 522:464–477

8. Podzuweit T, Lubbe WF, Opie LH (1976) Cyclic adenosine monophosphates, ventricular fibrillation and antiarrhythmic drugs. Lancet 1:341–342

9. Podzuweit T, Dalby AJ, Cherry GW, Opie LH (1978) Cyclic AMP levels in ischaemic and non-ischaemic myocardium following coronary artery ligation: relation to ventricular fibrillation. J Mol Cell Cardiol 10:81–94

10. Ueda I, Okumura F (1971) Effects of chloroform, diethylether, and a propiophenone derivative, 3-dimethylamino-2-methyl-2-phenoxypropiophenone hydrochloride upon cyclic nucleotide phosphodiesterase. Biochem Pharmacol 20:1967–1971

11. Worthington MG, Opie LH (1987) Forskolin, an adenylate cyclase activator, elevates cAMP without arrhythmogenic or positive inotropic effects (abstract). Cardiovasc Drugs Ther 1:304

Prevalence, Significance, and Control of Ventricular Arrhythmias in Patients with Heart Failure*

B.N. Singh, M.L. Schoenbaum, M. Antimisiaris, and C. Takanaka

Introduction

For many years it has been appreciated that patients surviving acute myocardial infarction experience an increased incidence of sudden death especially in the first 6 months to 1 year [1,2]. It is also known that the highest risk for such an event is in patients with markedly reduced ejection fraction particularly in association with complex ventricular ectopy [3,4]. There is also a suggestion that ventricular arrhythmias are associated with an enhanced mortality from sudden death independently of left ventricular dysfunction [3].

The so-called potentially lethal ventricular arrhythmias, occurring also in other forms of structural heart disease such as hypertrophic and dilated cardiomyopathies, are now increasingly recognized [5,6]. They too appear to be markers of increased mortality from sudden death. Of interest is the incidence and the prognostic significance of ventricular arrhythmias complicating heart failure from various causes [6,8–15]. The issue has become of major importance with the recognition that the mortality rate for patients with congestive heart failure is extremely high, being about 50% in the 1st year following referral for the treatment of patients with class III or IV NYHA functional disability [3]. About 40% of such deaths are sudden [16–18]. Sudden death is not influenced by vasodilator therapy, which does however exert a beneficial effect on deaths related to heart failure [19–21]. The implication is that sudden deaths in this setting are arrhythmic in nature, and that vasodilators are devoid of intrinsic antiarrhythmic properties. The purpose of this paper is to discuss, within a brief compass, the prevalence, prognostic significance, and the potential pharmacologic approaches to mortality reduction by the control of *asymptomatic* ventricular arrhythmias in patients with congestive heart failure.

Prevalence and Prognostic Significance

Numerous studies have documented a high incidence of potentially lethal ventricular arrhythmias – ventricular couplets, multiform complexes, and

*Supported by Medical Research Funds of Veterans Administration and the American Heart Association of the Greater Los Angeles Affiliate, California.

B.S. Lewis, A. Kimchi (Eds.)
Heart Failure Mechanisms and Management
© Springer-Verlag Berlin Heidelberg 1991

nonsustained ventricular tachycardia – in patients with dilated cardiomyopathy and in those with heart failure due to ischemic heart disease [6–15,22,23]. The incidence of complex ventricular ectopy has ranged between 12% and 95% [16]; the incidence of nonsustained ventricular tachycardia has been similar [16]. In contrast, the incidence of nonsustained ventricular tachycardia is about 10% 2 weeks after an acute infarction. In nearly every study, in patients with nonsustained ventricular tachycardia there was a higher total or sudden death rate compared to those who did not have the arrhythmia. Interestingly, patients having ventricular tachycardia ran three times the risk of dying as those without the tachycardia. Furthermore, during follow-up patients with ventricular tachycardia also had a higher mortality in every study. These data suggest that the effect on mortality is independent of the clinical severity of heart failure. This was also suggested by the preliminary data of the Veterans Administration Cooperative Study of the effect of vasodilator therapy on mortality in congestive cardiac failure [24]. The question has therefore arisen whether the suppression of such arrhythmias documented on Holter recordings may prolong survival over and above that induced by vasodilator therapy in patients with congestive cardiac failure.

Pathophysiological Considerations

The pathophysiological mechanisms underlying the development of ventricular arrhythmias in patients with congestive heart failure are complex and likely to be multifactorial [3,22,23]. In most cases of advanced cardiac failure, the interaction between significant electrolyte derangements and augmented activity of the sympathetic nervous system are likely to be involved [25,26]. The overall situation may be further compounded by the use of therapeutic regimens (such as cardiac glycosides, diuretics, and antiarrhythmic agents with proarrhythmic actions). There is also controversy regarding the precise nature of the preterminal events in the development of the sudden death syndrome in individual patients. However, from the analysis of Holter recordings in patients dying suddenly while wearing Holter monitors, a number of features have been identified [27]. There is evidence that although the largest number of patients dying suddenly have coronary artery disease, the initiating event does not appear to be triggered by episodes of myocardial ischemia [27]. Perhaps of the greatest interest has been the finding that most episodes are triggered by ventricular ectopic beats. In most cases the initial arrhythmia is ventricular tachycardia which deteriorates into ventricular fibrillation as a result of acceleration of the tachycardia [14,27].

It must be emphasized that while an episode of myocardial ischemia does not appear to be the immediate cause of the ventricular tachycardia, it may provide the basis for its degeneration into fibrillation especially in the setting of augmented adrenergic activity. These considerations are based on observations in patients experiencing out-of-hospital sudden death while wearing Holter monitoring. Although such patients almost invariably have reduced ventricular ejection fractions, rarely are they in frank heart failure. Thus, it is possible that the sequence of events mediating sudden death in patients with frank heart failure may differ. Indeed, in-hospital monitoring of heart failure patients awaiting cardiac transplantation has indicated that in many patients profound tachycardia and asystole rather than ventricular tachycardia or fibrillation constitutes the terminal event [28]. If this is indeed the most common mechanism of sudden death in patients with heart failure, it may have a significant bearing on the issue of attempts at mortality reduction by the use of antiarrhythmic drugs.

Pharmacologic Approaches and Impact on Survival: Reported Studies

A clear distinction should be made between the treatment of sustained ventricular arrhythmias associated with symptoms and those that are nonsustained and asymptomatic. In the former, treatment is for the relief of symptoms with the expectation of prolonging survival. The role of electrophysiological testing in the design of therapy is widely used although controversies remain. In the latter (the group under discussion here), the sole objective of therapy is enhanced survival by the suppression of spontaneously occurring ventricular arrhythmias. The role of electrophysiological testing in this subset of patients is questionable.

Significance of Vasodilator Therapy. It is known that vasodilators, angiotensin-converting enzyme inhibitors in particular, do increase serum potassium levels, reduce the augmented plasma catecholamine levels, and produce a concomitant decrease in premature ventricular contractions (PVCs) and runs of nonsustained ventricular tachycardia [29]. The fact that this does not lead to a reduction in the incidence of sudden death (versus cardiac and total deaths which are reduced) may suggest that a reduction in PVCs is unlikely to result in a fall in the rate of sudden deaths in this setting. Alternatively, vasodilators may not exert a primary anti-fibrillatory action in the setting of cardiac disease. Both these issues are of significance and are discussed below.

Role of Beta-Blockers and Mortality in Congestive Cardiac Failure. It is widely recognized that beta-blockers, at least those which exert a heart rate lowering effect under resting conditions [30], reduce the incidence of sudden death in the survivors of acute myocardial infarction. The precise mechanism underlying such a beneficial effect is not known, but to date this is the only modality of therapy that, in systematic controlled and blinded studies, has shown a salutary effect on sudden death. It is not known whether it is due to a change in ventricular fibrillation threshold, suppression of PVCs, a primary effect on ischemia, or to other factors such as prevention of fibrillation by their so-called class III effects resulting from physiological adaptation of the adrenergic system to prolonged beta-receptor blockade [31].

Although initially the use of beta-blockers in cardiac failure was viewed with a considerable degree of skepticism and concern, there appears to be little doubt that these agents can be given with safety in a subset of patients with cardiac failure [32]. The issue under question is whether these agents may exert a favorable effect on mortality in patients with heart failure. Undoubtedly, the markedly augmented adrenergic drive in patients with heart failure is of prognostic significance [25]. The hypothesis has been developed that the blunting of the sympathetic nervous system by beta-blockers in heart failure by up-regulating beta-receptor density in the myocardium may not only improve hemodynamic function but may prolong survival by reducing the arrhythmogenic actions of catecholamines. Three small trials (two using metoprolol and one acebutalol) have demonstrated that very small doses of beta-blockers appear to produce symptomatic improvement in a subset of patients with dilated cardiomyopathy [32–34]. The limited mortality data from these trials when pooled indicated a trend in favor of treatment, but no definitive conclusions can be reached [35]. A larger trial, the Multi-center Metoprolol in Dilated Cardiomyopathy Study, is currently ongoing with the aim of enrolling 320 patients to be randomized into metoprolol and placebo arms over a 2-year period. The results of this study will be of far-reaching importance. In the meantime, however, it remains uncertain whether this class of drugs have an effect on mortality from sudden death in patients with cardiac failure, and whether such an effect might be related to the suppression of ventricular arrhythmias.

Therapy and Mortality in Heart Failure. Although it appears to be relatively well established that the presence of complex ectopic activity in patients with heart failure significantly increases the risk for sudden arrhythmic deaths, no controlled trials have been conducted to test the hypothesis that the suppression of such arrhythmias in these patients reduces the incidence of sudden death. The results of uncontrolled albeit small studies are at variance.

Parmley and Chatterjee [36] analyzed the incidence of sudden deaths in a subgroup of patients with heart failure and complex ventricular ectopic beats. The patients were treated with quinidine or procainamide ($n = 26$) or with amiodarone ($n = 13$). The treated group had a cumulative survival rate of 90%–95% at 6 months compared with approximately 65% in patients not receiving antiarrhythmic therapy. The difference was significant ($p < 0.05$). In another study reported by Dargie et al. [26], it was clearly established that the presence of ventricular ectopic activity in patients with heart failure was a strong predictor for subsequent cardiac death. Furthermore, a comparison of groups of such patients on treatment with amiodarone with those not treated with antiarrhythmic agents showed a significant difference in favor of amiodarone which not only reduced ventricular ectopy but also prolonged survival. In contrast, Chakko and Georghiade [13] followed 43 patients with chronic heart failure due to dilated cardiomyopathy; 88% of the patients had complex ventricular ectopic activity, with 51% having nonsustained asymptomatic ventricular tachycardia. Of these patients 23 received long-term antiarrhythmic therapy with procainamide or quinidine, and 20 were not treated. The two groups were comparable. At a mean follow-up period of 16 months, there were 16 deaths, 62% sudden. There was no significant difference between the numbers of such deaths in the treated and untreated groups.

It must be emphasized that these studies are severely limited by the numbers of patients and the lack of adequate controls and standardization of therapy. They merely indicate that the data support the idea of a stringently controlled study with adequate sample size and statistical power that should be undertaken to test the hypothesis that antiarrhythmic therapy reduces the mortality from sudden death in patients with cardiac failure, and that such an effect is linked to a suppression of complex ventricular ectopic activity. However, there is no unanimity of opinion regarding the choice of antiarrhythmic agents that might be used as electropharmacologic probes to address these fundamental questions. Nonetheless, there are numerous considerations which bear on the issue, not the least being the preliminary data from the Cardiac Arrhythmia Suppression Trial (CAST) [37] in the United States in patients surviving acute myocardial infarction. [37]

Characteristics of a Desirable Antiarrhythmic Agent for Mortality Reduction in Cardiac Failure

In the design of an antiarrhythmic regimen for mortality reduction in patients with heart failure and potentially lethal ventricular arrhythmias two main factors merit consideration: the pathophysiological mechanisms of heart failure having a bearing on the genesis of arrhythmias and the electrophysiological and pharmacodynamic properties of antiarrhythmic compounds. Electrolyte disturbances and the derangements of the autonomic nervous system are clearly important. The electrolyte abnormalities may result not only from persistent diuretic therapy but also as a result of the stimulation of the renin-angiotensin system [25,26]. It has long been known that the sympathetic nervous system is activated in heart failure in proportion to the severity of cardiac failure [25,26], there being a relationship between plasma norepinephrine levels and survival in these patients. The choice of an antiarrhythmic compound in the setting of heart failure must clearly allow for the fact that it is nearly impossible to restore complete normality of homeostasis with respect to electrolytes and plasma norepinephrine levels. Electrolyte disturbances, especially hypokalemia and hypomagnesemia, may not only reduce the efficacy of certain antiarrhythmic agents (especially class I agents) but may aggravate the tendency for proarrhythmic effects both for class I (ventricular tachycardia and fibrillation) and class III (torsades de pointes) agents. The arrhythmogenic effects of elevated plasma catecholamines is well known; it is also known that attenuation of the effects of adrenergic stimulation by whatever means has beneficial effects in cardiac arrhythmias. Thus, in the choice of an agent it might be desirable to select one that does have the additional property of inhibiting adrenergic drive while eliminating either the trigger mechanisms for ventricular arrhythmias or conferring on the myocardium an antifibrillatory propensity by selectively prolonging refractoriness.

It is almost trite to emphasize that the side effects profile of the agent to be used in cardiac failure needs to acceptable. On the other hand, since the arrhythmia mortality is inordinately high in this group of patients, the spectrum and severity of side effects that might be acceptable for an effective antiarrhythmic agent in this setting are clearly different from those in subsets of patients with a lower potential for sudden cardiac death. It is nevertheless clear that antiarrhythmic agents for patients with heart failure should not have the proclivity to depress ventricular function and exacerbate cardiac failure.

Lessons from the Cardiac Arrhythmia Suppression Trial: To Depress Conduction or to Prolong Refractoriness

Although the preliminary results of CAST are from a different subset of patients with asymptomatic ventricular arrhythmias, they have an important bearing on the treatment of similar arrhythmias in patients with cardiac failure. The aim of CAST was to test the hypothesis that the suppression of PVCs by antiarrhythmic agents in the survivors of acute infarction reduces the incidence of sudden cardiac death. The test drugs were flecainide, encainide, and ethmozine.

Flecainide and encainide were selected for the trial because these drugs produce a predictable suppression of PVCs: in about 80% of patients there is over 75% suppression of total PVCs, over 90% suppression of ventricular couplets, and close to 100% suppression of ventricular tachycardia beats. Ethmozine was selected because of its favorable side effects profile and its modest PVC suppressant action. Thus, in the asymptomatic patient with complex PVCs with increased risk for sudden arrhythmic deaths, encainide and similar drugs provided the basis for CAST under the aegis of the United States National Heart Lung and Blood Institute's Clinical Trials Branch in Bethesda, Maryland. In the event, after 2 years into the study, it appeared that rather than reducing the incidence of death in the group with encainide or flecainide, there was an *increase* in mortality when compared to the effects of placebo. The preliminary results of the trial involving 1500 patients at 23 centers in the United States, Canada, and Sweden revealed that of the 730 patients assigned to encainide or flecainide and treated an average of 10 months, 56 died or suffered cardiac arrest, while among the 725 given a placebo 23 had died or suffered cardiac arrest. It also appeared that the effects of ethmozine (a less powerful PVC suppressant and a less powerful depressant of conduction) did not differ from those of the placebo. The difference in the case of encainide and flecainide is disturbing and cannot be ignored. They have been withdrawn from the trial, which is continuing. These results leave the clinician in considerable confusion regarding the role of PVC suppression by agents which selectively and markedly delay conduction as a modality of therapy of asymptomatic PVCs in the expectation of reducing sudden deaths in the survivors of acute infarction.

What are the implications of the results of CAST for design of studies to determine whether antiarrhythmic therapy might have an impact on sudden death in patients with cardiac failure? Several issues should be considered. First, it is clear that the degree of slowing of conduction induced by flecainide and encainide in patients with ventricular arrhythmias is perhaps excessive; while it clearly has a powerful suppressant effect on reducing the trigger mechanisms for the initiation of the sustained tachyarrhythmia, it appears to make the substrate more prone to develop focal reexcitation. It might be speculated that these drugs have little effect on the genesis of PVCs; it is likely that they merely prevent their propagation so they are not "seen" on the surface electrocardiogram. The excessive slowing of conduction induced by class 1c agents in concert with their differential effects on the action potential duration in the Purkinje fibers and ventricular muscle – shortening in the former and lengthening it in the latter [38,39] – might provide the background to their proarrhythmic actions. This overall action results in marked heterogeneity in excitability and refractoriness in the myocardium which is likely to be particularly significant in the context of disease. The CAST data indicate an urgent need to determine the mechanisms underlying the proarrhythmic actions of class I agents in general and to define the extent of slowing of conduction that might be beneficial, and when the effect is likely to become deleterious.

Second, the data raise the issue, suspected for sometime, that the reduction of PVCs (it being doubtful whether it is indeed possible to eliminate every PVC that is generated in the heart), may not lead directly to a reduction in sudden death. The CAST results support this premise, at least with respect to the drugs that have a marked propensity to slow conduction. On the other hand, the possibility is not excluded that reduction or elimination in repetitive beats by agents which have a different electrophysiological profile with no effect on conduction (e.g., beta blockers) or those with modest depressant effect on conduction (e.g., amiodarone) might be effective in altering mortality in patients with potentially life-threatening ventricular arrhythmias. It remains to be determined as to how much slowing of conduction in this setting is beneficial, and at what level of change in conduction in any subset of patients it begins to be deleterious. Finally, the results with encainide and flecainide in CAST do provide a further impetus for considering agents which modify the other "end" of the action potential (potassium channel blockers) in the control of malignant ventricular arrhythmias [39-44]. The focus here is on homogeneously increasing refractoriness by prolonging the action potential duration in the substrate but without the tendency for membrane oscillation leading to torsades de pointes [14]. Such an approach might lead to the development of effective pharmacological regimens for altering mortality from ventricular arrhythmias by their antifibrillatory properties without a *major* effect on conduction in the heart [44].

Class III Antiarrhythmic Drugs and Mortality Reduction from Sudden Death in Heart Failure: Future Studies

The available clinical and experimental electropharmacologic data indicate the potential importance of agents that appear to act by prolonging effective refractory period by a uniform lengthening of cardiac repolarization. The list of such agents is growing. The expanding appeal of these agents stems from a number of factors. First, because these agents as a class augment myocardial contractility [42], they are clearly desirable from the standpoint that the greatest number of patients at the highest risk for sudden arrhythmic deaths have reduced ventricular function. Second, this is also the subset of patients with the highest potential for developing proarrhythmic actions in the case of class I agents in general. Third, the fundamental action of class III drugs is unlikely to be linked solely to the suppression of PVCs [45]. CAST has suggested that such an approach based on a defined extent of PVC suppression is now in difficulties. It is possible and indeed likely that the potentially salutary antifibrillatory effects of class III compounds may occur entirely independently of the suppression of PVCs.

Finally, preliminary data that deal with the effects of amiodarone in heart failure [26] and the extensive results with the drug in patients with recalcitrant ventricular tachycardia and fibrillation [43] indicate its potential to curtail the rate of sudden deaths in patients with heart failure. It should be emphasized that the proarrhythmic effect of the drug is low compared to either class I agents or to other class III agents, most of which induce at least a 5% incidence of torsades de pointes [44]. In the case of amiodarone it appears to be less than 2%, occurring essentially in the setting of marked hypokalemia or when in association with drugs that further prolong cardiac repolarization or depress conduction. It is truly remarkable that despite the fact that the drug may prolong the QT interval to over 600 MS and produce a profound degree of tachycardia, the incidence of torsade de pointes remains low. The reason for this is not clear at present, but preliminary data recently reported by Takanaka and Singh [46] have suggested that it may be related to amiodarone's calcium-antagonistic effects, inhibiting the propensity for the development of early afterdepolarizations responsible for torsades (see Fig. 1).

The overall electrophysiological properties of amiodarone, despite its complex side effects profile, have therefore formed the basis for considering it the best antiarrhythmic agent for determining the effects of therapy on the incidence of sudden death in patients with arrhythmias complicating cardiac failure. Such a blinded, placebo-controlled study has recently been initiated under the aegis of the Veterans Administration Cooperative Study Section. The results will clearly be of importance in establishing whether antifibrillatory and antiarrhythmic therapy exert an influence on sudden arrhythmic deaths in patients with congestive cardiac failure.

Summary

The results of antiarrhythmic therapy in patients with ventricular arrhythmias in the setting of heart failure are controversial and uncertain. In patients with advanced heart failure, recent data obtained during in-hospital monitoring suggest the important role of bradycardia and asystole. It is not known whether the suppression of PVCs by highly potent class I agents (e.g., encainide and

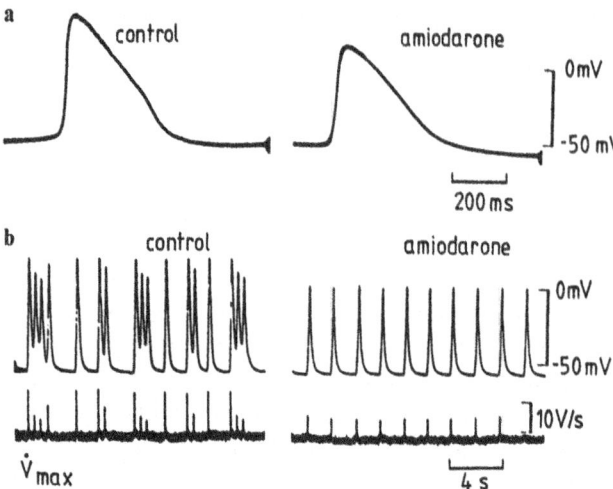

Fig. 1. a *Control*, an action potential due to abnormal automaticity recorded in control solution. *Amiodarone*, an action potential recorded 90 min after the initiation of amiodarone at 5.0×10^{-5} *M*. There was no significant change in the action potential duration although the amplitude of the action potential decreased considerably. **b** *Control*, action potentials and V_{max} in the control solution recorded from a preparation belonging to the "irregular group." *Amiodarone*, 90 min after the initiation of amiodarone at 5.0×10^{-5} *M*. Amiodarone totally precluded the development of additional depolarizations

flecainide) will reduce sudden death in these patients. If the data from CAST can be extrapolated to patients with heart failure, a similar or a higher rate of lethal proarrhythmic effects might be expected. The available data suggest that a placebo-controlled clinical trial in these patients with agents that prolong refractoriness and have either no effect or a minimal effect on cardiac conduction should be undertaken. The most promising agent for this purpose is amiodarone despite its complex side effect profile.

References

1. Ruberman W, Weinblatt E, Goldberg J (1977) Ventricular premature beats and mortality after acute myocardial infarction. N Engl J Med 293:750–755
2. Moss AJ, Davis HT, DeCamilla J (1977) Ventricular ectopic beats and their relation to sudden and non-sudden death after myocardial infarction. Circulation 60:998–1004
3. Bigger JT Jr, Fleiss JL, Kleiger R, Miller JP, Rolnitzky LM, the Multicenter Post-Infarction Group (1984) The relationship between ventricular arrhythmias, left ventricular dysfunction and mortality in the two years after myocardial infarction. Circulation 69:250
4. Mukharji J, Rude RE, Poole WK, Gustafson N, Thomas LJ Jr, Strauss HW, Jaffe AS, Muller JE, Roberts R, Raabe DS Jr, Croft CH, Passamani E, Braunwald E, Willerson JT, and the MILIS Study Group (1984) Risk factors for sudden death after acute myocardial infarction: two year follow-up. Am J Cardiol 54:31–37

5. McKenna WJ, England D, Doi YL, Deanfield JE, Oakley CM, Goodwin JF (1981) Arrhythmia in hypertrophy cardiomyopathy. Influence on prognosis. Br Heart J 46:168–172
6. Maskin CS, Siskind SJ, LeJemptel TH (1984) High prevalence of nonsustained ventricular tachycardia in severe congestive heart failure. Am Heart J 107:896–802
7. Sakurari T, Kawai C (1983) Sudden death in idiopathic cardiomyopathy. Jpn Circ J 47:581
8. Wilson JR, Schwartz P, Sutton MS-J, Ferrao N, Horowaitz LN, Reichek N, Josephson ME (1983) Prognosis in severe heart failure: relationship to hemodynamic measurements and ventricular ectopic activity. J Am Coll Cardiol 2:403
9. Von Olshausen K, Schafer A, Mehmel HC, Schwartz F, Senges J, Kubler W (1984) Ventricular arrhythmias in idiopathic dilated cardiomyopathy. Br Heart J 51:195
10. Franciosa JA, Wilen M, Ziesche SM, Cohn JN (1983) Survival in men with severe chronic left ventricular failure due to either coronary heart disease or idiopathic dilated cardiomyopathy. Am J Cardiol 51:831
11. Huang SK, Messer JV, Denes P (1983) Significance of ventricular tachycardia in idiopathic dilated cardiomyopathy: observations in 35 patients. Am J Cardiol 51:507
12. Francis GS (1983) Development of arrhythmias in the patient with congestive heart failure: pathophysiology, prevalence and prognosis. Am J Cardiol 51:507
13. Chakko CS, Gheorghiade M (1985) Ventricular arrhythmias in severe heart failure: incidence, significance, and effectiveness of antiarrhythmic therapy. Am Heart J 109:497
14. Meinertz T, Hofman T, Kasper W, Treese N, Bechtold H, Stienen U, Pop T, Leitner E-RV, Andersen D, Meyer J (1984) Significance of ventricular arrhythmias in idiopathic dilated cardiomyopathy. Am J Cardiol 53:902
15. Holmes J, Kubo SH, Cody RJ, Kligfield P (1985) Arrhythmias in ischemic and non-ischemic dilated cardiomyopathy: prediction of mortality by ambulatory electrocardiography. Am J Cardiol 55:146
16. Bigger JT (1987) Why some patients with congestive heart failure die: arrhythmias and sudden cardiac death. Circulation 75 (Suppl IV):28–35
17. Unverferth DV, Magorein RD, Moeschberger ML, Baker PB, Fetters JK, Leier CV (1984) Factors influencing the one-year mortality of dilated cardiomyopathy. Am J Cardiol 54:147
18. Bigger JT Jr, Weld RM, Rolnitzky LM (1981) The prevalence and significance of ventricular tachycardia detected by ambulatory ECG recording in the hospital phase of acute myocardial infarction. Am J Cardiol 48:815
19. Cohn JN, Archibald DF, Ziesche S, Franciosa JA, Harston WE, Tristani FE, Dunkman WB, Jacobs W, Francis GS, Flohr KH, Goldman S, Cobb FR, Shah PM, Saunders R, Fletcher RD, Loeb HS, Hughes VC, Baker B (1986) Effect of vasodilator therapy on mortality in chronic congestive heart failure. Results of a Veterans Administration cooperative study. N Engl J Med 314:1547
20. The Consensus Trial Study Group (1987) Effects of enalapril on mortality in severe congestive heart failure: result of the cooperative North Scandinavian enalapril survival study (CONSENSUS). N Engl J Med 316:1429–1435
21. The Captopril Multicenter Research Group I (1985) A cooperative multicenter study of captopril in congestive heart failure: hemodynamic effects and long-term response. Am Heart J 110:439–447
22. Francis GS (1986) Development of arrhythmias in the patient with congestive heart failure: pathophysiology, prevalence and prognosis. Am J Cardiol 57:3B–7B
23. Buxton AE, Marchlinski FE, Waxman HL, Flores MA, Cassidy DM, Josephson ME (1984) Prognostic factors in nonsustained ventricular tachycardia. Am J Cardiol 53:1275
24. Fletcher RD, Archibald D, Orndorff J, Cohn J (1986) Dysrhythmias on short-term Holter as an independent predictor of mortality in congestive heart failure (abstract). J Am Coll Cardiol 7:143 A
25. Packer M, Lee WH, Kessler PD, Gottlieb SS, Bernstein JL, Kukin ML (1987) Role of neurohumoral mechanisms in determining survival in patients with severe chronic heart failure. Circulation 75(Suppl IV):30–35
26. Dargie HJ, Cleland JGF, Leckie BJ, Inglis CG, East BW, Ford I (1987) Relation of arrhythmias and electrolyte abnormalities to survival in patients with severe congestive heart failure. Circulation 75(Suppl IV):IV-98–107

27. Bayes de Luna A, Coumel P, Leclerq JF (1987) Ambulatory sudden cardiac death: mechanisms of production of fatal arrhythmia on the basis of data from 157 cases. Am Heart J 117:151–159
28. Luu M, Stevenson WG, Stevenson LW, Baron K, Warden J (1989) Diverse mechanisms of unexpected cardiac arrests in advanced heart failure. Circulation 80:1675–1680
29. Cleland JGF, Dargie HJ, Hodsman GP (1984) Captopril in heart failure: a double-blind controlled study. Br Heart J 52:530–536
30. Kjekshus J (1987) Heart rate reduction – a mechanism of benefit? Eur Heart J 8(Suppl 1):115–122
31. Raine AEG, Vaughan Williams EM (1981) Adaptation to prolonged beta-blockade of rabbit atrial, Purkinje and ventricular potentials, and papillary muscle contraction. Time-course of development of, and recovery from, adaptation. Circ Res 48:804–812
32. Anderson JL, Lutz JR, Gilbert EM, Sorenson SG, Yanowitz FG, Menlove RL, Bartholomew M (1985) A randomized trial of low-dose beta-blockade therapy for idiopathic dilated cardiomyopathy. Am J Cardiol 55:471–475
33. Currie PJ, Kelly MJ, McKenzie A, Harper RW, Lim YL, Federman J, Anderson ST, Pitt A (1984) Oral beta-adrenergic blockade with metoprolol in chronic severe dilated cardiomyopathy J Am Coll Cardiol 3:203–209
34. Engelmeier RS, O'Connell JB, Walsh R, Rad N, Scanlon PJ, Gunnar RM (1985) Improvement in symptoms and exercise tolerance by metoprolol in patients with dilated cardiomyopathy: a double-blind, randomized, placebo-controlled trial. Circulation 72:536–546
35. Furberg CD, Yusuf S (1988) Effect of drug therapy on survival in chronic congestive heart failure. Am J Cardiol 62:41A–45A
36. Parmley WW, Chatterjee K (1988) Congestive heart failure and arrhythmias: an overview. Am J Cardiol 57:34B–37B
37. The Cardiac Arrhythmia Suppression Trial (CAST) Investigators (1989) Preliminary Report: Effect of encainide and flecainide on mortality in a randomized trial of arrhythmia suppression after myocardial infarction. New Engl J Med 321:406–412
38. Singh BN, Courtney K (1990) On the classification of antiarrhythmic mechanisms: experimental and clinical correlations. In Zipes DP, Jalife J (eds) Cardiac electrophysiology: from the cell to the bedside. Saunders, Philadelphia, pp 882–897
39. Singh BN (1987) Effects of antiarrhythmic compounds on the cardiac action potential: basis for the interpretation of their antiarrhythmic actions. In: Zipes DP (ed) Yu PN, Goodwin JF (Series eds) Progress of cardiology. Lea and Febiger, Philadelphia, pp 37–86
40. Singh BN, Vaughan Williams EM (1970) A third class of antiarrhythmic action. Effects on atrial and ventricular intracellular potentials and other pharmacologic actions on cardiac muscle of in MJ1999 and AH 3474. Br J Pharmacol 39:675–685
41. Singh BN, Vaughan Williams EM (1970) The effect of amiodarone, a new anti-anginal drug, on cardiac muscle. Br J Pharmacol 39:357–367
42. Singh BN, Nademanee K (1985) Control of arrhythmias by selective lengthening of cardiac repolarization: theoretical considerations and clinical observations. Am Heart J 109:421–430
43. Singh BN (ed) (1988) Control of cardiac arrhythmias by lengthening repolarization. Futura, Mount Kisco NY
44. Singh BN (editorial) (1988) When is QT prolongation antiarrhythmic and when is it pro-arrhythmic? Am J Cardiol 63:867–869
45. Singh BN (editorial) (1989) Controlling cardiac arrhythmias: to delay conduction or to prolong refractoriness? Cardiovasc Drugs Ther 3:671–674
46. Takanaka C, Singh BN (1990) Barium-induced non-driven action potentials as a model of triggered automaticity and early afterdepolarizations: differing effects of amiodarone and quinidine and significance of slow-channel activity. J Am Coll Cardiol 15(1):213–221

Exercise Physiology and Exercise Therapy
in Heart Failure

Exercise Testing and Training of Patients with Congestive Heart Failure and Left Ventricular Dysfunction

N.K.WENGER

Introduction

Major conceptual changes in the management of patients with congestive heart failure have assumed even greater importance as newer therapies have alleviated or limited disabling symptoms and prolonged survival [1,2]. Protracted bed rest is no longer the recommended approach, nor are usual well-tolerated activities restricted. Rather, there is emphasis on the benefits of judiciously applied prescriptive exercise training for appropriately selected patients, with the goal of enhancing activity tolerance. This parallels the evolution from exercise restriction to exercise prescription in the management of patients with coronary heart disease and myocardial infarction.

Exercise testing is also increasingly undertaken to provide an objective, replicable evaluation of the activity tolerance of the patient with heart failure, to assess the severity of the disease, to evaluate the responses of patients with heart failure treated with different pharmacologic agents to increasing levels of physical activity, and to determine the effect of exercise rehabilitation.

Most patients with compensated congestive cardiac failure are asymptomatic at rest. The occurrence of exertional dyspnea and fatigue with progressive levels of activity is the disabling feature. Premature onset of exertional symptoms limits the tolerance for physical activity. Because activity intolerance often occurs gradually, albeit progressively, the patient's perception of exercise impairment, based on the New York Heart Association functional classification delineation of the symptomatic response to "usual" levels of activity, may be faulty and misleading; as a patient's expectations of physical work capacity decline, the perception of the intensity of "usual" physical activity concomitantly decreases [3].

Exercise Capacity and Exercise Endpoints: Left Ventricular Dysfunction and Congestive Heart Failure

A variety of noninvasive test procedures have documented the poor correlation among resting left ventricular function (ejection fraction) or dimensions, hemodynamic measurements, symptomatic status, and exercise capacity [4,5]. Also, exercise capacity is substantially dependent on the pace at which physical

B.S. Lewis, A. Kimchi (Eds.)
Heart Failure Mechanisms and Management
© Springer-Verlag Berlin Heidelberg 1991

activity is performed [6]. Further, hemodynamic data appear comparable for patients whose exercise endpoint is dyspnea and those who terminate exercise owing to fatigue. Fatigue had previously been attributed to inadequate tissue perfusion, i.e., lack of nutritive blood flow to skeletal muscle, but fatigue appears not to be due solely to the decreased cardiac output and oxygen supply. With increasing levels of exercise, there is inability of the failing heart to concomitantly increase the cardiac output; skeletal muscle underperfusion promotes an increase in glycolysis, with a resultant increase in lactate levels that may produce fatigue. Impairment of blood flow alone is inadequate to explain all the abnormalities [7]; the components resulting in fatigue that are related to alterations in oxidative metabolism, changes in substrate utilization, inadequate vasodilator response, and abnormalities of autonomic autoregulation of the circulation remain uncertain. Following cardiac transplantation and restoration of a normal cardiac output, exercise tolerance fails to improve for weeks to months, with the mechanisms responsible for this delayed response not yet delineated [8].

Dyspnea or breathlessness was previously considered due to an increase in left atrial pressure but is now known not to correlate significantly with elevation of the pulmonary capillary wedge pressure. The patient with heart failure has an increased level of ventilation for any level of exercise; breathing is rapid and shallow, with increased ventilation of the dead space; minute ventilation is increased to maintain adequate alveolar ventilation. There is no consistent relationship between the exercise pulmonary capillary wedge pressure and ventilation; ventilation appears more closely related to the resting pulmonary capillary wedge pressure. Significant differences in oxygen uptake occur in patients with heart failure at the same workload, dependent in great part on the efficiency of exercising. Slow exercise has been described to be typically terminated owing to fatigue, whereas dyspnea is the activity-limiting feature with rapid exercise, despite a comparable peak pulmonary capillary pressure in each at termination of exercise [9].

Compensatory Mechanisms to Preserve Exercise Tolerance: Left Ventricular Dysfunction

Four features described to preserve the exercise tolerance in patients with ventricular dysfunction are (a) the maintenance of chronotropic competence, i.e., the ability to increase the heart rate to sustain the cardiac output when stroke volume cannot be further increased; (b) the ability to tolerate an elevated pulmonary capillary wedge pressure without experiencing dyspnea; (c) the capacity for ventricular dilatation to effect an increase in stroke volume; and (d) the capacity to decrease peripheral vascular resistance in response to upright exercise.

The Importance of Right Ventricular Function

Both pulmonary vascular resistance and resting right ventricular ejection fraction correlate with exercise capacity in patients with left ventricular dysfunction and heart failure [10]. The pulmonary vascular resistance in patients with heart failure fails to decrease with exercise, as is the case in individuals with normal ventricular function. Right ventricular function is predominantly afterload dependent; therefore, drugs that dilate the pulmonary vascular bed can improve the exercise capacity of patients with congestive heart failure.

Anaerobic Threshold Versus Lactate Threshold

There has been challenge to equating the lactate threshold with the anaerobic threshold. An increase in lactate production with exercise can occur without a change in blood lactate levels. Habitual activity levels also influence the lactate threshold, independent of changes in circulatory function. Inactivity decreases the lactate threshold, whereas exercise training increases lactate clearance, but not lactate production. Increased lactate production can occur under fully aerobic conditions, due to activation of fast-twitch muscle fibers and differences in substrate utilization. Further, change in oxygen consumption can occur without concomitant change in the anaerobic threshold; this often reflects changes in patient motivation rather than changes in functional capacity.

Exercise Training of Patients with Ventricular Dysfunction and Heart Failure

Although reports in the literature describe predominantly the exercise training of small, highly selected groups of these patients, often in a setting of considerable exercise supervision, both the safety and the benefits of exercise training for patients with ventricular dysfunction and heart failure have far exceeded initial expectations. Exercise-related complications have been limited, and training has effected a substantial improvement in exercise duration and peak oxygen consumption [11]. The oxygen pulse (maximal oxygen uptake/maximal heart rate) increases with training. Although the left ventricular ejection fraction at rest or with exercise does not improve, deterioration of ventricular function is generally not encountered [11-13].

The determinants of the safety of exercise training for patients with ventricular dysfunction and compensated heart failure include the stability of the cardiovascular status; the severity and etiology of the underlying cardiovascular disease; the occurrence and complexity of ventricular arrhythmias; the proximity to an acute event, particularly in patients with ischemic heart disease; and the intensity of the exercise training.

The mechanisms of improvement in functional capacity with exercise training include an improvement in the oxidative capacity of trained skeletal muscle; this is predominantly a muscle-specific effect. There is an increase in the arteriovenous oxygen difference, significantly due to a redistribution of blood flow; the relative contributions of the vasodilator capacity of exercising muscle versus the vasoconstriction in nonexercising muscle are uncertain and may vary with cardiovascular drug therapies. The capacity of exercising muscle to effect this increase in oxygen extraction is blunted with aging; therefore, greater exercise intolerance can be anticipated in elderly patients with congestive heart failure, owing to limitation of this compensatory response.

Exercise training increases the capacity for aerobic metabolism at any given muscle blood flow. Training produces an overall decrease in sympathetic tone; this may decrease vascular tone and increase the capacity for exercise vascular redistribution; it may also explain the improved vasodilator capacity of the muscular vasculature with training, permitting an increase in muscle blood flow at peak exercise. Exercise training thus appears to improve peripheral vasodilatation in patients with heart failure as it does in normal subject. The decrease in sympathetic tone decreases the heart rate, due to the upregulation of beta-receptors. Central adaptation appears particularly dependent on the severity of the myocardial failure; exercise training may increase ventricular enlargement and myocardial hypertrophy in some patients with mild or moderate ventricular dysfunction.

Mechanisms of the Exercise Training Effect

The mechanisms by which patients with heart failure improve their cardiac output with exercise may vary with the etiology of the congestive heart failure. In patients with underlying cardiomyopathy, the major increase in cardiac output (ejection fraction) appears due to an increase in stroke volume, with little or no change in the ventricular end-diastolic diameter. Patients with ischemic heart disease have little change in ejection fraction but increase their left ventricular end-diastolic diameter and systolic diameter to improve the cardiac output [14].

The decrease in myocardial oxygen demand at any level of submaximal work that occurs in response to exercise training is due to a decrease in the heart rate and systolic blood pressure responses to exercise. This training effect reflects predominantly peripheral adaptations, with an increase in peak blood flow to exercising muscles and improved peripheral oxygen extraction. Maximal oxygen uptake also increases. Decrease in the myocardial oxygen demand can lessen ischemia in patients whose etiology of heart failure is ischemic heart disease. Little or no improvement in ventricular function is generally described, suggesting primarily or exclusively a peripheral adaptation in most patients. Improvement in physical work capacity has been effected by long-term, low-intensity exercise training, a regimen well within the ability and safety guidelines for most patients with congestive cardiac failure. A significant improvement in quality of life has been associated both with actual improvement in exercise tolerance and with an improved perception of personal health status.

Recently, some central hemodynamic adaptations (in addition to peripheral adaptations) to exercise training have been suggested to result from longer term, higher intensity exercise training of patients with well-compensated, albeit severe, ventricular dysfunction [11]. Concomitantly, another recent report cautions that left ventricular function may deteriorate in patients with recent large anterior myocardial infarction subjected to early exercise training [15,16]. Clearly, these aspects require further clarification.

Exercise Training in Ventricular Dysfunction and Heart Failure: What we Must Learn

Exercise rehabilitation programs for cardiac patients currently include larger numbers of elderly patients, coronary patients with residual ventricular dysfunction, patients with cardiac enlargement and compensated congestive cardiac failure, medically complex patients with significant comorbidity treated with multiple cardiac drugs, patients after heart valve replacement or valvuloplasty, and patients following cardiac transplantation. A larger number of patients with compensated congestive heart failure or underlying ventricular dysfunction are thus likely to be involved in exercise training.

It remains uncertain whether comparable responses to exercise training occur in patients with different etiologies of ventricular dysfunction. Neither do we know whether the etiology of the heart failure influences the risk of exercise-related malignant ventricular arrhythmias. The optimal mode, duration, and surveillance of exercise training have yet to be determined, as does the relationship of exercise training to drug therapies for congestive heart failure, i.e., the exercise-drug interactions. Finally, the long-term functional and prognostic outcomes of exercise training must be ascertained. Important areas for research, in addition to the effect of exercise training on mortality and morbidity, are the effects on left ventricular function; the mechanism(s) of benefit also require delineation – do they differ with age, gender, etiology of the ventricular dysfunction?

Vasodilator Drugs, Positive Inotropic Drugs, and Exercise Capacity: Ventricular Dysfunction and Heart Failure

In patients with chronic congestive heart failure, the compensatory vasoconstriction and attendant increase in systemic vascular resistance may limit cardiac performance and decrease the delivery of blood to exercising muscles. Vasodilator therapy is designed to overcome this excessive compensatory vasoconstriction that places an increased workload on an already impaired left ventricle. Although many varieties of vasodilator drugs improve symptoms and produce hemodynamic benefit at rest in patients with heart failure, the improvement in exercise capacity and the change in the symptoms that occur with activity appear dependent on the type of vasodilator drug used [17–20]. Any drug that improves symptoms, both at rest and with activity, is likely to encourage an increased spontaneous activity level. The training effect of this spontaneous activity may improve the vasodilator capacity of exercising muscle and increase skeletal muscle oxidative enzymes.

The action of different vasodilator drugs involves different mechanisms of vasodilatation. Vasodilator preparations that act directly on arteriolar smooth muscle, such as hydralazine and calcium antagonist drugs, counteract the excessive compensatory resting vasoconstrictive response to congestive heart failure, thereby decreasing the workload on the left ventricle. However, vasoconstriction normally occurs with exercise in the renal and splanchnic beds; this exercise-induced redistribution of cardiac output is an important adaptation to provide optimal delivery of blood flow to exercising muscles. The nonspecific vasodilator drugs do not permit these regional changes in blood flow just noted to occur, with resulting suboptimal delivery of blood to exercising muscles. Further, since alpha-adrenergic vasoconstriction appears to be the most important mechanism enabling this redistribution of blood flow with exercise, alpha-adrenergic blocking vasodilator drugs, such as prazosin, that result in generalized vasodilatation increase the need for a greater cardiac output; energy output is wasted in perfusing the viscera during exercise, with a resultant lack or limitation of improvement in exercise capacity in patients with heart failure treated with this type of vasodilator agent.

Vasodilator therapy with the angiotensin-converting enzyme inhibitor drugs counteracts the excessive compensatory vasoconstriction of heart failure by decreasing levels of angiotensin II, vasopressin, and norepinephrine. Normal regulation of the sympathetic control of vascular tone during exercise is not impeded, permitting an increase in blood flow to exercising skeletal muscles and limitation of blood flow to the viscera during exercise. This may, at least in part, explain the dramatic improvement in the exercise capacity of patients with congestive heart failure treated with angiotensin-converting enzyme inhibitors [21].

Positive inotropic agents may improve myocardial contractility in patients with heart failure. However, in patients who are asymptomatic at rest, the inotropic effect may be desirable only during activity, i.e., avoiding the unnecessarily increased cardiac work at rest.

Exercise Testing in Ventricular Dysfunction and Heart Failure

Exercise testing can objectively assess the level of exercise tolerance, evaluate the severity of cardiocirculatory impairment or dysfunction, and monitor the changes of these parameters in response to therapy [22]. Contrary to prior concerns, the complications of exercise testing of patients with stable congestive heart failure were minimal in the Veterans Administration Cooperative Study – Vasodilator Heart Failure Trial [23]. No major adverse events occurred during repeated exercise testing of 607 patients in almost 3,000 tests; exercise-induced hypotension was rare, even after the application of vasodilator therapy. Further, exercise testing was terminated in only about 1.6% of all patients because of ventricular arrhythmias.

However, data derived from exercise testing do not predictably reflect the extent to which exercise-related symptoms limit the performance of usual daily activities. Exercise testing is typically terminated by the occurrence of severe symptoms, whereas far more modest symptoms provoke cessation of usual daily activities. Most exercise testing protocols involve continuous work of progressive intensity, whereas the performance of usual activities is intermittent, with marked variations in pace and intensity.

The optimal method for exercise testing of patients with heart failure is not known; and perhaps different methods are preferable for different purposes. For example, to evaluate the ability of a patient with compensated heart failure to return to work (or the converse, to determine that the degree of impairment is too severe to do so, as for disability determinations), an intermittent test protocol may more nearly mimic work activities. This may not be feasible for arm test protocols, as the resistance in the system to be overcome in initiating higher levels of arm exercise may discourage patients from attempting the next step or stage. A continuous test protocol, albeit with small incremental increases in exercise intensity, may adequately measure maximal performance, but it is uncertain whether small benefits from a therapeutic intervention could readily be detected. In patients with heart failure who have a reasonable exercise capacity, the need to perform a large number of exercise steps with small increments of intensity may engender muscle fatigue that does not represent a cardiovascular limitation. The addition of respiratory gas analyses may complement the exercise testing.

Summary

The goal of management of most chronic illnesses is improvement in symptomatic status and enhancement of functional capabilities. Exercise testing can effectively and objectively and with safety assess the activity capacity of patients with heart failure and document the response to therapeutic interventions. Exercise training, predominantly owing to peripheral adaptations, can improve the physical work capacity. The optimal mode(s), intensity, and duration of exercise training; and guidelines for the surveillance and ECG monitoring of this training have yet to be determined.

Acknowledgements. The author expresses appreciation to Julia Wright and Jeanette Zahler for assistance in the preparation of this manuscript.

References

1. The CONCENSUS Trial Study Group (1987) Effects of enalapril on mortality in severe congestive heart failure. Results of the Cooperative North Scandinavian Enalapril Survival Study (CONCENSUS). N Engl J Med 316:1429–1435
2. Cohn JN, Archibald DG, Ziesche S, Franciosa JA, Harston WE, Tristani FE, Dunkman WB, Jacobs W, Francis GS, Flohr KH, Goldman S, Cobb FR, Shah PM, Saunders R, Fletcher RD, Loeb HS, Hughes VC, Baker B (1986) Effect of vasodilator therapy on mortality in chronic congestive heart failure. Results of a Veterans Administration cooperative study. N Engl J Med 314:1547–1552
3. Goldman L, Cook EF, Mitchell N, Flatley M, Sherman H, Cohn PF (1982) Pitfalls in the serial assessment of cardiac functional status. How a reduction in "ordinary" activity may reduce the apparent degree of cardiac compromise and give a misleading impression of improvements. J Chron Dis 35:763–771
4. Franciosa JA (1986) Epidemiologic patterns, clinical evaluation, and long-term prognosis in chronic congestive heart failure. Am J Med 80 (Suppl 2B):14–21
5. Guyatt GH (1985) Methodologic problems in clinical trials in heart failure. J Chron Dis 38:353–363
6. Feinstein AR, Joseph BR, Wells CK (1986) Scientific and clinical problems in indexes of functional disability. Ann Intern Med 81:641–664
7. Massie BM, Conway M, Rajagopalan B, Yonge R, Frostick S, Ledingham J, Sleight P, Radda G (1988) Skeletal muscle metabolism during exercise under ischemic conditions in congestive heart failure. Evidence for abnormalities unrelated to blood flow. Circulation 78:320–326
8. Lipkin DP, Jones DA, Round JM, Poole-Wilson PA (1985) Maximal force, fibre type, and enzymatic activity in quadriceps of patients with severe heart failure: a mechanism for reduced exercise capacity (abstract). Br Heart J 54:622
9. Lipkin DP, Canepa-Anson R, Stephens MR, Poole-Wilson PA (1986) Factors determining symptoms in chronic heart failure: comparison of fast and slow exercise tests. Br Heart J 55:439–445
10. Baker BJ, Wilen MM, Boyd CM, Dinh H, Franciosa JA (1984) Relation of right ventricular ejection fraction to exercise capacity in chronic left ventricular failure. Am J Cardiol 54:596–599
11. Sullivan MJ, Higginbotham MR, Cobb FR (1988) Exercise training in patients with severe left ventricular dysfunction. Hemodynamic and metabolic effects. Circulation 78:506–515
12. Giordano A, Giannuzzi P, Tavazzi L (1988) Feasibility of physical training in post-infarct patients with left ventricular aneurysm: a haemodynamic study. Eur Heart J 9 (Suppl F):11–15
13. Cobb FR, Williams RS, McEwan P, Jones RH, Coleman RE, Wallace AG (1982) Effects of exercise training on ventricular function in patients with recent myocardial infarction. Circulation 66:100–108
14. Shen WF, Roubin GS, Hirasawa K, Choong C Y-P, Hutton BF, Harris PJ, Fletcher PJ, Kelly DT (1985) Left ventricular volume and ejection fraction response to exercise in chronic heart failure: differences between dilated cardiomyopathy and previous myocardial infarction. Am J Cardiol 55:1027–1031
15. Jugdutt BI, Michrowski BL, Kappagoda CT (1988) Exercise training after anterior Q wave myocardial infarction: importance of regional left ventricular function and topography. J Am Coll Cardiol 12:362–372
16. Iskandrian AS (1988) Exercise training after anterior Q wave myocardial infarction: harmful or beneficial. J Am Coll Cardiol 12:373–374
17. Leier CV, Huss P, Magorien RD, Unverferth DV (1983) Improved exercise capacity and differing arterial and venous tolerance during chronic isosorbide dinitrate therapy for congestive heart failure. Circulation 67:817–822
18. Franciosa JA, Wilen MM, Jordan RA (1985) Effects of enalapril, a new angiotensin-converting enzyme inhibitor, in a controlled trial in heart failure. J Am Coll Cardiol 5:101–107
19. Captopril Multicenter Research Group (1983) A placebo-controlled trial of captopril in refractory chronic congestive heart failure. J Am Coll Cardiol 2:755–763

20. Lipkin DT, Poole-Wilson PA (1985) Treatment of chronic heart failure. A review of recent drug trials. Br Med J 291:993–996
21. Tan LB (1987) Clinical and research implications of new concepts in the assessment of cardiac pumping performance in heart failure. Cardiovasc Res 21:615–622
22. Wilson JR (1987) Exercise and the failing heart. Cardiol Clin 5:171–181
23. Tristani FE, Hughes CV, Archibald DG, Sheldahl JM, Cohn JN, Fletcher R (1987) Safety of graded symptom-limited exercise testing in patients with congestive heart failure. Circulation 76 (Suppl VI):VI-54–VI-58

Hemodynamic Response to Exercise in Patients with Congestive Heart Failure

D.T. Kelly, S.D. Anderson, W.F. Shen, C.Y.P. Choong, and G.S. Roubin

Introduction

In normal subjects and athletes, exercise is limited mainly by fatigue which is thought to be due to metabolic changes that occur in exercising muscles [1]. In patients with chronic congestive heart failure (CHF), during exercise abnormal hemodynamics and pulmonary gas exchange patterns develop, but the mechanism of impaired exercise tolerance is thought to be due to the metabolic changes produced by exercising muscles, rather than the central effects of breathlessness arising from the rapidly rising pulmonary wedge pressure and the other abnormal hemodynamic responses [2]. During exercise in normals, there is not only increased total cardiac output, but a considerable redistribution of the cardiac output and an increasing percentage of blood flow goes to the exercising muscles, such that at maximal exercise approximately 75%–80% of the total cardiac output goes to the exercising muscles. This is accompanied by a splenic vasoconstriction.

Physiologically distribution of the cardiac output during exercise is apparently maintained unaltered in CHF [3].

Methods

Study Group. Twenty-three male patients with a mean age of 51 years and a range of 27–62 years, with heart failure in New York Heart Association class II or III were studied. The etiology of heart failure was ischemic in 13 and cardiomyopathy in 10. No patient developed angina or further ST segment changes during exercise, and there was no other evidence of active ischemia in any of the 13 patients whose failure was due initially to coronary disease. The mean left ventricular ejection fraction was 24% with a range of 14%–43%. Primary pulmonary disease was excluded by history and normal resting lung function by spirometry and expiratory flow rates. All patients were taking diuretics, 17 digoxin and 3 vasodilators.

Six men with a mean age of 48 years with normal left ventricular function and normal coronary arteries served as controls. They previously were catheterized because of atypical chest pain.

B.S. Lewis, A. Kimchi (Eds.)
Heart Failure Mechanisms and Management
© Springer-Verlag Berlin Heidelberg 1991

Study Protocol. Patients were exercised in a semi-upright position with an electronically braked bicycle ergometer. Continuous bicycle exercise, starting at 15 W and increasing 15 W every 3 min till exhaustion, was used. The final exercise workload was regarded as the individual patient's maximum workload. At rest and exercise, right atrial pulmonary artery and wedge pressure were measured, as was systemic arterial pressure. In addition, simultaneous gated blood pool radionuclide ventriculography was carried out at rest in each phase of exercise to measure left ventricular ejection fraction. Ventilation was directly measured at rest in all phases of exercise. Systemic and pulmonary resistance were calculated, as was stroke volume and stroke work, by conventional formulae. In all patients metabolic measurements were determined with samples from radial and pulmonary arteries and, in addition, in 13 patients from catheters inserted in the iliac vein. Oxygen transport, bicarbonate, pH, PO_2, and PCO_2, were measured, and from this arterial venous mixed oxygen difference and arterial venous oxygen content difference were calculated from both pulmonary artery and iliac vein. Ventilation was measured at rest and during exercise, and the respiratory exchange ratio R value was derived from the ratio of VCO_2 to VO_2.

Statistical Analysis. Results were expressed as mean and standard error of the mean. Student's *t* test was used to compare the difference between patients and normals at rest and at maximum exercise. The relationship between exercise response and workload was determined by regression analysis. To test the difference in response of each variable between patients and normals, the slope and interception of the regression lines were compared using the analysis of covariance [4]. A significant difference was achieved when the *p* value was less than 0.05. Comparisons of nonlinear relationships were carried out after logarithmic transformation of the data.

Results

The mean maximum workload achieved by controls was 125 ± 7 W and 75 ± 5 W by patients with heart failure. Although patients became breathless they stopped because of fatigue not breathlessness, and no patient developed angina or ST segment changes. Their hemodynamic and metabolic data are illustrated in the accompanying graphs.

Compared to controls, patients with CHF showed abnormal hemodynamic responses to exercise (Fig. 1), decreased oxygen utilization, increased anaerobic metabolism, and reduced exercise capacity. There was a difference between the systemic and pulmonary resistance changes during exercise. Systemic resistance fell in CHF patients although less than in the controls. In contrast, pulmonary resistance in the CHF patients already at a high resting level did not fall during exercise in comparison to controls, where it was markedly lower at rest and fell during exercise. This is an important observation and may partially explain the limitation of maximum exercise capacity in patients with CHF (Fig. 2). Pul-

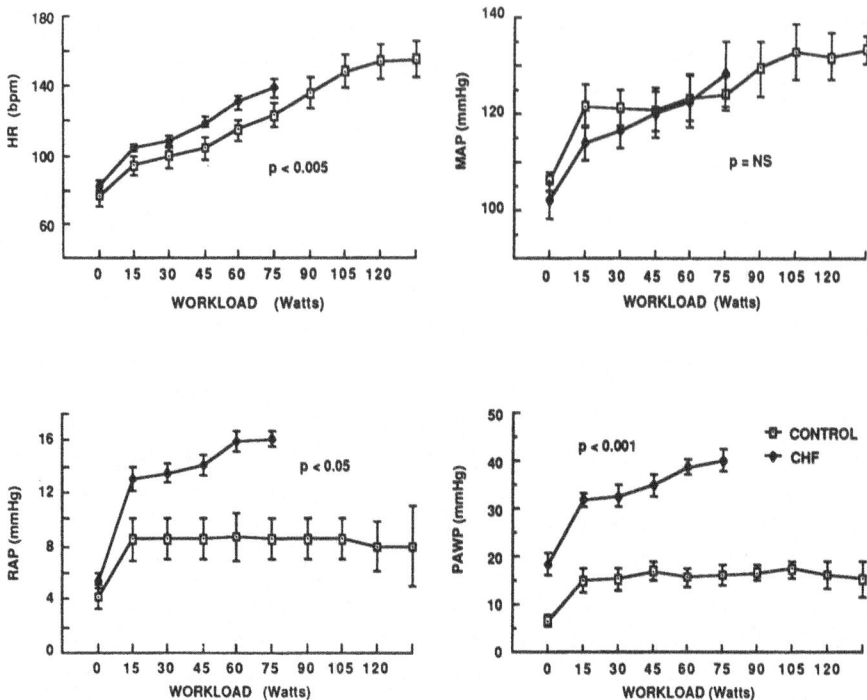

Fig. 1. Heart rate (*HR*), mean arterial pressure (*MAP*), right atrial pressure (*RAP*), and pulmonary wedge pressure (*PA WP*) at rest and during exercise in the control and the heart failure (*CHF*) groups. The *p* values refer to differences during exercise at identical workloads (i.e., the workloads of the CHF patients compared to that same workload of the controls)

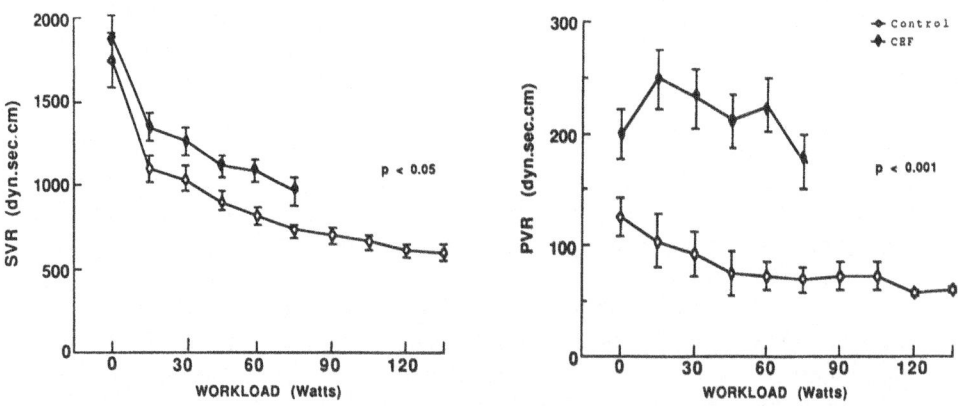

Fig. 2. Systemic vascular resistance (*SVR*) and pulmonary vascular resistance (*PVR*) at rest and during exercise in the control and cardiac heart failure (*CHF*) groups. Regarding *p* values, see Fig. 1

monary vascular resistance changes during exercise have not been well documented in patients with CHF.

When oxygen uptake, cardiac output, and arteriovenous oxygen content differences centrally and in the femoral vein were compared, it was apparent that in patients with CHF the relative arteriovenous oxygen content difference between the legs and the pulmonary artery did not change (Fig. 3). This suggests that in patients with heart failure, the physiological changes in the normal distribution of the cardiac output during exercise which increases blood flow to exercising leg muscle is not relatively altered in spite of the low cardiac output and therefore lower leg blood flow. This confirms previous studies [3].

At maximal exercise, although cardiac output in the CHF patient was much lower than in the controls, the femoral venous pH and PCO_2 were similar, suggesting that acidosis was a common factor that limited exercise by fatigue in both groups (Fig. 4).

The femoral venous PO_2 did not fall below the critical level of 10 mmHg, suggesting that muscle fatigue may not be determined solely by oxygen delivery. Some blood from tissues other than exercising muscle could have been present in our samples, but previous studies have shown that skin blood flow in patients with cardiac heart failure does not contribute significantly to femoral blood flow.

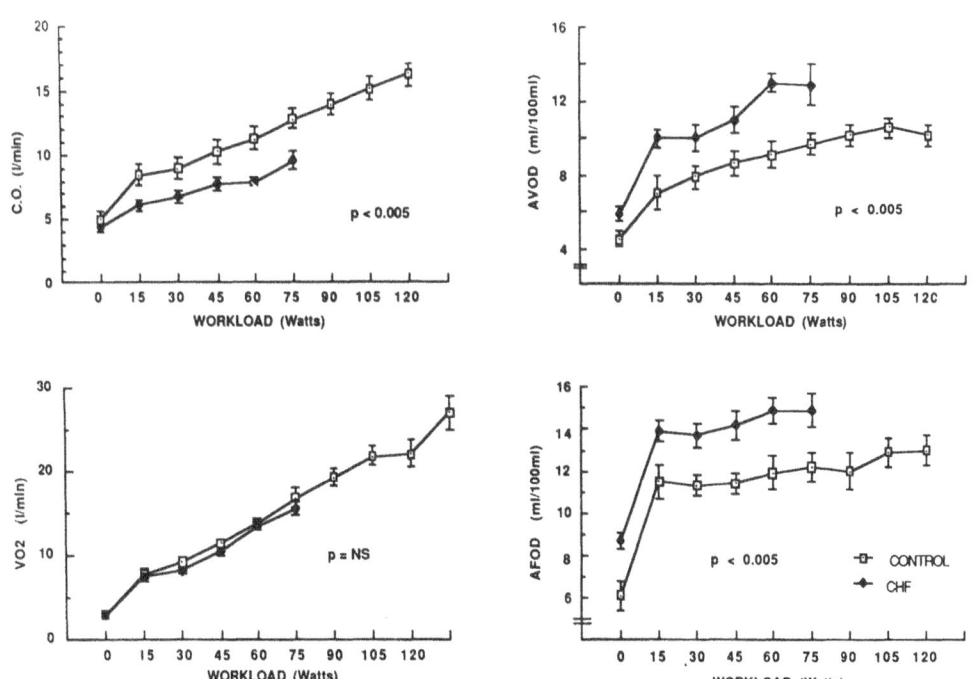

Fig. 3. Cardiac output (*CO*), arterial-mixed venous oxygen content difference (*AVOD*), oxygen consumption (*VO₂*), and arterial-femoral venous oxygen content difference (*AFOD*) at rest and during exercise in control and heart failure groups. Regarding *p* values, see Fig. 1

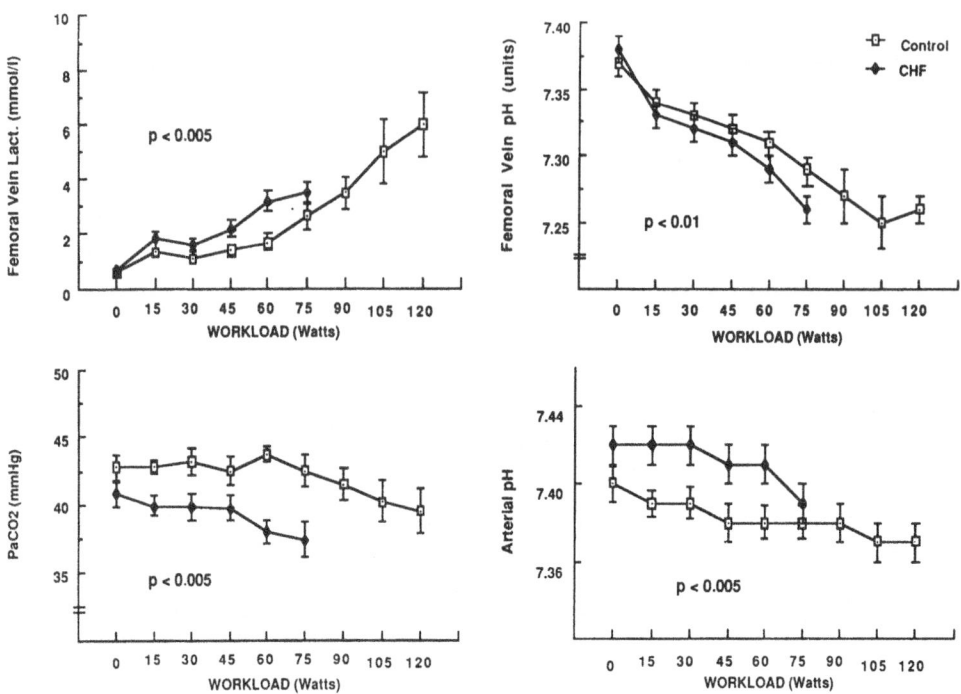

Fig. 4. Femoral venous lactate, femoral pH, arterial carbon dioxide tension ($PaCO_2$), and arterial pH at rest and during exercise in the two groups. Regarding p values, see Fig. 1

Discussion

During progressive exercise levels CHF patients had a lower femoral venous pH, but at maximum exercise, although cardiac output in CHF patients was much lower than the control, the femoral venous pH and PCO_2 values were not significantly different between the two groups. This suggested that acidosis was a common factor that limited exercise by fatigue in both groups, even though the two groups had different exercise capacities.

During exercise, ventilation was higher in the CHF patients. Although dyspnea increased progressively with exercise in both groups, it was not the limiting factor. Weber et al. [5] have shown that during exercise patients with CHF use only a small proportion of their predicted maximum voluntary ventilation, and this is in agreement with our study. Increased lactate and VCO_2 produced by exercising muscles is thought to produce hyperpnea in patients with CHF.

In patients with CHF, the wide femoral arterial-mixed venous oxygen content difference suggests leg blood flow was reduced during exercise and is due to the low cardiac output plus an inability to further redistribute this to exercising limbs. Both oxygen delivery and utilization in exercising muscles were reduced, while anaerobic metabolism was increased. Peripheral metabolic acids accumulating from the exercising muscles together with the increased pulmonary vascular resistance appear to be the factors that limit exercise capacity in patients with congestive heart failure.

References

1. Jones NL (1980) Hydrogen ion balance during exercise. Clin Sci 59:85–91
2. Higginbotham MB, Morris KG, Conn EW, Coleman RE, Cobb FR (1983) Determinants of variable exercise performance among patients with severe left ventricular dysfunction. Am J Cardiol 51:52–60
3. Franciosa JA, Leddy CL, Wilen M, Schwartz DE (1984) Relation between haemodynamic and ventilatory responses in determining exercise capacity in severe congestive heart failure. Am J Cardiol 53:127–134
4. Snedecor GW, Cochrane WG (1967) Statistical methods, 6th edn. Iowa State Univ Press, Ames
5. Weber KT, Kinasewitz GT, Janicki JS, Fishman AP (1982) Oxygen utilization and ventilation during exercise in patients with chronic cardiac failure. Circulation 65:1213–1223

Substrate Utilization During Exercise in Chronic Cardiac Failure

M. Riley, J.S. Elborn, C.F. Stanford, and D.P. Nicholls

Introduction

The classical definition of chronic cardiac failure (CCF) as a state in which the heart fails to maintain an adequate circulation for the needs of the body [1] does not refer to the numerous hormonal and metabolic adaptations to the condition [2]. Foremost amongst these are abnormal neurohumoral responses at rest and during exercise [3], such as increased activation of the sympathetic and renin-angiotensin-aldosterone system, which may in fact be counter-productive. In addition, there are abnormalities of peripheral circulation, perhaps related to the above, but not simply due to reduced cardiac output, as an acute rise in cardiac output does not necessarily result in functional improvement [4]. The use of ^{31}P nuclear magnetic resonance (^{31}P-NMR) has revealed metabolic abnormalities in skeletal muscle in patients with CCF [5]. The contribution of these various factors to the clinical picture in patients remains unclear.

Substrate utilization during steady-state submaximal (aerobic) exercise was studied in a group of patients with CCF and in normal controls. Such a test was chosen so as to reproduce daily activity, in that patients rarely exercise to their symptom-limited maximum, and also to minimize increases in blood lactate concentrations, which would have the effect of causing evolution of CO_2 not directly produced by oxidative processes [6].

Studies on Patients

We studied 15 patients with stable, non-oedematous CCF in NYHA functional classes II or III, comparing them with 14 age- and sex-matched sedentary controls. Substrate utilization was determined by indirect calorimetry, in which the amounts of O_2 consumed ($\dot{V}O_2$), CO_2 produced ($\dot{V}CO_2$) and N_2 excreted are used to assess the relative contributions of fat, carbohydrate and protein to energy expenditure [7,8]. Subjects, having been previously familiarized with the exercise equipment, presented to the laboratory after an overnight fast and, in the case of the patients, prior to their morning medication. A Teflon cannula was inserted into a vein in the antecubital fossa, and a 2-h urine collection commenced immediately before exercise began for measurement of urea excretion. We initially attempted to measure urea excretion in sweat as well by using covered filter paper patches, but none was detected due to the low workloads performed.

B.S. Lewis, A. Kimchi (Eds.)
Heart Failure Mechanisms and Management
© Springer-Verlag Berlin Heidelberg 1991

Subjects then performed a constant speed treadmill exercise test for 20 min. Throughout the test, respired gas analysis was performed. Subjects breathed through a mouthpiece with a noseclip in situ. Inspired air flow was measured by a vane turbine, and expired air O_2 and CO_2 concentrations determined by paramagnetic and infra-red analysis respectively. $\dot{V}O_2$, $\dot{V}CO_2$ and minute ventilation ($\dot{V}E$) were displayed on-line by a computer.

Responses were analysed for the steady-state period of $\dot{V}O_2$. The workload chosen corresponded to 56% ± 7% (mean ± SD) in patients, and 52% ± 4% in normals, of their predetermined peak achieved $\dot{V}O_2$ (Fig. 1). The heart rate and $\dot{V}E$ at steady-state did not differ in the two groups, in spite of the different absolute workloads. Blood lactate levels showed a small rise in both groups at the beginning of exercise but remained stable thereafter (Fig. 2). The overall lactate level was higher in patients, but no significant difference between patients and controls was detected at any given time point. Free fatty acid (FFA) and noradrenaline levels were higher in patients throughout exercise (Fig. 3). The respiratory exchange ratio ($\dot{V}CO_2/\dot{V}O_2$), equivalent to the respiratory quotient (RQ), was significantly lower in patients (Fig. 4). Along with small differences in urinary N_2 excretion, this enabled us to conclude that patients proportionately use more fat, less carbohydrate, and slightly more protein during exercise than do normals (Fig. 5).

Discussion

Our results confirm abnormal metabolism during exercise in patients with CCF. Several studies [9–11] have shown increased lactate responses during exercise

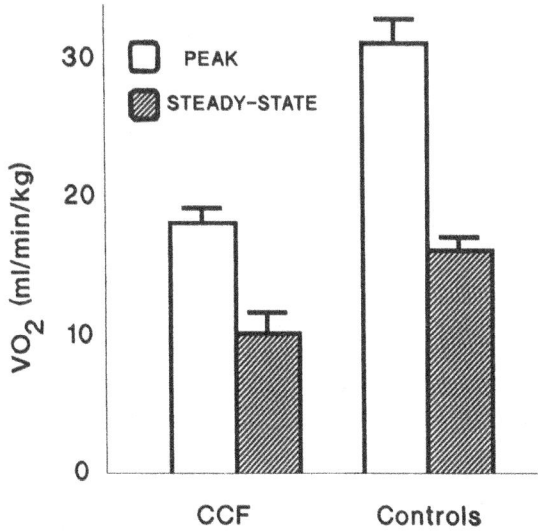

Fig. 1. Peak oxygen consumption (mean ± SEM; *open bars*) and steady-state oxygen consumption (*hatched bars*) in patients and controls. The ratio steady-state $\dot{V}O_2$: peak $\dot{V}O_2$ was 55.6 ±6.5% (mean ± SD) in patients and 52.0 ±4.4% in controls (NS)

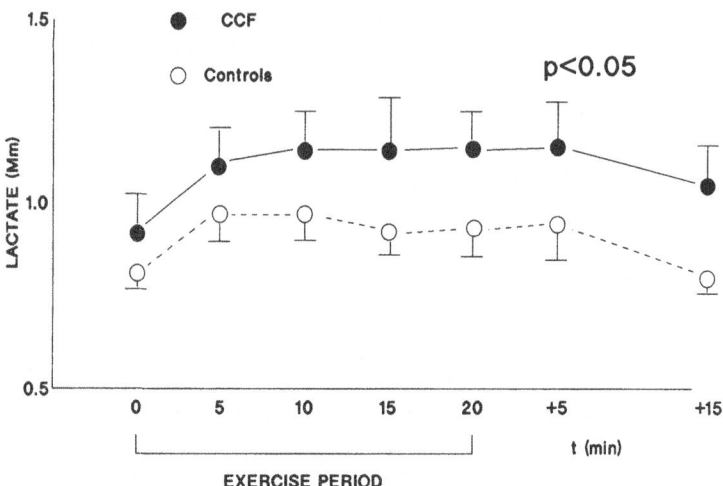

Fig. 2. Venous lactate (mean ± SEM) during the steady-state exercise test in patients (*filled circles*) and controls (*open circles*). Overall, lactate was higher in patients, but the difference was not significant at any individual time point

compared to controls, and this has been ascribed to poor cardiac output. Administration of amrinone, a positive inotrope, can delay the lactate response to exercise [12,13], but β-agonists such as dobutamine [4,14] and dopamine [15] increase cardiac output without increasing peak achieved $\dot{V}O_2$ or delaying the lactate rise. Other workers have also found a poor correlation between exercise tolerance and haemodynamic indices of cardiac function [16–18], which would point towards peripheral dysfunction. Using the technique of ^{31}P-NMR, recent work has suggested skeletal muscle abnormalities in patients with CCF [19,20], with the occurrence of excessive acidosis and a rise in the phosphate/ phosphocreatine ratio. These differences are observed at similar relative workloads to controls [5], despite similar levels of muscle blood flow. It is probable therefore that the changes observed in CCF are due to abnormalities of peripheral metabolism rather than simply due to poor blood flow to working muscle.

It might be expected that the metabolism in patients would resemble deconditioned individuals, in whom fat utilization is less than in controls [21–25], but in fact we observed greater fat utilization in patients. The key to this apparent paradox may lie in the elevated noradrenaline and FFA levels observed in our patients. Resting noradrenaline levels are known to be increased in CCF [26,27], and as in normal subjects [28,29] levels increase with exercise, although the peak response may be less [3,30,31]. Our data indicate that noradrenaline levels are elevated compared to normals during submaximal exercise. Noradrenaline is known to stimulate lipolysis [32–34], and the increased FFA levels observed in our patients are in keeping with this. Elevated FFA levels usually indicate greater fat utilization [33,35,36], and we have confirmed this by indirect calorimetry. Lactate inhibits lipolysis [37,38], but the small difference in lactate that we measured is probably insufficient to have any great effect.

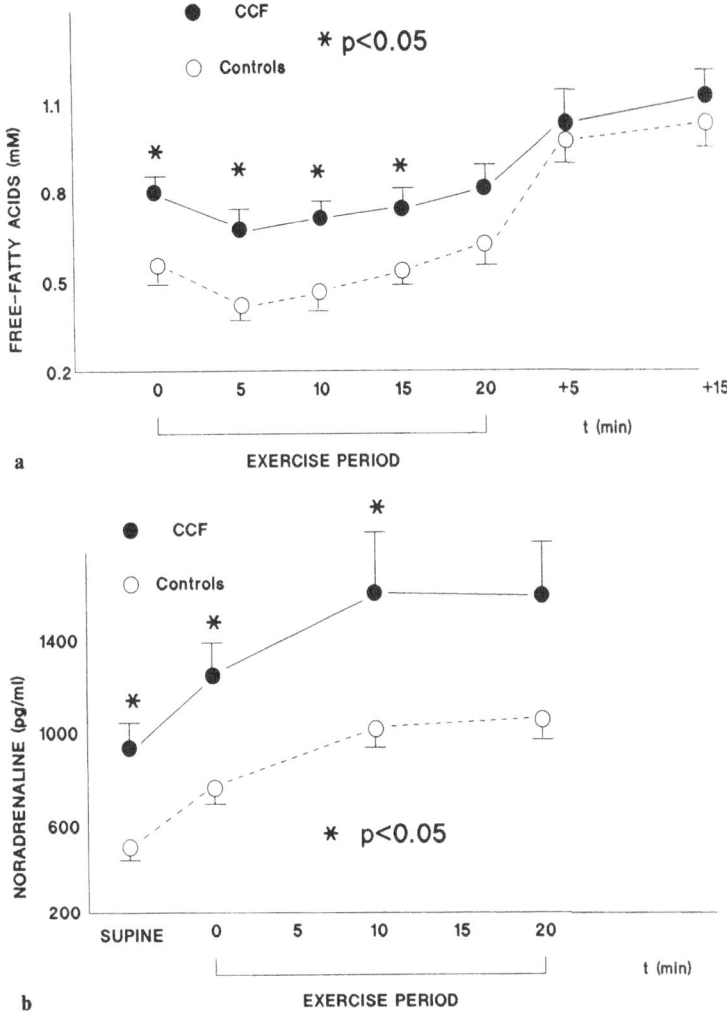

Fig. 3. Free fatty acids (**a**) and noradrenaline (**b**; mean ± SEM) during the steady-state exercise test in patients (*filled circles*) and controls. Analysis of variance showed both FFA and noradrenaline to be elevated in patients, the differences being significant at the individual time points shown

In addition to catecholamines, other factors may influence substrate utilization. Insulin may suppress fat utilization [39]. Levels fall during exercise in normals, but paradoxically levels are higher in the trained state [28,29]. This would cast doubt on the role of insulin as a regulator of substrate utilization patterns during exercise. Growth hormone may increase FFA levels [40] and shows a prolonged rise with exercise [28,29]. The significance of these observations in relation to patients with CCF has not yet been clarified.

Reduced muscle glycogen stores have been demonstrated in patients with CCF [41]. Elevated FFA levels and increased fat utilization may preserve muscle glycogen [39] by inhibiting its use [42]. This may be advantageous to the individual

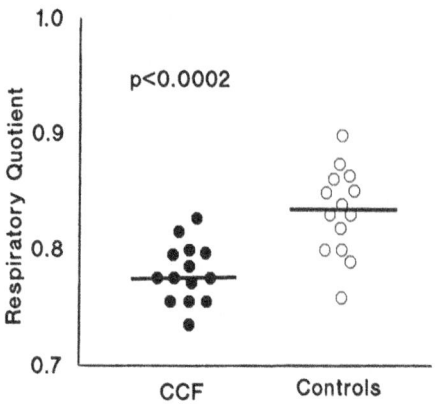

Fig. 4. Respiratory quotient ($\dot{V}CO_2 / \dot{V}O_2$) in patients (*filled circles*) and controls. The mean of each group is indicated by the *solid line*

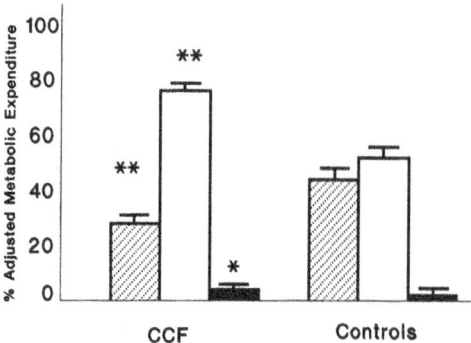

Fig. 5. Percentage (mean ± SEM) of carbohydrate (*hatched bars*), fat (*open bars*) and protein (*filled bars*) utilized during the steady-state exercise in patients and controls. Values are expressed as a percentage of adjusted metabolic expenditure. Significant differences in utilization between patients and controls are illustrated by * ($p < 0.05$) and ** ($p < 0.0002$)

with CCF, as depletion of muscle glycogen has been demonstrated to be closely associated with the development of fatigue [43]. Fatigue occurs less rapidly when the diet is rich in carbohydrate [44], so maximizing muscle glycogen stores. Fat stores are very much larger, and so depletion is not encountered [45]. A shift to fat metabolism may therefore be an adaptive process to attempt to conserve normal muscle function.

Protein is normally not utilized to any great extent during exercise [46,47], but when muscle glycogen stores are depleted, protein may contribute up to 10% of energy expenditure during maximal exercise [48]. We observed a small but unimportant increase in protein utilization in patients with CCF, although inaccuracies may have arisen both from the method of estimation, and possibly from the effects of drugs on urea excretion.

The increased dependency on fat utilization in patients with CCF may therefore be a net result of several complex neurohumoral and metabolic abnormalities. The overall result is less efficient use of delivered O_2, as $1\,1\,O_2$ when oxidizing glycogen alone yields 6.5 mol ATP, whereas when FFA is oxidized, only 5.6 mol ATP is produced [45]. As impaired O_2 delivery by the circulation is a fundamental problem in CCF [49], a shift to fat utilization would further reduce exercise capacity. It is not known whether a dietary increase in carbohydrate intake would change the substrate utilization profile [44] and so improve functional capacity.

Conclusion

This study has demonstrated abnormal metabolism during exercise in patients with CCF, with a shift towards fat utilization. This may occur as a compensatory mechanism, but the result is likely to be a further reduction in functional capacity. The exact cause of these metabolic changes has not yet been identified.

References

1. Wood PW (1956) Diseases of the heart and circulation. Lippincott, Philadelphia
2. Harris P (1983) Evolution and the cardiac patient. 6. Origins of congestive cardiac failure. Cardiovasc Res 17:440–445
3. Francis GS (1985) Neurohumoral mechanisms involved in congestive heart failure. Am J Cardiol 55:15A–21A
4. Wilson JR, Martin JL, Ferraro N (1984) Impaired skeletal muscle nutritive flow during exercise in patients with congestive heart failure: role of cardiac pump dysfunction as determined by the effect of dobutamine. Am J Cardiol 53:1308–1315
5. Massie B, Conway M, Yonge R, Frostick S, Ledingham T, Sleight P, Radda G, Rajagopalan B (1987) Skeletal muscle metabolism in patients with congestive heart failure: relation to clinical severity and blood flow. Circulation 76:1009–1019
6. Clode M, Campbell EJM (1969) The relationship between gas exchange and change in blood lactate concentrations during exercise. Clin Sci 37:263–272
7. Lusk G (1923) The elements of the science of nutrition, 3rd edn. Saunders, Philadelphia, pp 18–25, 468–472
8. Frayn KN (1983) Calculation of substrate oxidation rates in vivo from gaseous exchange. J Appl Physiol 55:628–634
9. Meakins T, Long CVH (1927) Oxygen consumption, oxygen debt and lactic acid in circulatory failure. J Clin Invest 4:273–293
10. Cotes JE (1955) The role of oxygen, carbon dioxide and lactic acid in the ventilatory response to exercise in patients with mitral stenosis. Clin Sci 14:317–328
11. Huckabee WE, Judson WE (1958) The role of anaerobic metabolism in the performance of mild muscular work. I. Relationship to oxygen consumption and cardiac output and the effect of congestive heart failure. J Clin Invest 37:1577–1592
12. Siskind SJ, Sonnenblick EH, Forman R, Scheuer T, Le Jemtel TH (1981) Acute substantial benefit of inotropic therapy with amrinone on exercise haemodynamics and metabolism in severe congestive heart failure. Circulation 64:966–973
13. Weber KT, Janicki TS (1985) Lactate production during maximal and submaximal exercise in patients with chronic heart failure. J Am Coll Cardiol 6:717–724
14. Maskin CS, Forman R, Sonnenblick EH, Frishman WH, Le Jemtel TH (1983) Failure of dobutamine to increase exercise capacity despite hemodynamic improvement in severe heart failure. Am J Cardiol 51:177–182
15. Maskin CS, Kugler J, Sonnenblick EH, Le Jemtel TH (1983) Acute inotropic stimulation with dopamine in severe congestive heart failure: beneficial hemodynamic effect at rest but not during maximal exercise. Am J Cardiol 52:1028–1032

16. Franciosa JA, Ziesche S, Wilen M (1979) Functional capacity of patients with chronic left ventricular failure: relationship of bicycle exercise performance to clinical and hemodynamic characterization. Am J Med 67:460–466

17. Litchfield RL, Kerber RE, Benge JW, Mark AL, Sopko J, Bhatnagar RK, Marcus ML (1982) Normal exercise capacity in patients with severe left ventricular dysfunction: compensatory mechanisms. Circulation 66:129–134

18. Szlachcic J, Massie BM, Kramer BL, Topic N, Tubau J (1985) Correlates and prognostic implication of exercise capacity in chronic congestive heart failure. Am J Cardiol 55:1037–1042

19. Wilson JR, Fink L, Maris J, Ferraro N, Power-Vanwart T, Eleff S, Chance B (1985) Evaluation of energy metabolism in skeletal muscle of patients with heart failure with gated phosphorus-31 nuclear magnetic resonance. Circulation 71:57–62

20. Ledingham J, Radda G, Rajagopalan B (1989) Phosphorus magnetic resonance spectroscopy of leg muscle in heart failure. Clin Sci 76:48P–49P

21. Issekutz B, Miller HI, Paul P, Ravatil K (1965) Aerobic work capacity and plasma FFA turnover. J Appl Physiol 20:293–296

22. Saltin B, Nazar K, Costill DL, Stein E, Jansson E, Essen B, Gollnick PD (1976) The nature of the training response: peripheral and central adaptation to one-legged exercise. Acta Physiol Scand 96:289–305

23. Henriksson J (1977) Training induced adaptations of skeletal muscle and metabolism during submaximal exercise. J Physiol 270:661–675

24. Gollnick PD, Saltin B (1982) Significance of skeletal muscle oxidative enzyme enhancement with endurance training. Clin Physiol 2:1–12

25. Gollnick PD (1985) Metabolism of substrates: energy substrate metabolism during exercise and as modified by training. Fed Proc 44:353–357

26. Chidsey CA, Harrison DC, Braunwald E (1962) Augmentation of plasma nor-epinephrine response to exercise in patients with congestive heart failure. N Engl J Med 267:650–654

27. Francis GS, Goldsmith SR, Pierpont G, Cohn JN (1984) Free and conjugated plasma cate-cholamines in patients with congestive heart failure. J Lab Clin Med 103:393–398

28. Hartley LH, Mason JW, Hogan RP, Jones LG, Kotchen TA, Mougley EH, Wherry FE, Pennington LL, Ricketts PT (1972) Multiple hormonal responses to graded exercise in relation to physical training. J Appl Physiol 33:602–606

29. Bloom SR, Johnson RH, Park DM, Rennie MJ, Sulaiman WR (1976) Differences in the metabolic and hormonal response to exercise between racing cyclists and untrained individuals. J Physiol 258:1–18

30. Francis GS, Goldsmith SR, Ziesche SM, Cohn JN (1982) Response of plasma norepinephrine and epinephrine to dynamic exercise in patients with congestive heart failure. Am J Cardiol 49:1152–1156

31. Francis GS, Goldsmith SR, Ziesche S, Nakajima H, Cohn JN (1985) Relative attenuation of sympathetic drive during exercise in patients with congestive heart failure. J Am Coll Cardiol 5:832–839

32. Steinberg D, Nestel PJ, Buskirk ER, Thompson RH (1964) Calorigenic effect of norepinephrine correlated with plasma free fatty acid turnover and oxidation. J Clin Invest 43:167–176

33. Issekutz B, Miller HI, Paul P, Rodahl K (1964) Source of fat oxidation in exercising dogs. Am J Physiol 207:583–589

34. Rodahl K, Miller HI, Issekutz B (1964) Plasma free fatty acids in exercise. J Appl Physiol 19:489–492

35. Fritz IB, Davis DG, Holtrop RH, Dundee H (1958) Fatty acid oxidation by skeletal muscle during rest and activity. Am J Physiol 194:379–386

36. Paul P (1975) Effects of long lasting physical exercise and training on lipid metabolism. In: Howald H, Poortmans TR (eds) Metabolic adaptation to prolonged physical exercise. Birkhäuser, Basel, pp 156–193

37. Fredholm BB (1971) The effect of lactate in canine subcutaneous adipose tissue in situ. Acta Physiol Scand 81:110–123

38. Issekutz B, Shaw WAS, Issekutz TB (1975) Effect of lactate on FFA and glycerol turnover in resting and exercising dogs. J Appl Physiol 39:349–353

39. Costill DL, Coyle E, Dalsky G, Evans W, Fink W, Hoopes D (1977) Effects of elevated plasma FFA and insulin on muscle glycogen usage during exercise. J Appl Physiol 43:695–699

40. Grunt JA, Crigler TF, Slone D, Soeldner JS (1967) Changes in serum insulin, blood sugar and free fatty acid levels four hours after administration of human growth hormone to fasting children with short stature. Yale J Biol Med 40:68–74

41. Broqvist M, Dehlstrom U, Karlsson E, Larsson J (1987) Electrolytes and energy metabolism in severe chronic congestive heart failure. Circulation 76 (Suppl IV): IV–357

42. Rennie M, Winder WM, Holloszy JO (1976) A sparing effect of increased free fatty acids on muscle glycogen content in exercising rat. Biochem J 156:647–655

43. Bergstrom J, Hermansen L, Hultman E, Saltin B (1967) Diet, muscle glycogen and physical performance. Acta Physiol Scand 71:140–150

44. Christensen E-H, Hansen O (1939) Arbeitsfähigkeit und Ernährung. Skand Arch Physiol 81:160–175

45. Åstrand P-O, Rodahl K (1986) Textbook of work physiology, 3rd edn. McGraw-Hill, New York

46. Crittenden RH (1904) Physiological economy in nutrition. Stokes, New York

47. Hedman R (1957) The available glycogen in man and the connection between rate of oxygen intake and carbohydrate usage. Acta Physiol Scand 40:305–321

48. Lemon PWR, Mullin JP (1980) Effect of initial muscle glycogen levels on protein catabolism during exercise. J Appl Physiol 48:624–629

49. Weber KT, Kinasewitz GT, Janicki JS, Fishman AP (1982) Oxygen utilization and ventilation during exercise in patients with chronic heart failure. Circulation 65:1213–1223

Neurohumoral Mechanisms

Metabolic and Neurogenic Determinants of Blood Flow in Congestive Heart Failure*

R. Zelis, L. Sinoway, T. Musch, D. Davis, B. Clemson, and U. Leuenberger

Introduction

One of the most striking regional blood flow abnormalities noted in congestive heart failure (CHF) is the inability of skeletal muscle blood flow to increase normally in response to a maximal metabolic vasodilator stimulus [1,2]. Whereas this is seen during systemic dynamic exercise, it is also demonstrable when a metabolic vasodilator stimulus is applied to a single limb, suggesting that the abnormality resides in the peripheral circulation not with the heart. As a substitute for exercise we have used another metabolic stimulus to evaluate the mechanisms responsible for this abnormality. When blood flow is interrupted to an extremity for 5-10 min, and the arterial occlusion is suddenly released, blood flow increases very rapidly, reaching a peak within 5-15 s. This is the peak reactive hyperemic blood flow response (RHBF), which is a good index of maximal metabolic vasodilator capacity. This is significantly reduced in CHF to levels that are 50% of normal [2]. This reduction is proportional to the maximal oxygen consumption that can be achieved with systemic dynamic exercise [3]. It has been suggested that the abnormality in vasodilator capacity was not with the precapillary resistance vessels but was more likely to be at the level of the small arterial resistance vessels. Previously these vessels had been thought to serve primarily a conductance function, but now they are recognized contributors to peripheral vascular resistance [4].

Mechanisms for Impaired RHBF

Although it has been suggested that the sympathetic nervous system restrains maximal skeletal muscle blood flow during exercise, nerve blockade and alpha blockade with intra-arterial phentolamine failed to increase peak RHBF to normal in CHF [1].

A number of lines of evidence have implicated sodium as contributing to stiffness of these vessels [2]. Increased vascular sodium has been noted in an animal model of heart failure [1]. Feeding salt and a mineralocorticoid reduced

*Supported by grants from the UP PHS (HL 30691, HL 34510, and HL 01744) and the American Heart Association, South Central Pennsylvania Chapter.

B.S. Lewis, A. Kimchi (Eds.)
Heart Failure Mechanisms and Management
© Springer-Verlag Berlin Heidelberg 1991

peak RHBF in normal individuals [1]. Sodium retention might also work by increasing tissue pressure (subclinical edema). Increasing venous pressure for a number of hours in an animal or human reduced peak RHBF concomitant with an increase in tissue pressure [1].

Moreover vigorous diuresis increased peak RHBF approximately 30% of the way to normal over a 24-h period [5]. However continued diuresis failed to increase peak RHBF further. Therefore it seemed clear that some additional factor must be operative in regulating maximal arterial blood flow. Recent studies have helped define this factor, which accounts for the remaining 70% of the abnormality [6] (Fig. 1).

To determine the relationship of cardiac function to the peak RHBF abnormality, maximal blood flow was measured before and at two time points following cardiac transplantation [6]. Just prior to discharge from the hospital, peak RHBF had increased only minimally despite the fact that the transplanted heart was functioning normally, and the patients were free of heart failure symptoms. When the subjects were studied a number of months later, after they had returned to normal activities, peak RHBF had returned completely to normal. This delay suggested that some element of exercise conditioning may have been playing a role.

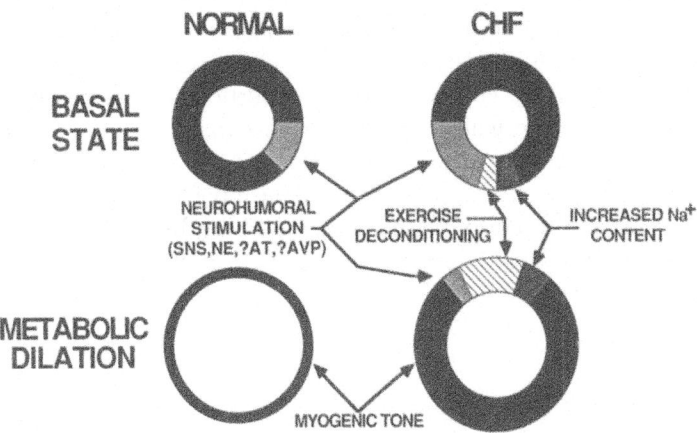

Fig. 1. Determinants of vasomotor tone in the basal state and under conditions of metabolic vasodilation. The lumen of each blood vessel is drawn to scale from data derived from studies of blood flow in human limbs. The relative contribution of neurohumoral stimulation and the two components of the "stiffness factor" (sodium and deconditioning) to a reduced blood flow noted in CHF are portrayed. *CHF*, congestive heart failure; *SNS*, sympathetic nervous system neuronal activity; *NE*, norepinephrine; *AT*, angiotensin; *AVP*, arginine vasopressin. (Reproduced from Modern Concepts in Cardiovascular Diseases 58:7–18, 1989 by permission of the American Heart Association [46])

Exercise Conditioning and RHBF

There are considerable data to support the contention that the vasculature participates in an exercise-conditioning response. One of the first studies to support this hypothesis was of tennis players [7]. In these individuals who have a high degree of conditioning of one upper extremity, maximal arterial conductance was considerably greater in the dominant limb. In a group of unconditioned normal volunteers a program of unilateral gripping exercise performed over a period of 4 weeks resulted in a significant increase in peak RHBF, whereas there was no significant change in the untrained limb [8]. Studies of individuals who had experienced upper limb immobilization due to placement of a cast following an orthopedic procedure, showed that the immobilized limb had a lower peak RHBF than a normally functioning limb, a process that was reversed after 1 month of normal bilateral upper arm activity [9]. These data make a compelling case that chronic activity can lead to an increased limb vasodilator capacity, whereas inactivity can lead to a reduced limb vasodilator capacity.

Endothelial Function in Small Arteries

Recent data suggest that the small arteries are really large resistance vessels that play a regulatory role coupling the heart and the precapillary resistance vessels [10–11]. With metabolic vasodilatation and accumulation of local tissue metabolites, precapillary resistance vessels relax. The dilation however extends proximal to the level of local metabolite production by a process of ascending vasodilation. This may be mediated by propagation of an action potential upstream over short distances. The function of this dilatation is to feed more blood to a muscle group that is metabolically active. As flow increases to this group the velocity along the course of the larger resistance vessels (small arteries) increases. An increase in endothelial sheer rate then leads to dilatation of these vessels by inducing the release of endothelially derived relaxing factor (EDRF) causing the adjacent vascular smooth muscle to relax. Recently, one EDRF has been identified and the metabolic process for its production has been defined. Nitric oxide (NO) synthase is the enzyme for production of NO from L-Arginine [12]. In addition, an endothelly derived hyperpolarizing factor has been postulated (EDHF) which can also mediate vasodilation.

It has been shown that a chronic change in blood velocity across a vascular segment can lead to an altered capacity of the endothelium to release EDRF in a response to an appropriate stimulus. An arterial-venous shunt leads to an increased EDRF release capacity [13]. Moreover, it was recently demonstrated that isolated vessels taken from an animal model of CHF have a reduced capacity to release EDRF [14]. The capacity to the vasculature in humans to respond stimuli that release EDRF has been demonstrated. In particular, flow-mediated relaxation of the brachial artery is readily demonstrable in humans by a process that has a time constant similar to that described in animals [11].

Recently, studies in humans have suggested that forearm resistance vessels and large arteries failed to dilate normally to intraarterial acetylcholine [15]. The small vessel abnormality was specific since the response to nitroglycerine was normal, suggesting that there was endothelial dysfunction. The large arteries failed to respond to the nitrate, suggesting that structural abnormalities were present. Flow mediated relaxation of large vessels was also noted. Some of these abnormalities are likely secondary to the chronic low flow state associated with heart failure and it can be reversed by exercising conditioning [4] (Fig. 1).

It is important to note that changes in the ability of vessels to alter their maximal vasodilator potential do not occur instantaneously. When a chronic low flow state is introduced, the deconditioning process develops slowly. When a high flow state is introduced, the favorable vascular changes are also slow to develop. These observations may help explain why there is a delay in the improvement of exercise tolerance with vasodilator therapy of patients with heart failure or following cardiac transplantation [4]. It might also explain why compensated patients with heart failure may not display this abnormality despite the with-holding of vasodilator drugs for a period of 1-2 days. To demonstrate this abnormality not only must decompensation of heart failure develop, but it must also be associated with a decrease in activity.

Skeletal Muscle Metabolism in CHF

The impairment in exercise tolerance in CHF implies that there is a reduction in maximal systemic oxygen consumption (VO_{2max}) or a reduction in exercise duration at a submaximal level of exertion [16-18]. Cardiac abnormalities alone can not explain this reduction in VO_{2max}. An acute improvement in resting or exercise cardiac output produced by a positive inotropic agent or a vasodilator fails to result in a major increase in VO_{2max} [19,20]. Rather, it is likely that part of the reduction in VO_{2max} is related to the vascular stiffness abnormality. With exercise of one arm at various submaximal levels of exertion, blood flow failed to increase normally in heart failure. Although this was accompanied by an increased oxygen extraction, it was not sufficient to normalize arm oxygen consumption during exercise [1].

Further evidence for the concept that the vascular stiffness factor may contribute to a reduced exercise VO_2 came from studies in an animal isolated exercising skeletal muscle preparation [1]. Two interventions were introduced which attenuated the exercise hyperemia. The intra-arterial infusion of no-repinephrine (NE) lowered skeletal muscle blood flow during exercise, however oxygen consumption was well maintained. It was suggested that an intramuscular redistribution of blood flow from inactive to active muscle fibers occurred. Thus, activation of the sympathetic nervous system in CHF could be playing a protective role which is favorable for the metabolic requirements of exercising skeletal muscle, thereby enhancing circulatory efficiency [1].

The second intervention used to attenuate the exercise hyperemia was restriction of blood flow at the large arterial level. Coincident with the fall in blood flow was a comparable reduction in oxygen consumption. From this study, it was proposed that the vascular stiffness factor in heart failure had metabolic consequences.

Recently it has been demonstrated that there is a significant intrinsic abnormality in skeletal muscle metabolism in CHF as well as a flow abnormality. In some patients with CHF, there appears to be a greater depletion in high-energy phosphates, increased glycolysis, and skeletal muscle acidosis during exercise which are not dependent on the level of exercise hyperemia [21,22]. Whether this is secondary to a chronic low blood flow state or secondary to inactivity and thus deconditioning, is not clear. Changes in mitochondrial structure have been noted in heart failure, suggesting a reduced content of oxidative enzymes similar to that seen with the deconditioning [23].

These skeletal muscle metabolic abnormalities can have significant systemic consequences during exercise, the most significant of which is the production of lactic acidosis. Moreover, the unfavorable metabolic status of exercising skeletal may be one of the factors triggering activation of the sympathetic nervous system.

Afferent Stimulus for Sympathetic Vasoconstriction

Multiple factors may incite the increases in sympathetic tone during exercise in CHF. Relative hypotension may be present due to an inappropriately low pressor response from failure of the heart to increase contractility or to respond appropriately to the increased venous return. Normally an increase in systemic arterial pressure causes arterial baroreceptors to restrain the sympathetic nervous system during exercise. In CHF, not only is blood pressure lower [16], but the baroreceptors do not respond normally [24]. In addition, the cardiopulmonary baroreceptor afferent response to the increased venous return may be blunted as well [24]. This usually modulates the increased sympathetic tone that accompanies exercise. Somatic afferent nerves in skeletal muscle that respond to metabolic stimuli (low pH, decreased PCr/Pi ratio) during exercise may be activated due to poor skeletal muscle perfusion [25]. There may also be an increased "central command" component of the exercise vasoconstrictor reflex. Central command is the reflex response elicited by the conscious volitional activity to exercise. This normally produces an increase in heart rate at the beginning of exercise. It may also increase sympathetic vasoconstrictor activity [26] at more strenuous levels of *perceived* exertion. Additionally the sudden increase in venous return of cold blood from the extremities can transiently decrease core temperature and lead to a cutaneous arteriolar constriction [1]. Lastly, venous congestion could initiate a venoarterial spinal reflex leading to sympathetic efferent nerve activation [27].

Sympathetically Mediated Vasoconstriction

The extent of "sympathetically mediated vasoconstriction" in CHF is difficult to quantify. That is because a number of processes are involved, any one of which could serve as an index of "sympathetic tone." Firstly there is sympathetic efferent nerve depolarization. This causes the release of NE, which then interacts with postjunctional alpha receptors to constrict vascular smooth muscle. These events, located at the vascular neuroeffector junction, are accompanied by a number of additional processes (Fig. 2). Some of these have been studied in CHF. It is important to note that the role of the sympathetic nervous system in regulating myocardial contractility may be different from that played in peripheral tissues [28]. In addition, the events occurring around vascular sympathetic nerves in different vascular tissues may also be different. In this discussion, no distinctions are made between data from individual vascular beds.

Neuronal Norepinephrine Release

Depolarization of the sympathetic nerves (1)[1] is accompanied by NE released (2) into the neuroeffector junction. The neurotransmitter interacts with post-

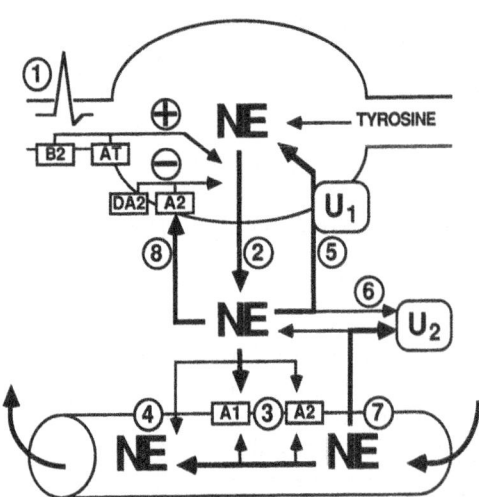

Fig. 2. Factors regulating norepinephrine (*NE*) release, uptake, and spillover into the circulation. These are indicated by circled numbers and are described in the text, with the numbers enclosed in parentheses. U_1, Neuronal NE uptake; U_2, nonneuronal NE uptake. Abbreviations for pre- and postjunctional receptors: *B2*, beta^{-2}; *A1*, alpha^{-2}; *A2*, alpha^{-2} adrenergic receptors; *DA2*, dopaminergic; *AT*, angiotensin II receptors. (Reproduced from Modern Concepts in Cardiovascular Disease 58: 7–18, 1989 by permission of the American Heart Association [46])

---

[1] The numbers in parentheses refer to the events in Fig. 2 that are represented by the circled numbers.

junctional alpha-1 and alpha-2 receptors (3) causing vasoconstriction [29]. Some NE in the neuroeffector junction (20%–25%) can spill over into the circulation (4) [30]. This can then be delivered to vessels elsewhere (3) and produce vasoconstriction. Neuronally released NE preferentially stimulates postjunctional alpha-1 receptors whereas humorally delivered norepinephrine can affect both populations of alpha receptors. This may be related to the location of postjunctional alpha-1 receptors within the neuroeffector junction. Postjunctional alpha-2 receptors appear to have an extrajunctional location. A number of abnormalities have been noted in these processes.

From microneurographic studies of the peroneal nerve of humans with heart failure, increased sympathetic nerve activity (1) has been demonstrated [31]. In some animal models of CHF (aortic stenosis), an increase in neurogenic vasomotor tone has been noted [32], whereas in others (banding of the pulmonary artery) humoral mechanisms account for the observed vasoconstriction [33]. Few studies have dealt with neuronal NE (2) release. In a rat myocardial infarction model of CHF in which an isolated neurovascular preparation preincubated with ^{3}H-labeled norepinephrine was studied, it was suggested that neuronal NE release was normal with multiple submaximal levels of electrical stimulation [34]. However, the maximal response in CHF was reduced. In a dog tachycardia model of heart failure, maximal stimulation of the lumbar sympathetic chain led to impaired vasoconstrictor response, whereas the response to infused intra-arterial NE was normal [35]. These data suggest that tissue NE levels are low, a phenomenon that has been recently confirmed [36]. Selective blockade of alpha receptors in humans has demonstrated that both postjunctional alpha-1 and alpha-2 receptors are involved in the vasoconstrictor response to heart failure (3) and that prejunctional alpha-2 receptors work normally (8) [37]. Together these data suggest that sympathetic nerve activation is increased in CHF (1). This leads to neuronal NE depletion and a reduction in maximal neuronal release of NE (2). However, during submaximal activation, neuronal release may be normal for the strength of the stimulus delivered. The postjunctional vasoconstrictor response (3) is probably normal for the amount of NE delivered.

Norepinephrine Kinetics in Clinical CHF

Studies of systemic NE kinetics in clinical CHF have demonstrated that spillover of NE from the neuroeffector junction into the circulation (4) is increased [30,38–39]. Although this is a better reflection of sympathetic efferent nerve activation than plasma NE levels alone, it still represents only a small fraction of the NE delivered to the neuroeffector junction. Moreover, it has been demonstrated that clearance of NE from the circulation (7) is markedly reduced in heart failure [30,38–39]. In fact, clearance abnormalities can account for approximately half of the elevated plasma NE concentration seen.

NE is cleared from the neuroeffector junction by neuronal uptake (uptake 1; 5) and nonneuronal uptake (uptake 2; 6). Neuronal uptake (5) appears to be the most important regulator of neuroeffector junctional NE concentration. It operates effectively at low NE concentrations, however it is an easily saturable process. Nonneuronal uptake accounts for less clearance of norepinephrine from the neuroeffector junction. The uptake 2 mechanism is much less sensitive than the uptake 1, however the capacity of the uptake 2 system is much greater than that for uptake 1. Although uptake 2 (6) is the most important mechanism for clearance of circulating NE (7), the uptake 1 mechanism (5) can account for a significant portion of the removal process of norepinephrine in a number of circulations [40]. In the heart, uptake 1 is the major mechanism for removal of NE from the circulation.

In clinical CHF, NE clearance is very sensitive to the effects of neuronal uptake blockade by desipramine. A dose of desipramine that does not affect norepinephrine clearance in normal subjects caused a significant reduction in clearance in CHF [41]. This suggests that the fraction of amine carriers on sympathetic nerves that are occupied by norepinephrine are significantly increased in CHF. In fact, uptake 1 blockade leads to an increased plasma NE in CHF, whereas it does not affect plasma NE in normal individuals [41]. Larger doses of desipramine reduces clearance in normals but also reduces NE spillover, presumably due to feedback inhibition of NE release via the prejunctional alpha-2 receptor (8). Studies utilizing ^{3}H-labeled isoproterenol kinetic techniques demonstrated that uptake 2 (6) is significantly reduced in CHF [42].

Norepinephrine Turnover

NE turnover involves the net effect of processes (2, 4-6). Studies of heart NE turnover has produced conflicting results. In the heart of cardiomyopathic hamsters NE turnover has been noted to be increased [28]. On the other hand, in a preliminary report using a rat myocardial infarction model of heart failure a different result was obtained [36]. NE turnover was studied by evaluating the rate of decline in tissue NE content following blockade of norepinephrine synthesis using alpha methyl-para-tyrosine. In this study tissue NE levels fell more in the sham operated animals than in the myocardial infarction rats. This suggests that turnover was reduced in this model of moderate compensated CHF. Only under conditions of exercise was NE turnover increased, and only in the heart.

The norepinephrine turnover data derived from studies with alpha methyl-para-tyrosine do not necessarily mean that sympathetic nerve activity is decreased; rather they suggest that the processes involved in control of neuronal NE release and reuptake seem to favor conservation of neuronal NE pools in heart failure. For example, neuronal NE uptake (5) might be increased. However, the finding of depleted tissue stores of NE would suggest that these mechanisms are not completely effective.

Prejunctional Receptors

In isolated studies using a neurovascular preparation, the response to prejunctional alpha-2 response with yohimbine was normal in a CHF model (8) [34]. Stimulation of intact postjunctional alpha-2 receptors does play a role in mediating forearm vasoconstriction in heart failure [37]. Thus the finding of down-regulated alpha-2 receptors on platelets in heart failure does not necessarily reflect prejunctional alpha-2 receptor down-regulation in vascular sympathetic nerves [43].

It is possible that other prejunctional receptors may be playing a physiological role in regulating NE release. Patients given an alpha-2 adrenergic agonist (guanabenz) [44] or a dopamine 2 agonist (bromocriptine) [45] demonstrate a reduction in plasma NE concentration. It is not known whether this reflects a peripheral effect of the drug on prejunctional receptors or a peripheral nervous system response to decreased central sympathetic outflow.

Other stimulatory prejunctional receptors could be enhancing neuronal NE release. A potent stimulus for the prejunctional beta-2 receptor is epinephrine. Epinephrine participates in uptake 1 (5) in a manner similar to NE. When sympathetic nerves are activated reflexively in heart failure by orthostatic stress, epinephrine can be released along with NE. The resultant stimulation of beta-2 receptors in skeletal muscle vessels may be one mechanism by which head-up tilting causes a paradoxical increase in forearm blood flow in CHF [27]. Neuronally released epinephrine has the potential for facilitating neuronal NE release. Prejunctional angiotensin II receptors have not been studied in heart failure. With activation of the renin angiotensin system in CHF these receptors could facilitate NE release.

Summary

The activity of the sympathetic nervous system appears to be increased in CHF. Although there is increased nerve activity, there are mechanisms operative to conserve neuronal norepinephrine in the face of this increased activity. Despite these mechanisms depletion of neuronal NE takes place. The concentration of NE is increased in the neuroeffector junction in a number of circumstances as is spillover of NE from this pool into the circulation. However, the elevated plasma NE levels in heart failure are equally dependent upon an increased spillover and a decreased clearance of NE. Since the decrease in NE clearance is predominantly due to decreased nonneuronal NE uptake, it is probably related to poor organ perfusion. Thus the abnormality of flow delivery to tissues seems to influence both major determinants of plasma NE. Low blood flow during exercise may serve as one of the afferent stimuli to increase sympathetic nerve traffic and NE release into the circulation. Once NE gets out into the blood stream, a sluggish circulation fails to deliver NE to the peripheral tissues where it can be cleared.

References

1. Zelis R, Flaim SF (1982) Alterations in vasomotor tone in congestive heart failure. Prog Cardiovasc Dis 24:437–459
2. Zelis R, Mason DT, Braunwald E (1968) A comparison of peripheral resistance vessels in normal subjects and in patients with congestive heart failure. J Clin Invest 47:960–969
3. Yancy CW Jr, Vissing S, Buckey JC, Bellomo JF, Firth BG, Blomqvist CG (1988) Maximal conductance versus maximal oxygen uptake in patients with congestive heart failure (abstract). J Am Coll Cardiol 11:72A
4. Zelis R, Sinoway LI, Musch TI, Davis D, Just H (1988) Regional blood flow in heart failure – the concept of compensatory mechanisms with short and long time constants. Am J Cardiol 62:2E–8E
5. Sinoway LI, Minotti J, Musch T, Goldner D, Davis D, Leaman D, Zelis R (1987) Enhanced metabolic vasodilation secondary to diuretic therapy in decompensated congestive heart failure secondary to coronary artery disease. Am J Cardiol 60:107–111
6. Sinoway LI, Minotti JR, Davis D, Pennock J, Burg J, Musch TI, Zelis R (1988) Delayed reversal of impaired peripheral vasodilation in congestive heart failure following orthotopic heart transplantation. Am J Cardiol 61:1076–1079
7. Sinoway LI, Musch TI, Minotti JR, Zelis R (1986) Enhanced maximal metabolic vasodilation in the dominant forearms of tennis players. J Appl Physiol 61:673–678
8. Sinoway LI, Shenberger J, Wilson JS, McLaughlin D, Musch T, Zelis R (1987) A 30-day forearm work protocol increases maximal forearm blood flow. J Appl Physiol 62:1062–1067
9. Sinoway LI, Minotti J, Sirio C, Musch TI, Matthews W, Zelis R (1986) The effects of prolonged unilateral forearm immobilization on maximal peripheral blood flow (abstract). J Am Coll Cardiol 7:224A
10. Vanhoutte PM (1987) Endothelium and the control of vascular tissue. NIPS 2:18–22
11. Sinoway LI, Hendrickson C, Zelis R (1989) The characteristics of flow mediated brachial artery vasodilatation in human subjects. Circ Res 64:32–34
12. Moncada S, Palmer RMJ, Higgs EA (1989) Biosynthesis of nitric oxide from L-arginine. A pathway for the regulation of cell function and communication. Biochem Pharmacol 38:1709–1715
13. Miller VM, Aarhus LL, Vanhoutte PM (1986) Modulation of endothelium-dependent responses by chronic alterations in blood flow. Am J Physiol 251:H520–H527
14. Kaiser L, Spickard RC, Olivier NB (1989) Heart failure depresses endothelial cell dependent relaxation to acetylcholine in the canine femoral artery. Am J Physiol 256:H962–H967
15. Drexler H, Hayoz D, Münzel T, Hornig B, Zeiher AM, Just H, Brunner HR, Zelis R (1990) Endothelial function of forearm conduit and resistance vessels in patients with chronic heart failure. (submitted)
16. Musch TI, Moore RL, Leathers DJ, Bruno A, Zelis R (1986) Endurance training in rats with chronic heart failure induced by myocardial infarction. Circulation 74:431–441
17. Musch TI, Moore RI, Riedy M, Burke P, Zelis R, Leo ME, Bruno A, Bradford GE (1988) Glycogen concentrations and endurance capacity of rats with chronic heart failure. J Appl Physiol 64:1153–1159
18. Weber KT, Kinasewitz GT, Janicki JS, Fishman AP (1982) Oxygen utilization and ventilation during exercise in patients with chronic cardiac failure. Circulation 65:1213–1232
19. Kugler J, Maskin C, Frishman WH, Sonnenblick EH, LeJemtel TH (1982) Regional and systemic metabolic effects of angiotensin converting enzyme inhibition during exercise in patients with severe heart failure. Circulation 66:1256–1261
20. Maskin CS, Kugler J, Sonnenblick EH, LeJemtel TH (1983) Acute inotropic stimulation with dopamine in severe congestive heart failure: beneficial hemodynamic effect at rest but not during maximal exercise. Am J Cardiol 52:1028–1032
21. Wiener DH, Fink PI, Maris J, Jones RA, Chance B, Wilson JR (1986) Abnormal skeletal muscle bioenergetics during exercise in patients with heart failure: role of reduced muscle blood flow. Circulation 73:1127–1136
22. Massie B, Conway M, Yonge R, Frostick S, Ledingham J, Sleight P, Radda G, Rajagopalan B (1987) Skeletal muscle metabolism in patients with congestive heart failure: relation to clinical severity and blood flow. Circulation 76:1009–1019

23. Drexler H, Riede U, Schafer H-E (1987) Reduced oxidative capacity of skeletal muscle in patients with severe heart failure (abstract). Circulation 76:IV-178

24. Abboud FM, Thames MD, Mark AL (1987) Role of cardiac afferent nerves in regulation of circulation during coronary occlusion and heart failure. In: Abboud FM, Fozzard HA, Gilmore JP, Reis DJ (eds) Disturbances in neurogenic control of the circulation. Williams and Wilkins, Baltimore MD, pp 65-86

25. Sinoway LI, Prophet SA, Gorman IN, Dolecki M, Briggs RW, Zelis R (1989) Muscle acidosis during static exercise is associated with calf vasoconstriction. J Appl Physiol 66:429-436

26. Mitchell JH (1985) Cardiovascular control during exercise: central and reflex neural mechanisms. Am J Cardiol 55:34D-41D

27. Kassis E, Jacobsen TN, Mogensen F, Amtorp O (1986) Sympathetic reflex control of skeletal muscle blood flow in patients with congestive heart failure: evidence for β-adrenergic circulatory control. Circulation 74:929-938

28. Sole MJ (1984) Sympathetic neurotransmitter activity and congestive heart failure. In: Usdin E, Carlsson A, Dahlström A, Engel J (eds) Cathecolamines: basic and peripheral mechanisms. Liss, New York, pp 309-317

29. Jie K, van Brummelen P, Vermey P, Timmermans PBPWM, van Zwieten PA (1984) Identification of vascular postsynaptic α_1- and α_2-adrenoceptors in man. Circ Res 54:447-452

30. Zelis R, Davis D (1986) The sympathetic nervous system in congestive heart failure. Heart Failure 2:21-32

31. Leimbach WN, Wallin BG, Victor RG, Aylward PE, Sundlof G, Mark AL (1986) Direct evidence from intraneural recordings for increased central sympathetic outflow in patients with heart failure. Circulation 73:913-919

32. Schmid PG, Mayer HE, Mark AL, Heistad DD, Abboud FM (1977) Differences in the regulation of vascular resistance in guinea pigs with right and left heart failure. Circ Res 41:85-93

33. McNamara RF, Schmid PG, Schmidt JA, Lund DD, Bhatnagar RK (1979) Humoral regulation of vascular resistance after 30 days of pulmonary artery constriction. Am J Physiol 236:H866-H872

34. Zelis R, Brunner H, Zelis K, Wichmann T (1988) Vascular sympathetic nerve function in congestive heart failure. Am J Cardiol 62:63E-67E

35. Wilson JR, Matthai W, Lanoce V, Frey M, Ferraro N (1988) Effect of experimental heart failure on peripheral sympathetic vasoconstriction. Am J Physiol 254:H727-H733

36. Clemson B, Hogeman C, Strzelecka D, Hoover D, Patel A, Davis D, Baily R, Zelis R (1988) Is sympathetic nervous system activity increased in the rat myocardial infarction model of moderate compensated heart failure (abstract)? Clin Res 36:539A

37. Kubo S, Rector TS, Heifetz SM, Cohn JN (1989) Role of alpha-2 receptor mediated forearm vasoconstriction in patients with congestive heart failure. Circulation 80:1660-1667

38. Hasking GJ, Esler MD, Jennings GL, Burton D, Korner PI (1986) Norepinephrine spillover to plasma in patients with congestive heart failure: evidence of increased overall and cardiorenal sympathetic nervous activity. Circulation 73:615-621

39. Davis D, Baily R, Zelis R (1988) Abnormalities in systemic norepinephrine kinetics in human congestive heart failure. Am J Physiol 254:E760-E766

40. Goldstein DS, Brush JE Jr, Eisenhofer G, Stull R, Esler M (1985) In vivo measurement of neuronal uptake of norepinephrine in the human heart. Circulation 78:41-48

41. Clemson B, Baily R, Davis D, Zelis R (1990) The effects of desipramine on norepinephrine clearance in congestive heart failure. Am J Physiol 259:E261-E265

42. Leuenberger U, Kenney G, Davis D, Deiling S, Strzelecka D, Zelis R (1990) Nonneuronal norepinephrine clearance is low in congestive heart failure (abstract). Clin Res 37:274A

43. Weiss RJ, Tobes M, Wertz CE, Smith CB (1983) Platelet alpha$_2$ adrenoreceptors in chronic congestive heart failure. Am J Cardiol 52:101-105

44. Francis CS, Goldsmith SR, Levine TB, Olivari MT, Cohn JN (1984) The neurohumoral axis in congestive heart failure. Ann Intern Med 101:370-377

45. Francis GS, Park R, Cohn JN (1983) The effect of bromocriptine in patients with congestive heart failure. Am Heart J 106:100-106

46. Zelis R, Sinoway L, Musch T, Davis D (1989) Vasoconstrictor mechanisms in congestive heart failure. Parts I and II. Modern concepts in cardiovascular diseases 58:1-18

Natriuretic Peptides from the Heart, Brain, and Kidney: Localization, Processing, Vasoactivity, and Proteolytic Degradation

S.M. Feller, A. Bub, M. Gagelmann, and W.G. Forssmann

Localization and Processing

Attempts at isolating natriuretic peptides from the mammalian heart resulted in the isolation of many bioactive fragments [1]. Later, modifications of the initial isolation methods led to identification of the native molecules in various tissues and body fluids [2]. Today it is well established that the mammalian heart stores a 126 amino acid molecule, known as atrial natriuretic factor (ANF) 126, γ-atrial natriuretic peptide (ANP), or, as we have named it in our laboratory, cardiodilatin (CDD) 126 (Fig. 1) [2]. This prohormone is stored in secretory granules and processed to a 28 amino acid molecule (CDD 28 or α-ANP; Fig. 1) during its secretion into the circulation [2]. Biochemical, immunochemical, and molecular biological studies have shown that CDD/ANP is synthesized in a distinct population of chromaffin cells in the adrenal medulla, where the 126 amino acid prohormone and CDD 28/α-ANP are colocalized [3–5]. Two shorter peptides of the CDD/ANP family, consisting of 24 and 25 amino acids, were isolated from the porcine brain [6]. Blot hybridization shows CDD/ANP specific mRNA in different brain areas [7].

Additionally, two different peptides with partial sequence homology to CDD/ANP were identified in peptide extracts from porcine brain (see Fig. 1) [8,9]. These peptides of 26 and 32 amino acids, were named brain natriuretic peptides (BNP) due to their biological activity and origin. They are derived from a 131 amino acid preprohormone as deduced from the sequence of a cloned porcine brain cDNA [10]. A recent publication documented that a BNP prohormone of 106 amino acids may be stored in the porcine heart, but that its concentration is much lower than that of the CDD/ANP prohormone [11].

CDD/ANP immunoreactivity (CDD/ANP-IR) is detectable in atrial myocytes with antibodies raised against different epitopes of the CDD/ANP prohormone. Most of the immunoreactivity material is located in the perinuclear region. A similar staining is obtained with antibodies against porcine BNP 26; simultaneous incubation of atrial sections with gold-labeled antibodies against CDD 28/α-ANP and porcine BNP 26 (gold particles of different sizes) indicates the costorage of different natriuretic peptides in atrial granules (unpublished observations). During the past 5 years, CDD/ANP gene transcription has been shown in many extra-atrial tissues, including heart ventricles, various blood vessels, and lung [7]. Besides these tissues, several other organs have been identified as sites of synthesis or storage of CDD/ANP and BNP peptides (Table

B.S. Lewis, A. Kimchi (Eds.)
Heart Failure Mechanisms and Management
© Springer-Verlag Berlin Heidelberg 1991

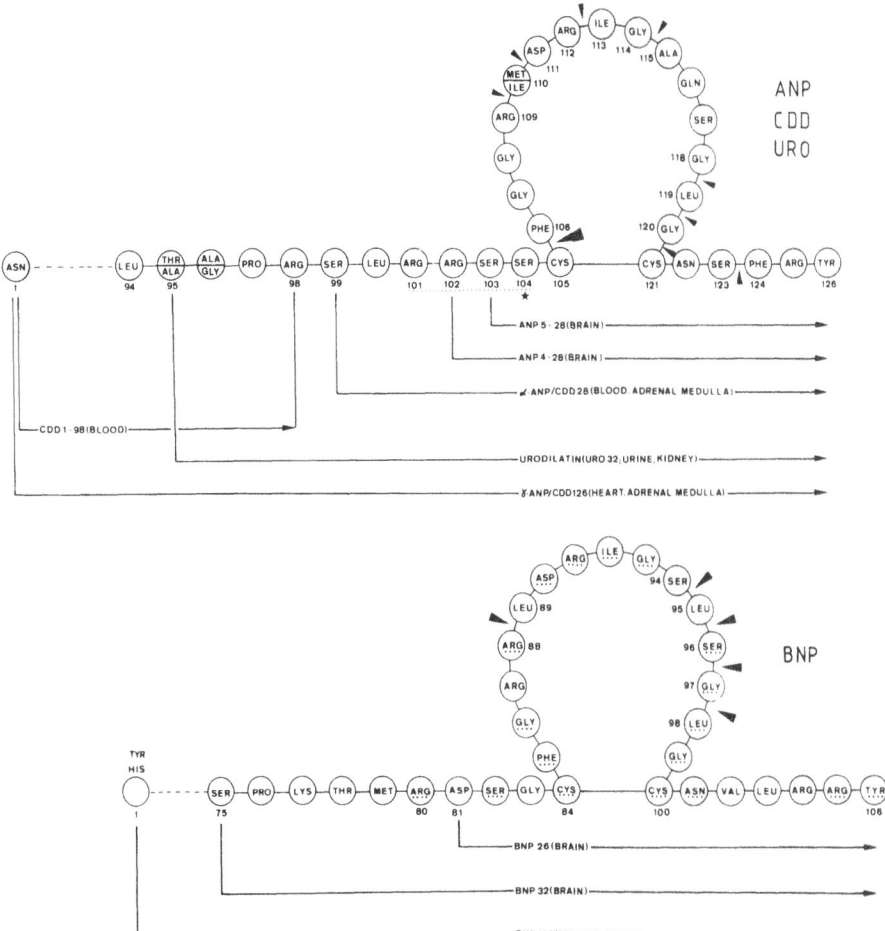

Fig. 1. Amino acid sequences and structures of mammalian natriuretic peptides. *Arrows*, molecular forms of natriuretic peptides isolated from different organs and body fluids; *arrowheads*, presently known cleavage sites of peptidases from blood and kidney; *long dotted line*, amino acids 101–104 of the CDD/ANP prohormone, the recognition sequence for cAMP-dependent protein kinase; *star*, phosphorylation site; *underlining dots*, amino acids of porcine BNP that are identical to the homologous position in CDD/ANP; *numbers*, amino acid position relative to the prohormone

1)[2,12,13]. Immunoreactive cells have been localized in different parts of the gut, in the pancreas, and in the kidney. However, uptake and storage of CDD/ANP-IR without a de novo synthesis has been reported, for example, in the pancreas and a neuronal cell line [14,15].

As early as 1985, CDD/ANP-IR material from the rat kidney was analyzed by Sakamoto et al. [16]. The renal concentration of CDD/ANP-IR, determined with radioimmunoassay (RIA, 5 ng/g wet weight tissue), was much higher than that in plasma. However, the renal immunoreactivity material showed no significant difference in its elution pattern on a gel filtration column when compared with circulating rat CDD 28/α-ANP. In the kidney, an important

Table 1. Storage and synthesis sites of mammalian natriuretic peptides

Organ/Tissue	ANP/Cardiodilatin/Urodilatin Methods			
	RIA	IH	IC	mRNA
Heart				
Atria	+ +	+ +	+ +	+ + (0.5%-2%)
Ventricles	+	+	+	+ (0.01%)
Septum (CS)	+	+	+	+
Vessels				
Aortic arch	+		+	
Vena pulmonalis	+	+		
Vena cava	+	+		
Cns				
Thalamus	+	+		+ (0.001%)
Hypothalamus	+	+		+ (0.00025%)
Bulbus olfactorius	+	+		
Pituitary gland	+	+		+ (0.001%)
Brain stem (different regions)	+	+		+ (0.005%-0.001%)
Cortex cerebri	+	+	+	
Spinal cord	+	+		
Pns				
Ganglia (different types)	+	+	+	
Intestinum				
Stomach	+	+		
Duodenum	+	+		
Jejunum	+	+		
Colon	+	+		
Lung	+	+		+
Adrenal medulla	+	+	+	+
Kidney	+	+		+
Pancreas	+	+		
Salivary glands	+	+	+	
Eye (retina, etc.)	+	+		

Organ/Tissue	Brain natriuretic peptide Methods				
	Pept.	RIA	IH	IC	mRNA
Heart	12 KD (106 ?)				
Auricles		+ +		+	+
Non auricle atria		+ +			
Ventricles		+			
Brain	(26, 32)				
Olfactory bulb		+	+		
Hippocampus		+	+		
Striatum		+	+		
Cortex		+	+		
Cerebellum		+	+		
Thalamus		+	+		
Pons		+	+		
Hypothalamus		+	+		
Septum		+	+		
Spinal cord		+	+		

RIA, Radioimmunoassay; *IH*, immunohistochemistry; *IC*, immunocytochemistry; *mRNA*, messenger ribonucleic acid hybridization; *Pept.*, peptide isolation; percentages are those of CDD/ANP specific mRNA in the mRNA pool of an organ/tissue.

target organ, CDD/ANP-IR was detected mainly in the renal cortex, where the majority of CDD/ANP receptors are present. No intrarenal synthesis of CDD/ANP or a related peptide could be proven at this time. In the following years, doubts were cast on the idea that high concentrations of CDD/ANP-IR in the kidney occur only due to high densities of receptors. Comparison of healthy subjects and patients with various diseases, peculiarly showed no correlation between CDD/ANP-IR levels in plasma and urine [17]. Various immunohistochemical studies indicated that at least an internalization could occur in some parts of the kidney [18-20].

In 1986, Schulz-Knappe et al. from our laboratory started to isolate bioactive CDD/ANP-IR from human urine. Surprisingly, sequence analysis of the purified material showed a CDD/ANP peptide which was four amino acids longer than the plasma form CDD 28/α-ANP [21]. This was named urodilatin. Although several isolations of circulating CDD/ANP had been performed by different groups, this molecule was never detected in blood [2]. Together with the data from RIA and immunohistochemistry an intrarenal synthesis of CDD/ANP peptides seemed possible, and we decided to clarify whether the kidney is a site of CDD/ANP synthesis or not. Immunohistochemical studies with antibodies against synthetic CDD 28/α-ANP in kidneys of different mammals, reveals a staining of cells in renal tubules or collecting ducts according to the analyzed species. In contrast, only a weak staining is obtained with antibodies against the N-terminus of the CDD/ANP prohormone [22,23]. This indicates that, if CDD/ANP peptides are intrarenally synthetized and stored, the CDD/ANP prohormone is not a major storage form. These results were confirmed by biochemical purification of CDD/ANP-IR from porcine kidney in combination with RIA and bioassay. The analysis of partially purified peptide extracts on a gel filtration column shows only small amounts of CDD/ANP-IR eluting earlier than CDD 28/α-ANP or urodilatin [23]. Additionally, low molecular weight forms of CDD/ANP-IR were further purified and the highly purified peptides were analyzed on a cation exchange HPLC column which separates CDD 28/α-ANP and urodilatin. Two immunoreactive peaks eluting similarly to synthetic CDD 28/α-ANP and urodilatin were detected. The CDD/ANP-IR eluting-like urodilatin represented at least 75% of the total CDD/ANP-IR in the kidney. The material eluting like CDD 28/α-ANP was probably, at least in part, derived from the blood contained in the renal tissue.

Enzymatic Phosphorylation

CDD 28/α-ANP and other CDD/ANP peptides containing the amino acids 101-104 of the CDD/ANP prohormone (Arg-Arg-Ser-Ser; Fig. 1), but not porcine BNP peptides, possess the recognition sequence (Arg-Arg-X-Ser) for phosphorylation by the cAMP-dependent protein kinase [24]. It has been shown that the phosphorylated CDD 28/α-ANP has a reduced vasoactivity [25,26] (Fig. 2) and a higher resistance against endopeptidase 24.11, the major CDD/ANP

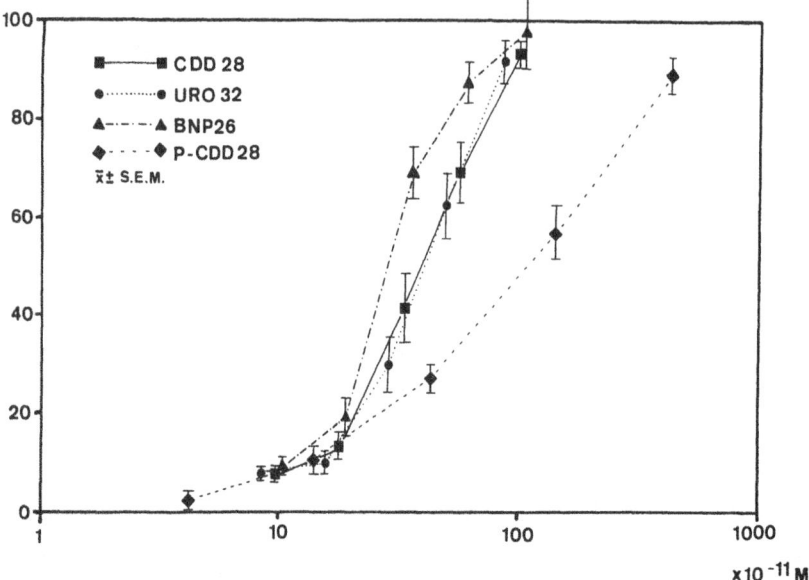

Fig. 2. Vasorelaxant potency of natriuretic peptides on rabbit aortic strips. Aortic strips from NZW rabbits in a standard bioassay system were pretensed with 2 *g*, equilibrated, and precontracted with norepinephrine (NE, 10^{-7} *M*). Peptides were added after the contraction induced by NE had reached a stable level. Vasoactivity (percentage relaxation) is given as the inverse of the contraction induced by NE. *URO 32*, urodilatin; *P-CDD 28*, CDD 28/α-ANP phosphorylated by cAMP-depedent protein kinase

degradating enzyme in the kidney [27,28]. However, an in vivo phosphorylation of CDD/ANP peptides by the cAMP-dependent protein kinase has not been demonstrated in the heart, although an in situ phosphorylation of a minor portion of the CDD/ANP prohormone contained in atrial tissue and in cultured cells can be obtained [29,30]. On the other hand, two very recent studies show that CDD/ANP peptides may be phosphorylated in vivo after their secretion from the heart. Shenolikar et al. have shown, that cAMP-dependent protein kinase activity is associated with kidney brush-border membranes [31], and Kübler et al. found that erythrocytes and some cell lines exhibit a cAMP-dependent ectoprotein kinase activity [32]. Future studies should show whether a phosphorylation of natriuretic peptides occurs in blood and kidney and maybe even in other organs and body fluids.

Vasoactivity

We have quantified the vasorelaxant activity of synthetic human CDD 28/α-ANP (unphosphorylated and phosphorylated forms), urodilatin, and porcine BNP 26 in physiological and pharmacological concentrations on precontracted vascular strips (10^{-7} M norepinephrine) of thoracic aorta from NZW rabbits. In this bioassay, CDD 28/α-ANP and urodilatin are equipotent while BNP 26 is more potent (Fig. 2). cAMP-dependent phosphorylation greatly diminishes the vasorelaxant activity of CDD 28/α-ANP. The greater smooth-muscle relaxation potency of high doses of BNP 26 in comparison to CDD 28/α-ANP was mentioned in the first publication on BNP, where the chick rectum assay was used [8]. Despite this, no major differences are observed between these peptides when tested on rabbit aortic strips at physiological concentrations.

In a second study, we defined the lowest doses of BNP 26, CDD 28/α-ANP and urodilatin necessary to induce vasorelaxation of different rabbit arteries. Two representative examples are shown in Fig. 3a and 3b. Significant differences are observed with the different arteries (Fig. 3c). Again, urodilatin is equipotent to CDD 28/α-ANP, and BNP 26 tends to be slightly more effective. Of the arteries tested, the mesenteric was the only nonresponsive one, suggesting it is not a target organ for natriuretic peptides. The consistent order of potency of these sequence-related peptides on different arteries indicates that they interact with the same receptors and utilize the same signaling system.

It is well known, that many biological activities of CDD/ANP peptides, for example vasodilatation, are mediated by an activation of particulate guanylate cyclase [33]. The majority of studies on this topic have been carried out using primary cultures of aortic smooth-muscle cells. However, this system has a disadvantage since it has been reported that CDD/ANP receptors are affected by the cultivation of these cells [34].

We measured the changes of cGMP and cAMP levels on application of natriuretic peptides directly to vascular tissue of the aorta. The incubation with peptides was carried out after dissection of the thoracic aorta, weighing of vascular rings, and equilibration in a physiological buffer. Cyclic nucleotide concentrations were measured by RIA after tissue homogenization and extraction with ice-cold ethanol. Application of 10^{-7} M BNP 26 results in a rapid increase of cGMP in aortic tissue (Fig. 4). This effect is potentiated by the addition of the phosphodiesterase inhibitor 3-isobutyl-1-methyl-xanthine (IBMX, 10^{-4} M), which decreases the breakdown of intracellular cGMP but has only minor effects on intracellular cAMP. cGMP increased to a maximum of approximately fivefold over control levels after 2 min in the presence or absence of IBMX. Prolonged incubation with BNP leads to a partial decrease in cGMP to approximately 50% of the maximum concentration. The levels of cAMP were not affected by BNP. Similar results are obtained with CDD 28/α-ANP and urodilatin. The effects of CDD 28/α-ANP, BNP 26, and urodilatin on cGMP in aortic tissue are dose dependent. Changes in cGMP levels are induced by pharmacological concentrations (10^{-7}–10^{-9} M) and concentrations that are observed in the plasma in various diseases or after experimental stimulation of CDD/ANP secretion (10^{-10} M).

In all experiments, we observed relatively large deviations in vasorelaxation and cGMP responses of different aortic samples, which could depend upon variations in the sensitivity of these samples. We compared the cGMP response in different areas of the aortic arch and thoracic aorta. Furthermore, we wanted

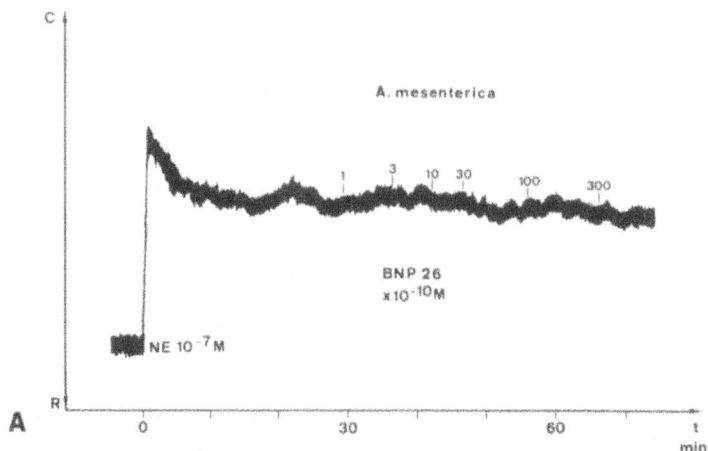

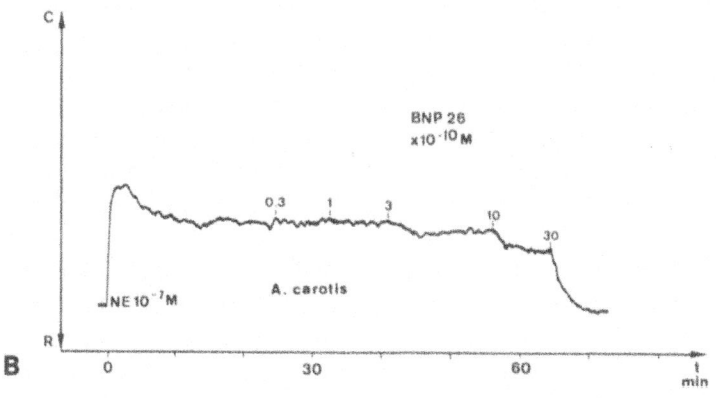

Type of artery	Tested peptide		
	CDD 28	Uro 32	BNP 26
	(Detection limit concentrations in molarity)		
Aorta	$1-3 \times 10^{-11}$	$1-3 \times 10^{-11}$	1×10^{-11}
A. renalis	$3-10 \times 10^{-11}$	$3-10 \times 10^{-11}$	3×10^{-11}
A. carotis	3×10^{-10}	3×10^{-10}	3×10^{-10}
A. axillaris	$1-3 \times 10^{-10}$	$1-3 \times 10^{-10}$	$1-3 \times 10^{-10}$
A. mesenterica [*]	none	none	none

C   * Tested up to 3×10^{-7} M

Fig. 3A-C. Detection of the minimum concentrations of CDD/ANP 28, urodilatin, and BNP 26 necessary to induce vasorelaxation of different rabbit arteries. Experiments were performed with arterial rings 0.5 cm long, as described in Fig. 2 (pretension 1 g). *C*, contraction; *R*, relaxation

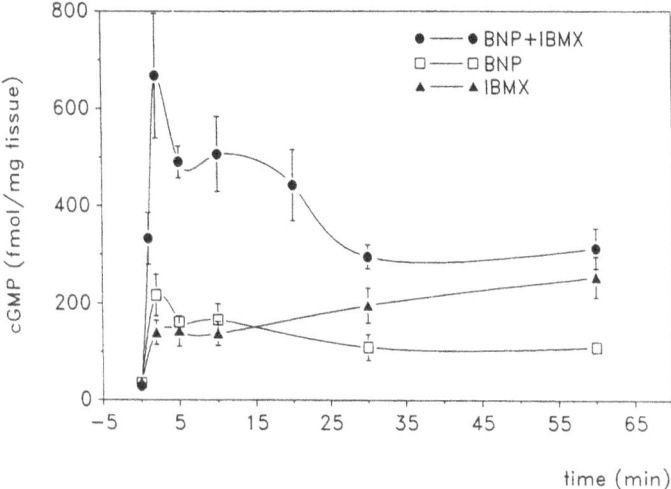

Fig. 4. Changes in cGMP concentrations in rabbit aortic rings after application of BNP 26 and/or IBMX for up to 60 min. *IBMX*, 3-isobutyl-1-methyl-xanthine (10^{-4} M; phosphodiesterase inhibitor); *BNP*, BNP 26 (10^{-7} M). Weight of vascular rings, 10–15 mg. cGMP was determined by RIA

to determine whether functional receptors for natriuretic peptides are present in the aortic arch, where the existence of CDD/ANP-synthetizing cells has been reported [35]. We found significant differences in sensitivity to natriuretic peptides along the thoracic aorta (Fig. 5) and cells with natriuretic peptide receptors in the aortic arch. At present, it is unclear whether BNP is also synthetized in the aortic arch, and whether the coexistence of cells that synthesize CDD/ANP and cells carrying natriuretic peptide receptors is more than an evolutionary relict.

Degradation

In contrast to the striking similarity of vasodilatative effects of BNP 26, CDD 28/α-ANP and urodilatin, major differences occur in the proteolytic inactivation of these peptides. The kidney is not only an important target organ but is of great importance in the inactivation of natriuretic peptides and their removal from the circulation. Today we know that the renal degradation of CDD 28/α-ANP is initiated by endopeptidase 24.11, an enzyme which is present in renal tubules at high concentrations [29]. After the incubation of CDD 28/α-ANP with endopeptidase 24.11 or purified membranes from renal cortex, a single cleavage product is detected by HPLC analysis [27,36]. This product lacks biological activity and was identified as a 28 amino acid molecule with a single cleavage between cystein 105 and phenylalanine 106 (Fig. 1). The disulfide bridge between cystein 105 and cystein 121 remained intact. In contrast, urodilatin is almost inert when incubated under the same conditions [27,36]. Besides the above-mentioned

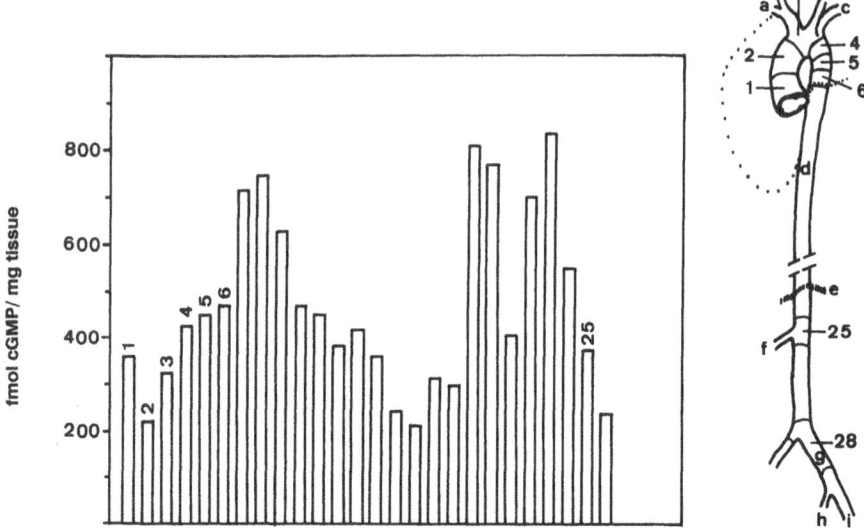

Fig. 5. Elevation of cGMP response in different parts of the rabbit aorta on application of BNP. Aortic rings were incubated with BNP 26 (10^{-7} M) and IBMX (10^{-4} M) for 10 min. Control rings (data not shown) were incubated only with IBMX (10^{-4} M); cGMP levels of controls were approximately 150 fmol/mg tissue. a, Truncus brachiocephalus; b A. carotis communis sinistra; c, A. subclavia sinistra; d, pars thoracicus aortae; e, diaphragma; f, A. renalis; g, A. ileaca communis; h, A. ileaca externa; i, A. ileaca interna

cleavage site, several other target sequences for peptidases present in plasma or kidney have been reported (Fig. 1). Currently it is unclear to what extent these peptidases influence the concentration of bioactive CDD 28/α-ANP in blood and glomerular filtrate in vivo.

The high concentration of endopeptidase 24.11 in renal brush-border membranes supports the hypothesis that CDD 28/α-ANP is inactivated after its filtration into the lumen of the nephron almost immediately and quantitatively. If this is true in vivo, CDD 28/α-ANP probably does not influence the functional receptors that have been shown to exist in renal collecting ducts [37,38]. Urodilatin is the only bioactive CDD/ANP-like peptide that has been isolated and sequenced from urine so far [21] and is resistant to endopeptidase 24.11. We therefore consider that urodilatin may be the native molecule that interacts with the natriuretic peptide receptors in renal collecting ducts after its secretion into the lumen of the nephron.

Very recently, BNP-IR has been detected in the blood [39]. An interaction with vascular and renal receptors may be expected. Our degradation experiments with porcine BNP 26, performed as in our previous studies with CDD 28/α-ANP and urodilatin, show several cleavage products, but no cleavage between cystein 84 and phenylalanine 85 was observed (Fig. 1). Only a few data are available on BNP, and its importance as a signal transmitter to the renal tubules and collecting ducts has not been investigated to date.

Summary

Several sites of synthesis of natriuretic peptides have been identified, and a co-existence of CDD/ANP and BNP peptides in some organs has been shown. The posttranslational processing by various, organ-specific, systems results in a variety of molecular forms with different biological activities. The distribution of functional receptors in many different organs and tissues indicates multiple target organs and possibly several, still unknown functions of the natriuretic peptides, besides their relevance in fluid homeostasis. The structural and sequential similarities between the natriuretic peptides, together with our own investigations and other publications [40], support the idea that they may, at least in some tissues, act via the same receptors. cGMP is the second messenger system used for the signal transfer into target cells in many cases. On the other hand, only CDD/ANP peptides contain a recognition sequence for an effective phosphorylation by cAMP-dependant protein kinase and significant differences are observed in proteolytic inactivation. Although a vast number of publications exists, many additional experiments are necessary to understand the "real" in vivo functions of the natriuretic peptides.

References

1. Forssmann WG (1986) Cardiac hormones. I. Review on the morphology, biochemistry and molecular biology of the endocrine heart. Eur J Clin Invest 16:439-451
2. Forssmann WG, Feller S, Meyer M, Rippegather G, Schulz-Knappe P (1989) Morphology of the myoendocrine cardiac cell and extra-auricular systems producing cardiac hormones. In: Kaufmann W, Wambach G (eds) Endocrinology of the heart. Springer, Berlin Heidelberg New York, pp 3-26
3. Ong H, Lazure C, Nguyen TT, McNicoll N, Seidah N, Chrétien M, De Lean A (1987) Bovine adrenal chromaffin granules are a site of synthesis of atrial natriuretic factor. Biochem Biophys Res Commun 147:957-963
4. Meyer M, Feller S, Gagelmann M, Hock D, Nokihara K, Forssmann WG (1988) Lokalisation von Cardiodilatin (CDD) im Nebennierenmark. Verh Anat Ges 83:429-432
5. Morel G, Chabot JG, Garcia-Caballero T, Gossard F, Dihl F, Belles-Isles M, Heisler S (1988) Synthesis, internalization and localization of atrial natriuretic peptide in rat renal medulla. Endocrinology 123:149-158
6. Ueda S, Sudoh T, Fukuda K, Kangawa K, Minamino N, Matsuo H (1987) Identification of alpha atrial natriuretic peptide (4-28) and (5-28) in porcine brain. Biochem Biophys Res Commun 149:1055-1062
7. Gardner DG, LaPointe MC, Wu J (1988) Expression and regulation of the gene for atrial natriuretic factor. In: Martini L, Ganong WF (eds) Frontiers in neuroendocrinology, vol 10. Raven, New York, pp 45-61
8. Sudoh T, Kangawa K, Minamino N, Matsuo H (1988) A new natriuretic peptide in porcine brain. Nature 332:78-81
9. Sudoh T, Minamino N, Kangawa K, Matsuo H (1988) Brain natriuretic peptide-32: N-terminal six amino acid extended form of brain natriuretic peptide identified in porcine brain. Biochem Biophys Res Commun 155:726-732
10. Maekawa K, Sudoh T, Furusawa M, Minamino N, Kangawa K, Ohkubo H, Nakanishi S, Matsuo H (1988) Cloning and sequence analysis of a cDNA encoding a precursor for porcine brain natriuretic peptide. Biochem Biophys Res Commun 157:410-416

11. Minamino N, Kangawa K, Matsuo H (1988) Isolation and identification of a high molecular weight brain natriuretic peptide in porcine cardiac atrium. Biochem Biophys Res Commun 157:402–409

12. Vollmar AM, Friedrich A, Sinowatz F, Schulz R (1988) Presence of atrial natriuretic peptide-like material in guinea pig intestine. Peptides 9:965–971

13. Itoh H, Nakao K, Saito Y, Yamada T, Shirakami G, Mukoyama M, Arai H, Hosoda K, Suga S, Minamino N, Kangawa K, Matsuo H, Imura H (1989) Radioimmunoassay for brain natriuretic peptide. Detection of BNP in canine brain. Biochem Biophys Res Commun 158:120–128

14. Chabot JG, Morel G, Kopelman H, Belles-Isles M, Heisler S (1987) Atrial natriuretic factor and exocrine pancreas: autoradiographic localization of binding sites and ultrastructural evidence for internalization of endogenous ANF. Pancreas 2:404–413

15. Morel G, Belles-Isles M, Heisler S (1987) Internalization of atrial natriuretic factor by AtT-20 corticotropin secreting cells. Biol Cell 59:233–238

16. Sakamoto M, Nakao K, Kihara M, Morii N, Sugawara A, Suda M, Shimokura M, Kiso Y, Yamori Y, Imura H (1985) Existence of atrial natriuretic polypeptide in kidney. Biochem Biophys Res Commun 128:1281–1287

17. Marumo F, Umetani N, Sakamoto H, Ando K, Ishigami T (1987) Characteristics of atrial natriuretic peptide (ANP) in human plasma and urine (abstr). Kidney Int 31:278

18. McKenzie JC, Tanaka I, Misono KS, Inagami T (1985) Immunohistochemical localization of atrial natriuretic factor in the kidney, adrenal medulla, pituitary and atrium of rat. J Histochem Cytochem 33:828–832

19. Flügge G, Inagami T, Fuchs E (1987) Atrial natriuretic peptide detected by immunocyto-chemistry in peripheral organs of Tupaia belangeri. Histochemistry 86:479–483

20. Feller S, Meyer M, Hock D, Forssmann WG (1988) Extraaurikuläre Lokalisation von Cardiodilatin (abstract). Acta Anat Basel 132:80

21. Schulz-Knappe P, Forssmann K, Herbst F, Hock D, Pipkorn R, Forssmann WG (1988) Isolation and structural analysis of "urodilatin", a new peptide of the cardiodilatin-(ANP)-family extracted from human urine. Klin Wochenschr 66:752–759

22. Forssmann WG, Nokihara K, Gagelmann M, Hock D, Feller S, Schulz-Knappe P, Herbst F (1989) The heart is the center of new endocrine, paracrine, and neuroendocrine system. Arch Histol Cytol 52 (Suppl):293–315

23. Feller SM, Gagelmann M, Forssmann WG (1988) Urodilatin: a newly described member of the ANP family. Trends Pharmacol Sci 10:93–94

24. Rittenhouse J, Moberly L, O'Donnell ME, Owen NE, Marcus F (1986) Phosphorylation of atrial natriuretic peptides by cyclic AMP dependent protein kinase. J Biol Chem 261:7607–7610

25. Olins GM, Metha PP, Blehm DJ, Patton DR, Zupec ME, Whipple DE, Tjoeng FS, Adams SP, Olins PO, Gieres JK (1987) Phosphorylation of high- and low-molecular mass atrial natriuretic peptide analogs by cyclic AMP-dependent protein kinase. FEBS Lett 224:325–330

26. Gagelmann M, Hock D, Forssmann WG (1987) Relaxation of smooth muscle by cardiodilatin/atrial natriuretic peptide is inhibited by cAMP-dependent phosphorylation. FEBS Lett 225:251–254

27. Gagelmann M, Feller S, Hock D, Schulz-Knappe P, Forssmann WG (1989) Biochemistry of the differential release, processing and degradation of cardiac and related peptide hormones. In: Kartmann W, Wambach G (eds) Endocrinology of the heart. Springer, Berlin Heidelberg New York, pp 27–40

28. Sonnenberg JL, Sakane Y, Jeng AY, Koehn JA, Ansell JA, Wennogle LP, Ghai RD (1988) Identification of protease 3.4.24.11 as the major atrial natriuretic factor degrading enzyme in the rat kidney. Peptides 9:173–180

29. Rittenhouse J, Moberly L, Ahmed H, Marcus F (1988) Phosphorylation in situ of atrial natriuretic peptide prohormone at the cyclic AMP-dependent site. J Biol Chem 263:3778–3783

30. Bloch KD, Jones SW, Preibisch G, Seipke G, Seidman CE, Seidman JG (1987) Proatrial natriuretic factor is phosphorylated by rat cardiocytes in culture. J Biol Chem 262:9956–9961

31. Shenolikar S, Fischer K, Chang L, Weinmann EJ (1988) Type II cAMP-dependent protein kinase is associated with the rabbit kidney brush border. Second Messengers Phosphoprot 12:95–104

32. Kübler D, Reinhardt D, Pyerin W, Kinzel V (1989) A new model of posttranslational processing of ANP: cAMP-dependent phosphorylation in extracellular sites (abstract). Eur J Cell Biol 48 (Suppl 26):37
33. Murad F, Leitman DC, Bennett BM, Molina C, Waldman SA Regulation of guanylate cyclase by atrial natriuretic factor and the role of cyclic GMP in vasodilatation
34. Uchida K, Mizuno T, Shimonaka M, Sugiura N, Hagiwara H, Hirose S (1989) Subtype switching of ANP receptors during in vitro culture of vascular cells. Am J Physiol 256:H311–H314
35. Gardner DG, Deschepper CF, Baxter JD (1987) The gene for atrial natriuretic factor is expressed in the aortic arch. Hypertension 9:103–106
36. Gagelmann M, Hock D, Forssmann WG (1988) Urodilatin (CDD/ANP-95–126) is not biologically inactivated by a peptidase from dog kidney cortex membranes in contrast to atrial natriuretic peptide/cardiodilatin (α-hANP/CDD-99–126). FEBS Lett 233:249–254
37. Sonnenberg H, Honrath U, Chong CK, Wilson DR (1986) Atrial natriuretic factor inhibits sodium transport in medullary collecting duct. Am J Physiol 250:F963–F966
38. Light DB, Schwiebert EM, Karlson KH, Stanton BA (1989) Atrial natriuretic peptide inhibits cation channel in renal medullary collecting duct cells. Science 243:383–385
39. Saito Y, Nakao K, Itoh H, Yamada T, Mukoyama M, Arai H, Hosoda K, Shirakami G, Suga S, Minamino N, Kangawa K, Matsuo H, Imura H (1989) Brain natriuretic peptide is a novel cardiac hormone. Biochem Biophys Res Commun 158:360–368
40. Oehlenschlager WF, Baron DA, Schomer H, Curie MG (1989) Atrial and brain natriuretic peptide share binding sites in the kidney and the heart. Eur J Pharmacol 161:159–164

Newer Interventional Techniques

Percutaneous Laser Angioplasty in the Treatment of Coronary and Peripheral Vascular Disease

G. Lee, J.L. Rink, D.L. Rink, M.H. Lee, and D.T. Mason

Due to the inherent problems of limited access and high restenosis rate with conventional balloon angioplasty a principal goal in vascular intervention is the removal of atheromatous obstruction. An important approach to the solution is the application of laser energy for photoablation of plaque mass. In 1977 during our observations that a heated soldering iron melted atheroma, the concept was conceived to use laser energy as the heat source for this purpose. At the Lawrence Livermore Laboratories in 1980 we were able to demonstrate laser dissolution of plaque in cadaver vessel segments, utilizing argon, neodymium yttrium-aluminum-garnet (Nd:YAG) and carbon dioxide laser beams [1].

The Coaxial Laser-Heated Metal Probe Delivery System

Since special optical fibers allow propagation of light, in 1982 we used flexible thin quartz silica fibers for the transmission of laser energies from argon and Nd:YAG sources to vascular target sites within the body of live experimental animals for the recanalization of atheromatous obstructions [2]. To diminish the associated risk of vascular damage employing the free-beam mode, a novel delivery system was developed in our laboratories in which a metal cautery cap was mounted at the distal fiberoptic tip [3]. This laser-heated metal cap device, which we originated during our 1980 experiments, was also demonstrated in 1982 to be methodologically efficacious by successful recanalization coaxially in whole human atheromatous vascular segments and in living animal arteries obstructed by plaque from anastomosed cadaver vessels.

While the fiberoptic laser-heated metal cap is an advancement in safety without compromise of effectiveness, the need for coaxial guidance was apparent to further deduce hazard and aid maneuverability. Thus by 1984 an engineering breakthrough in our laboratories provided the incorporation of a front-mounted fixed central guidewire into the laser-heated metal cap [4]. More recently, this coaxial thermal probe system has been advanced in design to include also a coaxial-guided over-the-wire probe. In addition, another technological milestone achieved in our laboratories was the development of a truly portable state-of-the-art Nd:YAG medical laser designed specifically for user-friendly cardiovascular applications. The coaxial-guided thermal probe delivery catheters combined with the dedicated Nd:YAG medical laser constitute the Unicorn system (Xintec Corporation, Oakland, California).

B.S. Lewis, A. Kimchi (Eds.)
Heart Failure Mechanisms and Management
© Springer-Verlag Berlin Heidelberg 1991

Intraoperative Coronary Laser Angioplasty

In 1985 the United States Food and Drug Administration approved clinical trials in coronary and peripheral vessels under Xintec Corporation sponsorship. To determine the feasibility and safety of the laser-heated metal cap delivery system for recanalization of vascular obstruction, the thermal probe catheter alongside a steerable guidewire [5] or with the fixed central guidewire [4] was initially used clinically to relieve coronary stenosis during open-heart surgery. Laser-effected alleviation of coronary obstruction (without the addition of balloon angioplasty) was documented by intraoperative angioscopy and/or by predischarge angiography [6–8]. Long-term improved patency of these lased areas was shown by repeat angiography at 4–6 months.

Percutaneous Peripheral Laser Angioplasty

Building upon this salutary clinical experience in coronary obstructions intraoperatively, as well as in severe peripheral vascular disease intraoperatively [9], the fixed central guidewire on-the-thermal probe was then effectively employed percutaneously to recanalize peripheral vascular obstructions and occlusions of iliac, femoral, and popliteal vessels in over 42 lessons in more than 32 patients without complications (no perforations, spasm, or significant adhesiveness) [10]. Laser therapy was the sole intervention in three patients (Fig. 1); the remainder were followed by balloon angioplasty [11]. Symptom relief and/or leg salvage was achieved with improved ankle/arm index in all patients.

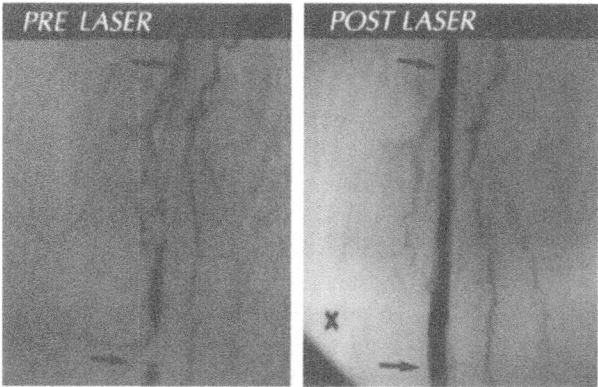

Fig. 1. In this 59-year-old woman with severe claudication, arteriography showed complete 4-cm occlusion of the left superficial femoral artery (*arrows, left panel*). The 2.6-mm Unicorn-Probe system was used to recanalize the total obstruction (*arrows, right panel*). No follow-up balloon angioplasty was required. Symptomatology was relieved, and the ankle-arm index improved considerably

Percutaneous Coronary Laser Angioplasty

Beginning in 1988, we have utilized percutaneously the coaxial-guided over-the-wire catheter probe to successfully recanalize obstructions in both the left and right coronary arteries in patients with angina pectoris [12]. Multiple intermittent bursts of laser energy achieved thermal vaporization of atherosclerotic plaque as the metal probe was advanced over the guidewire in an antegrade fashion. During laser firing, heart rhythm, electrocardiographic tracing, and arterial pressure remained stable. There also were no other untoward sequelae including chest discomfort, vessel perforation, or vasospasm. Total time from percutaneous insertion of the laser catheter to its withdrawal was less than 10 min. Angiography before and after laser delivery documented successful removal of plaque obstruction (Fig. 2). The laser procedure allowed easy access for subsequent balloon angioplasty.

Conclusions

Percutaneous laser angioplasty using the Unicorn central tracking steerable guidewire thermal probe catheter system provides rapid and safe plaque ablation of coronary and peripheral disease in appropriately selected patients. By virtue of the rapid rise and fall of temperature responses (average 18 W per pulse of 0.6-s duration) characteristic of the Unicorn probes, the obstructing atheroma is debulked without complications.

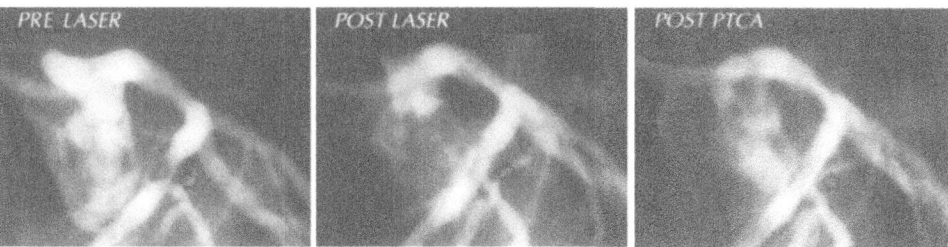

Fig. 2. In this 73-year-old man with refractory angina, cineangiography (left anterior oblique view) revealed proximal discrete obstruction (*arrow, left panel*) of the left anterior descending coronary artery. The Unicorn-Plus laser catheter system was introduced via a femoral artery, percutaneous guiding catheter positioned in the left coronary orifice. A 0.014-in. coaxial steerable guidewire was passed through the obstruction, and the 1.6-mm thermal probe was advanced over-the-wire to relieve the obstruction by thermal ablation (*arrow, middle panel*). Further treatment was carried out by balloon angioplasty (*arrow, right panel*)

References

1. Lee G, Ikeda RM, Kozina J, Mason DT (1981) Laser-dissolution of coronary atherosclerotic obstruction. Am Heart J 102:1074–1075
2. Lee G, Ikeda RM, Stobbe D, Ogata C, Theis J, Mason DT (1983) Laser irradiation of human atherosclerotic obstructive disease: simultaneous visualization and vaporization achieved by a dual fiberoptic catheter. Am Heart J 105:163–164
3. Lee G, Ikeda RM, Chan MC, Dukich J, Lee MH, Theis JH, Bommer WJ, Reis RL, Hanna ES, Mason DT (1984) Dissolution of atherosclerotic heart disease by fiberoptic laser-heated metal cautery cap. Am Heart J 107:777–778
4. Lee G, Chan MC, Rink DL, Beerline D, Lee MH, Reis RL, Mason DT (1987) Coronary revascularization by a new coaxially-guided laser-heated metal cap system. Am Heart J 113:1507–1508
5. Lee G, Chan MC, Ikeda RM, Rink JL, Lee MH, Dukich J, Reis RL, Mason DT (1985) Intravascular steerable guidewire for fiberoptic laser-heated metal cautery cap in dissolution of human atherosclerotic coronary disease. Am Heart J 110:1304–1306
6. Lee G, Garcia JM, Chan MC, Corso PJ, Bacos J, Lee MH, Pichard A, Reis RL, Mason DT (1986) Clinically successful long-term coronary recanalization. Am Heart J 112:1323–1325
7. Lee G, Reis RL, Chan MC, Boggan MD, Lee MH, Low RI, Argenal A, Hannah H, Mason DT (1986) Clinical laser recanalization of coronary obstruction: angioscopic and angiographic documentation. Chest 90:770–772
8. Lee G, Sommerhaug RG, Argenal A, Chan MC, Rink D, Mason DT (1987) Clinical laser revascularization of coronary obstruction with the coaxial-guided laser-heated metal cap catheter. Am Heart J 114:1524–1526
9. Lee G, Reis RL, Boggan MD, Chan MC, Lee MH, Low RI, Hannah H, Mason DT (1986) Laser recanalization in severe end-stage peripheral vascular disease. Am J Cardiol 59:386–387
10. Lee G, Masden R, Weiss JA, Falk R, Temes GD, Pool GE, Argenal A, Wixson D, Mason DT (1988) Percutaneous peripheral laser angioplasty: demonstration of the clinical safety and efficacy of a new coaxial-guided laser-heated cap system. Am Heart J 116:1640–1641
11. Lee G, Masden RR, Scharf D, Weiss JA, Falk RL, Temes GD, Pool GE, Coons H, Argenal AJ, Wixson D, Mason DT (1989) Percutaneous laser angioplasty of peripheral atherosclerotic obstructions by the Unicorn-cap(Tm) probe system: a multicenter study. J Am Coll Cardiol 13:14A
12. Lee G, Argenal AJ, Rink D, Lee MH, Mason DT (1988) Percutaneous coronary laser angioplasty: successful clinical application of a new thermal cap catheter coaxially guided over a steerable central guidewire. Am Heart J 116:1637–1638

The Influence
of Percutaneous Aortic Balloon Valvuloplasty
on Heart Failure in Elderly Patients
with Calcific Aortic Stenosis

E. Di Segni, A. Bakst, B. Beker, H. Dean, A. Levi, Y. Arbel, and H.O. Klein

Percutaneous balloon valvuloplasty was recently introduced in the treatment of calcific aortic stenosis, the leading valvular disease among the elderly in the Western world [1–4]. This paper reports results with percutaneous aortic balloon valvuloplasty in a group of elderly patients with congestive heart failure.

Patients and Methods

Between October 1986 and February 1989 percutaneous balloon aortic valvuloplasty was performed in 39 patients with calcific aortic stenosis. Thirty-four of these with congestive heart failure are the object of this report. Patients were referred for the procedure if they were considered very poor candidates for cardiac surgery, or if they refused surgery (six cases). Of these 34, 11 were men and 23 were women. Their age ranged from 60 to 87 years (mean 77 ± 5.9). Each patient had congestive heart failure: 23 were in New York Heart Association class IV, 10 in class III, and 1 in class II. In addition, 13 patients had angina pectoris and eight syncope. Six patients were moribund at the time that valvuloplasty was attempted.

The protocol for valvuloplasty changed during the study period with the introduction of technical improvements. A first group of 24 patients was treated with the protocol previously described [5]. After entering the left ventricle in a retrograde way a balloon dilatation catheter was advanced across the aortic valve over a 260-cm-long, 0.038- or 0.035-in. exchange wire. We used either Schneider-Shiley (Zurich) balloon dilatation catheters with balloon diameters of 15 mm or 19 mm, 4 cm or 5.5 cm in length, or Mansfield Scientific (Massachusetts, USA) balloon catheters with balloon diameters of 15 mm or 20 mm, 3 cm in length. Sequential dilations first with the 15-mm balloon catheter and then with the 19- or 20-mm balloon catheters were performed. Each balloon was inflated at least three times for 10–60 s. Hemodynamic measurements were performed before dilatation, after each series of dilatations, and at the end of the procedure. Cardiac output was measured either by the Fick method or by thermodilution in triplicate. Aortic valve area was calculated using the Hakki formula [6]. In the last group of ten patients the following modifications, according to the technique suggested by Cribier et al. [7], were used: a 14-F introducer sheath (Cook, Bloomington, Indiana, USA) positioned in the femoral artery was used for

B.S. Lewis, A. Kimchi (Eds.)
Heart Failure Mechanisms and Management
© Springer-Verlag Berlin Heidelberg 1991

catheter exchange; a 0.035-in. 300-cm-long back-up exchange guide wire (Schneider-Shiley) was used for keeping the balloon stable. Dilatations were performed using a Cribier-Letac 15- to 20-mm stepped-up balloon catheter or a 23-mm balloon catheter (Mansfield Scientific).

Noninvasive assessment of the aortic stenosis was performed by echo Doppler study in 30 patients before the procedure and repeated within 1 week of the procedure in 22 patients. Doppler peak aortic gradient was measured using the modified Bernoulli equation, and aortic valve area by the continuity equation using peak aortic and left ventricular outflow tract velocity. Gated radionuclide ejection fraction with technetium 99 (MUGA) was performed in 17 patients before valvuloplasty and in 13 after the procedure, but in only 9 patients was this parameter measured before and immediately after valvuloplasty. Patients were followed at the outpatient clinic at 1, 3, and 6 months following the valvuloplasty and every 6 months thereafter. Studies at visits included physical examination, echo Doppler study, and occasionally measurement of radionuclide ejection fraction.

Statistical analysis was performed using paired Student's t test.

Results

In the entire group of 34 patients, peak left ventricular aortic gradient was 76.6 $\pm$ 35.3 mmHg before valvuloplasty and 43.6 $\pm$ 25.4 mmHg after the procedure (Fig. 1). Average aortic valve area was 0.43 $\pm$ 0.21 cm^2 before and 0.72 $\pm$ 0.39 cm^2 after

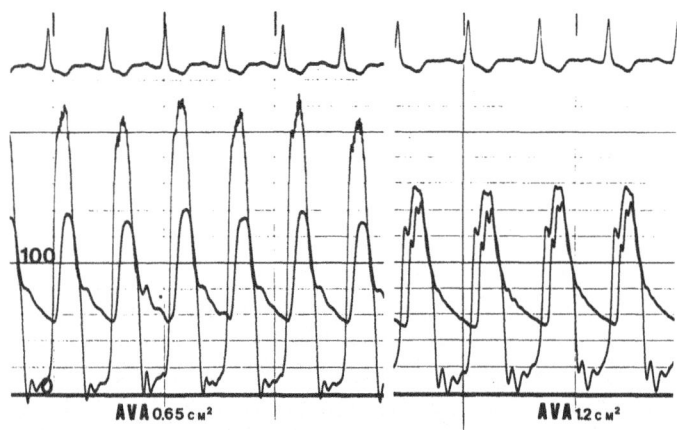

Fig. 1. Simultaneous recording of left ventricular and aortic pressures before (*left*) and after (*right*) balloon aortic valvuloplasty. At the end of the procedure, peak left ventricular aortic gradient decreased from 80 to 15 mmHg and aortic valve area (*AVA*) increased from 0.65 to 1.2 cm^2. Mechanical alternans, seen on the left tracing, disappeared immediately

the procedure. Cardiac output increased from 3.5 ± 1.6 l/min to 4.0 ± 1.7 l/min. All results were statistically highly significant ($p < 0.0001$; Table 1).

In the first group of 24 patients treated with the earlier technique, baseline peak left ventricular aortic gradient was 75.5 ± 37.9 mmHg, decreasing to 46.8 ± 25.7 mmHg after valvuloplasty ($p < 0.001$). Aortic valve area increased from 0.40 ± 0.17 cm^2 to 0.62 ± 0.38 cm^2 ($p < 0.005$), and cardiac output increased from 3.1 ± 1.9 l/min to 3.4 ± 1.2 l/min ($p < 0.03$). In the second group of ten patients treated with the newer technique, baseline peak left ventricular aortic gradient was 79.2 ± 30 mmHg, decreasing to 36 ± 24 mmHg ($p < 0.001$). Aortic valve area was 0.49 ± 0.28 cm^2 before and 0.93 ± 0.36 cm^2 after the procedure ($p ± 0.001$). Cardiac output increased from 4.2 ± 2.1 l/min before to 5.1 ± 2.1 l/min after the procedure ($p < 0.003$). No statistical difference was found between the first and the second groups for baseline left ventricular aortic gradient, aortic valve area, cardiac output, or postvalvuloplasty left ventricular aortic gradient. Increase in the aortic valve area and in cardiac output was statistically significantly better in the second group than in the first ($p < 0.03$ and $p < 0.04$ respectively, Table 1).

Table 1. Hemodynamic results of balloon aortic valvuloplasty

	Left ventricular aortic gradient (mmHg)		Aortic valve area (cm^2)		Cardiac output (l/min)	
	Baseline	After	Baseline	After	Baseline	After
All cases	76.6 ± 35.3	43.6 ± 25.4	0.43 ± 0.21	0.72 ± 0.39	3.5 ± 1.6	4.0 ± 1.7
Group I	75.5 ± 37.9	46.8 ± 25.7	0.40 ± 0.17	0.62 ± 0.38[a]	3.1 ± 1.9	3.4 ± 1.2[b]
Group II	77.2 ± 30	36 ± 24	0.49 ± 0.28	0.93 ± 0.36[a]	5.1 ± 2.1	4.2 ± 2.1[b]

Differences between all baseline values and values after valvuloplasty were statistically highly significant (see text).
[a] $p < 0.03$ between group I and group II for aortic valve area.
[b] $p < 0.04$ between group I and group II for cardiac output values.

For the entire group Doppler peak aortic valve gradient was 86 ± 26 mmHg before valvuloplasty and 53 ± 21 mmHg after the procedure ($p < 0.001$). Doppler-calculated aortic valve area was 0.51 ± 0.21 cm^2 before and 0.90 ± 0.37 cm^2 after the procedure ($p < 0.001$). Results of radionuclide ejection fraction were summarized only in the nine patients in whom this parameter was measured before and immediately after the procedure. In these cases, ejection fraction was 48% ± 16% before and 51% ± 13% after valvuloplasty. Although there was a trend toward increase in ejection fraction, the results were not statistically significant because of the small number of available data.

Twenty-six patients (76%) exhibited an immediate improvement of at least one New York Heart Association functional class following valvuloplasty, with the majority of them (19 cases) reaching the functional class I or II (Fig. 2). This improvement lasted at 1-month follow-up visit. Seven patients, all initially in

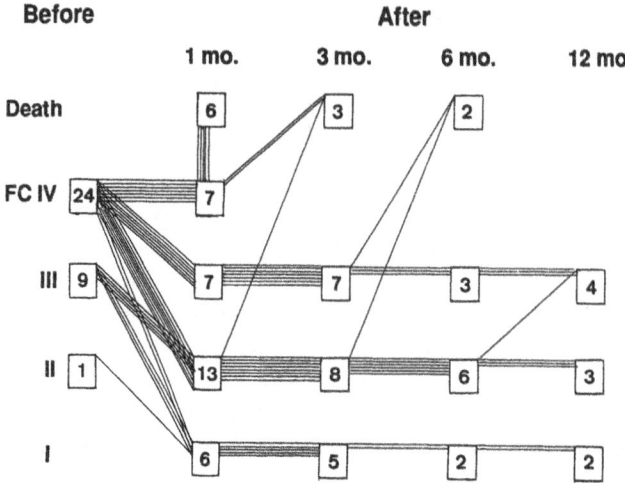

Fig. 2. Clinical follow-up after balloon aortic valvuloplasty (one patient was lost at 1-month follow-up). Patients surviving at 1 month were followed for a mean of 6.8 ± 3.8 months

functional class IV did not improve, and six of them died within 1 month of the procedure. The patients surviving at 1 month visit were followed for a mean of 6.8 ± 3.8 months. At 3 months three more patients had died, and 20 patients were still maintaining their initial improvement. Two additional patients with known coronary artery disease died within 6 months because of myocardial infarction. The remaining 11 patients followed for this period maintained their initial clinical improvement, with eight of them being in functional class I or II. At 12-month follow-up eight out of nine patients were in stable condition, and only one had clinical deterioration. Mortality cases are analyzed in Table 2. Six patients died within 1 month of the valvuloplasty (none during the procedure).

Table 2. Mortality after balloon aortic valvuloplasty

	Aortic valve area (cm²)		Rhythm
	Baseline	After	
Cases of mortality	0.6	0.6	NSR
within 1 month	0.3	0.3	NSR
	0.2	0.4	AF
	0.15	0.4	AF
	0.4	2	AF
	0.3	0.6	NSR, CVA
Cases of mortality	0.6	0.8	AF
within 3 months	0.4	0.98	AF
	0.6	0.9	NSR, CVA

NSR, normal sinus rhythm; *AF*, atrial fibrillation; *CVA*, cerebrovascular accident.

Five were intrahospital deaths. All but one were terminally ill patients. Four of them represent failure of valvuloplasty; in two, with bicuspid aortic valve, there was no change of aortic valve area, and in two, with extremely reduced baseline aortic valve area, postvalvuloplasty area increased by 100% at least, but remained only 0.4 cm^2. Two patients with good valvuloplasty results died at 1 and at 3 months, respectively, following a stroke. Three additional patients died within 3 months in spite of good valvuloplasty results with aortic valve areas of 2, 0.80, and 0.98 cm^2, respectively. Each of these patients had atrial fibrillation and poor echocardiographic left ventricular contraction. Two deaths that occurred between 3 and 6 months of follow-up were due to myocardial infarction.

The procedure was generally well tolerated by patients. Hypotension during balloon inflation was observed in each case; syncope, promptly reverted by balloon deflation, occurred in six patients. Bleeding requiring blood transfusion occurred in seven patients, all of them belonging to the first group. One patient of the first group treated by the femoral approach, required surgical repair of the iliac artery. Severe hemiplegia occurred in two patients, in one during the procedure and in the other 1 day later.

Discussion

Cribier et al. [2] initially reported on 92 cases in whom left ventricular aortic gradient decreased from 75 ± 26 to 30 ± 13 mmHg, and aortic valve area increased from 0.49 ± 17 to 0.93 ± 0.36 cm^2. A recent report of the same group [8], summarizing 300 cases, indicated an increase of aortic valve area from 0.53 ± 18 to 0.97 ± 0.34 cm^2. In the 170 patients of Safian et al. [9] transaortic gradient decreased from 71 ± 20 to 36 ± 14 mmHg and aortic valve area increased from 0.6 ± 0.2 cm^2 to 0.9 ± 0.3 cm^2. Comparable results were reported by others [10]. The hemodynamic changes induced by balloon aortic valvuloplasty were not always accompanied by corresponding clinical improvement, and thus the initial enthusiasm for balloon valvuloplasty as an alternative to surgery has been replaced by a more cautious approach.

In the Safian et al. series [9], 6/168 patients died in hospital and 25 (16%) died a mean of 6.4 ± 5.3 months after valvuloplasty. Other reports [11,12], based on relatively small series, aroused doubts about the effectiveness of balloon valvuloplasty in influencing the clinical course.

In analyzing the results reported in the literature, the influence of two factors should be taken into account: (a) the inclusion in the earlier series of extremely sick, moribund patients and (b) the improvement in hemodynamic results as a consequence of the introduction of new technical developments. Increasingly large balloon dilatation catheters have been recommended, with a double balloon technique used by some [12]; a back-up stiff guide wire was developed to overcome the frequent inability to keep the balloon in stable position across the aortic valve during balloon inflation; large introducer sheath and stepped-up balloon catheter to avoid local vascular trauma and repeated change of catheters for stepped up dilatation have been developed [7].

We found that the technique developed by Cribier et al. [7] greatly improved our valvuloplasty results, making the procedure easier, safer, and more reproducible. In our second group of patients treated with this technique, postvalvuloplasty aortic valve area was significantly wider (0.93 versus 0.62 cm^2), and nine of ten patients of the second group had 50% or more increase in the aortic valve area following valvuloplasty, compared to 48% in the first group.

An important factor limiting the widespread application of balloon aortic valvuloplasty is the reported high restenosis rate. In the Safian et al. series [9] there was recurrence of symptoms in 28% of patients at a mean of 7.5 ± 5.7 months after the procedure. In Block's [13] series 56% of patients had recurrence of symptoms, restenosis, or death at a mean of 5.6 months of the valvuloplasty. Twenty-six (76%) of our patients improved to at least one functional class, with the majority of them (19) reaching functional class I or II. This improvement was accompanied by a trend to improvement in left ventricular ejection fraction. A high rate of early deaths (17% at 1 month and 26% at 3 months) was observed, but among survivors followed for a mean of 6.8 ± 3.8 months the subsequent course was generally characterized by persistent clinical improvement. At 12-month follow-up there were two additional deaths (because of myocardial infarction), and only one case of clinical deterioration.

Two patients died at 1 and at 3 months following a stroke. Two late deaths were due to myocardial infarction – an event unrelated to the valvular disease itself or to the procedure. Three additional patients, who died in spite of a very satisfactory postvalvuloplasty aortic valve area, are of particular interest since each one presented with atrial fibrillation. It appears that atrial fibrillation in these patients was the expression of such advanced myocardial damage as not to allow recovery of myocardial function. Similar failings in improvement in extremely depressed myocardial function have been reported after aortic valve replacement [14].

None of the patients died during the procedure in our series. Nonetheless, aortic valvuloplasty is a procedure involving a substantial risk of serious complications. Two patients had hemiplegia – one during the procedure and one 1 day later. The incidence of reported strokes varied from 4 of 300 patients in the Letac et al. series [8] to 7.1% in the Acar et al. [15] series. Local vascular complications and bleeding requiring blood transfusion became rare when using the 14-F introducer sheath. In none of our cases was an appreciable increase in aortic insufficiency found.

Balloon aortic valvuloplasty proved to be effective in the majority of patients in dilating the aortic valve and improving the symptomatic status. These results may be considered satisfactory and the risks acceptable considering the highly selected population of elderly and very sick patients referred for the procedure. The prognosis in candidates for balloon aortic valvuloplasty is poor, with 1-year mortality of 43% and 2-year mortality of 63% [16]. For these patients, who carry a very high surgical risk, or for those unwilling to undergo aortic valve replacement, balloon aortic valvuloplasty represents a valid palliative treatment.

References

1. Cribier A, Saoudi N, Berland J, Savin T, Rocha P, Letac B (1986) Percutaneous transluminal valvuloplasty of acquired aortic stenosis in elderly patients: an alternative to valve replacement? Lancet I:63–67
2. Cribier A, Savin T, Berland J, Rocha P, Mechmeche R, Saoudi N, Behar P. Letac B (1987) Percutaneous transluminal balloon valvuloplasty of adult aortic stenosis: Report of 92 cases. J Am Coll Cardiol 9:382–386
3. McKay R, Safian RD. Lock JE, Diver DJ, Berman AD, Warren SE, Come PC, Baim DS, Mandell VE. Royal HD, Grossman W (1987) Assessment of left ventricular and aortic valve function after aortic balloon valvuloplasty in adult patients with critical aortic stenosis. Circulation 75:192–203
4. Isner JM, Salem DN, Desnoyers MR, Hougen IJ, Mackey WC, Pandian NG. Eichorn EJ, Konstam MA, Levine HJ (1987) Treatment of calcific aortic stenosis by balloon valvuloplasty. Am J Cardiol 59:313–317
5. Di Segni E, Bakst A, Levi A, Rosenschein U, Klein Z, Beker B, Dean H, Kaplinsky E (1988) Percutaneous balloon valvuloplasty for calcific aortic stenosis in the elderly. Harefuah 114:268–291
6. Hakki AH, Iskandrian AS, Bemis CE, Kimbris D, Mintz GS, Segal BL, Brice C (1981) A simplified valve formula for the calculation of stenotic cardiac valve areas. Circulation 63:1050–1055
7. Cribier GA, Grigera F, Eltchaninoff F, Lefebvre E, Berland J, Letac B (1989) New developments in aortic balloon valvuloplasty (abstract). J Am Coll Cardiol 13:17A
8. Letac B, Gerber LI, Koning R (1988) Insights on the mechanism of balloon valvuloplasty in aortic stenosis. Am J Cardiol 62:1241–1247
9. Safian RD, Mandell VS, Thurer RE, Hutchins GM, Schnitt SJ, Grossman W. McKay RG (1987) Postmortem and intraoperative balloon valvuloplasty of calcific aortic stenosis in elderly patients: mechanisms of successful dilation. J Am Coll Cardiol 9:655–660
10. Kleaveland JP, Hill J, Margolis J. Herrman H, Vetrovec G, Cowley M, Bass T. Nocero M, Pepine C (1988) M-HEART registry for percutaneous transluminal aortic valvuloplasty: follow-up report. Circulation 78 (4) II-533
11. Serruys PW, Luijten HE, Beatt KJ, Dimario C, De Feyter PJ, Essed CE, Roelandt JRTC. van den Brand M (1988) Percutaneous balloon valvuloplasty for calcific aortic stenosis – a treatment "sine cure"? Eur Heart J 9:782–794
12. Litvack F, Jakubowski AT, Buchbinder NA, Eigler N (1988) Lack of sustained clinical improvement in an elderly population after percutaneous aortic valvuloplasty. Am J Cardiol 62:270–275
13. Block PC (1988) Aortic valvuloplasty – a valid alternative? N Engl J Med 319:169
14. Carabello BA, Green LH, Grossman W, Conn LH, Koster JK, Collins JJ Jr (1980) Hemodynamic determinants of prognosis of aortic valve replacement in critical aortic stenosis and advanced congestive heart failure. Circulation 62:42–48
15. Acar J, Vahanian A, Slama M, Cormier B, Michel PL, Luxereau P. Farah E. Leborgne O, Dermine P (1988) Treatment of calcified aortic stenosis: surgery or percutaneous transluminal aortic valvuloplasty? Eur Heart J 9:163–171
16. O'Keefe JH Jr, Vlietstra RE, Bailey KR, Holmes DR Jr (1987) Natural history of candidates for balloon aortic valvuloplasty. Mayo Clin Proc 62:986–991

Newer Surgical Techniques in the Patient with Heart Failure

Cardiomyoplasty: A New Approach to Surgical Treatment of Heart Failure

V.S. Chekanov and A.A. Krakovsky

Introduction

Cardiomyoplasty occupies an important place among the recent problems in cardiac surgery. In 1932 Leriche and Fontaine [17] used an automuscle to determine experimentally the possibility of indirect myocardial revascularization after coronary artery ligation; in 1935 Beck introduced this method into clinical practice. By 1966 Petrovsky [25] had performed about 100 operations of this kind. However the method was not adopted; its results were doubtful, and the investigators were prepared to reject it.

The revolution in the method was brought about by electronics. The skeletal muscle, when stimulated, was transformed gradually from cross-striated to smooth muscle; it thus became possible to use this muscle constantly as a contractile element. Experimental investigations have been carried out in France and in the USA, and in the mid-1980s Carpentier and McGovern introduced the method into clinical practice [21,22,5,6]. They suggested that investigations of the cardiomyoplasty could be employed not only for the replacement of the diseased myocardium of various cardiac chambers, but with the aid of skeletal automuscle to create an extracardial contrapulsation system. Investigations on the automuscular neoventricle creation have been quite successful; the same can be said about an automuscular blood pump playing the role of an artificial heart.

This paper analyzes the hemodynamic function of the cardiomyoplasty method in experimental left ventricular (LV) aneurysm formation.

Material and Methods

Ninety mongrel dogs weighing 18–25 kg were studied experimentally. The animals were treated in strict conformity with international rules for experimental investigation.

The experiments can be divided into three series:

1. A series of 13 experiments to elaborate optimal variants of the surgical technique. A LV aneurysm with apical localization was created. We then evaluated hemodynamic parameters and realized the second stage of the operation – the cardiomyoplasty, consisting of the application of a latissimus

B.S. Lewis, A. Kimchi (Eds.)
Heart Failure Mechanisms and Management
© Springer-Verlag Berlin Heidelberg 1991

dorsi (LD) muscular flap on the aneurysmatic region of the heart with preliminary LV aneurysm resection and replacement of the resected region by the autopericardium. We elaborated the most adequate approach to the LD muscle – the atraumatic technique for its isolation, the method of its implantation into the thoracic cavity, and the optimal method for its application on the region of a preliminarily formed and resected LV aneurysm. At every stage of the investigation we carefully considered the muscular flap's optimal parameters and the selection of stimulation regimen.

2. A series of 36 experiments in which we analyzed the influence of the stimulated, non-pre-trained LD muscle flap, after application on the resected LV aneurysm region, according to various parameters of intracardiac hemodynamics.

3. A series of 41 experiments in which we analyzed the influence of the muscle-heart complex on intracardiac hemodynamics and contractile function of LV myocardium. Simultaneously, we elaborated the method of a training LD muscle stimulation and studied the influence of various stimulation regimens on the essential biochemical blood indices.

All surgical investigations were carried out after ketamine premedication (10–15 mg/kg) and with narcosis and standard neuroleptanalgesia (fentanyl, droperidol). Myorelaxants were not used because of their uncontrolled action on skeletal muscle contractility. No cardiotonics were used during hemodynamic studies.

Hemodynamic parameters were recorded on the Mingograph-7 (Siemens, Sweden) which provided an integral scheme of hemodynamic estimation "on line," including the first derivative of LV pressure dp/dt. The stroke ejection from the LV and the volume bloodflow velocity were measured with the electromagnetic flowmeter Statham-Gould-SP-2201 (USA) (Fig. 1). In the late postoperative period (3–24 h) and in the third series of experiments cardiac index (CI), stroke volume (SV), were determined with a cardiac output thermodilution apparatus (B. Braun, Melsungen AG, FRG) and a thermodilu-

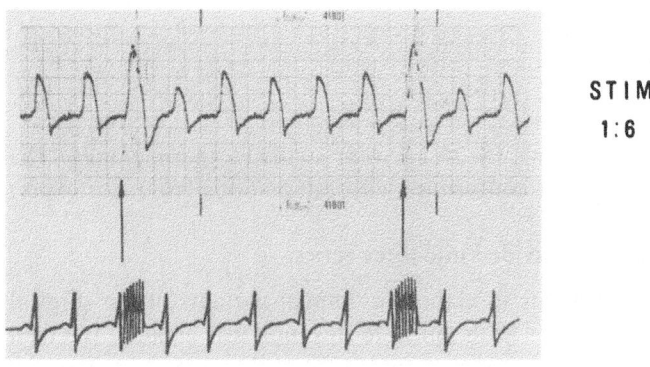

STIM
1:6

Fig. 1. Flowmetric curve registered during muscle stimulation (transducer is on the aorta)

tional balloon catheter Corodyn ID-E-JN (B. Braun, FRG) installed in the pulmonary artery trunk. Two-lumen catheters from the same firm were used for the monitoring of the aortic, left atrial, LV, and caudal venous pressures. All data were processed statistically by totalities comparison with paired variables. The homogeneity of values was confirmed statistically; the standard error for each experiment and for the group of experiments was 18%. The mean functions' significance was estimated with an error which did not exceed 10%.

Original electrostimulators were designed in conjunction with the Moscow Physical Engineering Institute. We used the electromyoneuro cardiostimulator Stiminak, which provides R-wave-synchronized automuscle guidance within the limits of a given rhythm (up to 150 beats/min), with an automatic transition in the rhythm division or doubling regimen and allowing automatic cessation in cases of cardiac rhythm increase or arrhythmias. An external magnetic device allows programming of the implantable neuromyostimulator to any synchronization ratio from 1:1 to 1:8.

The cardiosynchronized stimulation of the automuscle was achieved with bursts of impulses (tension, 2.8 V; burst duration, 217 ms; impulse duration, 0.52 ms; impulse frequency in the burst, 25–30 Hz). The number of impulses in the burst could be changed from 1 to 8 according to indications. The device sensitivity to the negative R wave (SR^-) is 3.2 V; for the positive R wave (SR^+), 2.1 V. The mass of the apparatus is 85 gm; its dimensions, $65 \times 47.5 \times 11$ mm. The calculated duration of the apparatus work with the mean rhythm of 70 beats/min and synchronization ratio of 1:1 is 10 years.

We would also like to emphasize the expediency of implantable radio-frequency stimulators with a guided influence and variable parameters in cardiomyoplasty, particularly in experimental work. An external transmitter with autonomous feeding allows variation in the frequency of impulse "volleys" from 10 to 120 imp/min; in addition, the number of impulses in the burst can be varied from 1 to 7, and their amplitude from 0 to 10 V. Some parameters of the radiofrequency stimulator used in our investigations possess a fixed value; these are the duration and the frequency of impulses in the burst (0.5 ms and 30 Hz, respectively).

Besides the radiofrequency stimulator, we have also employed original sensor and stimulating neuromuscular electrodes, the latter consisting of a cuffed carbonized cup applied directly on the nerve of the LD muscle. Where necessary we added another stimulating electrode which passed through all the muscle's thickness.

Operative Technique

In the right lateral position an incision was made in the 6th intercostal space from the interspinal muscles to the left lateral sternum border. The LD muscle was isolated completely; the main thoracodorsal neurovascular peduncle was preserved. In the second series of experiments the tendinous part of the muscle fixation to the brachial bone was intact. A long tendon band, fixed to the transverse vertebral appendices, was cut out of the muscular flap and released from the fat tissue. This band was used as an original layer in aneurysm formation. The stimulating electrode from the myostimulator was implanted in the region where the thoracodorsal neurovascular bundle enters the LD muscle.

After thoracotomy a window was formed in the region of the 3rd intercostal space for the introduction of the automuscular flap into the pleural cavity. During the main stage of surgical intervention the muscle was fed by means of the background stimulation with single impulses (40 imp/min; impulse duration, 150 ms; amplitude, 0.5–0.8 V).

For the first time, we tried a method using a vascular peduncle to protect the muscular graft from ischemic injury during the preparation and introduction. Myoplegia was performed under roentgenologic control by introducing a catheter into the thoracodorsal artery through the femoral artery or through the aorta immediately after thoracotomy. Oxygenated cold myoplegic solution was injected at a pressure of 200–250 mmHg. After the thorax was opened, a large pericardial patch was tailored. The ascending aorta was isolated and a flowmeter gauge set. A two-lumen catheter for the LV and pulmonary arterial pressure measurement was introduced through the left atrial appendage. The pericardium was opened, a curved clamp (Satinsky type) was applied on the LV apical region, and the apex dissected to the level of distal papillary muscles. The operation was carried out on the beating heart without extracorporeal circulation. An autopericardial patch, prepared beforehand, was sutured to the border of a formed myocardial defect with blanket sutures (Prolen 4.0), which passed through the entire myocardial thickness; the tendon band from the LD muscle, prepared during muscular flap mobilization, was taken into the stitches. The clamp was removed and after air embolization prophylaxis an enormous autopericardial saccular LV aneurysm was allowed to fill; the aneurysm was pulsating paradoxically (Fig. 2). After relative hemodynamic stabilization initial hemodynamic data were recorded. A sensing electrode from the electromyostimulator was implanted on the right ventricular outflow tract.

During the next operative stage the automuscular flap was transferred to the thoracic cavity and fixed to the LV myocardium; the flap had the slope shape and was fixed with 8–12 U-like sutures on the LV perimeter. The automuscle portion adjacent to the resected aneurysm region was fixed to the myocardial defect border as a "seal" with four U-like sutures. In this way a "new" apical portion of the LV with an inner autopericardial layer was formed (Fig. 2). Sensing and stimulating electrodes were connected to the Stiminak stimulator and a cardio-synchronized stimulation started.

Hemodynamic parameters were determined immediately after operation, on the 5th, 10th, 30th, 60th and 120th minutes, at 3, 6, 12 and 24 h, and in the late period after the beginning of the muscle-heart complex function. In order to test the myocytes' lesions in the trained muscle we took blood samples via a catheter introduced into a peripheral vein. The activity of serum creatine kinase, its isoenzyme MB, and the myoglobin concentration were evaluated.

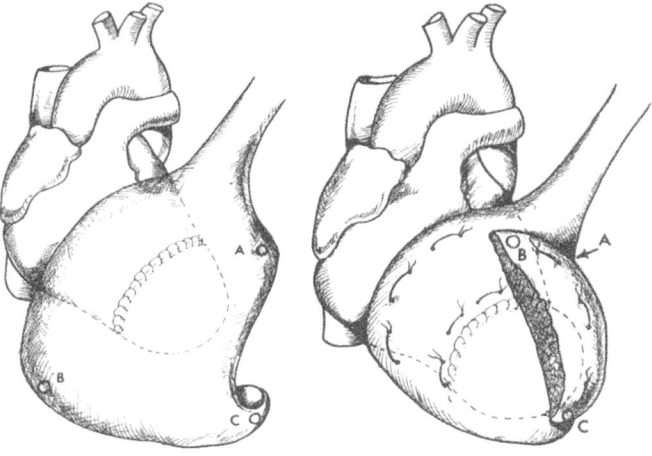

Fig. 2. First and second steps of the cardiomyoplasty operation

Comparisons were made between hemodynamic parameters measured at the 20th minute after formation of the autopericardial LV aneurysm (taken as initial values) and the mean values measured at the 10th, 30th, 60th and 120th min of functioning of the dynamic muscle-heart complex. At the other stages the hemodynamic picture was similar. All hemodynamic investigations were performed at various pulsation ratios.

Results

$\bar{p}_{LVmax}$ increased significantly during the muscle-heart complex function at different postoperative terms – by 64%–71%. This index correlates directly with LV power indices NL ($p = +0.93$) and with the LV pumping coefficient KLH ($p = +0.76$), which were increased by 87% and 63% respectively ($p < 0.01$).

LV end-diastolic pressure decreased ($p < 0.01$) in all stages of the newly formed muscle-heart complex by 74.5%. Ventriculography, performed in some cases, showed a significant increase of LV ejection fraction with a decrease in end-diastolic volume, as a result of skeletal muscle application on the aneurysm and liquidation of the aneurysmatic sac's pathological pulsation under the contracting muscle's influence. The comparison of functional characteristics showed a difference in SV, CI, saturation index (SI), and LV stroke work index (WLVS) from the baseline data ($p < 0.05$). SV increased by 36%–43%, CI by 32%–40%, and WLVS by 34%–50% the initial values in equally calculated circulating blood volume. The same tendency was seen in the late postoperative period. The maximal rate of increase (dp/dt max) and decrease (dp/dt min) of intraventricular pressure rose significantly, by 47% and 84% respectively (Fig. 3).

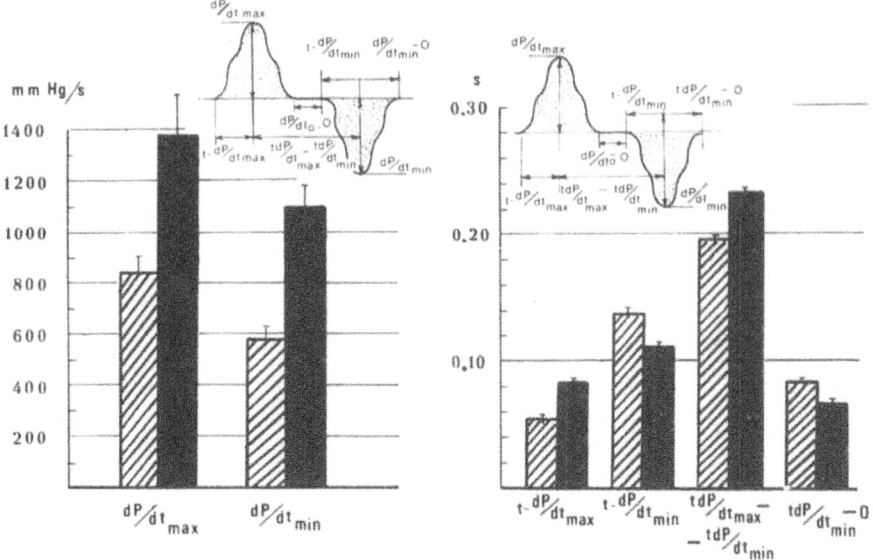

Fig. 3. Cardiomyoplasty – analysis of hemodynamie parameters (left ventricle)

The time needed for achievement of maximal velocity in LV pressure increase (active contraction time) increased by 34% as a result of contraction time lengthening – the skeletal muscle stimulation procedure and the creation of a subsequent hemodynamic effect are possible only when a tetanic contraction is formed in response to the defined variants of burst impulsation. The decrease in active relaxation time and increase in duration of the LV ejection period after cardiomyoplasty was not significant.

The time for LV passive filling, dp/dt_{min-0}, in the postoperative period decreased by 18%–21%. In the late postoperative period the ratio of the maximal valocities for pressure increase and decrease:

$$\frac{dp/dt\ max}{dp/dt\ min} = \frac{V\ max}{V\ min}$$

was greater than 1 in 74% of our observations. This testifies to the progressive increase of the postload which limits mechanically the pressure increase velocity. There was a direct correlation between $\bar{p}_{LVmax}$ and LVPTI values and the maximal velocity of pressure increase ($p = \pm0.86$). It is noteworthy that in 47% of our observations we recorded a zero velocity interval dp/dt (0-0), which is uncommon in dogs. This sign is considered by many to indicate a normal contractile capacity for the LV.

Discussion

In order to treat heart failure, different methods of cardiac function support have been elaborated for more than 25 years [4,13,14]. A more recent approach to the question of cardiac support has been to use skeletal muscle [24,26,27], a method which was initially subjected to a very large spectrum of investigations [1,16,28,29]. Different muscles have been transplanted on the heart with different goals: augmentation of cardiac cavity, reinforcement of the region of myocardial infarction or postinfarction aneurysm, augmentation of cardiac ejection, and synchronous imposition of the muscle's contraction rhythm by utilizing its contractile capacities [2,3,11,18,19,23]. Various muscles have been used: the diaphragmatic muscle, the LD, the rectus abdominis, intercostal gracilis, the sternohyoideus, and others [5-9,15,27]. The transplants were of different types: free, pedunculated, or, in some cases, free transplants with microvascular anastomoses (innervated, denervated, stimulated, and nonstimulated).

Nakamura [24] formed a muscular pedunculated graft from the diaphragmatic muscle and implanted it on the right atrium, so that atrial dimensions were almost doubled. He used prolonged stimulation, but did not achieve an important hemodynamic effect. However, during two experiments with the muscle wrapped around the heart and stimulated for 8 min by the Kantrowitz method, a 20 mmHg pressure rise was achieved, though irreversible muscle fatigue subsequently developed.

The experimentally proven hemodynamic effect of cardiomyoplasty [10,19,20] made it possible for Carpentier [5] and McGovern [21,22] to perform cardiomyoplasty; however, until recently, there was almost no indication of possible long-term cardiac function support [9]. The automuscle's advantages, compared to synthetic materials used in cardiac surgery, are explainable and clear, but only the creation of a hemodynamic effect could make this method competitive. Investigation of the skeletal LD muscle's use as a neoventricle and an experimental hydraulic approbation of this model occupy an important place in the solution of this problem [12,20].

Conclusions

The skeletal muscles have been investigated from the point of view of cardiac function support for the last 50 years. At a time when biological heart transplantation entails many problems and artificial hearts need serious improvement, the more recent, reassuring results in the use of skeletal muscle perhaps herald a new era in the surgical management of severe congestive heart failure.

References

1. Acker MA, Hammond RL, Mannion JD, Salmons SS, Stephenson LW (1986) An autologous biologic pump motor. J Thorac Cardiovasc Surg 92:733-746
2. Acker MA, Anderson WA, Hammond KL et al. (1987) Skeletal muscle ventricles in circulation. One to eleven weeks experience. J Thorac Cardiovasc Surg 94:163-174
3. Andersen JS, Anderson WA, Hammond RL, Gale D, Stephenson LW (1988) Cardiac augmentation with skeletal muscle. Heart Failure 4:23-31
4. Beck CS (1935) The development of a new blood supply to the heart by operation. Ann Surg 102:801
5. Carpentier A, Chachques JC (1985) Myocardial substitution with a stimulated skeletal muscle: first successful clinical case. Lancet II:1267
6. Carpentier A, Chachques JC (1987) Latissimus Dorsi cardiomyoplasty to increase cardiac output. In: Rabago G, Cooley DA (eds) Heart valve replacement and future trends in cardiac surgery. Future, New York, pp 473-486
7. Chachques JC, Mitz V, Hero M et al. (1985) Experimental cardiomyoplasty using the Latissimus Dorsi muscle flap. J Cardiovasc Surg 26:457
8. Chachques JC, Grandjean P, Taumasi JJ, Pekler P, Chauvaud S, Bourgeois I, Carpentier A (1987) Dynamic cardiomyoplasty: a new approach to assist chronic myocardial failure. Life Support S Syst 5:323-327
9. Chachques JC, Grandjean P, Schwartz K, Mihaileanu S et al. (1988) Effect of Latissimus Dorsi dynamic cardiomyoplasty on ventricular function. Circulation 78 (Suppl III): N 5 (III-203)-(III-216)
10. Chiu RC-J (1986) Biomechanical cardiac assist. Cardiomyoplasty and muscle-powered devices. Futura, Mount Kisco, New York
11. Dewar ML, Drinkwater DC, Wittnich C et al. (1984) Synchronously stimulated skeletal muscle graft for myocardial repair: an experimental study. J Thorac Cardiovasc Surg 87:325
12. Dewar M, Walsh G, Abraham E, DeSimon BS, Foot E, Stewart J, Fraser R, Chiu RC-J (1987) Left ventricular full-thickness cardiomyoplasty with pericardial neoendocardium: experimental development of a surgical procedure. Ann Thorac Surg
13. Kantrowitz A (1960) Functioning autogenous muscle used experimentally as an auxillary ventricle. Trans Am Artif Intern Organs 6:305-310
14. Kantrowitz A, McKinnon WMP (1959) The experimental use of the diaphragm as an auxillary myocardium. Surg Forum 9:266-268
15. Kusaba E, Schraut W, Sawatani S, Jaron D, Freed P, Kantrowitz A (1973) A diaphragmatic graft for augmenting left ventricular function: a feasibility study. Trans Am Soc Artif Intern Organs 19:231-257
16. Kusserow BK, Clapp JF (1964) A small ventricle-type pump for prolonged perfusions, construction and initial studies, including attempts to power a pump biologically with skeletal muscle. Trans Am Soc Artif Intern Organs 8:74-78
17. Leriche R, Fontaine R (1933) Essai expérimental de traitement de certains infarctus du myocarde et de l'anevrisme du coeur par une greffe de muscle strié. Bull Soc Nat Chir 59:229-232
18. Macoviak JA, Stephenson LW, Spielman S, Greenspan A, Likoff M (1981) Replacement of ventricular myocardium with diaphragmatic skeletal muscle. J Thorac Cardiovasc Surg 81:519-527
19. Macoviak JA, Stephenson LW, Alavi A, Kelly A, Edmunds LH (1981) The effect of electrical stimulation on diaphragmatic muscle used to enlarge right ventricle. Surgery 90:271
20. Macoviak JA, Stinson EB, Starkey TD, Hansen DE, Cabill PD, Miller DC, Shumway NE (1986) Myoventriculoplasty and neoventricle myograft cardiac augmentation to establish pulmonary blood flow. J Thorac Cardiovasc Surg 93:212-220
21. Magovern GS, Parc SB, Magovern GJ Jr, Benckart DH, Tullis G, Rozar E, Kao R, Christlieb I (1986) Latissimus Dorsi as a functioning synchronously paced muscle component in the repair of a left ventricular aneurysm. Ann Thorac Surg 41:116

22. Magovern GJ, Heckler FR, Park SB, Christlieb I, Magovern GJ Jr, Kao RL, Bencart DH, Tullis G, Rozar E, Liebler GA, Burkholder JA, Maher TD (1987) Paced Latissimus Dorsi used for dynamic cardiomyoplasty of left ventricular aneurysms. Ann Thorac Surg 44:379–388

23. Molteni L, Almada H, Ferrpira R (1989) Synchronously stimulated skeletal muscle graft for left ventricular assistance. J Thorac Cardiovasc Surg 97:439–446

24. Nakamura K, Glenn WWL (1964) Graft of the diaphragm as a functioning substitute for the myocardium. J Surg Res 4:435–439

25. Petrovsky BV (1966) Surgical treatment of cardiac aneurysms. J Cardiovasc Surg 2:87–91

26. Salmons S, Henricson J (1981) The adaptive response of skeletal muscle to increased use. J Muscle Nerve 4:94–105

27. Sheperd MP (1969) Diaphragmatic muscle and cardiac surgery. Ann Coll Surg Engl 45:212–231

28. Sola OM, Dillard DH, Ivey TD et al. (1985) Autotransplantation of skeletal muscle into myocardium. Circulation 71:341

29. Walsh GL, Dewar ML, Khalafalla et al. (1986) Characteristics of transformed fatigue-resistant skeletal muscle for long-term cardiac assist by extra-aortic balloon counterpulsation. Surg Forum 37:201

Left Ventricular Aneurysmectomy and Ventriculoplasty: Early Angiographic Results and Long-Term Follow-Up

C. Vassanelli, G. Morando, G. Menegatti, M. Turri, L. Zanolla,
G. Besa, and P. Zardini

Introduction

The formation of an aneurysm (An) of the left ventricle (LV) is a not infrequent complication of a myocardial infarction, with an incidence between 3% and 38% (average 15%) [1–3]. LV An is identified on contrast cineangiography as a thinned and dilated portion with akinetic or dyskinetic contraction pattern [4,5]. Early diagnosis is important for the management of this disease, since surgical treatment of postinfarction LV An is now a well-established procedure [3,4,6–9]. However, the effect of scar resection on functional recovery of cardiac performance and on long-term survival is still controversial. Among the surgical techniques aimed to improve results, Jatene [10] recently proposed a method of reconstruction in order to (1) restore the normal size and shape of the LV cavity, (2) reduce the workload of the residual myocardium, and (3) improve the function of tissue adjacent to resected scar.

Material and Methods

Patients

From January 1987 to September 1988, 22 consecutive male patients (mean age 54.6 ± 9.3 years, range 35–67, group I) were operated on for resection of a chronic, anterolateral postinfarction LV An associated with ventriculoplasty. In three patients saphenous vein bypass grafting was performed. Patients who had already had an additional repair of a ventricular septal rupture were excluded from this evaluation.

Angiographic Evaluation

All patients underwent coronary and LV angiography preoperatively and before hospital discharge (average 2 weeks). Contrast LV angiography was performed at 30° right anterior oblique view, injecting 40–50 ml of iopamidol in 2 s and filming at 40 frames/s. Postextrasystolic beats were excluded from analysis. A LV An was defined as a regional dilatation associated with systolic akinesis or dyskinesis,

B.S. Lewis, A. Kimchi (Eds.)
Heart Failure Mechanisms and Management
© Springer-Verlag Berlin Heidelberg 1991

anatomically or functionally distinct from the remaining myocardium. Significative mitral rigurgitation was absent in all patients. End-systolic and end-diastolic frames were projected and LV silhouettes digitized. Long axis was traced from the mid-aortic plane to the apex. Global LV volumes were calculated using the area-length method [11]. After having traced a line dividing the aneurysm and the contractile portion of the LV, end-diastolic and end-systolic volumes of the contractile section were calculated according to the hemispheroid model [12]. The morphology of ventricular cavity was assessed by a distortion index (DI), calculated from end-diastolic and end-systolic contours, as the ratio between the areas obtained from the intersection of LV silhouette and long axis. To obtain a normal range, the same analysis was performed on the left ventriculogram of 10 normal male subjects (mean age 52 ± 9.5 years, range 38–63) studied for atypical chest pain, with normal LV function and absence of significative coronary artery disease (group II).

Operative Technique

A standard median sternotomy is made and the pericardium is opened, exposing the heart. Cardiopulmonary bypass is established and the LV is vented via a right superior vein cannula. In the beating heart, the negative pressure exerted by the vent catheter usually delineates the margins of the An. After ventriculotomy, LV is explored, and mural thrombi removed. The noncontractile area is identified and resected. Two purse-string sutures are stitched on scarred endocardial tissue layer. Twelve to fifteen mattress sutures are stitched through a preclotted dacron patch shaping a round area of 15–20 mm. These sutures are then passed through the contractile wall edges and two long teflon strips. After aortic cross-clamping and cardioplegic arrest, the two purse-string sutures are tightened to reduce the left ventriculotomy to a circular area of the same size as the dacron patch. Mattress sutures are tied to anchor the patch to the edges of the resected wall and to the septal contractile area. One layer continuous suture is then used to connect the dacron patch and the ventriculotomy rims. When coronary artery revascularization is indicated, the distal graft anastomoses are performed under cardioplegic arrest, and the proximal ones during rewarming.

Follow Up

One-year postoperative follow-up was performed by direct phone call to patients, enquiring about symptoms (exertional or resting chest pain, dyspnea, orthopnea, fatigue), the level of physical activity achievable, and current medications.

Statistical Analysis

All data are reported as mean ± one standard deviation. Continuous variables were compared by *t*-test for paired and unpaired data when appropriate. To correlate variables with unknown distribution, Spearman correlation coefficients were computed.

Results

The interval between the acute myocardial infarction and the operation ranged from 26 days to 18 months (mean 9.2 ± 5.3 months). One patient was excluded from the study because he had electrocardiographic (new pathologic Q waves in inferior leads) and enzymatic evidence of an acute myocardial infarction following operation; this patient underwent orthotopic heart transplantation 7 months after aneurysmectomy, because of refractory congestive heart failure. Coronary artery bypass grafts in the three patients who received additional revascularization were patent at predischarge angiography. After aneurysm repair and ventriculoplasty, LV volumes were significantly reduced (end-diastolic volume from 158.4 ± 37.1 to 111.9 ± 21.8 ml/m^2, $p < 0.001$; end-systolic volume from 118.8 ± 33.3 to 62.5 ± 20.6 ml/m^2, $p < 0.001$), and global ejection fraction increased from 0.25 ± 0.09 to 0.44 ± 0.12 ($p < 0.001$). No change was observed in LV end-diastolic pressure after operation (from 21.8 ± 7.5 to 21.2 ± 5.7 mmHg).

The shape of the LV of patients with aneurysm was markedly abnormal (Table 1): in fact the DI was significantly higher than in the control group both in diastole (0.95 ± 0.24 vs 0.79 ± 0.10, $p = 0.01$) and in systole (1.17 ± 0.48 vs 0.66 ± 0.11, $p < 0.001$). However, after surgical repair no differences were found between the two groups for the diastolic and systolic DI (0.61 ± 0.20 vs 0.79 ± 0.10, and 0.59 ± 0.20 vs 0.66 ± 0.11 respectively).

Changes in ejection fraction correlated significantly with improvement of the distortion index in diastole (Spearman's rho = –0.463, $p = 0.017$) and in systole

Table 1. Comparison of distortion index in diastole and in systole

	II	before VPL	after VPL
		Groups	
		I	
Distortion index			
Diastole	0.79 ± 0.10[a]	0.95 ± 0.24	0.61 ± 0.20[b]
Systole	0.66 ± 0.11[c]	1.17 ± 0.48	0.59 ± 0.20[b]

VPL = Ventriculoplasty.
[a] p = 0.01 group II vs group I before VPL.
[b] P < 0.001 group I before VPL vs group I after VPL.
[c] p < 0.001 group II vs group I before VPL.

(Spearman's rho $= -0.447$, $p = 0.021$). The increase of global ejection fraction after ventriculoplasty directly correlated to the preoperative ejection fraction of the contractile section of the LV ($r = 0.59$, $p = 0.002$, Fig. 1).

All patients were discharged from the hospital. Nineteen patients were still alive at 1-year follow-up. Two patients died of congestive heart failure, 4 and 9 months after hospital discharge, respectively. Most patients had a good clinical outcome, improving at least one functional class (Fig. 2). Two patients (who did not receive coronary artery bypass grafting) complained of nocturnal chest pain.

Discussion

This study indicates that the resection of postinfarction LV scars followed by ventricular reconstruction results in a significant decrease in cardiac volumes. The significative reduction of end-diastolic and particularly of end-systolic volumes induces a marked improvement in overall ventricular function as evidenced by an increase of global ejection fraction at rest. This improvement is associated with a normalization of ventricular shape.

LV An may be expected to develop between 3% and 38% of patients surviving a transmural acute myocardial infarction. The reported variation in incidence

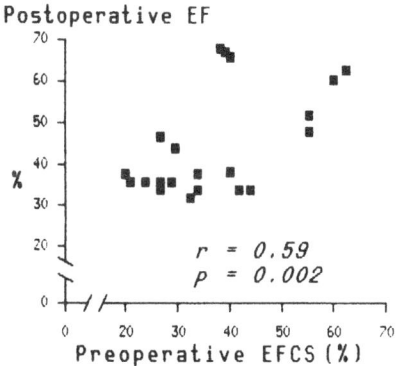

Fig. 1. Correlation between preoperative ejection fraction of contractile section (*EFCS*) and postoperative global ejection fraction (*EF*)

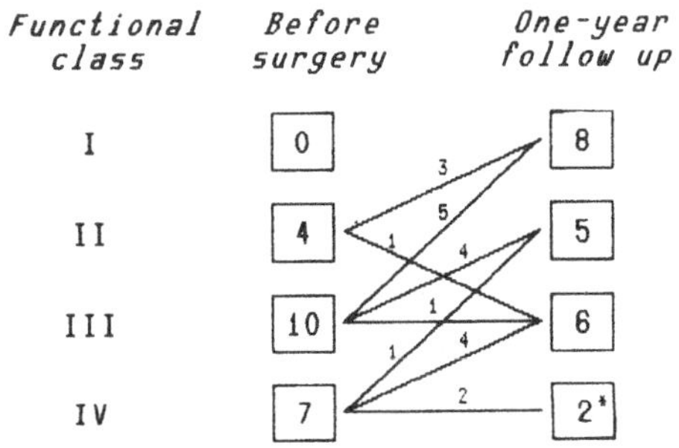

Fig. 2. Functional class before and 1 year after aneurysmectomy and ventriculo-plasty

might be due to the different diagnostic criteria utilized [1,3,13,14]. Some studies suggested that An formation is likely related to changes in wall stress [15–17]. Powerful contraction of the noninfarcted muscle may produce stretching and loss of geometric integrity in the weakened necrotic and fibrous tissue. The hemodynamic consequences of LV An are not only due to loss of contractile tissue, but also to changes in the shape of the ventricle and in the direction of fiber shortening. Physiologic ventricular contraction is the result of synergic activation of all units of myocardium [18]. According to this view and to Laplace's law, the abnormality in shape and in regional wall motion, by interrupting the coordination, impairs the effectiveness of contraction [19]. Moreover, the An may show a paradoxical expansion with backwards and forwards movement of blood in the sac. All these factors have a detrimental effect on diastolic and systolic function of the nonaneurysmal portion of the LV, which has an higher workload (higher wall stress) and an increase in oxygen requirements. The hemodynamic improvement observed in our series is likely to be the result not only of the resection of the scar, but also of the correct geometric reconstruction of the LV. Some authors have suggested the importance of ventricular shape in operative results of patients with postinfarction An [19,20]. Hutchins et al. [21] showed that the shape of the normal ventricle corresponds to that expected according to the principle of minimal work with the best efficiency. In fact, the normal ventricular configuration is a compromise between a spherical and a tubular shape: the first would need the least energy for diastolic filling and the second would permit maximal conversion of systolic muscle tension into cavitary pressure. The same author [22], studying the geometry of 18 hearts of patients who died after repair of ventricular An, found that postoperative shock might be explained by an inadequate ventricular reconstruction causing an excessive reduction in wall curvature.

Conclusions

The surgical technique used in our study has advantages over the classical linear suture in that it allows a complete resection of aneurysmal tissue without compromising the ventricular geometry. The size of the cavity is reduced and the correct direction of fibers is preserved.

References

1. Olearchyk A, Lemole GM, Spagna PM (1984) Left ventricular aneurysm. J Thorac Cardiovasc Surg 88:544–553
2. Forman MB, Collins HW, Kopelman HA, Vaughn WK, Perry JM, Virmani R, Friesinger GC (1986) Determinants of left ventricular aneurysm formation after anterior myocardial infarction: a clinical and angiographic study. J Am Coll Cardiol 8:1256–1262

3. Reddi SB, Cooley DA, Duncan JM, Norman JC (1981) Left ventricular aneurysm. Twenty-year surgical experience with 1572 patients at the Texas Heart Institute. Cardiovasc Dis Bull Texas Heart Inst 8:165–186
4. Barrat Boyes BG, White HD, Agnew MB, Prembertpn JR, Will CJ (1984) The results of surgical treatment of ventricular aneurysm. J Thorac Cardiovasc Surg 87:87–98
5. Cohen M, Packer M, Gorlin R (1983) Indications for left ventricular aneurysmectomy. Circulation 4:717–722
6. Cooley DA, Collins HA, Morris GC JR, Chapman DW (1958) Ventricular aneurysm after myocardial infarction: surgical excision with use of temporary cardiopulmonary bypass. JAMA 167:557–560
7. Keenan DJM, Monro JL, Ross JK, Manners JM, Conway N, Johnson AM (1985) Left ventricular aneurysm. The Wessex experience. Br Heart J 54:269–272
8. Kiefer SK, Flaker GC, Martin RH, Curtis JJ (1983) Clinical improvement after ventricular aneurysm repair: prediction by angiographic and hemodynamic variables. J Am Coll Cardiol 2:3037–3043
9. Tebbe U, Kreuzer H (1989) Pros and cons of surgery of the left ventricular aneurysm: a review. Thorac Cardiovasc Surg 37:3–10
10. Jatene AD (1985) Left ventricular aneurysmectomy. Resection or reconstruction. J Thorac Cardiovasc Surg 89:321–331
11. Greene DG, Carlisle R, Grant C (1967) Estimation of left ventricular volume by one-plane cineangiography. Circulation 35:61–69
12. Watson LE, Dickhaus DW, Martin RH (1975) Left ventricular aneurysm: preoperative hemodynamics, chamber volume, and results of aneurysmectomy. Circulation 52:868–873
13. Aranda JM, Befeler B, Thurer R, Vargas A, El-Sharif N, Lazzara R (1977) Long-term clinical and hemodynamic studies after ventricular aneurysmectomy and aorta-coronary bypass. J Thorac Cardiovasc Surg 73:772–779
14. Cohen DE, Vogel RA (1986) Left ventricular Aneurysm as a coronary risk factor independent of overall left ventricular function. Am Heart J 111:23–30
15. Arvan S, Badillo P (1985) Contractile properties of the left ventricle with aneurysm. Am J Cardiol 55:338–341
16. Grondin P, Kretz JG, Bical O, Donzequ-gouge P, Petitclerc R, Campeau L (1979) Natural history of saccular aneurysm of the left ventricle. J Thorac Cardiovasc Surg 77:57–64
17. Robbins SL, Cotran RS (1979) Pathologic basis of disease. Saunders, Philadelphia, p 657
18. Wiggers CJ (1964) Physiology in health and disease. Lea and Febiger, Philadelphia, p 461
19. Gorlin R, Klein MD, Sullivan JM (1967) Prospective study of ventricular aneurysm. Mechanistic concept and clinical recognition. Am J Med 42:512–531
20. Dor V, Saab M, Coste P, Kornaszewska M, Montiglio F (1989) Left ventricular aneurysm: a new surgical approach. Thorac Cardiovasc Surg 37:11–19
21. Hutchins GM, Bulkley BH, Moore GW, Piasio MA, Lohr FT (1978) Shape of the human cardiac ventricles. Am J Cardiol 41:646–654
22. Hutchins GM, Brawley RK (1980) The influence of cardiac geometry on the result of ventricular aneurysm repair. Am J Pathol 99:221–230

Cardiac Assist Devices, Heart Transplantation

Hemodynamic Effect of the Jarvik 7-70 Total Artificial Heart: The Minneapolis Heart Institute Experience

D.E. Burns, M.R. Pritzker, L.D. Joyce, D. Hunn, M.R. Mooney,
J.D. Madison, K. Johnson, C. Madison, W. Pedersen, T.A. Carlson,
M. Gordon, M. Walker, C.R. Jorgensen, F.L. Gobel,
and I.F. Goldenberg

Introduction

In the short period of time since it has been introduced, the Jarvik 7-70 total artificial heart (TAH) has become the most utilized and arguably the most successful prosthetic cardiac replacement device when used as a bridge to orthotopic cardiac transplantation (OCT). In this paper, the drive parameters of the Utah Drive and the hemodynamic performance of the Jarvik 7-70 TAH are evaluated in detail and compared to performance of the failing heart prior to implantation. At this writing, seven implants of this device have been undertaken at the Minneapolis Heart Institute as bridges to orthotopic cardiac transplantation since Food and Drug Administration approval was received in September 1985. This report summarizes pre- and postimplant Utah drive settings and hemodynamic parameters in six consecutive patients (the first ever recipient of the Jarvik 7-70 TAH has been reported previously) [1].

Methods

Data were obtained by retrospective examination of each patient's hospital record. Hourly recordings of Utah drive settings and hemodynamic parameters were made by nursing staff on the intensive care unit flow sheet. These recordings were taken from electrocardiograms, pressure tracings (systemic, pulmonary artery, and right and left atrial), the Utah driver, and the Cardiac Output Monitor and Diagnostic Unit (COMDU). Particular attention was paid to hemodynamic recordings made in the period just before artificial heart implantation was performed, and the period just after surgery was completed. These values were chosen to represent the degree of circulatory failure before and extent of recovery immediately upon implantation of the Jarvik 7-70 TAH.

Equipment

Jarvik 7-70 Total Artificial Heart. This TAH is a pneumatic device that consists of two separate ventricles whose blood surface is made of segmented polyu-

B.S. Lewis, A. Kimchi (Eds.)
Heart Failure Mechanisms and Management
© Springer-Verlag Berlin Heidelberg 1991

rethane [2]. The diaphragms within the ventricle consist of highly flexible four-layer sheets of biomer, which makes the diaphragm extremely pliable. There are four clinical grade, pyrolytic carbon disk valves (Medtronic-Hall). The Jarvik 7-70 holds 70 ml. The overall shape is spherical with anatomical transitions to the great vessels and the atrium. This device is connected to the pneumatic Utah driver by two drive lines (one drive to each ventricle).

Utah Pneumatic Heart Driver. The Utah pneumatic heart driver controls the rate and output of the Jarvik 7-70 TAH [2]. Each ventricle of the TAH is connected to this pneumatic heart driver by a special polyurethane drive line that exits from the patient's chest. The pneumatic driver is connected to a source of compressed air, a vacuum, and an electrical source. The heart driver may be adjusted to regulate the number of beats per minute (heart rate), the driving pressure that expands the diaphragm in both the right and left ventricle, and the percent of time spent in systole.

Cardiac Output Monitor and Diagnostic Unit (COMDU). This device continuously monitors and records the cardiac output from each ventricle of the TAH.

Patient Population

Records of six consecutive patients (four males, two females) who received the Jarvik 7-70 TAH as a bridge to OCT at the Minneapolis Heart Institute were analyzed. Mean age was 29 ± 6 years, with a range from 15 to 50 years. Indications for implantation included acute myocarditis ($n = 1$, age 28 years), failure to wean from cardiopulmonary bypass after cardiac surgery ($n = 2$; ages 50 and 45 years, ischemic heart disease and valvular heart disease), acute failure of a grafted organ at OCT ($n = 1$, age 19 years, idiopathic cardiomyopathy), and rapid deterioration while awaiting OCT ($n = 2$; ages 17 and 15 years, idiopathic cardiomyopathy). Body surface areas ranged from 1.40 to 2.15 m², with a mean of 1.80 ± 0.11 m².

Each patient was judged to be hopelessly ill and in end-stage cardiogenic shock. In all patients, deterioration of cardiac function persisted even during treatment with high doses of inotropic and vasopressor agents. In addition, three patients received intra-aortic balloon counterpulsation, and in two patients biventricular support systems were used. Cardiac function was judged unable to maintain life and the deterioration of vital organ function due to circulatory hypoperfusion led the medical and surgical staff to unanimously conclude that death was almost certain in each patient within a few hours. Following education of the patient and/or family members, informed consent was obtained.

Statistics

Results are reported as mean ± standard error of the mean. Student's paired t test was used to ascertain significant differences between pre- and postimplant values where appropriate. Probabilities reported are two-tailed. P values < 0.05 were considered statistically significant.

Results

The mean duration of implantation for the six patients in this study was 14 ± 3 days (range 4–26 days; total 81 days). There was no mechanical failure of the Jarvik 7–70 TAH, the Utah Drive system, or the COMDU.

Immediate Hemodynamic Effects. With implantation of the Jarvik 7–70 TAH, there was an immediate and significant increase in mean arterial pressure (compared to that during the last two readings prior to TAH implantation) from 49 ± 11 mmHg to 81 ± 6 mmHg ($p < 0.01$). Cardiac output increased from 2.4 ± 0.5 l/min to 4.8 ± 0.7 l/min ($p < 0.01$). Cardiac filling pressures also improved rapidly and dramatically: right atrial pressure decreased from 16 ± 3 mmHg to 11 ± 1 mmHg, and left atrial pressure decreased from 22 ± 5 mmHg to 11 ± 2 mmHg. The Jarvik 7–70 obviated the need for continued vasopressor support or other mechanical support in all patients. In fact, five patients required Nitroprusside to lower their blood pressure. This hemodynamic response with the Jarvik 7–70 was obtained using the following initial drive settings in these patients: heart rate 98 ± 5 (range 84–118), left drive pressure 177 ± 6 mmHg (160–200 mmHg), right drive pressure 55 ± 6 mmHg (40–75 mmHg), percent systole $47\% \pm 3\%$ (39%–55%).

Long-Term Hemodynamic Effects. Detailed analysis was performed on all postimplant drive settings and hemodynamic variables over the entire period of implantation. Over the entire course of implantation, mean drive settings were maintained as follows: heart rate 108 ± 8 per minute (75–125), left drive pressure 194 ± 19 mmHg (150–230 mmHg), right drive pressure 48 ± 8 mmHg (25–75 mmHg), percent systole $51\% \pm 4\%$ (37%–55%). These resulted in mean hemodynamic values as follows: mean arterial pressure 89 ± 7 mmHg (65–135 mmHg), left cardiac output 5.6 ± 0.6 l/min (3.0–8.0 l/min), right cardiac output 5.8 ± 0.5 l/min (3.1–8.3 l/min), right atrial pressure 15 ± 3 mmHg (7–26 mmHg), left atrial pressure 12 ± 3 mmHg (5–23 mmHg). Any hemodynamic instability occurring during TAH implantation was controlled by varying the drive settings.

Orthotopic Cardiac Transplantation and Long-Term Follow-Up. All patients subsequently received human OCT. Four patients are alive at home and have returned either to work or school, and two patients died. The first patient who died was a 45-year-old female who had the TAH for 5 days. She had an OCT for 25 days and died from rejection. The second patient was a 28-year-old female who had the TAH implanted for 4 days and had an OCT for 861 days. Her cause of death was also rejection.

Discussion

Although the first Jarvik 7 TAH (100 ml) was implanted in December 1982, the first use of the smaller Jarvik 7-70 (70 ml) was not until December 1985 at the Minneapolis Heart Institute [1]. After Food and Drug Administration approval was obtained for urgent use of the smaller artificial heart due to the small thoracic volume of the patient, this implantation was successful and a satisfactory fit was achieved. As reported previously, over a 45-day period, the Jarvik 7-70 TAH proved to be very adequate both in its ability to support the circulation and its lack of tendency to generate thromboemboli. Organ function eventually recovered and infection was controlled so that human heart transplantation was accomplished. Indeed, this initial experience with the Jarvik 7-70 TAH as a bridge to heart transplantation prompted Joyce et al. to comment that "this heart is equal to (if not superior to) the Jarvik 7[1]. Further, in a recent comparison of the Jarvik 7 with the smaller Jarvik 7-70 in patients with different chest sizes, Herland et al. concluded that the Jarvik 7-70 "has supported small and large recipients, and its ease of implantation warrants its preferred use" over the 100 ml Jarvik 7 [3]. In fact, the Jarvik 7-70 is now the most commonly implanted TAH [4]. The data reported here further support that the Jarvik 7-70 along with the Utah Driver can adequately support the circulation. Indeed, after implantation, no further inotropic or vasopressor agents or mechanical devices other than the TAH was needed.

Summary

The TAH and Utah driver can adequately support the circulation and can be used as a bridge to OCT in patients with cardiogenic shock.

References

1. Joyce LD, Pritzker MR, Kiser JC, Nicoloff DM, Kersten TE, Von Rueden TJ, Eales F, Johnson KE, Jorgensen CR, Gobel FL, Van Tassel RA (1986) Use of the mini Jarvik-7 total artificial heart as a bridge to transplantation. J Heart Transplant 5:203–209
2. DeVries WC, Joyce LD (1983) The artificial heart. CIBA Clinical Symposia 35(6)

3. Herlan DB, Kormos RL, Wei L, Borovetz HS, Hardesty RL, Griffith BP (1987) Hemodynamic and functional considerations of the Jarvik total artificial heart (TAH). Trans Am Soc Artif Intern Organs 33(3):147–150

4. Joyce LD, Johnson KE, Cabrol C, Griffith BP, Copeland JG, DeVries WC, Keon WJ, Solner E, Frazier OH, Bucherl ES, Semb B, Akalin H, Aris A, Carmichael MJ, Cooley D, Dembitsky W, English T, Halbrook H, Hetzer R, Herbert Y, Keon WJ, Loisnace D, Noon G, Pennington G, Peterson A, Phillips SJ, Pierce WS, Unger F, Pifarre R, Tector A (1988) Nine year experience with the clinical use of total artificial hearts as cardiac support devices. Trans Am Soc Artif Intern Organs 34:703–707

Selection of Therapy for Patients with Advanced Heart Failure: Tailored Afterload Reduction or Cardiac Transplantation?

L.W. Stevenson

Introduction

At the time of the first heart transplant in 1967, patients with severe symptoms of heart failure rarely survived 6 months [1]. Although the initial results of cardiac transplantation were dismal, the determination of the Stanford program eventually led to the recognition of cardiac transplantation as effective therapy for selected patients [2]. The current survival statistics after cardiac transplantation are 80%–90% at 1 year for established programs [3]. However, the shortage of donor hearts limits transplantation to a minority of the 15 000 potential candidates with congestive heart failure in the United States [4]. The number of cardiac transplants in the United States increased from 60 in 1982 to 1500 in 1986 but is no longer increasing due to the limited donor pool. The national waiting list currently contains 1000 patients, and each month 60% more new patients are added than are transplanted.

Concurrent improvement in medical therapy has accompanied the improvement in cardiac transplantation. Afterload reduction tailored specifically to hemodynamic goals for the population with advanced heart failure was originally designed to allow hospital discharge for ineligible patients and for patients on the waiting list [5]. However, such therapy has led to better status and survival than expected for many patients without transplantation. Comparison of relative survival curves and functional status with and without transplantation allows identification of those with the greatest expected benefits from transplantation compared to tailored medical therapy.

Spetrum of Heart Failure

Progression of Ventricular Dysfunction

Chronic heart failure resulting from systolic dysfunction with resultant ventricular dilatation is the indication for transplantation in 92% of recipients, resulting about equally from coronary artery disease and nonischemic cardiomyopathy with occasional primary valvular disease [3]. Before consideration for transplantation, those patients with ischemic disease should be evaluated for potentially reversible myocardial dysfunction due to ischemia, even in the

B.S. Lewis, A. Kimchi (Eds.)
Heart Failure Mechanisms and Management
© Springer-Verlag Berlin Heidelberg 1991

absence of angina [6]. Patients with less than 6 months of symptoms from nonischemic cardiomyopathy should be followed without transplantation if at all possible, as almost 50% will demonstrate significant recovery within the next 6 months [7,8]. In the remaining patients with irreversible myocardial injury, prognosis remains relatively good despite decreasing objection fraction (EF) until the advanced stages of disease, as shown on the shoulder curve for survival (Fig. 1), which reflects survival with heart failure, assuming coronary anatomy has been appropriately addressed.

Once the EF is < 25%, severity of heart failure may be better reflected by clinical parameters, although patients with EF over 20% generally fare better than those under 10% [9]. Many patients function relatively normally despite EF < 25% and decreased maximal exercise tolerance, and can be maintained without hospitalizations or frequent medical adjustments to prevent symptoms of pulmonary or systemic venous congestion. The prevalence of this compensated state is probably underestimated, many patients being unrecognized unless a ventricular arrhythmia, an embolic event, or a routine chest X-ray causes further investigation. Patients who have never decompensated despite low EF have a 1-year survival of about 80% [10,11], and are not generally referred for transplantation. However without systematic therapy and follow-up, symptomatic patients with cardiomyopathy and EF < 25% referred for transplantation had a worse outcome even if they were considered "too well" at the time of evaluation; their mortality without transplantation was 39% (82% of the deaths occurring suddenly), with an additional 11% requiring transplantation [7].

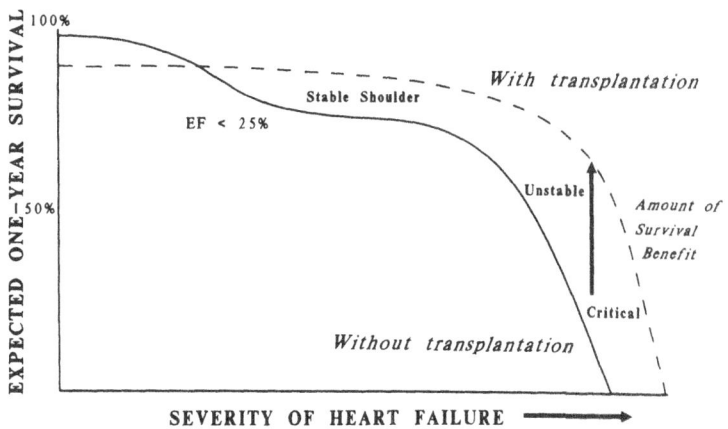

Fig. 1. The shoulder curve of relative survivals for patients with chronic heart failure who undergo transplantation (*dotted line*) or remain on medical therapy (*solid line*), based on the clinical status achieved during medical therapy. Survivals reflect those currently published for transplantation [3] and medical therapy [5,9,42]

Clinical Profile of the Potential Transplant Candidate

The majority of patients considered for transplantation are those with EF < 20% in whom clinical deterioration is occurring [9], and survival is shown on the falling limb of the relative survival curve. What is the survival for such patients who do not undergo transplantation? The 10% 6-month survival described in 1978 for candidates who died on the waiting list characterizes an era in which transplantation was offered only to the sickest patients. Survival for cardiomyopathy patients without transplantation in 1982 was 20% at 1 year [12]. Survival for patients with nonmedical contraindications to transplantation was 25% at 1 year [13] and was also compromised by the variability of the follow-up care provided by local physicians and the high proportion of noncompliant patients [13].

Nonsurgical survival in this group of potential transplant patients may be estimated on the basis of clinical and hemodynamic prognostic factors. For comparison to previous populations investigated, the initial clinical profile was determined for 152 consecutive patients with EF ≤ 20% who were discharged after referral for cardiac transplantation (Table 1). Applying known prognostic factors to this profile, survival is again predicted to be very poor, with 1-year survival of < 50%. The EF of ≤ 20% has been associated with survival as low as 27% at 6 months [14]. In patients with coronary artery disease and mean EF 18%, 1-year survival was 34% [15]. In heart failure patients with overall 65% 1-year survival, the average EF of nonsurvivors was 24% [11,15]. Patients with class IV symptoms had 34%-38% 1-year survival [11,15]. The potential transplant candidates were frequently evaluated during a period of deterioration, reflected by the referral itself and by an average of two hospitalizations in the preceding 6 months. In addition, the deteriorating status in our population occurred despite previous therapy which included vasodilators in 75% of patients referred to our program.

Hemodynamic predictors for mortality among patients with advanced heart failure have included a cardiac index < 2.25 l/min/m² [17] with the cardiac index for nonsurvivors averaging 2.0 l/min/m² in two series [17,18] with overall 50%

Table 1. Profile of 152 patients with ejection fraction ≤ 20%, when referred for transplantation

Age (years)	45 ± 13
Male gender	85% of patients
Coronary artery disease	49% of patients
Ejection fraction	15 ± 3%
Clinical class (NYHA)	3.6 ± .5
Orthopnea (0–4 scale)	3 ± 1
Hospitalizations (number in previous 6 months)	2 ± 2
Cardiac index (l/min/m²)	2.0 ± .6
Pulmonary wedge pressure (mmHg)	28 ± 9
Pulmonary arterial pressure (mmHg)	55 ± 16
Right atrial pressure (mmHg)	13 ± 9
Mean arterial pressure (mmHg)	84 ± 10
Systemic vascular resistance (dynes s cm⁻⁵)	1700 ± 700
Left ventricular diameter (diastolic, mm)	76 ± 10

1-year survival. Pulmonary capillary wedge pressure > 25–27 mmHg has been a poor prognostic factor [16,17], as has right atrial pressure > 10 mmHg [16], and mean arterial pressure < 88 mmHg [10,17]. Serum sodium ≤ 137 was associated with 1-year survival of 37% in a population slightly older than ours [18]. Thus this population would previously have been predicted to have less than 50% 1-year survival without transplantation.

Tailored Therapy After Referral for Transplantation

Definition and Achievement of Hemodynamic Goals

As very few of these patients can be transplanted urgently and the majority cannot be transplanted at all, efforts must be directed to providing at least symptomatic relief. While reduction of cardiac filling pressures was initially instituted only to provide short-term symptomatic improvement, it has subsequently been shown to provide more complete afterload reduction and sustained clinical benefit [5].

Aggressive therapy with vasodilators and diuretics to lower left ventricular filling pressure in heart failure has been limited by concern that cardiac output will be compromised. However, the chronically dilated ventricle frequently achieves maximal cardiac outputs simultaneously with normal filling pressures [19] (Fig. 2), beyond which effective sarcomere length is unlikely to increase further. The major improvement in cardiac output during afterload reduction does not result from overall increase in ventricular ejection, as EF rarely increases and ventricular volume decreases [20] (Fig. 3). Instead, the major benefit of afterload reduction in advanced heart failure results from the increased forward stroke volume, reflecting the decrease in mitral regurgitation, which is significant

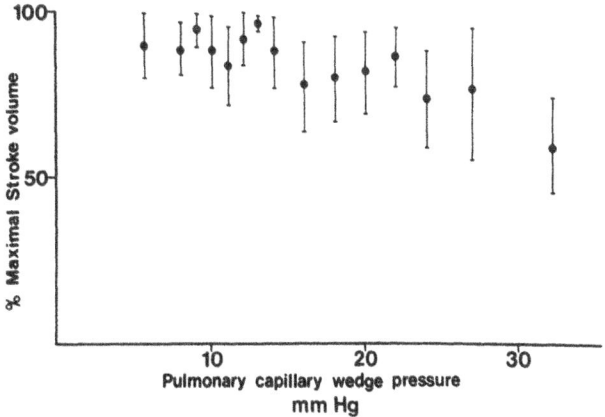

Fig. 2. Maintenance of stroke volume at normal pulmonary capillary wedge pressures, expressed as percentage of maximal stroke volume for each of 15 patients with chronic heart failure (average ejection fraction 18%) undergoing acute therapy with nitroprusside and diuretics [19], over a wide range of pulmonary capillary wedge pressures after initial average pressure of 31 mmHg

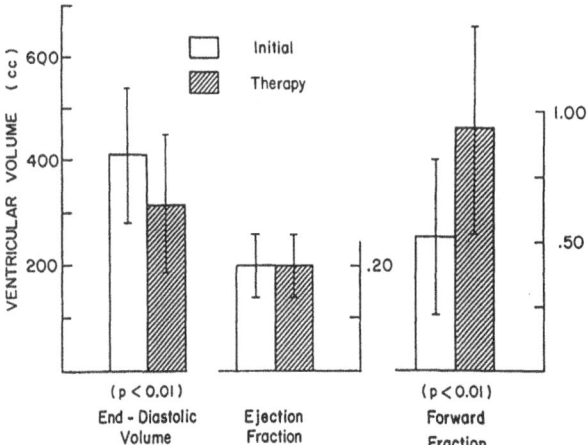

Fig. 3. Ventricular volumes and ejection fractions measured by radionuclide ventriculography before and after therapy tailored to reduce pulmonary capillary wedge pressure and systemic vascular resistance in 15 patients with chronic congestive heart failure [20]. The thermodilution stroke volumes (not shown) increased by 53% during therapy, resulting from the decrease in mitral regurgitation, shown as an increase in forward ejection fraction

in almost all patients [21]. The decreases in ventricular volume and mitral regurgitation which result from total afterload reduction in the supine position persist during upright exercise [22]. Maintenance of low filling pressures may thus not only minimize congestive symptoms, but decrease myocardial energy demands and retard ventricular decompensation. In addition, the concomitant reduction in right ventricular pressures and tricuspid regurgitation [23] may allow better nutritional status [24].

Our therapeutic goals in patients with advanced heart failure are achieved first with intravenous agents, then with oral vasodilators and a flexible diuretic regimen (Table 2). This therapy has allowed hospital discharge in 80% of patients transferred for urgent transplantation after previous medical therapy was considered ineffective, and a 1-year survival of 63% without transplantation (Fig. 4). At the time of discharge, the best hemodynamic predictor of survival for patients with EF $\leq$ 20% and initial pulmonary capillary wedge pressure $>$ 16 mmHg was the pulmonary capillary wedge pressure achieved on therapy, with those achieving $\leq$ 16 mmHg having a 1-year survival of 80%, compared to 40% survival with a higher pulmonary wedge pressure on tailored therapy despite mean initial pulmonary wedge pressure of 31 mmHg and initial cardiac index of 1.9 l/min/m² in each group (Fig. 5).

The approach to these patients, as outlined in Table 2, requires that hemodynamic status be measured, since routine physical assessment is too insensitive for elevated filling pressures to allow achievement of minimal ventricular volume [25]. While the value of hemodynamic measurements has been unclear during vasodilator studies from which most deteriorating and hospitalized patients were excluded [26,27], the achievement of specific hemodynamic

Table 2. The tailoring of therapy for advanced heart failure

---

1. Measurement of baseline hemodynamics
2. Intravenous nitroprusside and diuretics tailored to hemodynamic goals
   PCW $\leq$ 15 mmHg
   SVR $\leq$ 1200 dynes/s^{-cm}
   RA $\leq$ 9 mmHg
   SBP $\geq$ 80 mmHg
3. Definition of optimal hemodynamics by 24–48 h
4. Titration of high-dose oral agents as nitroprusside weaned
5. Ambulation, diuretic adjustment for 24–48 h
6. Maintain digoxin if no contraindication
7. Detailed patient education
8. Discharge with flexible diuretic regimen
9. Progressive walking program
10. Vigilant follow-up

RA, right atrial pressure; *PCW*, pulmonary capillary wedge pressure;
SBP, systolic blood pressure; *SVR*, systemic vascular resistance.

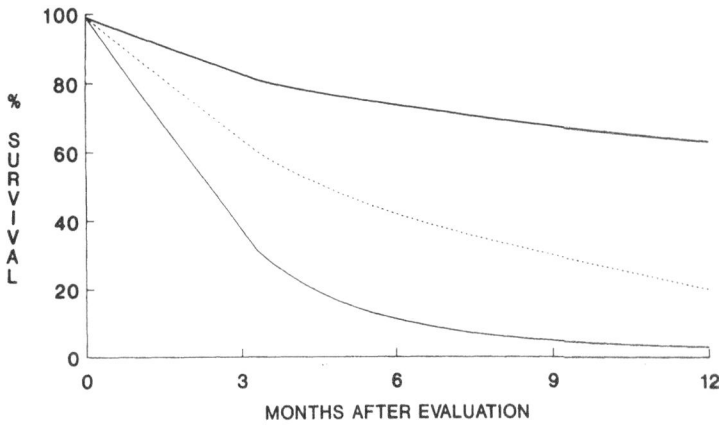

Fig. 4. Prognosis for patients not undergoing transplantation, based on previously published survival statistics and current results of tailored therapy for advanced heart failure (see text). *Solid line*, 1978; *dotted line*, 1982; *bold line*, 1988

goals (including minimal filling pressures) during acute therapy may be more important in the population referred for transplantation. Our approach to therapy involves intravenous nitroprusside [28] and subsequent high-dose oral vasodilators, and diuretics [29,30]. The benefits of nitroprusside, hydralazine/isordil and angiotensin converting-enzyme inhibition have previously been individually shown [28–32]. The power of tailored therapy incorporating all of the above principles has not until now been demonstrated for the population with advanced heart failure referred to transplantation which had previously been given a prognosis of < 6 months on medical therapy (Fig. 4).

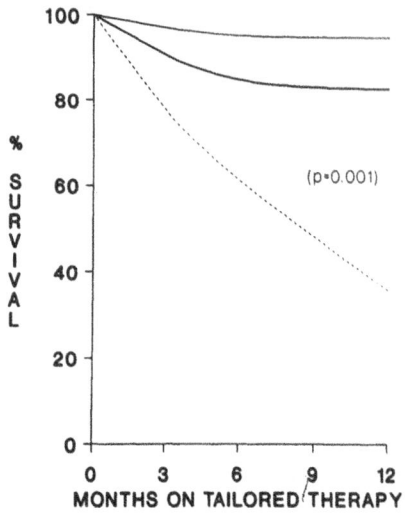

Fig. 5. Relationship of pulmonary capillary wedge pressure (PCW) to survival with advanced heart failure in 152 patients with ejection fraction ≤ 20%. Initial pulmonary capillary wedge pressure < 16 mmHg was associated with the best survival. For patients with initial higher pulmonary capillary wedge pressure, survival was predicted by the pulmonary capillary wedge pressure achieved on tailored therapy, but *not* by the initial elevated pulmonary capillary wedge pressure (31 ± 6 mmHg in both the high and low survival groups). *Solid line*, initial PCW ≤ 16; *bold line*, initial PCW > 16, final ≤ 16; *dotted line*, initial PCW > 16, final > 16mmHg

The Stable Shoulder

While overall survival for patients discharged after tailored therapy is approximately 60% at 1 year without transplantation, prognosis can be further defined by pulmonary capillary wedge pressure achieved and on the basis of early clinical follow-up after discharge. At 1 month following discharge on tailored medical therapy, 60% of referred patients who were potentially eligible for transplantation (without major noncardiac illness or high noncompliance risk) have demonstrated stability, as defined by stable weight on oral diuretics, stable sodium ≥ 130 meq/l, stable blood urea nitrogen ≤ 60 mg/dl, systolic blood pressure > 80, and absence of intolerable drug side effects [33]. In a study of 43 such patients, actuarial survival without transplantation was 76% at 1 year, despite EF 15 ±3% and previous decompensation on empiric afterload reduction. Therefore, tailored medical therapy can potentially raise 60% of patients eligible for transplantation from the falling limb back up to the shoulder of the survival curve (Fig. 1) where survival is similar to that described for patients without any history of decompensation.

For stable patients who undergo transplantation, the 1-year survival is 85%–95% [3], offering a survival benefit of 5%–25% compared to tailored medical therapy for that first year. While exercise capacity is good following transplantation [34,35], progressive improvement in exercise capacity also occurs over 2–6 months in patients responding to vasodilators [26,36]. There were no significant differences (Table 3) between the transplant and medical groups for parameters of functional capacity [33,37], despite a large difference in EF, suggesting that the functional benefit of transplantation may not be as large as anticipated for the majority of patients demonstrating early stability on tailored medical therapy.

Table 3. Functional capacity for survivors of cardiac transplantation or sustained medical therapy for stable heart failure

	Cardiac transplantation		Sustained medical therapy
	22[a]		20[a]
Initial ejection fraction	15 ± 3%		15 ± 3%
Late ejection fraction[b]	62 ± 7%	(p < 0.01)	22 ± 9%
Max oxygen uptake (cc)	1360 ± 340		1440 ± 350
% predicted max O_2[c]	60 ± 14%		62 ± 9%
Max O_2 pulse (cc/beat)	10 ± 2		10 ± 2
Six-minute walk (feet)	1460 ± 180		1430 ± 190
Adjustment to illness[d]	47 ± 11		52 ± 8
Anxiety[e]	9 ± 4		7 ± 4
Depression[e]	14 ± 8		12 ± 7
Medication doses/day	16 ± 6		13 ± 4
Unexpected hospital days	15 ± 17	(p < 0.01)	2 ± 4

[a] Survivors at > 6 months for potential transplant candidates who were stable at 1 month on tailored therapy.

[b] 14 ±6 months.

[c] Predicted from age, gender, height, and weight.

[d] From PAIS total score possible 0–138, high scores represent greater impairment.

[e] From multiple affective adjective checklist.

Selection and Priority for Transplantation After Tailored Therapy

Evaluation for cardiac transplantation includes right-heart catheterization to evaluate pulmonary vascular resistance, at which time the hemodynamic efficacy of previous medical therapy can be assessed, with revision of diuretic and vasodilator therapy as described (Table 2). The systematic provision of tailored therapy to all patients allows identification of patients least likely to succeed on medical therapy and thus most likely to benefit from transplantation.

Contraindications to Transplantation

The improved outcome after transplantation during the last 5 years [3] reflects increasing expertise as well as the widespread use of cyclosporin. Criteria for transplantation have evolved relatively uniformly at various transplant centers [37] (Table 4). Patients over 50 years of age (even 60–65 years) now do well if carefully selected [38], and patients with adult-onset diabetes mellitus may be accepted if there is no evidence of noncardiac end-organ compromise [39]. Debate continues regarding the criteria for pulmonary vascular resistance, but aggressive therapy to maintain lower left ventricular filling pressures demonstrates acceptable pulmonary vascular resistance in all but a small minority of patients, most of whom have had symptomatic pulmonary congestion for at least

Table 4. UCLA standard criteria for heart transplantation

Indications
Severe heart disease despite adequate medical therapy.
   a) Unacceptable quality of life because of disabling symptoms of congestive heart failure.
   OR
   b) Unacceptable risk of cardiac death within the next year, despite limited symptoms of
      congestive heart failure.
No other reasonable surgical option.

General eligibility
The patient must be without any noncardiac condition that would itself shorten life expectancy or
increase the risk of death from rejection or from complications of immunosuppression, particularly
infection.

Specific contraindications
Age over 65. Age over 55 is a relative contraindication.
Active infection.
Active ulcer disease.
Severe diabetes mellitus with end-organ damage.
Severe peripheral vascular disease.
Pulmonary function < 60%[a] or history of chronic bronchitis.
Creatinine > 2 mg/dl; creatinine clearance < 50 ml/min.[a]
Bilirubin > 2.5 mg/dl, serum glutamic-oxaloacetic transaminase > 2x normal.[a]
Pulmonary artery systolic pressure > 60 mmHg.[a] Mean transpulmonary gradient > 15 mmHg.[a]
High risk of life-threatening noncompliance.

[a] May need to provide optimal hemodynamics with nitroprusside, dobutamine, or both for 72 h to
determine reversibility of organ dysfunction caused by heart failure.

5 years, often due to primary valve disease. Optimization of hemodynamic status
for > 72 h may also be required to demonstrate adequate pulmonary, hepatic, or
renal function. Intrinsic renal function remains very difficult to assess in the
presence of hemodynamic compromise, in which situation a low creatinine
clearance may be accepted if renal size is normal and proteinuria is absent.
Compliance remains a major factor in long-term success of either medical therapy
or transplantation. Prolonged assessment of compliance during carefully
supervised medical trials has allowed late acceptance of some patients who would
otherwise have been ineligible for transplantation [40].

Priority for Transplantation

For all patients evaluated with left ventricular failure, approximately 10% cannot
be discharged without transplantation, some of whom die in the hospital. An
additional 10% may be ambulatory but require frequent hospital readmission for
maintenance of fluid balance, sometimes with the support of brief inotropic
infusions. Outpatient dobutamine infusions at low doses may allow some patients
to remain at home [41].

As waiting lists grow longer, a greater proportion of donor hearts are
allocated to urgent priority patients. A five-center study showed that overall

survival for urgent priority patients was 80%, compared to 90% for regular priority patients, with most of the difference resulting from higher postoperative mortality in the sicker recipients [42] (Table 5). While the survival is thus lower than that for regular priority patients, the urgent priority patients have negligible predicted survival without transplantation, thus giving them almost 75% predicted 1-year survival benefit. Survivors of urgent transplantation exercise to the same levels achieved by survivors of regular transplantation, approximately 60% of normal. Thus the potential survival and functional benefit of transplantation is much greater for the urgent population, although the absolute survival is slightly reduced. However, to award all donor hearts to the *most* critical patients would compromise both absolute survival *and* survival benefits, as shown on the tail end of the transplantation survival curve (Fig. 1). This issue has been raised in reference to the implantation of artificial hearts and other bridging devices, which automatically move candidates to the front of the waiting line.

Table 5. Impact of preoperative status on survival after transplantation

	Urgent priority (%)	Regular priority (%)
1 month survival after Tx	88	97
3 month survival after Tx	82	94
Overall survival	80	90
1 year expected survival without Tx	< 10	60–80
Expected survival benefit with Tx	> 70	10–30

Therapy for "Stable Patients"

For the 60% of stable patients or those stable after tailored therapy, the decision regarding transplantation depends on the availability of donor hearts and the individual patient preference. Those patients to whom survival is paramount may elect transplantation [7], while those who are oppressed by the prospect of frequent procedures and immunosuppressive drug side effects may elect tailored therapy initially. Some patients choose transplantation when sufficient time has elapsed for the maximal benefit of effective afterload reduction to be assessed. One group for whom observation is particularly desirable prior to transplant selection is those with less than 6 months of symptoms of nonischemic cardiomyopathy. Even in the absence of biopsy evidence of myocarditis, significant improvements in ventricular function occur in half of such patients, who may then be able to resume a normal life without either transplantation or intensive medical therapy [7,8].

For most patients stabilized on tailored therapy, the major risk during the next 12 months is sudden death, whether transplantation or sustained medical therapy is intended. Outpatient jeopardy for both groups is highest in the first 3 months after evaluation [43]. Waiting list mortality in the past has been approximately 20%. The average waiting time for cardiac transplantation in the United States has continued to increase, and as of the end of 1988, was over 4 months [44]. Thus for those patients without high priority, the intention to transplant may have less impact on 1-year survival than in the early days of transplantation, when the waiting time was usually < 3 months. As waiting lists grow longer, the dilemma of the waiting list survivor becomes more common. In the absence of acute ischemic syndromes or symptomatic ventricular arrhythmias, patients who have remained stable on the waiting list for over 6 months have a better chance of medical survival over the next year than when initially selected. It may be appropriate to re-evaluate 6-month waiting list survivors to determine whether their current risk profile and functional status still warrant cardiac transplantation.

For the majority of patients referred with advanced heart failure, transplantation is not possible [4] and tailored therapy is the only option. Transplantation should be allocated to maximize survival of the population, not to maximize survival of the donor hearts. Continual compromise needs to take place between survival standards which guarantee that transplantation is performed competently, and standards which preclude transplantation for the sicker patients who are most likely to benefit in terms of survival and functional status.

Future Selection of Therapy

Future progress toward understanding, predicting, and preventing sudden death would improve survival before or without transplantation in hemodynamically stable patients. Thus far, electrophysiologic study has not improved identification of high-risk patients without previous history of sudden death [45]. Empiric antiarrhythmic therapy has not been shown to improve survival [46]. Progress in this area may be stimulated by wider recognition of the role of bradyarrhythmias in the sudden death of advanced heart failure [47] which has previously been attributed primarily to ventricular tachycardia.

Development of newer oral inotropic agents may allow more patients to move to the stable shoulder of the survival curve [48,49]. It is unlikely that the drugs currently available will significantly improve survival for stabilized patients, whose major risk is not of hemodynamic decompensation, but of sudden death.

Advances in cardiac transplantation will include a better understanding of rejection, which will allow decreased biopsy frequency and fewer drug side effects. Immunosuppressive regimens are already much reduced compared to 5 years ago. Identification of the causes of accelerated graft atherosclerosis and chronic restrictive physiology following transplantation may lead to improved long-term survival and function following transplantation.

Summary

Cardiac transplantation and medical therapy for advanced heart failure have both evolved over the past 10 years. The 1-year survival after transplantation has improved to 80%-90%. However, afterload reduction tailored to hemodynamic goals for advanced heart failure now raises 60% of patients previously considered failures of medical therapy to the "stable shoulder" of the relative survival curve, where 1-year survival without transplantation can be over 70% during vigorous follow-up, despite average initial ejection fraction 15%, pulmonary wedge pressure 30 mmHg, and cardiac index 2.0 l/min/m². For these patients, the primary risk is of early sudden death whether transplantation or sustained medical therapy is intended. Patients stabilized on this therapy who survive 6 months without transplantation demonstrate exercise capacity equivalent to that achieved after transplantation (approximately 60% of normal) and similar quality of life. Public interest in cardiac transplantation and the decreasing validity of many former contraindications have enlarged the pool of potential candidates, while the donor shortage limits transplantation to a minority of those eligible. Those patients who remain unstable *after* tailored afterload reduction should receive priority as having the greatest expected benefit in both survival and function from cardiac transplantation.

References

1. Clark D, Stinson E, Griepp R (1971) Cardiac transplantation in man-VI. Prognosis of patients selected for cardiac transplantation. Ann Intern Med 75:15-21
2. Jamieson SW, Oyer PE, Reitz BA, Baumgartner WA, Bieber CP, Stinson EB, Shumway NE (1981) Cardiac transplantation at Stanford. Heart Transplant 1:86-91
3. Fragomeni LS, Kaye MP (1988) Registry of the international society for heart transplantation: fifth official report 1988. J Heart Transplant 7:249-253
4. Evans RW, Mannihen DL, Garrison LP, Maier AM. Donor availability as the primary determinant of the future of heart transplantation. JAMA 255:1892-1898
5. Stevenson LW, Dracup KA, Tillisch JH (1989) The efficacy of medical therapy tailored for severe congestive heart failure in patients transferred for urgent transplantation. Am J Cardiol (in press)
6. Tillisch JH, Brunken RB, Marshall R, Schwaiger M, Mandelkern M, Phelps M, Schelbert H (1986) Reversibility of cardiac wall-motion abnormalities predicted by positron tomography. N Engl J Med 314:884-888
7. Stevenson LW, Fowler MB, Schroeder JS, Stevenson WG, Dracup KA, Fond V (1987) Poor survival of patients with idiopathic cardiomyopathy considered too well for transplantation. Am J Med 83:871-876
8. Figulla HR, Rahig G, Nieger M, Luig H, Kreuzer H (1985) Spontenous hemodynamic improvement or stabilization and associated biopsy findings in patients with congestive cardiomyopathy. Circulation 71:1095-1104
9. Keogh AM, Freund J, Baron DW, Hickie JB (1988) Timing of transplantation in idiopathic dilated cardiomyopathy. Am J Cardiol 61:418-422
10. Massie B, Ports T, Chatterjee K, Parmley W, Ostland J, O'Young J, Haughom F (1981) Long-term vasodilator therapy for heart failure: clinical response and its relationship to hemodynamic measurements. Circulation 63:269-278

11. Wilson JR, Schwartz JS, St. John Sutton M, Ferraro N, Horowitz LN, Reichek N, Josephson ME (1983) Prognosis in severe heart failure: relation to hemodynamic measurements and ventricular ectopic activity. 2:403–409

12. Oyer PE, Jamieson SW, Stinson EB (1982) Cardiac transplantation for end-stage congestive heart failure. In: Braunwald E, Mock MB, Watson J (eds) Congestive heart failure. Grune and Stratton, New York, pp 324

13. Stevenson LW, MacAlpin RN, Drinkwater D, Clark S, Dracup K, Laks H (1986) Cardiac transplantation at UCLA: selection and survival. J Heart Transplant 5:62–64

14. Likoff MJ, Candler SL, Kay HR (1987) Clinical determinants of mortality of chronic congestive heart failure secondary to idiopathic dilated or to ischemic cardiomyopathy. Am J Cardiol 59:634–638

15. Califf RM, Bounous P, Harrell FE, McCants B, Lee KL, McKinnis RA, Rosati RA (1982) The prognosis in the presence of coronary artery disease. In: Braunwald E, Mock MB, Watson J (eds) Congestive heart failure. Grune and Stratton, New York, pp 34

16. Unverferth DV, Magorien RD, Moeschberger ML, Baker PB, Fetters JK, Leier CV (1984) Factors influencing the one-year mortality of dilated cardiomyopathy. Am J Cardiol 54:147–152

17. Franciosa JA, Wilen M, Ziesche S, Cohn JN (1983) Survival in men with severe chronic left ventricular failure due to either coronary heart disease or idiopathic dilated cardiomyopathy. Am J Cardiol 51:831–836

18. Lee WH, Packer M (1986) Prognostic importance of serum sodium concentration and its modification by converting-enzyme inhibition in patients with severe chronic heart failure. Circulation 73:257–267

19. Stevenson LW, Tillisch JH (1986) Maintenance of cardiac output with normal filling pressures in dilated heart failure. Circulation 74:1303–1308

20. Stevenson LW, Belil D, Grover-McKay M, Brunken RC, Schwaiger M, Tillisch JH, Schelbert HR (1987) Effects of afterload reduction on left ventricular volume and mitral regurgitation in severe congestive heart failure. Am J Cardiol 60:654–658

21. Strauss RH, Stevenson LW, Dadourian BJ, Child JS (1987) The predictability of mitral regurgitation detected by Doppler echocardiography in patients referred for cardiac transplantation. Am J Cardiol 59:892–894

22. Stevenson LW, Brunken RC, Grover-McKay M, Belil D, Schelbert HR, Tillisch JH (1990) Afterload reduction decreases ventricular volume and mitral regurgitation during upright exercise in advanced heart failure. J Am Coll Card 15:174–180

23. Hamilton MA, Stevenson LW, Woo M, Child JS, Tillisch JH, Dadourian B (1988) Thermodilution over-estimation of cardiac output change with heart failure therapy is not from the decrease in tricuspid regurgitation. Circulation 78:II-625

24. Carr JG, Stevenson LW, Walden JA, Heber D (1989) Prevelance and hemodynamic correlates of malnutrition in severe congestive heart failure secondary to ischemic or idiopathic dilated cardiomyopathy. Am J Cardiol (in press)

25. Stevenson LW, Perloff JK (1989) The limited reliability of physical signs for estimating hemodynamics in chronic heart failure. JAMA (in press)

26. Franciosa JA, Dunkman WB, Leddy CL (1984) Hemodynamic effects of vasodilators and long-term response in heart failure. J Am Coll Cardiol 3:1521–1530

27. Massie BM, Kramer BL, Topic N (1984) Lack of relationship between the short-term hemodynamic effects of captopril and subsequent clinical response. Circulation 69:1135–1141

28. Pierpont GL, Francis GS (1982) Medical management of terminal cardiomyopathy. J Heart Transplant 2:18–27

29. Chatterjee K, Parmley WW (1983) Vasodilator therapy for acute myocardial infarction and chronic congestive heart failure. J Am Coll Cardiol 1:133–153

30. Packer M, Meller J, Medina N, Gorlin R, Harman MV (1980) Dose requirements of hydralazine in patients with chronic congestive heart failure. Am J Cardiol 45:655–659

31. Cohn JN, Archibald DG, Ziesche S, Franciosa JA, and the Veterans Administration Study Group (1986) Effect of vasodilator therapy on mortality in chronic congestive heart failure. N Engl J Med 314:1547–1552

32. Consensus Trial Study Group (1987) Effects of enalapril on mortality in severe congestive heart failure. N Engl J Med 316:1429–1435

33. Stevenson LW, Sietsema K, Tillisch JH, Walden JA, Kobashigawa J, Drinkwater D, Laks H (1988) Cardiac transplantation compared to sustained medical therapy for stable heart failure: Exercise capacity is not different. Circulation 78:II-27
34. Savin WM, Haskell WL, Schroeder JS, Stinson EB (1980) Cardiorespiratory responses of cardiac transplant patients to graded, symptom-limited exercise. Circulation 62:55-60
35. Kavanaugh T, Yacoub MH, Mertens DJ, Kennedy J, Campbell RB, Sawyer P (1988) Cardiorespiratory responses to exercise training after orthotopic cardiac transplantation. Circulation 77:162-168
36. Rubin SA, Chatterjee K, Parmley WW (1980) Metabolic assessment of exercise in chronic heart failure patients treated with short-term vasodilators. Circulation 61:543-548
37. Carrier M, Emery RW, Riley JE, Levinson MM, Copeland JC (1986) Cardiac transplantation in patients over 50 years of age. J Am Coll Cardiol 8:285-288
38. Walden JA, Stevenson LW, Dracup K, Wilmarth J, Kobashigawa J, Moriguchi J (1988) Cardiac transplantation may not improve quality of life for patients with stable heart failure. Circulation 78:II-217
39. Rhenman MJ, Rhenman B, Icenogle T, Christensen R, Copeland J (1988) Diabetes and heart transplantation. J Heart Transplant 7:356-358
40. Stevenson LW, Laks H, Terasaki PI, Kahan BD, Drinkwater DC (1988) Cardiac transplantation: selection, immunosuppression, and survival. West J Med 149:572-582
41. Herrick CM, Mealey PC, Tischner LL, Holland CS (1987) Combined heart failure transplant program: advantages in assessing medical compliance. J Heart Transplant 6:141-146
42. Miller LW (1987) Ambulatory inotropic therapy as a bridge to cardiac transplantation. J Am Coll Cardiol 9:89A
43. Stevenson LW, Donohue BC, Tillisch JH, Schulman B, Dracup KA, Drinkwater DC, Laks H (1987) Urgent priority transplantation: when should it be done? J Heart Transplant 6:267-272
44. Stevenson LW, Westlake C, Drinkwater D, Tillisch JH, Laks H (1988) Identification of outpatients at high risk for death prior to transplantation (abstract). J Heart Transplant 7:84
45. UNOS Update (1988) 4:1-11
46. Stevenson WG, Stevenson LW, Weiss J, Tillisch JH (1988) Programmed ventricular stimulation in severe heart failure: high, short-term risk of sudden death despite noninducibility. Am Heart J 116:1447-1454
47. Nicklas JM, Mickelson JK, Das SK, Morady F, Schork MA, Pitt B (1988) Prospective randomized double-blind placebo-controlled trial of low-dose amiodarone in patients with severe heart failure and frequent ventricular ectopy. Circulation 78:II-29
48. Luu M, Stevenson WG, Stevenson LW, Baron K, Walden J (1989) Ventricular tachycardia is not the predominant cause of monitored sudden death in heart failure. J Am Coll Cardiol (in press)
49. Packer M, Leier CV (1987) Survival in congestive heart failure during treatment with drugs with positive inotropic actions. Circulation 75:IV55-63
50. Cody RJ, Packer M, Colucci WS (1988) Do positive inotropic agents adversely affect the survival of patients with chronic congestive heart failure? J Am Coll Cardiol 12:559-569

Current Problems in Heart and Heart-Lung Transplantation for Heart Failure

C. Cabrol, I. Gandjbakhch, A. Pavie, V. Bors, J. Szefner, M. Desruennes, A. Cabrol, P. Leger, E. Vaissier, J.P. Levasseur, B. Aupetit, and G. Chomette

Heart Transplantation

Since our initial orthotopic heart transplant (OHT) in 1968 [3], 1250 patients aged from 8 to 70 years have been referred to our unit because of irreversible heart failure. The causes of this irreversible myocardial damage were idiopathic cardiomyopathy in 62% of the patients, ischemic heart disease in 31%, and left ventricular failure after valvular replacement in 7%. Contraindications (pulmonary artery hypertension, age over 65, diabetes, infection, peptic ulcer disease, severe multiple organ failure) were found in 20% of the patients. Among the remaining, 25% died before the operation could be performed. On December 1988, a total of 563 transplantations had been performed (85% men, aged 3 months to 63 years).

Donor selection has involved several conditions: age under 55, absence of infection or transmissible disorders and cardiac disease, stable hemodynamic status without high-dose inotropic support, ABO blood group compatibility and negative lymphocyte cross-match and approximate size compatibility.

The surgical technique used was orthotopic heart transplantation in 510 patients (according to Lower and Shumway [9]) and heterotopic transplantation (HHT) in 53 (Barnard and Losman). Distant procurement of graft was 71%.

Our immunosuppressive therapy, since 1981, consists immediately preoperatively of azathioprine (AZA) (5 mg/kg) and methylprednisolone (mPred) (8 mg/kg), and postoperatively of rabbit antithymocyte globulin (ATG) (6 mg/kg/day) given for 3 days, AZA (3 mg/kg/day) for 1 or 2 days, then cyclosporine (Cy) (5 mg/kg/day). Cy doses were increased over a 2-week period to achieve a Cy serum level of 100–150 ng/ml. mPred was decreased from 6 to 2 mg/kg/day over 3 days. Prednisone (PRED) was then tapered over 6 weeks from 1–0.3 mg/kg/day. Moderate rejection was treated by increased doses of PRED (5 mg/kg/day) for 5 days. Severe rejection was treated with a 3-day course of mPred (1000 mg/day) and ATG (6 mg/kg/day). In one-third of our transplanted patients AZA was used at doses of 2 mg/kg/day (triple therapy). Monoclonal antibody OKT3 is used in refractory rejection episodes.

Present postoperative therapy consisted of 3 days of antibiotic therapy, isoprenaline infusion for 8 days in order to counteract the hemodynamic instability of this first week, reverse isolation for 10 days, and 1 month hospitalization.

B.S. Lewis, A. Kimchi (Eds.)
Heart Failure Mechanisms and Management
© Springer-Verlag Berlin Heidelberg 1991

The main cause of mortality (15%) was during the first postoperative week and due to low cardiac output, multiple organ failure as a result of a wrong choice of recipients (too old, or with borderline pulmonary artery hypertension, severe renal or hepatic dysfunction, systemic disease), or a wrong choice of donor (important size mismatch with the recipient or impaired hemodynamic function of the graft). Later complications include rejection and side effects of immuno-suppressive therapy mainly infection [2,7]. Acute rejection is a constant threat and must be detected early and surely by the classical and regularly repeated en-domyocardial biopsy and with echo Doppler examination, which is now the basic detection method in our center. "Chronic" rejection is responsible for late graft arteriosclerosis usually preceeded by an early acute immunologic vasculatis which must be detected and treated without delay. Cy toxicity [10] was respon-sible in 60% of the cases of diastolic hypertension, in 55% of renal dysfunction [5,12], in 22% of hirsutism, in 16% of hyperplasia of the gingiva, in 7% of hepatic dysfunction. The actuarial survival rate was 65% at 7 years and 234 transplanted patients are alive, the longest 14 years after the operation. All lead virtually normal social and family lives. Half of them have resumed their professional activity.

Recently, in patients in acute irreversible cardiac failure and who cannot have a transplant in time we implant *a total artificial heart* (JARVIK 7) (from April 1986, 40 patients have had such an implantation). Ages varied from 19 to 56 years. All patients were in terminal congestive cardiac failure due to idiopathic cardiomyopathy (15), viral myocarditis (1), postpartum myocarditis (2), valvular disease (1), acute rejections (4), graft failures (3) and ischemic diseases with a life expectancy of few hours (14). There was hepatic and renal functional insufficiency in all cases, subacute pulmonary oedema in 20 cases, and a cardiac arrest at the beginning of anesthesia in three cases. The cardiac prosthesis used was a Jarvik 7 100 cc in 21 cases, and 70 cc in 19 cases. Mechanical circulatory support lasted from 1 day to 5 months. There was no mechanical failure, no hemolysis, no thromboembolism, and only two right ventricular device malpo-sitions. Twenty-two patients died before transplantation, from multiple organ failure or infection. Sixteen were successfully transplanted, two of which still have an artificial heart. When reversible, hepatic and renal dysfunctions improved in a few days, and left atrial pressure was continuously monitored to avoid pul-monary edema, which disappeared in few hours when present before the im-plantation. The atrial and ventricular pressure curves given by the computer permitted us to obtain the appropriate cardiac output and systemic arterial pressure by adjusting the various parameters: drive pressure, heart rate, and percent systole, which had to be modified only during the first days. The Jarvik 7 total artificial heart appeared in our experience to be a very safe device, easy to drive, offering the best conditions to the acutely ill patients who can recover in this way a stable and correct physiological status, to be successfully transplanted without an emergency or priority status on the transplant waiting lists.

Heart and Lung Transplantation

Following our first European heart-lung transplant in March 1982 [4], we have performed 39 such operations on 22 men and 17 women, aged from 8 to 52 years, mainly for primary pulmonary hypertension (13 cases) and for Eisenmenger syndrome (17 cases) but also for cystic fibrosis (six cases), chronic thromboembolism of the pulmonary artery (one case), diffuse bronchectasis (one patient), and diffuse emphysema (one patient).

We encountered in our early series many important problems, but experience has taught us to be more precise in selecting recipients (avoiding too advanced disease with profound right heart failure, large ascites, severe coagulation problems, and hemorrhagic pleuropulmonary adhesions from previous operations), to also be more careful in selecting donors (good functioning lungs, clear on chest X-rays without infection, a PO2 $\geqslant$ 100 torr with FiO_2 of 40%, the same size of lung) and to improve our method of lung preservation (a 4 l EuroCollins flush after pulmonary artery injection of prostacyclin to obtain efficient vasodilatation) permitting long-distance procurement. We have also improved our surgical technique, avoiding mediastinal nerve injury and trauma of the donor's lungs, looking for meticulous hemostasis of the surgical field, and careful performing tracheal anastomosis. The post operative care was specially devoted to intensive pulmonary management because the lungs are the main causes of post-operative problems. Indeed, aside from the problems mentioned in cardiac transplantation, these special pulmonary complications are: (a) fistula of the tracheal anastomosis (infrequent), (b) early pulmonary dysfunction due to imperfect preservation, and (3) during the first 2 weeks, the "reimplantation sydrome of the lung," marked by a more or less severe pulmonary edema due to denervation of the lung, deprivation of bronchial arterial flow, and lack of lymphatic drainage. Pulmonary infections are more severe in these patients, and lung rejection, which is very difficult to ascertain, is rarely contemporary with heart rejection [6]. Lastly the patients may present a progressive and lethal form of obliterative bronchiolitis, [1] the physiopathology of which remains unclear (chronic infection, rejection, bronchial denervation).

These complications explain why the survival rate in such operations remains lower than in heart transplantations: 60% at 1 year, 50% at 2 years, and 40% at 5 years in the best series [8–11].

The results of heart-lung transplantation are improving. In our series one-third of the patients are still alive, among them an 8-year-old girl who presented with cystic fibrosis. In two patients a heart and unilateral lung transplant was performed to avoid unilateral lung adhesions due to a previous lateral thoracotomy. Our longest survival time is now 3 years, but this patient is presenting first symptoms of an obliterative bronchiolitis.

Summary

After 20 years of clinical application, although some problems remain, cardiac transplantation is now a safe and reliable treatment for patients in irreversible cardiac failure untreatable by other medical or surgical means.

a) Heart lung transplantation, although still to be improved, offers a serious hope to the patients for whom it is the only available therapy.
b) Since submission of this manuscript 801 heart and 112 heart lungs transplantations were performed in our unit (October 29, 1990).

References

1. Allen MD, Burke CM, McGregor CGA et al. (1986) Steroid-responsive bronchiolitis after human heart-lung transplantation. J Thorac Cardiovasc Surg 92:449–451
2. Baumgartner WA (1983) Infection in cardiac transplantation. J Heart Transplant 3 (I):75–80
3. Cabrol C, Gandjbakhch I, Pavie A, Cabrol A, Mattei MF, Leger P (1985) Heart transplantation in Paris, at "La Pitie" Hospital. Heart Transplant 4:476–480
4. Cabrol C, Gandjbakhch I, Pavie A, Laskar MJ, Cabrol A, Mattei MF (1984) Heart and heart-lung transplantation: technique and safeguards. Heart Transplant 3:110–114
5. Chomette G, Auriol M, Beaufils H, Rottembourg J, Cabrol C (1985) Morphology of cyclosporine nephrotoxicity in human heart transplant-recipients (abstract). Heart Transplant 4:617
6. Griffith BP, Hardesty RL, Trento A et al. (1985) Asynchronous rejection of heart and lungs following cardiopulmonary transplantation. Ann Thorac Surg 40:488–493
7. Hunt SA (1983) Complications of heart transplantation. J Heart Transplant 3 (I):70–74
8. Jamieson SW, Opunnaike HA (1986) Cardiopulmonary transplantation. Surg Clin North Am 63:2
9. Lower RR, Stoffer RC, Hurley EJ et al. (1961) Complete homograft replacement of the heart and both lungs. Surgery 50:842–845
10. Oyer PE, Stinson EB, Jamieson SW et al. (1983) Cyclosporin A in cardiac allografting: a preliminary experience. Transplant Proc 15:1257–1262
11. Reitz BA, Burton NA, Jamieson SW et al. (1980) Heart and lung transplantation: auto and allotransplantation in primates with extended survival. J Thorac Cardiovasc Surg 80:360–372
12. Rottembourg J, Mattei MF, Cabrol A, Leger P, Aupetit B, Beaufils H, Gluckman JC, Pavie A, Gandjbakhch I, Cabrol C (1985) Renal function and blood pressure in heart transplant recipients treated with Cyclosporine. J Heart Transplant 4:404–407

Transplant Coronary Disease

H.A. VALANTINE and J.S. SCHROEDER

Introduction

Accelerated coronary artery disease of the human cardiac allograft (transplant CAD), initially recognized at Stanford, has emerged as the major factor limiting long-term survival[1–2]. Though clinical and experimental heart transplantation have enabled detailed description of the morphologic and histologic features of this often clinically silent form of coronary disease, its pathogenesis remains unknown, and premorbid diagnosis continues to challenge physicians. Lack of afferent innervation of the allograft renders heart transplant recipients incapable of experiencing angina. The diffuse distribution and morphology of transplant CAD render it inamenable to conventional methods of revascularization, and retransplantation is currently the only therapy available. The need for clinical monitoring of transplant CAD determined the rigorous policy of annual coronary arteriography in all recipients at Stanford since 1970. From these data we have defined the prevalence, clinicopathologic correlates, and angiographic morphology of transplant CAD. Our 20 years' experience has enabled us to analyze changes in the epidemiology of this disease as immunosuppression has evolved. We have explored the pathogenetic mechanism which may give rise to this disease in experimental and clinical heart transplantation in an attempt to develop preventive and therapeutic modalities. Currently, our efforts are directed toward two major challenges: (1) developing quantitative methods for monitoring transplant CAD, to enable early diagnosis and provide a sensitive means for testing therapeutic and preventive interventions; and (2) identifying the cells, molecules, and mechanisms involved in the proliferative process characteristic of transplant CAD.

Prevalence

The prevalence of transplant CAD, initially reported from our experience of 81 patients surviving beyond 1 year [1], remains unchanged despite improved immunosuppression. Prior to the introduction of cyclosporine into clinical heart transplantation, we reported a 25% prevalence of angiographically diagnosed transplant CAD in 81 patients surviving beyond 1 year; graft failure occurred in 50% of these patients. Comparison of serial coronary arteriograms from 103

B.S. Lewis, A. Kimchi (Eds.)
Heart Failure Mechanisms and Management
© Springer-Verlag Berlin Heidelberg 1991

patients treated initially with azathioprine-based immunosuppression and in 78 patients for whom cyclosporine was the major immunosuppressive agent has shown the time-related incidence of transplant CAD to be unchanged by the use of cyclosporine [2]. The percent of patients free of angiographically visible transplant CAD at 1 year was 89% for the azathioprine group vs 86% for the cyclosporine group. At 3 years, 74% of the azathioprine group vs 63% of the cyclosporine group were free of visible disease (p = ns). By the 5th postoperative year, 58% of the azathioprine and 50% of the cyclosporine group were free of transplant CAD (p = ns). Although rejection incidence was higher in the azathioprine group, there was no apparent difference in the prevalence of transplant CAD. The inhomogeneity between the two groups for conventional risk factors such as hypertension, glucose intolerance, and prednisone dose may have masked any relationship between rejection incidence of transplant CAD. Nevertheless these data indicate that immunosuppression with cyclosporine has not decreased the time-related prevalence of transplant CAD.

Clinical Features and Risk Factors of Transplant CAD

Transplant CAD is characteristically unassociated with angina, and the most frequent modes of presentation are sudden death, progressive graft failure, and myocardial infarction. Pathologically proven myocardial infarction was documented in 26% of 202 heart transplant recipients surviving beyond 1 year, and 43% of these events occurred within 3 years of transplantation [3]. The presenting symptoms included congestive cardiac failure, palpitations, syncope, and asymptomatic electrocardiographic changes. In the Stanford experience, the cumulative percentages of graft loss as a consequence of transplant CAD (death or retransplantation) at 2–5 years are 23%, 32%, 36%, and 41% respectively (Table 1). This experience demonstrates the propensity of transplant CAD to remain silent, progress rapidly, and defy premorbid diagnosis.

In an attempt to identify possible risk factors for transplant CAD, we examined the relationship of multiple clinical and demographic variables to

Table 1. Cumulative ratio of CAD-related deaths or retransplantation to total number of deaths or retransplantations

Year	Azathioprine group (%)		Cyclosporine group (%)		All patients (%)	
2	31	(4/13)	13	(1/8)	23	(5/21)
3	35	(8/23)	29	(4/14)	32	(12/37)
4	33	(11/33)	40	(8/20)	36	(19/53)
5	35	(16/45)	52	(13/25)	41	(29/70)

No 1-year results are presented because only 1-year survivors are included in the analysis.

serial coronary angiographic findings in 132 patients who received cardiac transplants between 1970 and 1985. Donor age and fasting triglycerides at 1 year post-transplantation were the only factors significantly associated with angiographically documented CAD. There was no correlation between transplant CAD and other indices, including prior CAD in the recipient's native heart, number of rejection episodes during the first post-transplant year, number of HLA mismatches, level of maintenance steroids, fasting blood glucose, and cholesterol subfractions. These data indicate that the conventional risk factors associated with nontransplant CAD may not be applicable to transplant CAD.

Owing to the diffuse distribution and characteristic absence of collateral vessels, transplant CAD cannot be treated by revascularization. Currently, retransplantation is the only effective therapeutic option. The results of retransplantation are markedly inferior to those after the first transplant, with survival at 1 year of only 60% compared to 85% for the first transplant [4].

Angiographic Features of Transplant CAD

Review of more than 1000 arteriograms from 400 patients enabled a detailed angiographic characterization of transplant CAD which closely correlates with the histopathologic changes [5]. Three distinct types of lesions were identified: type A, discrete or tubular stenosis; type B, diffuse concentric narrowing, and type C, irregular vessels with occluded branches. When compared to arteriograms from patients with nontransplant CAD, a distinct difference in the frequency and distribution of each type of lesion was noted. In patients with transplant CAD, most of the concentric and distal obliterative lesions (types B and C) appeared in secondary and tertiary vessels. In contrast, no type B or C lesions were seen in nontransplant CAD. Comparison of the site of total occlusion of vessels and the quality of collateral vessel formation revealed a striking difference between the groups. In transplant CAD, proximal occlusions occurred less frequently, and collateral vessel formation was typically poor, while in nontransplant CAD, proximal occlusions and collateral vessel formation were frequent. Thus, angiographic findings in transplant CAD comprise a mixture of both typical atherosclerotic lesions, and unusual, but presumably transplant-related, progressive diffuse distal obliterative disease without collateral vessel development. Recognition of the characteristic concentric narrowing as an early manifestation of transplant CAD has prompted the use of quantitative methods for analyzing and monitoring this disease. Using calibrated coronary artery catheters and computerized edge-detection methods, we have documented a significant decrease in lumen diameter in all patients 1 year after transplantation.

Morphology and Histologic Features

The angiographic characteristics of transplant CAD can be related to the morphologic and histopathologic changes seen on examining the explanted or autopsy allograft, as described in the initial 12 heart transplant recipients at Stanford [6]. Two distinct types of lesions are recognized. The typical early lesion consists of circumferential and longitudinal increase in fibrous tissue and myointimal cells limited to coronary arteries with muscular media. This characteristic proliferative lesion results in a diffuse decrease in vascular lumen, and is consistent with the early angiographic appearance. The severity of intimal hyperplasia is proportional to the age of the graft, occurs as early as 9 days post-transplantation, and is characteristically found in grafts studied early after transplantation. A second type of lesion consisting of focal intimal plaques [7], indistinguishable from that found in nontransplant CAD, is recognized. This lesion, which contains large numbers of lipophages and lipid droplets, characteristically occurs in larger epicardial vessels and appears in grafts studied later in the course of the disease. Focal lesions which are apparent angiographically are late manifestations, and typically reflect more complex lesions with thrombotic components. Pathologic examination frequently reveals occlusion of smaller branches preceding that of larger epicardial vessels, which may account for occurrence of sudden death from infarction when larger coronary arteries appear unaffected on surveillance angiograms [7,8].

Pathogenesis and Prevention of Graft Atherosclerosis

The histopathologic findings at autopsy examination of patients who died of transplant CAD during the early Stanford experience gave rise to a hypothesis for this disease [9]. Griepp and colleagues [9] proposed that "the initial event is immune injury to the arterial endothelium, which results in loss of endothelial integrity and exposure of a thrombogenic surface. Formation and organization of microthrombi and proliferative repair of the injured endothelial myointimal cells result in a thickened hyperplastic intima. Infiltration of plasma lipids into this hypertrophied intima initiates the formation of atheromatous plaques which, by releasing free lipids into the intima, stimulate additional cellular proliferation."

Role of Lipids in the Pathogenesis of Transplant CAD

Abnormal blood lipid concentrations have been investigated as potential candidates in the pathogenesis of transplant CAD because of the histologic composition of lesions, the established role for impaired lipid metabolism as a significant risk factor in nontransplant CAD, the frequent finding of elevated blood lipids in cardiac transplant recipients, and the observation that transplant CAD may be accelerated by hypertriglyceridemia and hypercholesterolemia in experimental heart transplantation. Our early experience revealed no demonstrable association between transplant CAD, serum triglyceride, or cholesterol levels at 1, 2, and 3 years post-transplantation [9]. On subsequent analysis of 85 patients surviving beyond 1 year and transplanted between 1970 and 1979, we found raised serum triglyceride levels measured 1 year post-transplantation to be significantly associated with the development of transplant CAD [1]. More recent experience, including patients treated with cyclosporine, confirmed the link between transplant CAD and high serum triglyceride level at 1-year post-transplantation [10]. Patients with diffuse concentric distal disease had higher triglyceride levels than those with proximal and mid-vessel stenosis. No significant association between transplant CAD and cholesterol levels was discernible in the group as a whole. However, patients undergoing retransplantation for severe transplant CAD had significantly higher values of total plasma cholesterol and low-density lipoprotein compared to those without CAD, indicating a significant association between abnormal lipids and severe transplant CAD [4]. Hence, elevated plasma lipids may play an important role in the pathogenesis of advanced transplant CAD. However, data from experimental and clinical transplantation suggest that abnormal lipid concentrations are not the initiating factors, but rather that they may potentiate vascular injury initiated by an immune phenomenon.

Thrombosis

The earliest clinical investigation to explore the role of antithrombotic agents in transplant CAD was reported in 1977 [9]. Comparison of the time-related incidence of CAD in a group of patients undergoing cardiac transplantation prior to the use of endomyocardial biopsy for monitoring rejection, with a later group in whom rejection was monitored by histologic criteria, was reported. The latter group, who were treated with warfarin and dipyridamole, had a significantly lower incidence of CAD. Evidence supporting an important effect of platelet aggregation was presented in a subsequent experimental study [11]. In their work from Stanford, Lurie and colleagues [11] showed that cyclosporine A suppressed acute rejection in a rat model, but did not prevent the development of atherosclerotic lesions. In this rat model, the combination of cyclosporine A and dipyridamole successfully prevented transplant CAD up to 50 days post-transplantation. However, these encouraging experimental results have not been borne out in clinical heart transplantation. Despite autopsy studies showing that thrombosis does occur in patients dying of transplant CAD [9], clinical experience with the prophylactic use of anticoagulants and platelet antagonists does not support a primary role for thrombogenesis in human transplant CAD.

Immune Hypothesis

The hypothesis of immune injury to the arterial endothelium as the initiating event in human transplant CAD has been neither confirmed nor refuted despite over 10 years of investigation. However, recognition of accelerated atherosclerosis in renal transplants [12,13] and its ubiquitous presence in all other organ transplants lends it credence.

Experimental heart transplantation has provided good evidence to support the immune hypothesis for transplant CAD. The typical lesions affecting large and medium-sized coronary arteries were first described by Lower et al. [15] in long-surviving canine transplants. Minick and Murphy [14] demonstrated that repeated injections of horse serum into rabbits result in proliferative intimal thickening in coronary arteries as well as other major vessels. They postulated that the mechanism involved endothelial damage by immune complexes. These changes were worsened by concomitant lipid-rich diets.

Intimal hyperplasia was induced by Lurie et al. [11] in inbred, untreated AgB mismatched heterotopic rat cardiac allografts. In this experimental model, cyclosporine A was shown to suppress acute rejection, but not to prevent vascular disease. An indirect relationship to cytotoxic antibodies was postulated. Evidence from human cardiac transplants supporting the immune hypothesis for transplant CAD has been limited to only a few reports. Hess et al. [15] documented the association of cytotoxic B-cell antibodies with development of severe diffuse, tubular atherosclerosis in six cardiac transplant recipients. Uretsky et al. [16] reported that the occurrence of two or more major rejection episodes was associated with the development of CAD.

Acute vascular rejection in association with electron microscopic evidence of endothelial damage and immune complex deposition was reported by Palmer et al. [17] Vascular deposition of IgM and complement [C_3] and proliferative arteriolar occlusion occurred in a patient who developed progressive graft dysfunction and ultimately died of extensive myocardial infarction. In both cases biopsies performed just prior to death were unassociated with histologic evidence of acute cellular rejection. Such observations indicate that immune-mediated vascular injury may proceed in the absence of histologic evidence of acute rejection on endomyocardial biopsy. Our initial retrospective analysis suggested an association of rejection incidence with transplant CAD, but this has not been confirmed in further analysis [10].

In vitro studies of acute rejection indicate that the allograft response involves contributions from all major elements of the immune system. Activation of T-helper cells by class II major histocompatibility (MHC) antigens allows the release of lymphokines (macrophage-stimulating factor, IL-1, IL-2), which in turn result in activation of B cells, cytotoxic T cells, macrophages, and gamma interferon, with further expression of class II molecules on endothelial cells. Hence the absence of a demonstrable association between rejection incidence and subsequent development of transplant CAD may readily be explained. For example, modification of the host response by immunosuppressive agents currently used in cardiac transplantation could account for the absence of histologic evidence of rejection despite ongoing antigen-specific endothelial injury.

Experimental studies showing absence of class II antigen induction in allografts where rejection is adequately suppressed with cyclosporine, and increased antigen expression during histologic evidence of rejection, have been reported. These data suggest that after transplantation, class II antigens on the vascular endothelium provide the major stimulus for induction of host responses, and their induction may be suppressed by immunosuppressive drugs or, conversely, amplified by other factors. Viral infections may provide this additional stimulus for MHC expression.

Von Willebrand et al. [18] reported that in 12 of 14 renal transplant recipients with proven cytomegalovirus (CMV) disease the display of class II antigens was associated with a cytologic and a clinical episode of rejection. Epidemiologic analysis has revealed a similar relationship in heart transplant recipients at Stanford (unpublished data). Rejection incidence, time-related incidence, and death from transplant CAD were significantly higher in patients who developed evidence of CMV disease during the first postoperative year. Furthermore, in the absence of transfusion-transmitted disease, CMV infection has not been documented when both recipient and donor are CMV antibody negative. This provides indirect evidence that CMV is transmitted in the heart at the time of transplantation. The mechanisms by which CMV infections are linked to rejection and CAD are unknown, but the process may be related to enhanced immunogeneity and mediated by increased gamma interferon production.

Future Directions

Currently much research effort is directed at identifying the primary mediator of transplant CAD and elucidating the role of secondary factors such as lipids in the development of advanced disease. The cells and molecules currently being investigated include: those which are known to be produced by the host in response to antigen stimuli, mitogens such as growth factors which can result in intimal hyperplasia, and the effect of calcium overload on the smooth muscle and endothelium.

Clinical research is directed toward developing quantitative methods to improve detection of transplant CAD, and to provide sensitive methods of testing therapeutic and preventive interventions.

Summary

Accelerated coronary artery disease of the human cardiac allograft (transplant CAD) is now the major factor limiting long-term survival. Of the last 50 retransplants at Stanford, 25 have been for severe transplant CAD. The introduction of cyclosporine has had little impact on its prevalence, with only 86%, 63%, and 50% of patients being free of transplant CAD as detected by annual coronary arteriography at 1, 3, and 5 years post-transplantation. Since the heart remains denervated, transplant CAD frequently presents as myocardial infarction or sudden death. Coronary arteriographic characteristics of transplant CAD demonstrate a diffuse process, affecting distal vessels with little development of collaterals. This diffuse nature makes it difficult to detect transplant CAD early without quantitative arteriographic techniques. Attempts at prevention with antiplatelet drugs or coumadin have had little impact on prevalence. Multivariate analyses of potential risk factors have demonstrated a positive relationship to total and LDL cholesterol and number of rejection episodes in the first year. Cytomegalovirus infections are also associated with a higher prevalence of transplant CAD. Newer approaches to prevention include improved immunosuppression, calcium blockers, and antiviral agents.

References

1. Bieber CP, Hunt SA, Schwinn DA, Jamieson SA, Reitz BA, Oyer PE, Shumway NE, Stinson EB (1981) Complications in long-term survivors of cardiac transplantation. Transplant Proc 13:207-211
2. Gao S-Z, Schroeder JS, Alderman EL, Hunt SA, Valantine HA, Wiederhold V, Stinson EB (1989) Prevalence of accelerated coronary artery disease in heart transplant survivors: comparison of cyclosporine and azathioprine regimens. Circulation 80(Suppl III):III-100-105
3. Gao SZ, Schroeder J, Hunt H, Billingham M, Stinson E (1988) Myocardial infarction in cardiac transplant patients (abstract). Circulation 78 (Suppl II):II-438
4. Gao SZ, Schroeder JS, Hunt S, Stinson EB (1988) Retransplantation for severe accelerated coronary vascular disease in heart transplant recipients. Am J Cardiol 62:876-881
5. Gao S-Z, Alderman EL, Schroeder JS, Silverman JF, Hunt SA (1988) Accelerated coronary vascular disease in the heart transplant patient: coronary arteriographic findings. J Am Coll Cardiol 12:334-340
6. Bieber CP, Stinson EB, Shumway NE et al. (1970) Cardiac transplantation in man: cardiac allograft pathology. Circulation 41:753
7. Billingham ME (1987) Cardiac transplant atherosclerosis. Transplant Proc 19 (Suppl 5):19-25
8. Nitkin RS, Hunt SA, Schroeder JS (1985) Accelerated atherosclerosis in a cardiac transplant patient. J Am Coll Cardiol 6:243-245
9. Griepp RB, Stinson EB, Bieber CP, Reitz BA, Copeland JG, Oyer PE, Shumway NE (1977) Control of graft arteriosclerosis in human heart transplant recipients. Surgery 81:262-269
10. Gao SZ, Schroeder JS, Alderman EL, Hunt SA, Silverman JF, Wiederhold V, Stinson EB (1987) Clinical and laboratory correlates of accelerated coronary artery disease in the cardiac transplant patient. Circulation 76 (Suppl V):56-61
11. Lurie KG, Billingham ME, Jamieson SW, Harrison DC, Reitz BA (1981) Pathogenesis and prevention of graft arteriosclerosis in an experimental heart transplant model. Transplantation 31:41-47
12. Busch GJ, Galvanek EG, Reynolds ES (1971) Human renal allografts: analysis of lesions in long-term survivors. Human Pathol 2:253-298
13. Rowlands DT, Hill GS, Zmijewski CM (1976) The pathology of renal homograft rejection. Am J Pathol 85:774-804
14. Minick CR, Murphy GE (1973) Experimental induction of atheroarteriosclerosis by the synergy of allergic injury to arteries and lipid-rich diet. II. Effect of repeatedly injected foreign protein in rabbits fed a lipidrich, cholesterol poor diet. Am J Pathol 73:265

15. Hess ML, Hastillo A, Mohanakumar T, Cowley MJ, Vetrovac G, Szentpetery S, Wolfgang T, Lower RR (1983) Accelerated atherosclerosis in cardiac transplantation: Role of cytotoxic B-cell antibodies and hyperlipidemia. Circulation 68 (Suppl II):94–101

16. Uretsky BF, Murali S, Reddy PS, Rabin B, Lee A, Griffith BP, Hardesty RL, Trento A, Bahnson HT (1987) Development of coronary artery disease in cardiac transplant patients receiving immunosuppressive therapy with cyclosporine and prednisone. Circulation 76:827–834

17. Palmer DC, Tsai CC, Roodman ST, Godd JE, Miller LW, Sarafian JE, Williams GA (1985) Heart graft arteriosclerosis: an ominous finding on endomyocardial biopsy. Transplantation 39:385–388

18. von Willebrand E, Pettersson E, Ahonen J, Hayry P (1986) CMV infection, class II antigen expression, and human kidney allograft rejection. Transplantation 42:364–367

The manufacturer's authorised representative in the EU is Springer
Nature Customer Service Centre GmbH, Europaplatz 3, 69115 Heidelberg,
Germany. If you have any concerns regarding our products, please
contact ProductSafety@springernature.com

Printed and bound by CPI Group (UK) Ltd, Croydon, CR0 4YY
28/04/2026
02098503-0003